An Emergency Physician's Path

Robert P. Olympia
Elizabeth Barrall Werley
Jeffrey S. Lubin
Kahyun Yoon-Flannery
Editors

An Emergency Physician's Path

What to Expect After an Emergency Medicine Residency

Springer

Editors
Robert P. Olympia
Emergency Medicine
Penn State Milton S. Hershey
Medical Center
Hershey, PA, USA

Elizabeth Barrall Werley
Emergency Medicine
Penn State Milton S. Hershey
Medical Center
Hershey, PA, USA

Jeffrey S. Lubin
Emergency Medicine
Penn State Milton S. Hershey
Medical Center
Hershey, PA, USA

Kahyun Yoon-Flannery
MD Anderson Cancer Center at Cooper
Cooper Medical School of Rowan
University
Camden, NJ, USA

ISBN 978-3-031-47872-7 ISBN 978-3-031-47873-4 (eBook)
https://doi.org/10.1007/978-3-031-47873-4

This Springer imprint is published by the registered company Springer Nature Switzerland AG
The registered company address is: Gewerbestrasse 11, 6330 Cham, Switzerland

Printed on acid-free paper

Preface

> "When you do everything you can, sometimes more than you thought you could, you've got to walk away knowing you fought the good fight. You fought the good fight, and tomorrow you'll fight another one."—Dr. John Carter (NBC television series, *ER*)

I would be lying to you if I said that my first exposure to emergency medicine (EM) was based on experiences that normally fill a curriculum vitae and residency application. In fact, my first exposure to EM was in the mid-1990s alongside my medical school buddies, watching the triumphs and failures, the saves and misses, and the disease and trauma experienced by Drs. Mark Greene, Doug Ross, Susan Lewis, and John Carter on the television series, *ER*. Initially drawn to the fast-paced and heart-pounding world associated with EM depicted on the TV screen, I soon discovered early in my career the breadth that a career in EM could offer beyond the walls of the ED, including leadership opportunities, mentorship, education, research, advocacy, service, and collaboration. Despite the long grueling shifts, the sadness associated with death and delivering bad news, the crisis of ED overcrowding, the lack of staff and available beds, and the daily conflict with patients and their families, consultants, and staff, I can confidently say that my career in EM has been a blessing. I am overwhelmed with pride and gratitude when I think of the impact my career has had on my patients and their families, my students and residents, and my colleagues and staff. My hope is that your journey in EM is as rewarding and successful as well.

My first experience with the *Path Series* was several years ago when I was asked to write a few chapters for *A Pediatrician's Path: What to Expect after a Pediatrics Residency*. Previously I had been involved with medical textbooks that focused on the clinical side of medicine, but was immediately drawn to *Path's* focus on the steps to becoming a successful, well-rounded, and happy physician as written by experienced authors in the field. I am blessed to embark on this journey with two Penn State University colleagues whom I admire and respect tremendously. Elizabeth Werley is a board-certified EM physician, working both clinically and administratively in the arenas of emergency medicine, medical education, and the patient experience/satisfaction. Jeffrey Lubin is a board-certified EM physician, balancing his professional career with clinical emergency medicine and prehospital emergency care, education, leadership, administration, and research. Finally, we enlisted the leadership and experience of Kay Yoon-Flannery, a breast surgeon at the MD Anderson Cancer Center at Cooper, who has been involved as Editor with several previously published books in the *Path Series*. Along with my experience as a pediatric EM physician, we feel we have assembled an editorial staff with decades of clinical, administrative, research, educational, and leadership experience to fulfill the mission of this endeavor.

The editors felt it was important to develop a book that focuses on the choices that EM physicians make throughout their careers, regardless of their level of experience, and on practical skills that are important for the success and survival of EM physicians. We searched far and wide for contributors who have demonstrated clinical excellence and scholarship in their careers. Our contributors represent varied backgrounds and experience, covering general emergency medicine and subspecialty emergency medicine. Beginning with the history of emergency medicine (Chapter 1), the focus of *An Emergency Physician's Path* guides the medical student interested in a career in EM (Part I), the EM resident who may be interested in pursuing an emergency medicine fellowship (Part II), and the EM resident in their choice of a community or an academic emergency medicine career (Parts III and IV). Furthermore, we aim to assist junior EM physicians in their pursuit of a niche in emergency medicine (Part V), in their development of skills necessary to navigate through an ED shift (Part VI), and in establishing a footprint in research/scholarship (Part VII) and education (Part VIII). Lastly, Part IX discusses aspects important to the EM physician, from your first shift as an ED attending physician to your last shift before retirement.

The editors hope that *An Emergency Physician's Path* provides you a valuable tool that you will refer to during your career in emergency medicine, leading to professional success, optimal wellness, and a lifetime of fulfillment and satisfaction.

Hershey, PA, USA Robert P. Olympia
September 11, 2023

The original version of the book has been revised: The list of contributor's have been included. A correction to this book can be found at https://doi.org/10.1007/978-3-031-47873-4_105

Acknowledgments

Robert P. Olympia

> *"To know even one life has breathed easier because you have lived. This is to have succeeded."*—Ralph Waldo Emerson

The impact that I have had during my career in Emergency Medicine would not have been possible without the following people:

To all of the emergency department staff that I have worked with over my 25-year career, at the DuPont Hospital for Children, Christiana Care Hospital, Thomas Jefferson University, Children's Hospital at Montefiore, Newark Beth Israel Medical Center, and Penn State Hershey Medical Center. I am the physician I am today because of the compassion, dedication, hard work, and selflessness that I have learned from each and every one of you.

To my mentors, Drs. Magdy Attia, Steven Selbst, Waseem Hafeez, and Jeff Avner. Thank you for believing in me.

To my parents (Manuel and Delia), Coco, my sisters (Patricia, Catherine), and extended family from all over the world. Thank you for your unwavering love and support, and for being amazing role models. I hope I have made you all proud. Maraming salamat po, mahal kita.

To my wife, Jodi, and my children, Abigail and Madelyn. There is a reason why your beautiful faces are scattered throughout this book. Thank you for supporting me with an unconditional love and for allowing me to pursue my professional and personal dreams. You inspire me every day to be the best person that I can be. Any success in my life is because of you guys, and your belief in me has allowed me to overcome any obstacle in life. Love you to infinity and beyond!

Jeffrey S. Lubin

A career in medicine is hard, and life as an Emergency Physician brings its own unique challenges. I would like to express my sincerest gratitude to all those who have supported and guided me along the way. Starting as a member of Cornell University's student-run EMS all the way through today, it's been quite a journey! I am deeply thankful for the invaluable support and guidance provided by my mentors, colleagues, and friends. I want to thank my family (especially my wife Jill and my kids) and loved ones for their unwavering support and understanding. It remains an honor and a privilege to be a physician.

Elizabeth Barrall Werley

"Did you know freedom exists in a school book."—Jim Morrison, The Doors

I am filled with tremendous thanks to...

My parents who instilled in me a love of learning

My entire family growing up, who always encouraged and supported my dream of becoming a doctor

And my family now, who continues to support (and tolerate) me and all of my endeavors

Kahyun Yoon-Flannery

This book is our third in the path series and the most comprehensive thanks to my wonderful co-editors and contributing authors.

This book is dedicated to all the tirelessly working physicians of all our Emergency Rooms, particularly one Dr. Claudio Fernandez. His positive energy has always been endearing but all the more impressive during the pandemic when we were faced every day with doubt, uncertainty, and unexpected losses. We have all learned so much in the past several years about each other, ourselves, and the world. I am grateful for all of it, but most of all for his friendship.

Contents

Contributors

Sapana P. Adhikari, MD Atrium Mercy Hospital, Charlotte, NC, USA

Al'ai Alvarez, MD Emergency Medicine, Stanford University, Palo Alto, CA, USA

Joseph Andrie, MD Departments of Family and Community Medicine and Orthopedics and Rehabilitation, Penn State Milton S. Hershey Medical Center, Hershey, PA, USA

Maryam Arshad, MD Emory University, Atlanta, GA, USA

Jeff Baker, MD Associate Professor, Department of Emergency Medicine, University of Louisville, Louisville, KY, USA

John R. Barrett, MD Department of Emergency Medicine, Medical College of Georgia at Augusta University, Augusta, GA, USA

Erica Bates, MD Penn State Hershey Medical Center, Hershey, PA, USA

Nicole Battaglioli, MD Agnes Scott College, Atlanta, GA, USA

Monisha Bindra, MD Department of Emergency Medicine, Tower Health-Reading Hospital, West Reading, PA, USA

Christine Binkley, MD Department of Emergency Medicine, Northwestern Medicine, Kishwaukee Hospital, DeKalb, IL, USA

Eliot Blum, MD Emory University School of Medicine, Atlanta, GA, USA

Julia Bonanno, MD St. Luke's Bethlehem, Bethlehem, PA, USA

Michael J. Burla, MD Department of Emergency Medicine, Southern Maine Health Care, MaineHealth, Tufts School of Medicine, Biddeford, ME, USA

Tara Cassidy-Smith, MD Department of Emergency Medicine, Cooper Medical School of Rowan University, Camden, NJ, USA

Harvey Castro, MD Trusted ER, Coppell, TX, USA

Mathew Cherian, MD Department of Emergency Medicine, Carle Foundation Hospital, Urbana, IL, USA

Eric Chin, MD Department of Emergency Medicine, Brooke Army Medical Center, JBSA-Ft. Sam Houston, TX, USA

Arlene S. Chung, MD Department of Emergency Medicine, University of Vermont Health Network, Burlington, VT, USA

Monica Corsetti, MD Department of Emergency Medicine, Penn State Health, Harrisburg, PA, USA

Farah Z. Dadabhoy, MD Brigham and Women's Hospital, Harvard Medical School, Boston, MA, USA

Hillary E. Davis, MD Department of Emergency Medicine, University of Tennessee Medical Center, Knoxville, TN, USA

Kristin Davis, MD Emergency Medicine, West Virginia University Medicine, Morgantown, WV, USA

Eleanor Dunham, MD Department of Emergency Medicine, Penn State Hershey Medical Center, Hershey, PA, USA

Michael Ernst, MD Alabama College of Osteopathic Medicine, Dothan, AL, USA

Brenna M. Farmer, MD Weill Cornell MedicineNew York, NY, USANew York Presbyterian Brooklyn Methodist Hospital, Brooklyn, NY, USA

Laura J. Fil, MD Department of Emergency Medicine, Vassar Brother's Medical Center, Poughkeepsie, NY, USA

Charles Finch, MD Department of Integrated Medicine, Midwestern University—Arizona College of Osteopathic Medicine, Glendale, AZ, USA

Avram Flamm, MD Department of Emergency Medicine and Public Health Science, Penn State College of Medicine, Hershey, PA, USA

Theresa Forty, MD Department of Emergency Medicine, LewisGale Medical Center, Salem, VA, USA

Daniel Freess, MD Department of Emergency Medicine, Hartford Hospital, Hartford, CT, USA

Integrated Residency in Emergency Medicine, University of Connecticut, Hartford, CT, USA

Brian Freeze, MD Cooper University Hospital, Camden, NJ, USA

Linda Gangai, MD Emergency Medicine, Penn State Health-Milton S. Hershey Medical Center, Hershey, PA, USA

Joshua Ginsburg, MD Department of Emergency Medicine, UT Southwestern Medical Center, Dallas, TX, USA

Scott Goldstein, MD Department of Emergency Medicine' Chief, EMS and Disaster Medicine, Temple University Hospital, Philadelphia, PA, USA

Ravindra Gopaul, MD Department of Emergency Medicine

Penn State Milton S. Hershey Medical Center, Hershey, PA, USA

H. Michelle Greene, MD Nationwide Children's Hospital, Columbus, OH, USA

Justin Grill, MD Department of Emergency Medicine, Trinity Health Muskegon, Muskegon, MI, USA

Joshua Guttman, MD Emory University School of Medicine, Atlanta, GA, USA

Joseph Hansroth, MD Emergency Medicine, West Virginia University Medicine, Morgantown, WV, USA

C. James (Jim) Holliman, MD Emergency Medicine and Public Health Sciences, Pennsylvania State University M. S. Hershey Medical CenterHersheyPAUSA

Military and Emergency Medicine, Uniformed Services University of the Health Sciences, Bethesda, MD, USA

Blake Isom, MD Department of Emergency Medicine, UPMC Harrisburg, Harrisburg, PA, USA

Angela F. Jarman, MD University of California-Davis, Sacramento, CA, USA

Daniel Johnson, MD Department of Emergency Medicine, Penn State College of Medicine, Hershey, PA, USA

Kelly Johnson-Arbor, MD MedStar Georgetown University Hospital, Washington, DC, USA

Jason Jones, MD Department of Emergency Medicine, University of Florida, Gainesville, FL, USA

Annahieta Kalantari, MD Department of Emergency Medicine, Penn State Health Milton S Hershey Medical Center, Hershey, PA, USA

Lawrence E. Kass, MD Department of Emergency Medicine, Penn State Hershey Medical Center, Hershey, , PAUSA

Jonathan Ken, MD Department of Emergency Medicine, Penn State Hershey Medical Center, Hershey, PA, USA

Sajid Khan, MD University of Missouri–Kansas City, Kansas City, MO, USA

Tae Eung Kim, MDCorona Regional Medical Center, Corona, CA, USA

Erol Kohli, MD Attending Physician, Department of Emergency Medicine, BronxCare Health System, Bronx, NY, USA

Chadd K. Kraus, MD Department of Emergency and Hospital Medicine, Lehigh Valley Health Network (LVHN), Allentown, PA, USA

Aaron R. Kuzel, MD Department of Emergency Medicine, University of Louisville School of Medicine, Louisville, KY, USA

Diana V. Labrada, MD University of Kentucky, Lexington, KY, USA

Adam Landman, MD Brigham and Women's Hospital, Mass General Brigham, Boston, MA, USA

Harvard Medical School, Boston, MA, USA

Chaiya Laoteppitaks, MD Department of Emergency Medicine, Sidney Kimmel Medical College, Philadelphia, PA, USA

Michael LeWitt, MD Berwyn, PA, USA

Andrew Little, MD Advent Health East Orlando, Orlando, FL, USA

Jeffrey S. Lubin, MD Departments of Emergency Medicine and Public Health Sciences, Penn State Health Milton S. Hershey Medical Center, Hershey, PA, USA

Jennifer Maccagnano, MD Division of Emergency Medicine, Department of Clinical Specialties, New York Institute of Technology College of Osteopathic Medicine, Old Westbury, NY, USA

Nicholas W. Macklin, MD Department of Emergency Medicine, Wake Forest University School of Medicine, Winston-Salem, NC, USA

Kassem Makki, MD Department of Emergency Medicine-Brooklyn, New York Presbyterian Brooklyn Methodist Hospital, New York, NY, USA

Jessica Mann, MD Department of Emergency Medicine, Penn State Hershey Medical Center, Hershey, PA, USA

Andrew Marshall, MD Brigham and Women's Hospital, Harvard Medical School, Boston, MA, USA

Carmen Julia Martínez Martínez, MD Department of Emergency Medicine, University of South Alabama, Mobile, AL, USA

Department of Emergency Medicine, AdventHealth, Orlando, FL, USA

Laura H. Mattia Atlas Fiduciary Financial, LLC, Sarasota, FL, USA

Kathryn McCans, MD Penn State Hershey Medical Center, Hershey, PA, USA

Dan McCollum, MD Department of Emergency Medicine, Medical College of Georgia at Augusta University, Augusta, GA, USA

Alyson J. McGregor, MD University of South Carolina, Greenville, SC, USA

Eric M. Melnychuk, MD Department of Critical Care, Geisinger Medical Center, Danville, PA, USA

Michael Mesisca, MD Department of Emergency Medicine, Riverside University Health System, Moreno Valley, CA, USA

Aisha Mirza, MD Grey Nuns Community Hospital, University of Alberta, Edmonton, AB, Canada

Caroline Molins, MD Department of Emergency Medicine, University of South Alabama, Mobile, AL, USA

Department of Emergency Medicine, AdventHealth, Orlando, FL, USA

Martin Musi, MD Department of Emergency Medicine, University of Colorado, Boulder, CO, USA

Joan Naidorf, DO Alexandria, VA, USA

Ngoc-Anh Nguyen, MD Houston Methodist Hospital, Houston, TX, USA

Drew Nyce, MD Cooper University Hospital, Camden, NJ, USA

Mark F. Olaf, MD Department of Emergency Medicine, Geisinger Medical Center, Danville, PA, USA

Abigail Olympia, MD Harrisburg Christian School, Harrisburg, PA, USA

Robert P. Olympia, MD Department of Emergency Medicine and Pediatrics, Penn State Hershey Medical Center, Hershey, PA, USA

Nkeiruka N. Onyenekwu, MD Department of Diagnostic Medicine, Second Opinion Consultants, New Orleans, LA, USA

Olga M. Otter, MD Department of Emergency Medicine, University of North Carolina, Chapel Hill, NC, USA

Rachel Patterson, MD St. Luke's Bethlehem, Bethlehem, PA, USA

Faye Pedersen, MD Emergency Physician (Independent), Pittsburgh, PA, USA

Alexis Pelletier-Bui, MD Department of Emergency Medicine, Cooper Medical School of Rowan University, Camden, NJ, USA

Kimberly M. Rathbun, MD Department of Emergency Medicine, AU/UGA Medical Partnership, Athens, GA, USA

Lilia B. Reyes, MD Department of Emergency Medicine and Pediatrics, Penn State Children's Hospital, Hershey, PA, USA

Jessica Ryder, MD The University of Colorado Anschutz Medical Campus, Denver, CO, USA

Christopher E. San Miguel, MD Ohio State University Wexner Medical Center, Columbus, OH, USA

William Saunders, MD University of Toledo Medical Center, Toledo, OH, USA

Timothy J. Schaefer, MD University of Illinois College of Medicine at Peoria, Peoria, IL, USA

Callie Schnitker, MD University of Minnesota, Minneapolis, MN, USA

Department of Emergency Medicine and Hospice and Palliative Care, Regions Hospital, Saint Paul, MN, USA

Nick Schoenmann, MD Department of Emergency Medicine, Medical College of Georgia at Augusta University, Augusta, GA, USA

Jordan B. Schooler, MD Department of Emergency Medicine and Heart and Vascular Institute, Penn State Health Hershey Medical Center, Hershey, PA, USA

Angel L. Schuster, MD Department of Emergency Medicine and Pediatrics, Penn State Children's Hospital, Hershey, PA, USA

Katherine Selman, MD Department of Emergency Medicine, Cooper University Healthcare, Camden, NJ, USA

Judy B. Shahan, MD Department of Emergency Medicine, Geisinger Medical Center, Danville, PA, USA

Matthew Silvis, MD Departments of Family and Community Medicine and Orthopedics and Rehabilitation, Penn State Milton S. Hershey Medical Center, Hershey, PA, USA

Philippa Soskin, MD Department of Emergency Medicine, MedStar Georgetown University Hospital and Washington Hospital Center, Washington, DC, USA

Holly Stankewicz, MD St. Luke's Bethlehem, Bethlehem, PA, USA

Steven VanRees, MD Department of Emergency Medicine, Trinity Health Muskegon, Muskegon, MI, USA

Jeremy Webb, MD Department of Emergency Medicine, LewisGale Medical Center, Salem, VA, USA

Elizabeth Barrall Werley, MD Emergency Medicine, Penn State Health Milton S. Hershey Medical Center, Hershey, PA, USA

Harrison Wermuth, MD Department of Emergency Medicine, Saint Barnabas Hospital, Bronx, NY, USA

John Westhoff, MD Department of Internal Medicine, University of Nevada, Reno School of Medicine, Reno, NV, USA

Warren Wiechmann, MD UC Irvine Health School of Medicine, Irvine, CA, USA

Christopher J. Wilson, MD Department of Emergency Medicine, Geisinger Medical Center, Danville, PA, USA

Robert W. Wolford, MD Department of Emergency Medicine, University of Illinois College of Medicine at Peoria, Peoria, IL, USA

Samuel Wood, MD Department of Pain Management and Rehabilitation, University of Minnesota, Minneapolis, MN, USA

Kahyun Yoon-Flannery, MD MD Anderson Cancer Center at Cooper, Cooper Medical School of Rowan University, Camden, NJ, USA

Lydia Younger, MD Penn State Hershey Medical Center, Hershey, PA, USA

Chapter 1
History of Emergency Medicine

Michael Ernst and Abigail Olympia

There has always been a significant need in the world for emergency medical care. The French physician Dominique Jean Larrey (1766–1842), often regarded as the first modern military surgeon and the father of emergency medicine, was keenly aware of this prevalent need for emergency medical care. During his time in the French Revolutionary Wars, his attention was drawn to the French flying artillery (a strategy in which a team of horses pulled a cannon) and how quickly they could travel. He also noticed the need for faster transport of wounded soldiers from the battlefield to field hospitals. Larrey designed the ambulance volante ("Flying ambulance"), which was essentially an adaptation of the flying artillery, to transport soldiers more quickly to field hospitals. His work did not stop with the "Flying ambulance" though; Larrey also developed ways to make field hospitals more mobile and more similar to what we are familiar with as MASH units in the modern era [1]. He is also considered the first person to successfully perform a pericardiocentesis on a trauma patient. The patient was an Imperial Guard soldier who developed cardiac tamponade due to a thoracic knife wound [2]. Larrey embodied what the field of emergency medicine aims to this day to accomplish, to bring acutely ill patients the highest level of care in the most efficient way possible. He also believed in the idea that every soldier should be treated equally and with the highest level of care regardless of his or her rank. This principle of caring for all patients in their time of need regardless of status would also come to be one which emergency medicine would be founded upon. Consistent with the character of emergency medicine physicians today, Larrey used what knowledge and skills he did have to solve

M. Ernst (✉)
Alabama College of Osteopathic Medicine, Dothan, AL, USA
e-mail: ernstm@acom.edu

A. Olympia
Harrisburg Christian School, Harrisburg, PA, USA
e-mail: abigail.olympia@csagh.org

R. P. Olympia et al. (eds.), *An Emergency Physician's Path*, https://doi.org/10.1007/978-3-031-47873-4_1

complex issues and promote justice and equality in the care of patients. Larrey was just one example of a physician who knew that something needed to be done to improve the access to quality emergency medical care.

Notable advances in emergency care throughout the years:

The Revolutionary War (1776)

- Practiced medicine based on theories instead of truths
- Prescribed bloodletting to induce vomiting to restore balance
- Treated soldiers with serious ailments in a tent
- Lacked necessary supplies, as most medicines came from England

The American Civil War (1861)

- Used quarantine to eliminate yellow fever
- Used trains and boats to transport patients
- Established general hospitals
- Created specialty hospitals

The First Motorized Ambulance (1899)

- Replaced horse-drawn ambulances
- First used by the Michael Reese Hospital in Chicago
- Created a quicker and more efficient way for patients to receive medical care
- Used during World War One

World War One (1914)

- Began using ambulances, antiseptics, and anesthetics
- Learned how to store blood from donors until needed
- Used the Thomas Splint to increase the chances of a soldier surviving a bone fracture

The First Defibrillator (1930)

- Originally designed by Jean-Louis Prévost and Frédéric Batelli
- Tested the idea of using electrical shocks to change the rhythm of a heartbeat
- Created by William Kouwenhoven
- First tested on dogs
- First successful test on human in 1947

World War Two (1939)

- Administered morphine and serum albumin
- Eventually administered a blood substitute rich in oxygen-carrying red cells
- Tagged each casualty
- Treated casualties in a battalion aid station, and treated other casualties in a divisional hospital if stabilization was required
- Used army hospital ships as ambulances, and later used air evacuation to transport patients

As World War II ended, a period of industrialization ensued. Millions of World War II veterans had returned to the United States following the war and the energy that came from having won a war was evident throughout the country. Societies throughout the country began to expand and become more mobile. Families began to uproot and move to new locations. Gone were the days of physicians taking house calls as this form of medical practice was quickly overtaken by large hospitals with more advanced equipment. Federal funding for medical research was on the rise which promoted the development of novel disease treatments such as the Polio vaccine. During this time the public became much more dependent on local hospital emergency rooms [3]. In 1954, Robert H. Kennedy MD, chairman of the Committee on Trauma of the American College of Surgeons, delivered what is known as the "Oration on Trauma." In his speech, he addressed inadequacies in the care of trauma patients and referred to the emergency room as being the weakest part in the care for ill patients. Clearly something needed to be done to improve access to quality emergency medical care in the United States [4]. In 1961, James Mills Jr., MD, worked with Alexandria hospital in Virginia to create the "Alexandria Plan" which was a full-time emergency practice. The "Pontiac Plan" was also created in Michigan and was instituted as a part-time emergency practice. Prior to the institution of these plans, resident physicians or other medical staff were often the primary medical staff providing care for those in the emergency room. These plans helped ensure that patients in the emergency room were receiving around the clock care from attending physicians [3]. While these plans were a huge step in the right direction, an issue with this system remained. The physicians taking on these responsibilities and shifts in the emergency room were physicians from various specialties, some of which did not provide much of a background of knowledge or skill in the care of the acutely ill patient.

It was not until August 1968 that the American College of Emergency Physicians (ACEP) was formed by John Wiegenstein, MD along with seven other physicians from Michigan. The next 2 years involved multiple ACEP meetings including the first ACEP *Scientific Assembly* which took place in Denver, Colorado, in 1969. 1970 was a landmark year in the history of emergency medicine. Bruce Janiak became the first emergency medicine resident in the United States and was a resident at the University of Cincinnati which became the first emergency medicine residency program in the world [5]. The following year in 1971, the University of Southern California became the first academic department of emergency medicine in the United States [3]. These programs helped lay the foundation for the hundreds of emergency medicine residency training programs throughout the country today (Fig. 1.1).

Initially, emergency medicine was vetoed as an official specialty by the American Board of Medical Specialties. At the time, many on the board did not see the utility in having the specialty. It required much persistence from the pioneering physicians in emergency medicine in the late 1960s and early 1970s in showing the utility of emergency medicine as a specialty. Often times these physicians were ridiculed and professionally humiliated by colleagues in other specialties who did not see emergency medicine as a true medical specialty because other physicians had already

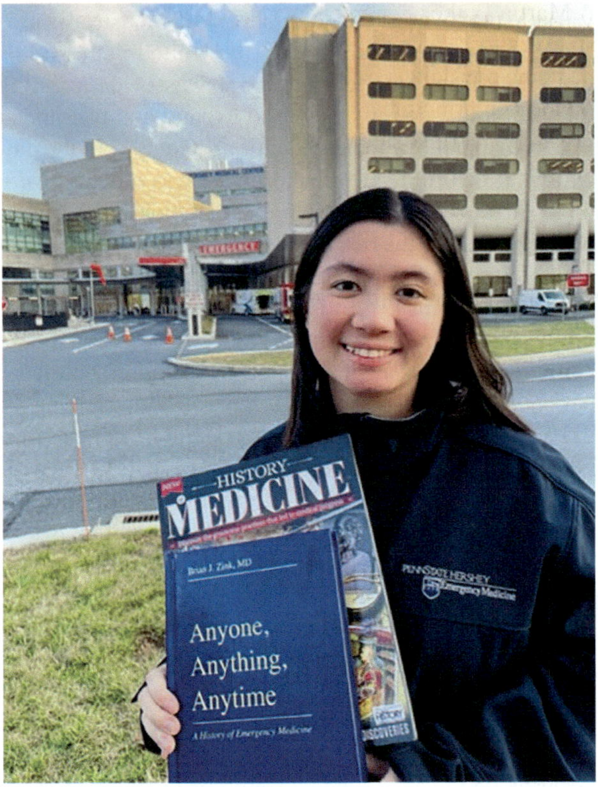

Fig. 1.1 Abigail Olympia celebrating the History of Emergency Medicine at the Penn State Hershey Medical Center Emergency Department

been taking on the management of critically ill patients as well as a lack of contribution to research from the emergency medical community. In 1972, 4 years after Wiegenstein and his colleagues formed ACEP, emergency medicine became officially recognized by the American Medical Association (AMA) as a medical specialty. Then, in 1974, the Emergency Medicine Residents' Association (EMRA) was formed. Finally, after much effort a historic vote by the American Board of Medical Specialties in 1979 took place which named emergency medicine an official medical specialty [6]. In the following year, the first American Board of Emergency Medicine (ABEM) Certification Examination was administered allowing the very first board-certified emergency physicians to be officially approved. It was another 3 years after the first board-certified emergency physicians were approved that emergency medicine began participating for the first time in the National Resident Matching Program (NRMP) [3]. Much has been accomplished in the emergency medicine field since this time and there are now several fellowship opportunities within emergency medicine as well as opportunities to train in emergency medicine all over the country and even globally. Thanks to the efforts of those who continue to teach and serve in emergency medicine, the field continues to expand to this day.

Martin Luther King Jr. has been quoted as saying "Not everybody can be famous but everybody can be great, because greatness is determined by service." Emergency medicine physicians truly are "great" individuals and physicians. This specialty was founded on principles of service and justice. Emergency medicine truly is the medical safety net of society. Everyday emergency medicine physicians take on some of the most complex medical, social, and ethical problems. They do it selflessly and out of a sincere care for their patients who are coming to them in some of their worst moments. It is in those moments where a patient comes to physicians in their hour of need that emergency medicine physicians can make a lifelong impact in the life of an individual. Emergency medicine provides a unique opportunity to leave a lifelong impact in the life of a patient in just minutes or hours. As the field of emergency medicine continues to expand, so does the opportunity to improve the quality of care of acutely ill patients. Like those who pioneered the field of emergency medicine, emergency medicine physicians today continue to advocate for the highest quality of care for their patients and the ability to make a positive impact in society and in the world.

References

1. ACEP. The Revolutionary Flying Ambulance of Napoleon's Surgeon. n.d.. https://web.archive.org/web/20131105230341/http://www.acep.org/About-Us/The-Revolutionary-Flying-Ambulance-of-Napoleon-s-Surgeon. Accessed 1 Sept 2022.
2. Baron Dominique-Jean Larrey: Founder of military surgery and Trauma Care—Hektoen International. Hektoen International—an on-line medical humanities journal. 2017, January 22. https://hekint.org/2017/01/22/baron-dominique-jean-larrey-founder-of-military-surgery-and-trauma-care/. Accessed 1 Sept 2022.
3. Zink BJ. Timeline. In: Anyone, anything, anytime: a history of emergency medicine. Mosby Elsevier; 2006. p. ix–x.
4. The American College of Surgeons | ACS. n.d.. https://www.facs.org/media/vqyhn5fn/1954_kennedy.pdf. Accessed 1 Sept 2022.
5. "Emergency medicine". Emermed.uc.edu. Accessed 9/1/2022.
6. "What is emergency medicine?". Yale School of Medicine. Archived from the original on 19 November 2010. Accessed 9/1/2022.

Part I
Choosing a Career in Emergency Medicine: A Medical Student's Perspective

Chapter 2
Why Should You Choose a Career in Emergency Medicine: The Pros and Cons

Jessica Mann

Early emergency medicine exposure prior to medical school or early in medical school often motivates medical students' choice of a career in emergency medicine [1]. This statement is an interesting concept for me. I started medical school after working 2 years as a research coordinator in an Emergency Department. When I began medical school, I was confident I was going to pursue a career in pediatrics despite the amazing experiences I encountered as a research coordinator. I went through the required clinical rotations during medical school and realized that every day I got up to go to the different rotations, I was just not that excited or motivated. I did not enjoy rounding daily on inpatients, discussing the same concerns and treatments. Going to the operating room during my surgical rotation was exciting, but I could not stand the long hours in the operating room. The pediatric clinic became repetitive and sometimes even boring for me. It was not until I did my first emergency medicine rotation that I realized I wanted to be at the hospital all the time. I also did not want to go home after my shifts were over in the emergency department and I was eager to wake up before every shift and get back to the emergency department. It was at that time I knew my future career was as an emergency physician. I look back now and wonder if I knew all along I was made for emergency medicine, considering the 2 years where I put medical school on hold to work in an emergency department and enjoyed my daily work environment.

J. Mann (✉)
Department of Emergency Medicine, Penn State Hershey Medical Center, Hershey, PA, USA
e-mail: jmann3@pennstatehealth.psu.edu

R. P. Olympia et al. (eds.), *An Emergency Physician's Path*,
https://doi.org/10.1007/978-3-031-47873-4_2

What Are the Benefits of a Career in Emergency Medicine?

Emergency medicine is the fourth-selected specialty match among US senior medical students [2]. There are many reasons that EM is pursued as a career. Those reasons vary from alliance with life goals to the duties of an emergency physician.

The length of residency can be an important factor in deciding what medical specialty to pursue. Some individuals are focused on starting a family. Other individuals are focused on gaining finances to not only pay off debt, but also to start building a savings for future life goals. An emergency medicine residency takes 3–4 years to complete. This is much more ideal for doctors wanting to start on their life goals compared to a surgical, radiologic, or medical subspecialty residency that can take anywhere from 5 to 7 years to complete.

Another attraction to becoming an emergency physician is the opportunity to subspecialize under this path. Numerous fellowship opportunities are discussed in length later in this book. It is very enticing to not only be able to certify in emergency medicine, but go on to have a variety of options to obtain a subspecialty certification. The options for fellowships after completing an emergency medicine residency include toxicology, pediatrics, emergency medical services, critical care, ultrasound, geriatrics, and more.

The career expectations of an emergency physician are also very enticing for individuals. A multitude of skills are required to be an emergency physician. These include procedural skills (suturing, lumbar puncture, chest thoracostomy), airway skills (intubation, emergent cricothyrotomy), ultrasound skills, interpreting EKGs, interpreting radiologic studies, and many more. In addition to the variety of skills, emergency patients are evaluated from a different perspective than say an inpatient or clinic patient. There will be limited to no follow-up with the majority of emergency patients, and the focus of the patient evaluation is on the immediate emergency/concern. This means that emergency physicians have the excitement of immediate interventions to stabilize a patient and then hand the daily care/follow-up to other services. There is no expectation of follow-up or rounding on patients (Fig. 2.1).

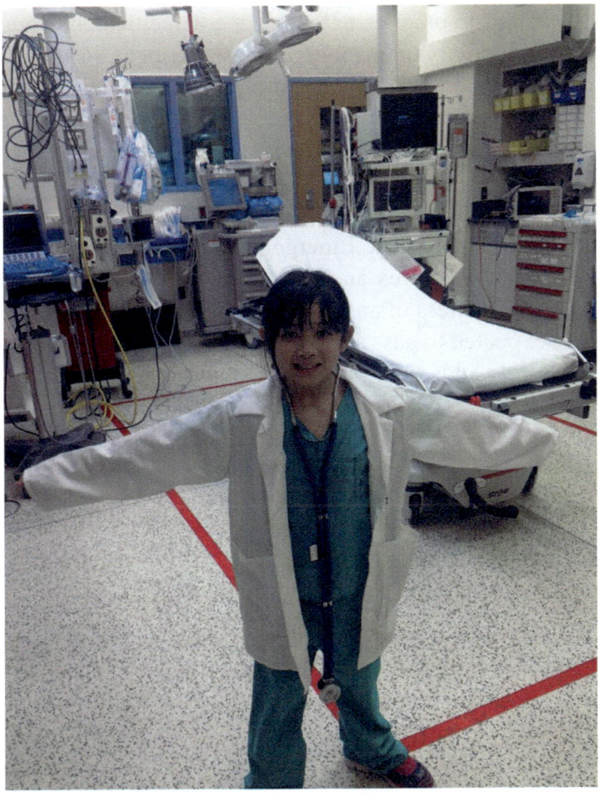

Fig. 2.1 Being exposed to the field of Emergency Medicine at an early age. Resuscitation Bay at the Penn State Hershey Medical Center Emergency Department

What Are the Negative Aspects of a Career in Emergency Medicine?

A recent Medscape report indicates that emergency medicine is the fifth most burned-out specialty behind urology, neurology, physical medicine and rehabilitation, and internal medicine [3]. The high burnout rate in emergency medicine can lead to a multitude of problems for a physician, both professionally and personally. Burnout consequences include an increase in mental health issues, dissatisfaction in the working environment and career, poor work-life balance, and even early retirement. In addition to these concerns, there have been studies to show this burnout starts as early as residency. Working in emergency medicine can be rewarding as discussed before, but starting with burnout as early as residency can lead to difficulties performing job responsibilities, exhaustion both at work and with home life, and overall attitude changes.

Annually emergency physicians face malpractice claims at a slightly higher rate than the average physician with each litigation episode possibly lasting years, and the emergency physician having a lack of support during this time [4]. The fear alone of a malpractice claim in the environment of emergency medicine leads many physicians to practice defensive medicine, which is not always ideal for a patient or the productivity of an emergency department. In addition, it causes most emergency physicians to always worry about mistakes they may make while treating patients. Most emergency physicians are constantly concerned about the higher risk of malpractice claims and how the institution they work for would support or help them through the process. This leads to a more stressful work environment.

Another point of concern with becoming an emergency physician is the board certification process. Emergency medicine is one of fourteen medical specialty boards that requires an oral examination for board certification [5]. This process adds to the stress of an emergency physician becoming board certified. Not only are they expected to pass a thorough written test, but they must also pass the oral boards. It not only adds to the stress, but it also adds to the cost of becoming board certified. On average, the oral examination costs an additional $1500 [5].

Some Aspects of a Career in Emergency Medicine Are Both Positive and Negative

The work environment can both be exciting and increase the stress level of an emergency physician. There is always going to be a variety of patients presenting to the emergency department. Patients may have an exciting or thrilling injury, they may be medically complex that causes critical thinking skills, or they may be so interesting that a physician will want to talk about the case for weeks. In addition, the rewarding feeling an emergency physician gets when they know they have impacted or saved a life is priceless. However, this variety of presentation and pressure to save lives can also lead to an intense and stressful work environment. It is a challenging and exhausting environment that likely contributes to the burnout rate.

The shift work that comes with being an emergency physician can be viewed as both a pro and a con. With shift work, an emergency physician leaves the shift with no duties to perform at home (unless they have an on-call program at their respective department/institution). Emergency physicians will not have any expectations to perform follow-up care on patients. However, most institutions expect emergency physicians to cover all shifts in a day. There are also numerous studies that show shift work can lead to sleep deprivation and sleep loss, which may have a detrimental impact on the overall health of an emergency physician.

The schedule of an emergency physician can lead to benefits and dissatisfaction. The schedule is flexible and most of the time emergency physicians are able to request time off that they will need to accommodate personal and/or professional events. Emergency physicians do not work excessive hours compared to other specialties. Most shifts are somewhere between 8 and 12 hours. An emergency physician's schedule is also usually predictable. The bad news about an EM schedule is that the emergency department is open 365 days a year, 24 hours a day. Emergency physicians will be expected to work holidays. Emergency physicians also are usually expected to work overnight shifts, which can disrupt the circadian rhythm. At some institutions, there are designated nocturnists, which can help avoid this negative aspect of the schedule.

I do not think there is a career in the world that does not face obstacles or negative aspects. The important thing to do when deciding on a career in emergency medicine is first figure out the goals you have for your future, both professionally and personally. Considering those goals, review the negative and positive aspects of a career as an emergency physician and determine if your own goals align with what a career in emergency medicine would be. Critical thinking, flexibility, and adaptation skills are only a few of the requirements to be an emergency medicine physician. The excitement of never knowing what one will encounter with the next patient makes this career a daily adventure. Most emergency physicians can balance the stress, burnout feelings, and demanding work environment by knowing the impact they make on each patient encounter.

References

1. Ray JC, et al. Choosing emergency medicine: influences on medical students' choice of emergency medicine. PLoS One. 2018;13(5):e0196639. https://doi.org/10.1371/journal.pone.0196639.
2. Keith KC, et al. Lifestyle factors and other influences on medical students choosing a career in emergency medicine. AEM Educ Train. 2020;5(1):37–42. https://doi.org/10.1002/aet2.10440.
3. Peckham C. Medscape National Physician Burnout & Depression Report 2019. Medscape 2019. https://www.medscape.com/slideshow/2019-lifestyle-burnout-depression-6011056#2. Accessed 25 Aug 2022.
4. Stehman C, et al. Burnout, drop out, suicide: physician loss in emergency medicine, part I. West J Emerg Med. 2019;20(3):485–94. https://doi.org/10.5811/westjem.2019.4.40970.
5. Brendan Murphy Senior News Writer. Licensing and board certification: what residents need to know. American Medical Association; 22 May 2019. http://www.ama-assn.org/medical-residents/transition-resident-attending/licensing-and-board-certification-what-residents.

Chapter 3
Preparing Yourself To Be the Best Candidate You Can Be

Jessica Ryder

Introduction

So now that you have decided that EM is the career for you, how do you get there? If you are reading this as a first-year medical student, congratulations! You are planning for the future and are already ahead of the game. That being said, I would caution not to get too far ahead of yourself. Medical school is a journey, and it is important to take your time and learn from each stop along the way without skipping straight to the destination. This is particularly important if your goal is to become the best emergency physician that you can be for your patients and your community. The following are general tips and advice that will help you create a solid foundation on which to build your EM career and, in doing so, make you an excellent candidate for the residency of your choosing.

The First 2 Years

It should go without saying that these first 2 years of medical school are your opportunity to build a vast medical knowledge bank. As an emergency physician, you will need to know a great deal about each of the different specialties, so it is important to start with a solid foundation. Put in the work, engage in your classes, and learn the material. This isn't college anymore, the information that you are learning is directly applicable to your career and patient care (with the exception of the Krebs Cycle that you'll memorize for the sixth time in your life). Take the time to get your bearings during the first few months and ace your courses. As you get into the latter half of your first year and into your second year, keep an ear out for research and

J. Ryder (✉)
The University of Colorado Anschutz Medical Campus, Denver, USA

R. P. Olympia et al. (eds.), *An Emergency Physician's Path*,
https://doi.org/10.1007/978-3-031-47873-4_3

volunteer opportunities that you are particularly interested in but do not let these opportunities distract you from the most important part of medical school: your medical knowledge.

During these first 2 years, join your school's Emergency Medicine Interest Group (EMIG) and learn from your upper classmen who will have a plethora of advice for rising EM physicians. Your EMIG will be able to assist you in finding an advisor in EM which is important to find early to help guide your academic planning. When you have available time and feel on-top of your course work, find shadow shifts in the emergency department to get a feel for whether EM is really right for you. This is a good way to build rapport with and show your commitment to your EM advisor. Become a member of national EM organizations: the American College of Emergency Physicians (ACEP) and your respective state chapter, the Emergency Medicine Residents' Association (EMRA), the Society for Academic Emergency Medicine (SAEM)'s Residents and Medical Students (RAMS) section, and the American Academy of Emergency Medicine (AAEM)'s Resident and Student Association (RSA). Explore the various benefits and opportunities that these organization have to offer.

Clinical Rotations

This is the part of medical school that so many wait for: the first stage of your boards may be behind you, you are finally part of a health care team, and you get to regularly see patients. This is your chance to apply your medical knowledge to the art of practicing medicine. Go into each rotation with an open mind, soak everything in, and connect with your preceptors and your patients. EM does not discriminate: we see any patient with any complaint at any time! These rotations are also helping you prepare for the more clinically oriented board exams as well as your EM rotations, both of which are key to a successful residency application. Doing well in your core clerkships will improve your class rank and play a significant role in the residency application screening process.

During the end of your third year and the beginning of your fourth year, you will spend the majority of your time preparing your EM residency application through the Electronic Residency Application Service (ERAS). You will complete your EM rotations, submit your ERAS application, and prepare for and go on interviews for residency. Plan your year carefully and use this time to explore areas of medicine in which you are interested. Take electives in medical fields in which an emergency physician can benefit from having additional knowledge. Many residency interviewers like to discuss how you will be spending the second half of your fourth year so find something that interests you. Explore the EM subspecialties and select elective rotations that will build your EM foundation and prepare you for your intern year. Table 3.1 shows a list of some of the EM subspecialties and helpful non-EM elective rotations.

Table 3.1 ACGME and non-ACGME accredited subspecialties and helpful elective rotations

EM Subspecialties		Helpful Elective Rotations
ACGME Accredited [1]	Non-ACGME Accredited	Anesthesia
Addition Medicine	Disaster Medicine	Cardiology
Clinical Informatics	Global Health and International Emergency Medicine	Critical Care
Emergency Medical Services	Ultrasound	Dermatology
Undersea and Hyperbaric Medicine	Wilderness Medicine	Ophthalmology
Palliative Emergency Care		Orthopedics
Pediatric Emergency Medicine		Otolaryngology
Sports Medicine		Radiology
Toxicology		Trauma

Finally, make the rotations work for you: let your preceptors know that you plan to go into EM. Chances are they will be excited to teach you about the aspects of their specialty that they want all emergency physicians to know. Even though these preceptors may be in different fields, they may have connections with EM faculty and can also help expand your network.

The Gatekeeper: USMLE/COMLEX

Many programs will use board exam results as a filter when initially sorting through hundreds of applications in ERAS [2]. You need to do well if you want your choice of residency programs. For allopathic students, the United States Medical Licensing Exam (USMLE) Step 1 results are reported only as pass or fail for everyone taking the test after January 24, 2022 [3], and a failing result is a red flag on residency applications. The same can be said for a failing score on the Comprehensive Osteopathic Medical Licensing Examination of the United States (COMLEX) Level 1 exam for osteopathic students, which changed to a pass/fail reporting system as of May 2022 [4]. With this change, many residency programs are placing higher emphasis on the USMLE Step 2 Clinical Knowledge (CK) and the COMLEX Level 2 Cognitive Evaluation (CE) scores [2]. Luckily for us, the majority of material tested on these exams is what we do every shift in the emergency department so studying for these board exams will help you on your EM rotations and vice versa. Reserve dedicated time to study for the second stage of your boards if you are able to. This may be challenging to balance with rotations so start planning early. With Step 1 and Level 1 results reported as pass/fail, it is best to have your CK or CE results by the time your ERAS applications becomes available to programs (usually in October) as many programs either require a passing score or screen applications based on a target score prior to offering interviews [2]. Know your learning style and do what works best for you in regard to the timing of these tests and your rotations.

If you fail or do not do well on these tests, it is not the end of your EM career. It just means that you will need to work hard to strengthen the other aspects of your application. Talk with your EM advisor, build your EM network, and blow your away rotations out of the water!

The Audition: EM Rotations

This is your time to shine and put everything you have learned into practice. Arguably the most important part of your application [6], home and away rotations in EM give you an opportunity to see what it is like to be a practicing emergency physician and show programs what kind of intern you will be in July. Through these EM rotations, you will get a Standardized Letter of Evaluation (SLOE). I highly recommend looking at a sample of this type of letter prior to your rotations, which can be found on the Council of Residency Directors in Emergency Medicine (CORD) website. It is a standard form that all EM clerkship directors fill out for rotating student which allows receiving programs to compare your performance between other rotators while adjusting your performance for the number of EM rotations you have completed at the time of the clerkship. Programs will designate where you would fall on their rank list and provide personalized comments based on your performance. These letters were cited as the most important factor in an application when deciding which applicants to offer an interview and was the only factor that was cited by all surveyed program directors when asked which factors play a role in applicant ranking from the 2020 National Residency Match Program's Program Director Survey [5].

It is recommended that you complete two EM rotations [4]. Both should be at hospitals with an EM residency program to allow for a more competitive SLOE. There is a section of the SLOE that asks how many students have completed an EM rotation at the letter writer's institution. It is difficult for programs to get a reliable sense of your capabilities if your letter writer has only ever evaluated three students. One of your rotations should ideally be completed at your home institution if your medical school has an associated EM residency program, leaving you with one home and one away rotation.

When selecting your away rotations, consider the type of program where you would want to train. If you want to stay in a particular geographic region, find rotations within that area to demonstrate interest and commitment. Find rotations at hospitals with similar clinical environments to your desired training environment (county, academic, community, rural, etc.). If you are not sure what region you want to end-up in or what kind of clinical environment you want to train in, use these rotations to figure that out. Be able to discuss what you learned about the different clinical environments when interviewing with programs, especially when your rotations differ from the clinical environment of the program with whom you are interviewing.

During your EM rotations, you should expect to be treated like an intern. It is important to let your team know how many EM rotations you have completed so that they can evaluate your performance based on your expected level of competency. When you pick up a patient, take ownership of that patient. Prior to entering the room, have a differential in mind based on the patient's chief complaint. Perform a focused history and physical exam, formulate a differential and plan, execute that plan after discussion with your team, and consistently reassess your patient. You should be safely independent. If the patient looks sick when you enter the room, do not hesitate to get help! If you do not know something, look up the answer before asking the residents or attending. Take time to gather your thoughts and have a solid management plan prior to presenting your patient. Your oral presentation is your moment to show the residents and attendings what kind of intern you will be. Keep it concise and focused. Present your history and physical exam with pertinent positives and negatives to demonstrate the differentials that you were considering as you evaluated the patient. Verbalize these differentials and justify why you do or do not think those are the primary diagnosis. Discuss the investigations you would like to order and where you think this patient is going to end up (discharged, observation, admitted, ICU, etc.). This entire presentation should take you about 2–3 min in total. It is ok to be wrong. Most programs want to see you demonstrate the appropriate thought process and that you can present a well thought-out evaluation of the patient [6]. Follow up on your investigations, have an idea of what the results mean for the patient's disposition and diagnosis, then notify your team. Ask if you can speak to the consultant about your patient and, when doing so, be sure to identify yourself as a medical student taking care of the patient.

When you are not evaluating a patient or documenting, be helpful and present. If you are asked to do something by any member of the team, say yes responsibly. If you do not know how to do something or if you have never done a procedure, let your team know. Look up the procedure and be able to verbalize the needed equipment and steps prior to performing it. Your team will be more inclined to offer you the chance to do the procedure if you can do so. Do not lie, ever! It is not safe for your patients, and you build more trust with your team when you say you do not know the answer or forgot to perform a specific physical exam rather than saying it was normal. Find the balance between being annoyingly eager and unnoticeably quiet. You want to pass the "3am test!" Programs are not necessarily looking for the smartest student or the student who gets every answer right. They are looking for someone that they want to work with on shift. Be a team player, be personable, be respectful, and learn how to read the room. During a resuscitation, help get the patient undressed without getting in the way of the nurse who is putting in an IV. If a patient asks for a blanket or pillow, be the one to bring it to them. Get to know where various supplies are kept in the department and bring your resident the procedure kit they need when they ask. Help your nurse or tech clean up the room so that the next patient can be seen faster.

Do not forget to ask for feedback. Asking for feedback in the middle of the shift during a lull allows for the opportunity to adjust and improve on shift. Ask for feedback again at the end of the shift from both residents and attendings that you worked with, and when someone offers advice for the future, take it to heart. If they give you their contact information, take it and reach out with questions. This is another opportunity to build your network with both attendings and residents. The residents at the program you are rotating with went through this same process just a few years before and can speak to other programs and experiences.

Research, Presentations, and Publications

This is an important box to check on your application but do not do research just to do research. Find something that interests you even if it is not directly in the field of EM. Remember, we see all patients and complaints so that stroke project with your favorite neurologist is still applicable to your EM career. Start looking for opportunities during your first year and be involved in projects during your second year, aiming to have a final product published or in review during your third and early fourth year.

Look for other opportunities to present and participate in national EM conferences. If you saw an interesting patient during a rotation, find an advisor and write up a case report. If you saw an interesting radiograph or ultrasound, find an image series to publish in. These can be low-hanging fruit that are easy and quick to write up, get your name published, but also, and more importantly, help you learn from interesting patients that you cared for firsthand. The national EM organizations each have an annual national conference with a multitude of presentation opportunities from abstracts and poster presentations to clinical case competitions to educational lecture opportunities. Participate in these conferences and gain experience in public speaking and presenting while surrounding yourself with the experts in the field.

EM programs tend to place less emphasis on the number of research projects that you are involved in [7]. Programs value commitment and longevity over sporadic involvement, so choose your projects carefully and have a true interest in what is being investigated. Make sure you know your project(s) inside and out. Be able to intelligently discuss your involvement as anything listed on your ERAS application and curriculum vitae (CV) is free game for interviewers.

Beyond Academics

Demonstrate a commitment to emergency medicine and explore the various niches within the specialty. Take time to volunteer, both medically and non-medically, in your local community. Volunteer in a medical tent at the local Rock'n'Roll Marathon and put IV's in dehydrated runners. On your away rotation, ask about volunteer opportunities in the community and spend a few hours at the local student-run refugee clinic. Be an active member of your school's EMIG and apply for leadership positions by the time you are a third- or fourth-year student. It is not enough to simply hold the position though. Have a plan for your EMIG with proposals for improvement and student engagement. Be able to elaborate on your role and vision for the organization as a leader.

There are numerous EM conferences throughout the year, both regionally and nationally. When planning your third and fourth years, schedule time to attend these conferences if feasible. Both SAEM and AAEM have medical student ambassadors at their national conferences, while EMRA, which is closely intertwined with ACEP, has leadership positions available for medical students. Apply for these positions and you will have the opportunity to network with experts in EM at these conferences while building relationships with mentors outside of your local institution. Volunteer as an ultrasound model at your local conference or be an actor in the SIM Wars competition. If available in-person, plan to attend the residency fairs where program leadership and current residents may be available to answer any questions you have about their programs. Do your research prior to attending this fair, whether virtual or in-person. Approach programs with specific questions and discuss something unique that interests you about that program. Have updated copies of your CV available to hand out if asked. Dress professionally. Collect contact information and business cards. The impression that you make at these conferences and events can influence how your application is screened. Know that when you attend the kickoff parties and EMRA parties, there are eyes everywhere so have fun responsibly. When you get home from the conference, wait a few days then reach out to some of the connections you made. Current residents are particularly helpful contacts to have as they can speak about their personal experiences with the program and what they feel the weaknesses or strengths of the program are.

A running theme throughout this chapter is networking: EM is a very small world. Start making connections early in medical school and maintain those relationships. Build these networks at every opportunity you have and lean on your mentors but do not expect them to do the work for you. Come to them with specific questions. Do not be afraid to ask different people the same question. Each person may approach your question from a different perspective. Engage your mentors during the application cycle. Have a variety of people edit your personal statement and ask for opinions on various training programs. Ask your mentors to reach out to programs on your behalf if there is a particular program from whom you have not heard but do this cautiously. Do not abuse your relationships. Have a candid conversation with your mentors about what you want out of training and which programs are at the top of your list. If they have contacts, ask if they would mind reaching out to advocate on your behalf. This should truly be reserved for your top programs if necessary.

Final Thoughts

While building your foundational medical knowledge and exploring EM, be sure to make time for yourself. Medical school is a stressful time and this only increases during the residency application season. Get outside, make time for your friends and family, bake those cupcakes you have been meaning to try, sit down, and finally finish that puzzle. You will find that the EM community values your personality outside of medicine and we want to be able to connect with you on a personal level so do not let that part of yourself get lost during medical school.

This chapter serves as a guide for making yourself a competitive candidate, but it is by no means comprehensive. Ask your mentors and upper classman for advice and explore the various resources available through the national EM organizations. This is an exciting time in your life so make every minute count.

Recommended EM Resources

- EMRA and CORD Student Advising Guide—a great overall guide to matching into EM

  Website: https://www.emra.org/books/msadvisingguide/msag/

- CORD's Emergency Medicine Medical Student Planner—a general outline of the four years in medical school for a successful EM match
- AAEM/RSA's Rules of the Road for Medical Students—another guide for a career in EM
- EMRA Match Tool—for searching residency programs and away rotations

  Website: https://webapps.emra.org/utils/spa/match#/search/map

- EMRA Resident-Student mentorship program—for finding resident mentors

  Website: https://www.emra.org/students/advising-resources/student-resident-mentorship-program/

- ALIEM's 3-minute EM Student Presentation—a general guide for oral patient presentations

  Website: https://www.aliem.com/the-3-minute-em-student-presentation/

- EM basic and EM:Rap's C3 series—podcasts with core EM knowledge to help prepare for away rotations
- Tintinalli's Emergency Medicine Just The Facts—a digestible version of one of the main EM textbooks
- Pre-Test Emergency Medicine—practice questions for the EM shelf exam

References

1. Accreditation Council for Graduate Medical Education. Overview. Emergency Medicine; n.d.. https://www.acgme.org/specialties/emergency-medicine/overview/. Accessed 20 Jan 2023.
2. National Resident Matching Program Data Release and Research Committee. Results of the 2022 NRMP Program Director Survey. https://www.nrmp.org/wp-content/uploads/2022/09/PD-Survey-Report-2022_FINALrev.pdf.
3. Examination results and scoring. USMLE. n.d.. https://www.usmle.org/scores transcripts/examination-results-and-scoring. Accessed 1 Oct 2022.
4. National Board of Osteopathic Medical Examiners. Scoring & reporting. National Board of Osteopathic Medical Examiners; n.d.. https://www.nbome.org/assessments/comlex-usa/comlex-usa-level-1/scores-transcripts/. Accessed 20 Jan 2023.
5. National Resident Matching Program Data Release and Research Committee. Results of the 2020 NRMP Program Director Survey. https://www.nrmp.org/wp-content/uploads/2022/01/2020-PD-Survey.pdf.
6. Emergency Medicine Residents' Association. Consensus statement for the emergency medicine 2022–2023 residency application cycle regarding emergency medicine away rotations. EMRA; n.d.. https://www.emra.org/be-involved/be-an-advocate/working-for-you/statement-for-residency-application-cycle-em-away-rotations/. Accessed 2 Oct 2022.
7. National Resident Matching Program. Charting Outcomes in the Match: U.S. Allopathic Seniors. 2022. https://www.nrmp.org/wp-content/uploads/2022/07/Charting-Outcomes-MD-Seniors-2022_Final.pdf.

Chapter 4
Making Sense of the Match

Christopher E. San Miguel

What Is the Match?

The Match is the process by which soon-to-be medical school graduates are assigned to graduate medical education programs called residencies. The initial phases of the application process are similar to applying to medical school. Applicants complete a common application and apply to individual programs through the Electronic Residency Application Service (ERAS). Programs review applications and offer interviews to applicants they think will be a good fit for their respective program. Applicants are free to accept and decline interviews as they receive them. At the end of interview season however, students do not receive admission decisions from individual programs. Instead, every applicant submits a preferred rank list of programs, and every program submits a preferred rank list of applicants to the National Residency Matching Program (NRMP). Using a complex algorithm, applicants and programs are matched. This is a binding agreement and backing out of a match is not allowed except under extreme circumstances.

How Does the Match Work?

The Match seeks to pair residency applicants and residency programs in such a way that it provides the same results as if every applicant accepted a position with their most preferred program which made them an offer of acceptance. Utilizing the match algorithm avoids the uncertainty and prolonged timeline of a traditional application system. There is no need for early acceptances, waitlists, or last-minute

C. E. San Miguel (✉)
Ohio State University Wexner Medical Center, Columbus, OH, USA
e-mail: Christopher.sanmiguel@osumc.edu

R. P. Olympia et al. (eds.), *An Emergency Physician's Path*,
https://doi.org/10.1007/978-3-031-47873-4_4

withdrawals. Except for extraordinary circumstances, every residency program knows exactly which newly minted doctors they will be training in just a few months, and conversely every medical school graduate knows where they will be training.

If you are the type of person who wants to know all the details of how the sausage is made, please read further. For everyone else, the summary statement is this: The only strategy you should employ in ranking programs is to list programs based solely on your preference. While a program's competitiveness and how much they like you will certainly influence the final match, these factors are independent of where you place them on your rank list. We'll re-examine this after we describe The Match Process.

Since 1998, The Match has utilized an applicant proposing algorithm [1]. This means the algorithm attempts to create all the matches by systematically working its way down each applicant's rank list. This is best seen in an example in Table 4.1. Imagine Adam is an Emergency Medicine applicant who has submitted a rank list of three emergency medicine programs in the following order: County, Community, and University Hospitals. Each program has four spots to fill in the Match. For this example, we are going to say that the algorithm has started to work on Adam's match about halfway down the list of total applicants; however, it is worth noting that the algorithm functions the exact same for each applicant regardless of their order.

The algorithm first attempts to match Adam at his top choice, County Hospital. As you can see in the table, four other applicants have already been tentatively matched at County Hospital. The algorithm then compares Adam's position on the County Hospital's rank list to the positions of the tentatively matched applicants. Unfortunately for Adam, he was ranked lower on County's rank list (84) than all the tentatively matched applicants (7, 9, 13, and 25), and so Adam will not match at County Hospital. In Match terms, a higher ranking is associated with a lower number, e.g., the highest ranked and most desirable applicant is rank number 1.

At this point, the algorithm attempts to place Adam at the next program on his rank list, Community Hospital. In Table 4.2, you can see that once again four applicants have already tentatively matched at Community Hospital. However, this time Adam (64) is ranked higher than Elizabeth (77). This means Adam is tentatively matched at Community Hospital! As for Elizabeth, the algorithm will now attempt to match her at whatever program she ranked right below Community Hospital on

Table 4.1 Rank order lists at the start of Adam's match

	Tentatively matched applicants' and Adam's position on program rank list		
Adam's rank list	County hospital	Community hospital	University hospital
1. County	7. Bryan	2. Brendan	4. Brooke
2. Community	9. Carla	33. Casey	14. Carson
3. University	13. Debra	49. Danielle	28. David
	25. Eleanor	77. Elizabeth	31. Ella
	84. Adam	64. Adam	7. Adam

her list. As seen in Table 4.3, Adam will stay tentatively matched at Community Hospital unless he is displaced by an applicant who was higher on Community Hospital's rank list, in the same way that he displaced Elizabeth.

Unfortunately, Adam is eventually displaced by Frank in Table 4.4. The algorithm now returns to Adam's rank list and attempts to place him at this his third ranked program, University Hospital. Adam is quite high on University Hospital's rank list (7), so he has once again been tentatively matched in Table 4.5. This time,

Table 4.2 Rank order lists after Adam's first attempted match—currently unmatched

	Tentatively matched applicants and position on program rank list		
Adam's rank list	County hospital	Community hospital	University hospital
2. Community	7. Bryan	2. Brendan	4. Brooke
3. University	9. Carla	43. Casey	14. Carson
	13. Debra	49. Danielle	28. David
	25. Eleanor	77. Elizabeth	31. Ella
		64. Adam	7. Adam

Table 4.3 Rank order lists after Adam's second attempted match—tentatively matched at community hospital

	Tentatively matched applicants and position on program rank list		
Adam's rank list	County hospital	Community hospital	University hospital
2. Community	7. Bryan	2. Brendan	4. Brooke
3. University	9. Carla	33. Casey	14. Carson
	13. Debra	49. Danielle	28. David
	25. Eleanor	64. Adam	31. Ella
		64. Adam	7. Adam

Table 4.4 Rank order lists after Frank's attempted match—Adam is currently unmatched

	Tentatively matched applicants and position on program rank list		
Adam's rank list	County hospital	Community hospital	University hospital
3. University	7. Bryan	2. Brendan	4. Brooke
	9. Carla	33. Casey	14. Carson
	13. Debra	49. Danielle	28. David
	25. Eleanor	52. Frank	31. Ella
			7. Adam

Table 4.5 Rank order lists after Adam's third attempted match—tentatively matched at university hospital

	Tentatively matched applicants and position on program rank list		
Adam's rank list	County hospital	Community hospital	University hospital
3. University	7. Bryan	2. Brendan	4. Brooke
	9. Carla	33. Casey	7. Adam
	13. Debra	49. Danielle	14. Carson
	25. Eleanor	52. Frank	28. David
			7. Adam

it was Ella (31) who was removed from her tentative match, and the algorithm must attempt to place her at her the next program on her rank list. Adam's rank list was quite short, so if he is displaced again, there are no further programs for the algorithm to attempt to match with him. If this occurs, Adam will go unmatched. This process continues until every applicant is either matched or has exhausted their list of ranked programs. Once this occurs, all the tentative matches become permanent.

Can I Use the System to My Advantage or Game the System?

The Match algorithm is already set up in favor of applicants. Because it works down each applicant's rank list rather than working down programs' rank lists, it is weighing the applicants' preferences heavier than the programs' preferences. The only thing which should influence a program's position on an applicant's rank list is the applicant's desire to train there relative to the other programs on the applicant's list.

You will have noticed as we worked through Adam's match process, that once the algorithm was attempting to match Adam at a program, the process was exactly the same, regardless of whether this was the first program on Adam's list or the last program on Adam's list. His spot on each program's rank list is set before the Match occurs and is unchanged by anything that happens during the Match. Adam did not miss the chance to match at University Hospital because he ranked two other programs higher. Both applicants and programs have no ability to change or influence their rank order lists after the submission deadline. Both sides simply wait a few weeks for the Match process to take place and be verified before the results are revealed during Match week.

You may have also noticed that University Hospital ranked Adam quite highly. Despite this high ranking, Adam only tentatively matched at University Hospital after he had already failed to match at the two programs which were higher on his rank list. Applicants are not pulled away from programs they prefer simply because another program finds them highly desirable. Applicants should not adjust their rank lists based on their perceived competitiveness at their programs of interest.

What Is the Process Like for Applicants Who Are Couples' Matching?

For those applicants attempting to start residency in the same year as their significant other, they may consider entering the Match as a couple. While this option is typically utilized by romantic partners, it is worth noting that any two applicants can participate in the Match as a couple. When coupled, the algorithm links the two applicants' rank order lists. As an individual, the only way to lose a tentative match is if a higher ranked applicant is placed at that program. As a couple, you can also

Table 4.6 Couples matching rank list

Adam's rank order list	Allison's rank order list
1. County Hospital (Chicago)	1. Community Hospital (Chicago)
2. County Hospital (Chicago)	2. County Hospital (Chicago)
3. Community Hospital (Chicago)	3. Community Hospital (Chicago)
4. Community Hospital (Chicago)	4. County Hospital (Chicago)
5. University Hospital (Philadelphia)	5. University Hospital (Philadelphia)
6. County Hospital (Chicago)	6. University Hospital (Philadelphia)
7. University Hospital (Philadelphia)	7. Community Hospital (Chicago)
8. Unranked	8. Community Hospital (Chicago)
9. County Hospital (Chicago)	9. Unranked
10. Unranked	10. University Hospital (Philadelphia)
11. University Hospital (Philadelphia)	11. Unranked
12. Community Hospital (Chicago)	12. Unranked
13. Unranked	13. County Hospital (Chicago)

lose a tentative match if your partner is displaced from their tentative match. In creating their rank order lists, each member of the couple may duplicate programs, but they cannot duplicate the pair of programs. See Table 4.6 for an example of rank order lists for Adam and Allison. Adam and Allison's ideal placements are Adam at County and Allison at Community. If either of them is unable to be matched at their number one program, the algorithm moves down to both of their second choices and attempts to place Adam at County and Allison at County. The next pair on the lists would attempt to place them both at Community. This process continues all the way down the list until the algorithm finds a tentative match for both applicants. As you can see, you can rank programs based on any criteria that is important to you as a couple. Any program can be paired with any other program on a couple's rank order list regardless of geography or specialty. A common strategy for couples is to apply in geographic areas with multiple programs for both applicants to increase the number of match possibilities which would result in them living in the same area.

How Well Does the Algorithm Work?

The algorithm does remarkably well in placing applicants at their most preferred program which has space for them. In fact, it would produce perfect results if the only way that any applicant was moved off of a tentative match was because they were displaced by a higher ranked applicant. However, because of couples matching and preliminary year matching, there are scenarios in which individuals are displaced for other reasons, e.g., their partner was displaced off their tentative match or the applicant was displaced off of their preliminary year match. Because of these possibilities, the processing order can have an impact on the final matches. The magnitude of this impact has been studied and is thankfully minimal. In experiments run on data from matches in the early 1990s, the largest impact which could be created was a change in program match for only 4 out of 22,353 applicants [1]. Regardless there is nothing the individual applicant can do to influence their processing order, so this does not change any of our recommendations.

When Do Applicants and Programs Find Out the Results of The Match?

The results of The Match are revealed in mid-March [2]. On the Monday of Match Week, programs find out if they have filled all their spots with incoming residents, and applicants find out if they have successfully matched to a residency program. On Thursday, programs find out which applicants have matched with them, but they have to keep it confidential for another day. On Friday, applicants find out where they will be completing residency. Most (if not all) medical schools have a Match Day ceremony for their students with varying formats and methods by which applicants discover their matches. If a public celebration is not your thing, all applicants are notified of their match by email as well.

What If I'm Unsuccessful in the Match/Don't Match?

For those applicants who don't match and programs that don't fill, Match week is quite busy. Between Monday and Thursday, programs and applicants can take part in the Supplemental Offer and Acceptance Program (SOAP) [3]. On Monday, unmatched applicants are able to review and modify their residency applications in ERAS and submit the updated applications to unfilled programs. Starting on Tuesday and continuing through Wednesday, programs can review applications, interview applicants, and develop their SOAP preference list. Unlike in The Match, applicants do not submit a preference or rank list in the SOAP. On Thursday, there are four offer rounds which last two hours each. In each round, offers are extended to applicants based on the number of positions available within a program and the applicant's position on the program's SOAP preference list. For instance, if County Hospital has three residency spots to fill, offers will be extended to the top three applicants on their preference list. Applicants can accept, decline, or allow offers to expire at the end of the round. Applicants may receive multiple offers in each round but can only accept one offer throughout the entire SOAP process. Once the applicant accepts an offer, they are committed to the program which made the offer and are not able to receive further offers. Continuing the above example, if only one applicant accepts County Hospital's offer in the first round, the second round will begin with offers being extended to the next two applicants on County Hospital's SOAP preference list who did not accept an offer in round one. There is certainly a lot more strategy for applicants and programs in the SOAP system than in The

Match. Any applicant who finds themselves needing to take part in the SOAP is strongly encouraged to work closely with their specialty advisors and Deans' offices to make sure they are optimizing their chances to receive and accept an offer.

References

1. Roth AE, Peranson E. The redesign of the matching market for American physicians: some engineering aspects of economic design. Am Econ Rev. 1999;89(4):748–80. https://doi.org/10.1257/aer.89.4.748.
2. 2023 main residency match applicants calendar. NRMP. n.d.. https://www.nrmp.org/match-calendars/main-residency-applicants/. Accessed 2 Feb 2023.
3. Soap. NRMP. n.d.. https://www.nrmp.org/residency-applicants/soap/. Accessed 2 Feb 2023.

Chapter 5
Letters of Recommendation, SLOEs, Applications, Personal Statements, and Interviews

Kristin Davis and Joseph Hansroth

Applications

The application process for Emergency Medicine (EM) residency can be intimidating. There are several things to consider including: obtaining letters of recommendation (LORs), writing a personal statement, and filling out/submitting the actual application. Then come the interviews and all the challenges associated with those. It may seem overwhelming at first, but with proper preparation, the process can go smoothly.

Most specialties, including EM, use the Association of American Medical Colleges' (AAMC) Electronic Residency Application Service (ERAS) application [1]. The ERAS platform allows applicants to submit all the components of their application to the participating programs of their choice [2]. ERAS consists of the following sections: personal and biographic information, curriculum vitae, personal statement, letter(s) of recommendation, USMLE transcript and/or COMLEX-USA transcript, medical student performance evaluation (MSPE or "Dean's Letter"), medical school transcript, and an optional photo. The ERAS Applicant Worksheet and ERAS Residency Applicant Checklist found on the AAMC website highlight all the information that must be included on your ERAS application [3]. Applications typically open in early June and may be submitted as early as September. Typically, the final deadline for submission varies from program to program, but with Emergency Medicine becoming more competitive, it is recommended that you submit your application as early as possible. This will give program directors (PDs) time to review your application and extend an invitation to interview. If your application is submitted too late, it may not be reviewed by PDs before all their interview

K. Davis (✉) · J. Hansroth
Emergency Medicine, West Virginia University Medicine, Morgantown, WV, USA
e-mail: kristin.davis@hsc.wvu.edu; jahansroth@hsc.wvu.edu

R. P. Olympia et al. (eds.), *An Emergency Physician's Path*,
https://doi.org/10.1007/978-3-031-47873-4_5

spots have filled. It is possible that you might still be waiting for a letter of recommendation on the submission date. In this case, it would be best to submit your application without this information so that PDs can begin reviewing the rest of your application. In a survey of PDs, only 15% stated it was "highly likely" that they would review an application if it were completed after the ERAS opening date [4]. Most of the information cannot be updated or changed after submission, but you may submit the missing letters as you receive them.

The number of emergency medicine residency programs has grown rapidly in the last decade, and in 2022, there are 277 training locations available with 2921 total positions [5–7]. This can create significant angst for the student pursuing a career in EM—*How many programs should I apply to? Does it matter how many programs I apply to? Are there differences in the types of programs?* Research shows that the average allopathic student applies to 46 programs and osteopathic students apply to an average of 50 programs. The average student will attend 12 interviews and having that same number on a rank list provides a 99% chance of a successful match [8]. When evaluating the list of programs for which to send your application, there are many things to consider.

- Does this program match what I am looking for in my residency? Consider the length of the program (3 versus 4 years), academic or community-based location, specific interests in the department, and opportunities for rotations at other sites.
- Is this in a location I would enjoy living? Although residency is a busy time, you will still have free time to do things besides work. Since resident wellness is important, find a place you can see yourself living. If you only like warm weather, a residency program in a far northern state may not be for you. If you can't see yourself living in a big city, there are plenty of programs outside of major urban areas—spend your time applying there instead.
- There are financial costs associated with the application process. Each application has a fee for submission. Travel for each interview also costs money and should be something you consider. The COVID pandemic changed a lot of this with online interviews and no in-person pre-interview dinners. When a pre-pandemic interview format returns, consider your time and financial costs when creating your interview list.
- Create a logical road trip if possible. Keep a running list of interviews and dates and try to interview at programs in the same region in order to maximize your travel efficiency.

Letters of Recommendations and Standardized Letters of Evaluation (SLOEs)

There are two types of Letters of Recommendation (LORs) that can be submitted as part of your ERAS application for EM residency. The traditional LOR can be written by anyone who knows you well, but should ideally be written by someone within the field of academic EM. Some students may also choose to have a close advisor such as a dean or a preceptor with whom the student worked extensively, write them a letter. It is a narrative-format letter that typically describes how hard you work and why you will be an asset in whatever program you are working. The Standardized Letter of Evaluation (SLOE) is a form developed by the Council of Residency Directors in Emergency Medicine (CORD) to provide a "global perspective" of an applicant to allow for standardized, concise, and a discerning way to compare candidates for EM residency [9]. The SLOE was created in the 1990s and has undergone several updates since its inception. According to one study, the SLOE has consistently been named the most important component of the EM residency application by program directors [10]. Most emergency medicine rotations for students applying to the field will provide a SLOE at the end of the rotation; just be sure to ask about this before the rotation starts. The information in the SLOE will typically be collected from on-shift evaluations and compiled by the clerkship director. The SLOE may be written as a single author letter or by a panel of attendings. This panel creates what is known as a departmental SLOE. The SLOE has four sections—Background Information, Qualifications for EM, Global Assessment, and Written Comments.

- Background Information provides some description of the program writing the letter (number of students on rotations, breakdown of grading in the past) and how well you are known by the department.
- Qualifications for EM asks a series of EM-rotation specific questions about performance and requests that the writers compare you to your peers (above level, at level, or below level). Most of the questions in this section focus on more intangible aspects of your rotation. Can you work with a team? Do you work hard? Can you care for patients with compassion? How much guidance will you need in residency?
- Global Assessment asks two big questions. First, how do you rank as compared to your peers in the same year as you—in the top 10%, top-third, middle-third, or lower-third? Second, where are you predicted to be on the program's rank list. Although the questions seem similar, and they are, there can be some important differences in where a student ranks. Someone who has all the answers but does not mesh well with the program and can't work on a team may rank high on the first question but may not be high on a program's rank list. Research has shown that the most important predictor of not matching in emergency medicine is a lower-third ranking on the SLOE. A single lower-third ranking is less than ideal but may not be devastating in regard to match outcomes. Multiple lower-third rankings though, especially across programs, do not portend well for a match in emergency medicine. If a student knows they are ranking significantly below peers, they should strongly consider contingency planning in order to increase their odds in matching. Contingency planning may mean applying to more programs or applying to newer programs in less competitive locations, but may also mean considering applying to other specialties.

- Written Comments will provide narrative feedback from your rotation. These may include anecdotes of things you did well on the rotation, attributes that made you stand out amongst your peers, areas where you are working, and explanations of how you were ranked on the global assessment.

A key part to your application will be your letters of reference. For EM, the most influential letters are SLOEs written by EM faculty who have worked with you clinically. SLOEs are typically written by your home department and by EDs where you have done rotations. Classic letters of recommendation can be uploaded too and may be a nice ancillary piece of information for program leaders to use when reviewing your application.

Personal Statements

The personal statement is designed to explain your journey to this point. Why did you choose medicine? How did you settle on emergency medicine? Is there a story that defines you? These are all topics you could consider covering in your personal statement. The personal statement is a required section of your application but is, by no means, the most important aspect. It may be easier to stand out for the wrong reasons when it comes to the personal statement. Be sure your grammar and spelling are correct. Being too "weird" or "witty" might raise a red flag on your application. Keep your personal statement to a single page and don't spend an exorbitant amount of time on this; program directors will read your work but your test scores, SLOEs, and MSPE are all considered more impactful [11].

Interviews

The interview is the final step in the application process for EM residency and is crucial to determine which program(s) will be a good fit for you. It typically has two parts: the interview day itself and a social gathering with the residents, which may be before or after the interview. Though it may seem less important because it is informal, the social gathering should still be taken seriously. It is a time to get to know the residents and get a feel for their well-being. It is more relaxed than the formal interview day, but a bad first impression could still negatively impact your chances of matching with the program. Some things to consider about the social gathering:

- Be on time and dress appropriately (typically business casual).
- Talk to as many of the residents as you can. Talk with your fellow applicants as well. Watch to see how the residents interact with each other and how they talk about the program off campus.

- Spend some time asking about the non-medical aspects of the program—What do residents do for fun? Are there specific neighborhoods that most people seem to like?
- There will typically be alcohol available; don't be the one who drinks too much.
- Enjoy the time interacting with your peers. Once you get the hang of the dinners, the food is typically very good, and you can get a great feel for the program before starting the formal interview day.

The formal interview day is typically the morning or afternoon after your interview dinner. At most programs, you will have interviews with the program director, other faculty members, and sometimes even the chief residents. This is the time to really sell yourself and leave a great impression. Many of your peers will also have excellent CVs but the interview is where you can really stand out. Rank lists are often made based on interviews. Here are some tips for the formal interview day:

- Practice your answers to some common interview questions beforehand. There will undoubtedly be questions that you have not prepared for, but you should be able to answer basic interview questions quickly and confidently.
- Review your own application before the interview day and be comfortable talking about any aspect of it. If you list that you speak three languages, be prepared to show your skills.
- Show up on time in professional attire.
- Engage with the other applicants.
- Ask questions that show your interest in the program.
- If you are very interested in the program, it is ok to say so, but be genuine. Feigned interest is quickly detected and will cause you to appear less desirable.
- Be respectful to ALL members of the team, including administrative staff. They have close relationships with PDs and current residents.
- After the interview, thank you notes (also sometimes called "love letters") are optional. They will rarely make or break your spot on the rank list, but if you have a favorite program, it's ok to tell them so.
- Most importantly, be yourself. You are interviewing at programs in an attempt to find the best fit for you. You will be working at this program for the next 3–4 years, so it's important to find somewhere you will be happy.

Applying to Emergency Medicine residency can be an exciting process. It takes time and effort to compose your application, but the reward is finding the program that is the best fit for you and where you will be happy. Work hard on your rotations to earn favorable SLOEs. Submit your application as soon as possible to programs where you would like to interview. On interview day, be the person with whom everyone wants to work—be personable, know your application, and be interested in the program and their unique characteristics. Although it may seem daunting now, the residency match process works and you can be successful, just like so many of the residents you meet along the way.

References

1. Association of American Medical Colleges. ERAS 2022 Participating Specialties & Programs 2022. https://services.aamc.org/eras/erasstats/par/index.cfm. Accessed 10 Mar 2022.
2. Association of American Medical Colleges. About ERAS. 2022. https://students-residents.aamc.org/applying-residencies-eras/about-eras. Accessed 10 Mar 2022.
3. Association of American Medical Colleges. ERAS Tools and Worksheets for Residency Applicants. 2022. https://students-residents.aamc.org/eras-tools-and-worksheets-residency-applicants/eras-tools-and-worksheets-residency-applicants. Accessed 10 Mar 2022.
4. Hillman E, Lutfy-Clayton L, Desai S, Kellogg A, Zhang XC, Hu K, Hess J. Student-advising recommendations from the council of residency directors student advising task force. West J Emerg Med. 2017;18(1):93–6.
5. Lutfy-Clayton L, Morrissey T, Pelletier-Bui A, Zhuang C, Zhang XC, Hu K, Desai S, Hess J, Tillman D, Hillman E. The emergency medicine applying guide. 2018. https://www.cordem.org/globalassets/files/committees/student-advising/2018-applying-guide-cord-cdem-emra-rsa.docx.pdf. Accessed 16 Mar 2022.
6. Emergency Medicine Residents' Association. EMRA Match. https://webapps.emra.org/utils/spa/match#/search/map. Accessed 16 Mar 2022.
7. National Resident Matching Program. Advance Data Tables 2022 Main Residency Match. 2022. https://www.nrmp.org/wp-content/uploads/2022/03/Advance-Data-Tables-2022-FINAL.pdf. Accessed 27 Apr 2022.
8. Van Dermark JT, Wald DA, Corker JR, Reid DG. Financial implications of the emergency medicine interview process. AEM Educ Train. 2017;1(1):60–9. https://doi.org/10.1002/aet2.10011.
9. Keim SM, Rein JA, Chisholm C, Dyne PL, Hendey GW, Jouriles NJ, King RW, Schrading W, Salomone J III, Swart G, Wightman JM. A standardized letter of recommendation for residency application. Acad Emerg Med. 1999;6(11):1141–6.
10. Hansroth JA, Davis KH, Quedado KD, Davis SM, Kiefer AS, Shaver EB, Kiefer CS, Cottrell S, Ferrari ND. Lower-third SLOE rankings impede, but do not prevent, a match in emergency medicine residency training. J Med Educ Curric Dev. 2020;7:1–7. https://doi.org/10.1177/2382120520980487.
11. Negaard M, Assimacopoulos E, Harland K, Van Heukelom J. Emergency medicine residency selection criteria: an update and comparison. AEM Educ Train. 2018;2(2):146–53. https://doi.org/10.1002/aet2.10089.

Chapter 6
Finding a Residency Program That Fits You

Elizabeth Barrall Werley

When determining the best fit between a residency program and an applicant, there are a lot of factors at play, several of which will be reviewed. However, it is important to first ensure that applicants understand the process that ultimately results in their entering residency training. Applicants should be aware of the various tools available to them to assist with the search process. Finally, various factors that impact the "fit" between a program and applicant will be discussed.

The Residency Application Process

The Electronic Residency Application Service (ERAS) is managed by the Association of American Medical Colleges (AAMC) and provides one central location to which all relevant application materials are housed and can be securely viewed [1]. MyERAS is the version that applicants will use to complete applications, upload relevant documents, and select programs to which they are applying. There are other subsets of ERAS specific to medical school deans, letter of recommendation writers, and residency programs, which they will use to upload additional files or review data [2].

After reviewing application materials, programs will determine if they will be offering an interview to an applicant or not. Next, interviews take place, and once the interview phase is complete, applicants and programs review their impressions of these encounters. Both applicants and programs develop their respective rank order list within the National Resident Matching Program (NRMP), or The Match.

E. B. Werley (✉)
Emergency Medicine, Penn State Health Milton S. Hershey Medical Center, Hershey, PA, USA
e-mail: ewerley@pennstatehealth.psu.edu

R. P. Olympia et al. (eds.), *An Emergency Physician's Path*,
https://doi.org/10.1007/978-3-031-47873-4_6

The NRMP utilizes a complex algorithm that pairs applicants "into the most preferred residency and fellowship positions at programs that also prefer them," meaning applicants can only be matched at programs that they rank and by whom they are ranked [3]. If either an applicant does not rank a program, or a program does not rank an applicant, a match cannot be made.

This information explains a large portion of how applicants and programs are paired together, with the timeline determined by the NRMP [3]. There are plans if an applicant does not match with a program or a program does not fill all their open positions. Although less common, there are also ways for programs to fill open residency positions outside the Match. This information is more nuanced and beyond the scope of this chapter, and these situations leave less flexibility in ensuring fit between candidates and programs as options are often very limited.

Reviewing Available Data

It is always best for applicants to have the most accurate information available about programs when determining to which programs they may want to apply, interview, and potentially match. While not exhaustive, below is a comprehensive list of resources available to applicants to help them gather information about programs.

Residency Explorer™ Tool

The Residency Explorer™ Tool is a database that permits applicants to investigate and compare programs, with a unique ability permitting applicants to compare their personal profiles to applicants who have matched at a respective program in the past. It represents multiple national organizations collaborating together to provide as much data as possible in one location, including AAMC, NRMP, Accreditation Council for Graduate Medical Education (ACGME), National Board of Medical Examiners (NBME), Federation of State Medical Boards (FSMB), National Board of Osteopathic Medical Examiners (NBOME), and the National GME Census Survey. Programs provide information to the National GME Census Survey annually, and this data, as well as content from the ACGME and ERAS, is updated at least annually [4]. As stated on the website, "Residency Explorer is the only resource with original, source-verified data from the reputable organizations involved in the transition to residency."

Residency Explorer delivers insights and information based on:

- *Residency applicant data from AAMC (ERAS)*
- *Matched applicant data from NRMP*
- *USMLE data from the USMLE Program*
- *COMLEX-USA data from the NBOME*
- *Residency program directory information from ACGME*

- *Program characteristics from the National GME Census Survey, jointly administered by the AAMC and AMA, to which 95% of residency programs self-report information about their programs*

The participating organizations "embrace the belief that our shared constituents—students, advisors, deans, program directors, and others—will benefit if we work together to develop a single resource that helps students understand historical outcomes, assess their candidacy, and make informed decisions" [4].

AMA FREIDA™

The American Medical Association's (AMA) Fellowship and Residency Electronic Interactive Database (FREIDA™) is an online tool that permits users to search for residency and fellowship programs accredited by the ACGME. Once an applicant identifies a specialty or subspecialty, the search can be further narrowed down by geographic locations, application type, program type, and presence of specialty tracks. Further details pertaining to visa acceptance, total and first year positions, percentage of United States allopathic medical school graduates, percentage of osteopathic medical school graduates, percentage of international medical graduates, first year salary, and average weekly work hours can all be delineated [5]. This data is supplied by programs and updated regularly. Other features include listings of vacant positions, an institution directory with hospital demographics and medical school affiliations, as well as additional features if you are a member of the AMA [5].

EMRA Match

The Emergency Medicine Residents' Association (EMRA) hosts an interactive residency search site called EMRA Match. It is a collaborative effort between EMRA, Clerkship Directors in Emergency Medicine (CDEM), Council of Residency Directors in Emergency Medicine (CORD), and American College of Emergency Physicians (ACEP) [6]. Interactive features including geographic zoom functions, search functions by program name, location, or region, as well as program length, accreditation, and primary training site. Data is submitted by programs, and not all questions require answers. Other variables that can be used to filter programs include board exam cut-off scores, percentage of osteopathic residents, emergency department annual volumes, shift length, shifts per month, the amount of time interns spend on off-service rotations, percentage of international medical graduates, moonlighting availability, number of intern positions, United States Medical Licensing Examination (USMLE)/Comprehensive Osteopathic Medical Licensing Examination (COMLEX) preferences, if board exam failures are permitted, secondary training sites, time permitted for elective rotations and critical care rotations, military program, visa sponsorship, number of required Standardized Letter of

Evaluation (SLOEs) required, as well as dual training programs. Highlighting a specific program provides a pop-up window with program demographics, the ability to mark the program as a favorite, links to any relevant social media sites held by the program (official or unofficial), as well as links to the program's website [6].

Texas STAR

Texas Seeking Transparency in Application to Residency (STAR) is another useful database, but it differs from the aforementioned sites because it is driven from the medical school and student perspective. It was started by the University of Texas (UT) Southwestern Medical Center, and is meant to be a resource for medical school deans, student advisors, and senior medical students [7]. Fourth year medical students from participating medical schools who just completed the match process are requested to complete an annual survey, providing data about their own application including board scores, class rank quartiles and other factors, as well as to which programs they applied, from which programs they received interview offers or rejections, as well as to which program they matched. This data subsequently becomes available to deans, advisers, and students of those participating medical schools. Some viewable data is specific to the institution, while other data is a composite broken down by geography [7].

SAEM Residency Directory

The Society for Academic Emergency Medicine (SAEM) has several directories available for searching clerkships, residencies, and fellowships. The SAEM Residency Directory has an interactive map with geographic zoom function, as well as search functions by institution name, location, geographic region, primary setting, and program length. Highlighting a specific program provides a pop-up window with more detailed information about the program, as well as links to the program's website. In addition to the map, there is also an alphabetical list view, to which the same filters can be applied [8].

Program Websites

Once an applicant has narrowed down their list of potential programs, it is imperative that they do research on individual programs. Even if applicants apply to numerous programs, ultimately they will need to determine if they will accept an interview offer, and, after interviewing, where that program will reside on their rank order list, if at all. Additionally, getting to know more information about the program, current residents, faculty, and other information can generate discussion and questions

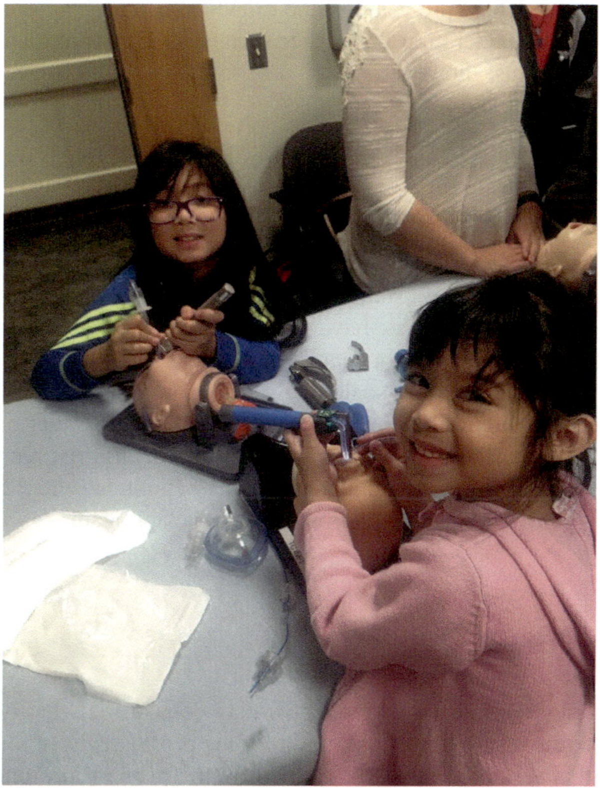

Fig. 6.1 Pediatric simulation lab, intubation, for kids by kids

during the interview day. Reviewing program websites can provide a wealth of information to applicants (Fig. 6.1).

Program and Applicant "Fit"

There are multiple factors that can be considered in determining fit between programs and applicants. When completing an initial search of programs using the aforementioned tools, an applicant will need to consider their personal preferences and priorities, as well as the overall estimated strength of their application. Several of these factors, not all-inclusive, are listed below.

3- Versus 4-Year Programs

One of the easiest factors to search or filter by includes length of training. All Emergency Medicine residency programs are either 3 or 4 years in length; both options are held to the same set of standards required by their ACGME accreditation status. There are benefits and drawbacks to each approach, and this should be taken into consideration with other variables. The large majority of programs are 3-year programs; however, there are some geographic areas where 4-year programs predominate.

Geography

Just like in real estate, for many applicants, location may mean everything. Most residency databases have a filter function by either geographic region or state to help narrow down a search. Applicants should reflect on their geographic preferences on the large scale, as well as consider the more local environment, such as urban, suburban, or more rural environments. Other environmental considerations include access to major highways, trains, airports, recreational activities, places of religious worship, childcare options, reputable school districts, as well as any other resources relevant and important to the applicant.

Program Type

Another factor that applicants may consider is what type of program they want in terms of the home institution. Some programs have more than one training site, so this variable is usually defined by the primary training site. For example, EMRA Match delineates three types of programs, namely community, county, or university; AMA FREIDA™ defines program types as university-based, community-based, community-based/university-affiliated, military-based, plus additional descriptors [5, 6]. While this discussion goes beyond the scope of this chapter, medical and academic/educational resources of the home institution, acuity and pathology mix of the patient population, ability to teach, and competition from other learners are all factors at play depending on the type of program.

Scholarly Activity

It is an ACGME requirement that all programs require their residents and faculty to participate in some aspect of scholarship, but how that is defined or set up is determined by the program [9]. Reviewing program websites may be useful, as many programs highlight the scholarship of their current and former residents as well as faculty. This information could be useful in helping the applicant determine if their own scholarly activity, volume of scholarship, or research interests matches that of a specific program.

Graduate Placement

An applicant does not need to know their long-term career plans at this stage in their medical training, but they may have some inkling as to what their future holds. If an applicant is interested in additional fellowship training, they may want to target programs that have demonstrated success in graduates progressing onto fellowships. Many programs will provide information on recent graduates, whether they moved on to community practice, academics, or additional training, and applicants may want to seek out a program that produces graduates similar to their own personal career interests.

Academic Focus/Scholarly Tracks

Some programs are well known for a specific niche of Emergency Medicine whether that is by virtue of specialized resources available at the program or institution, faculty with expertise on this topic, or extensive research on a given topic. Applicants with similar interests may want to target these programs. Many programs also offer scholarly tracks providing opportunities to focus on specific areas of Emergency Medicine (i.e., Critical Care, Pediatric Emergency Medicine, etc.), in addition to targeted faculty mentors and guidance for additional rotations. If an applicant has specific interests, finding programs that share this interest or provide additional exposure to it via a scholarly track may contribute to a good fit.

Board Scores

Medical school board scores may not make or break a candidate; it is just one piece of information in an otherwise large application full of data. That being said, board scores are still relevant. Some programs may openly state if they have an absolute or relative board score cutoff, either on their program website or if they provide this information in one of the residency search tools, such as EMRA Match [6]. If an applicant is a few points below a relative or recommended board cutoff value, and there are other elements that otherwise strengthen the application, then it may still be worth applying to that program. If a program defines an absolute cutoff value or if they do not accept failures, since these elements on applications can easily be filtered by programs, an applicant may need to seriously consider if they are going to apply to a program with those criteria, as it is very likely to be low-yield in generating an interview offer.

It remains to be seen how programs will interpret applications since USMLE Step 1 scoring went pass/fail after January 2022, and if a passing score will be sufficient or if programs are going to rely more heavily on USMLE Step 2 scores instead [10].

Another consideration is that of USMLE versus COMLEX scores. Some programs will accept and review applications including either or both scores, whereas other programs openly state they only accept USMLE scores. Discussion about this practice representing bias against osteopathic candidates is beyond the scope of this chapter, but osteopathic candidates should consider if they want to take USMLE Step 1 to counter this issue, or risk applying to these programs without USMLE and only COMLEX scores as it is less likely to generate interview offers.

Allopathic and Osteopathic Applicants

Previously there were ACGME-accredited and American Osteopathic Association (AOA)-accredited residency programs, but dual accreditation now negates this. Unfortunately, some residual bias may remain at the program, department, or institutional level against osteopathic candidates applying at traditionally allopathic programs. This should not discourage osteopathic candidates from applying to whichever programs they want, but they should also look at current program demographics on the program's website and consider the likelihood of being offered an interview.

International Medical Graduates

International Medical Graduates (IMGs) who are not citizens of the United States should look closely at any data about visas accepted by programs. This data may be denoted in one of the residency search tools and can often be found on a program's website or the sponsoring institution's GME website. If a sponsoring institution does not accept certain visas, and that is the visa held by the applicant, then it becomes a moot point and there is essentially a zero chance of that applicant matching at that program. Independent of the visa issue, there may be some bias against IMGs. Applicants should review residency search tools if IMGs are accepted at respective programs, as well as review current program websites to look and see how many current and recent residents are IMGs to better gauge their chances of being offered an interview and matching.

Diversity, Equity, and Inclusion

Awareness of this topic has fortunately increased in recent years. Applicants may look at program websites to view resident and faculty diversity, especially if program and faculty demographics are noted. Additionally, program websites, department websites, or institutional GME websites may highlight efforts to improve diversity, equity, and inclusion as it pertains to learners, faculty and staff, and the patient population.

Outreach

Some applicants may prioritize service to their local community beyond the requirements of the residency program. Community outreach efforts of the program or department are likely visible on a program website, department website, or even social media posts.

Extenuating Circumstances

Applicants should work closely with their medical school and Emergency Medicine-specific advisors to better understand the overall strength of their application. Some circumstances require compromises to be made. For example, if an applicant is participating in the couples match with a partner, they will need to determine their individual and collective priorities pertaining to the above factors and others. If an applicant has any academic red flags, such as a failed course or failed boards, it is not the end of the world. However, that applicant may need other elements on their application that speak to more positive attributes. Additionally, if an applicant has an explanation as to why there is an academic blemish (e.g., death in the family, illness, etc.), then they should explain this in their application, especially if the remainder of the application is without issue. Applicants with a less than ideal application still have a chance to match successfully, but they need to be realistic about their competitiveness as an applicant, and may need to consider a broader selection of programs.

Conclusion

No program will necessarily "check all the boxes" for every applicant so it is imperative that an applicant assess their list of personal priorities. It helps if applicants do their homework early on to help determine which programs are potentially a good fit. Residency search tools and program websites provide a wealth of useful information, but program make-up is ultimately a result of the incredibly complex NRMP Match algorithm. "Fit" is unique to the individual person; there is no one-size-fits-all answer.

References

1. Applying to residencies with ERAS®. Students & Residents. Association of American Medical Colleges. https://students-residents.aamc.org/applying-residencies-eras/applying-residencies-eras. Accessed 4 July 2022.
2. About ERAS®. Students & Residents. Association of American Medical Colleges. https://students-residents.aamc.org/applying-residencies-eras/applying-residencies-eras. Accessed 4 July 2022.
3. NRMP. The Match National Resident Matching Program. https://www.nrmp.org/. Accessed 4 July 2022.
4. Residency explorer™ tool. Residency Explorer™ Tool: Home. https://www.residencyexplorer.org/. Accessed 25 July 2022.
5. Tools to help you. American Medical Association. https://freida.ama-assn.org/. Accessed 25 July 2022.
6. EMRA Match. Emergency Medicine Residents' Association. https://webapps.emra.org/utils/spa/match#/search/map. Accessed 25 July 2022.
7. Texas STAR. UT Southwestern Medical Center. https://www.utsouthwestern.edu/education/medical-school/about-the-school/student-affairs/texas-star.html. Accessed 25 July 2022.
8. Residency directory—map view. Society for Academic Emergency Medicine. https://member.saem.org/SAEMIMIS/SAEM_Directories/ResidencyMap/SAEM_Directories/P/ResidencyMap.aspx?hkey=1e134970-ec57-4862-87fb-6971bad7a77b. Accessed 25 July 2022.
9. ACGME Program Requirements for Graduate Medical Education in Emergency Medicine. Accreditation Council for Graduate Medical Education https://www.acgme.org/globalassets/pfassets/programrequirements/110_emergencymedicine_2022.pdf. Accessed 1 Aug 2022.
10. USMLE Step 1 transition to pass/fail only score reporting. United States Medical Licensing Examination. https://www.usmle.org/usmle-step-1-transition-passfail-only-score-reporting. Published September 15, 2021. Accessed 2 Aug 2022.

Chapter 7
Combined Emergency Medicine Residency Programs: EM/Pediatrics, EM/Internal Medicine, EM/Internal Medicine/Critical Care, EM/Family Medicine, EM/Anesthesiology

Erica Bates

Introduction

The majority of emergency medicine residency programs provide "categorical," or traditional, training in emergency medicine (EM). However, a small number of programs also offer a dual training pathway that combines complete emergency medicine residency training with a second specialty, such as internal medicine, family medicine, pediatrics, or anesthesiology. These combined training programs are offered by institutions with categorical residency programs in both specialties and allow candidates to participate in both programs concurrently. Trainees in a combined residency program complete all of the same ACGME-mandated requirements as a categorical resident for each specialty; for example, they have the same procedural experience requirements as a "regular" emergency medicine candidate and must do the same amount of required primary care clinic time as a regular internal medicine resident. These combined programs are longer residencies than categorical programs, but overlapping requirements between specialties generally allow a year or two of saved time compared to doing each residency separately. Graduates may then become double board-certified to practice both specialties with the same privileges and credentials of a traditionally trained physician in each field. Graduates of a combined program are also eligible for any subspeciality fellowships available to either field.

People go into combined training programs for a variety of reasons. Some plan to divide their clinical time practicing both specialties, some want to practice internationally or in resource-poor environments where those extra skills are in high demand, and some see their dual training as a good foundation for further

E. Bates (✉)
Penn State Hershey Medical Center, Hershey, PA, USA
e-mail: Ebates1@pennstatehealth.psu.edu

R. P. Olympia et al. (eds.), *An Emergency Physician's Path*,
https://doi.org/10.1007/978-3-031-47873-4_7

specialization, such as a critical care fellowship. While there is not one "right" reason to pursue combined residency training, it is important to have a personal reason to pursue dual training. Combined residency is not designed for students who are simply having trouble deciding between two specialties, as a way to put off that decision further. It is a serious commitment to additional years of residency training and to undertaking significant additional demands in terms of knowledge and certification requirements. Combined program residents will still be in training as their categorical classmates from intern year are graduating, starting fellowships, and getting their first attending jobs. Combined training can be a fantastic opportunity for the right person, but it is important to consider what it is about the combined training option that will make those extra years in residency worth it to you.

A good applicant for a combined emergency medicine residency is a good applicant for each of the individual categorical programs involved. Students who are considering applying to a combined program should complete an acting internship rotation in each specialty and request letters of recommendation as if they are applying to categorical programs. Combined training programs tend to be small, with many offering only two spots per year. There are far fewer combined training programs than regular emergency medicine residencies. It is important for applicants to combined programs to also apply to an appropriate number of categorical residency programs to ensure they have a reasonable chance of matching. Applicants for combined residency programs interview with faculty and staff from both specialties as part of the process, and it is important to make sure that both departments at a prospective residency feel like a good fit. After all, you will be spending half of your residency time there!

EM/Internal Medicine

Combined emergency and internal medicine programs are the most common dual EM residency, with 12 programs nationally as of this writing. Due to some overlapping requirements, these programs prepare residents for dual certification in 5 years instead of the 6 or 7 years it would take to do the individual programs separately (with a 3- or 4-year EM program). Programs are small, with most accepting only two or three residents per year. Training in both specialties is integrated longitudinally, with residents alternating back and forth between rotations in both departments throughout the course of each post-graduate year on a schedule set by each individual residency program.

Residents who complete an EM/IM residency have a wide range of interests and career opportunities with this broad training. They are eligible for the full range of EM- and IM-based subspeciality fellowships, and many go on to complete further training in critical care. They are also uniquely qualified to participate in emergency-department based observation medicine units, which bridge the divide between the EM workup and inpatient care of many disease processes. Some graduates choose to practice both specialties clinically, often dividing their time between working as an emergency medicine physician and a hospitalist. Even if graduates ultimately decide to practice full time as emergency physicians, they often find that their deeper understanding of inpatient and outpatient care of common diseases seen in the ED is useful. Finally, EM/IM training offers benefits to physicians who work in international settings, where emergency and primary care conditions may all need to be managed at the same medical facility by a limited number of staff due to resource constraints.

EM/Internal Medicine/Critical Care

Dual trained EM/IM residents have a wide range of additional critical care fellowship training options available to them. Some, but not all, combined residency programs offer a dedicated EM/IM/critical care pathway, which allows a trainee to add a sixth year of training in order to complete the requirements of a critical care fellowship and sit for the medical critical care board exam. Medical students can apply to these combined EM/IM residency programs normally, and usually decide part way through their residency training whether to commit to the additional critical care fellowship pathway, or they may commit to a combined training program incorporating all three disciplines from the start. These 6-year programs and other independent critical care fellowship programs open to all EM applicants provide critical care training but do not include a formal pulmonology certification. Due to their internal medicine background, EM/IM graduates also have the option to pursue a separate traditional 3-year critical care/pulmonology fellowship after residency if they would like to become board certified pulmonologists.

Critical care is a natural fit for many EM/IM graduates. Combined residents typically enjoy the resuscitation of critically ill patients as part of what drew them to emergency medicine and have strong procedural training, including extensive airway experience, throughout residency. At the same time, their internal medicine training offers experience with the ongoing care of complex medically ill patients through substantial time on inpatient medicine, oncology, and cardiology rotations.

EM/Pediatrics

A combined emergency medicine and pediatrics residency is a 5-year program that prepares leaners to dual certify as a pediatrician and as an emergency physician. It is important to note that this is different from the process for completing a pediatric emergency medicine fellowship. Residents in a combined EM/pediatric program alternate between required pediatric and emergency medicine rotations during their training, which includes both inpatient and outpatient care for children, as well as core training in the care of pediatric emergencies that all EM physicians receive. Pediatric emergency medicine fellowship is an additional training program after either an EM or pediatrics residency that includes further training in pediatric-specific emergency care as well as additional pediatric critical care experiences. Pediatric emergency medicine fellowships are open to both EM and pediatrics applicants, so an EM/pediatrics trained physician would technically be eligible to go on to complete this fellowship if desired at the end of their residency. Most EM/pediatrics trained physicians go on to practice seeing pediatric emergency department patients without doing a further fellowship. Unlike a pediatrician who completes a pediatric emergency medicine fellowship, EM/pediatric combined residents are also fully qualified to care for adult patients of any age.

Dual trained EM/pediatrics graduates are eligible for a wide range of career options; they can practice outpatient primary care pediatrics, pursue a pediatric hospitalist position, apply to any pediatric or EM based fellowship, and see both adult and pediatric patients in the emergency department. While all emergency physicians are trained and credentialed to treat pediatric emergencies, the additional pediatric training and experience of a dual trained physician make them uniquely qualified to care for children.

EM/Family Medicine

Emergency medicine and family medicine combined residency programs consist of a 5-year dual training curriculum that prepares graduates to take the board certification exams for both specialties. Categorical EM residencies take either 3 or 4 years, while a regular family medicine residency is 3 years, with the overlap in certain shared rotations allowing the combined program to save trainees one additional year compared to completing each program separately. Trainees fulfill all of the core training requirements of each individual specialty program, including outpatient primary care clinic.

This dual training offers one of the broadest skillsets and allows a physician to provide a very wide range of services to their community, including routine prenatal care not otherwise included in EM/IM or EM/pediatric training. The breadth of this training may be especially attractive to those interested in practicing international medicine or in remote/critical access or austere environments. While there is a significant overlap in the acute and chronic disease processes managed by these two specialties, a dual trained physician receives significantly more training in procedures such as airway management, trauma, and resuscitation of the critically ill than a categorical family medicine resident and has a greater understanding of the long term management and outpatient workup of stable patients than a traditional emergency physician. The ability to work emergency department shifts, provide obstetric care and women's health, practice in an outpatient clinic, or in an inpatient hospital setting offers a high degree of career flexibility.

EM/Anesthesiology

Johns Hopkins University School of Medicine created the first, and currently only, combined residency program in emergency medicine and anesthesiology. Residents in this combined training program undergo 6 years of residency training in both emergency medicine and anesthesiology and are eligible to sit for both specialty board examinations at the conclusion of their training. The categorical emergency medicine residency at this institution is 4 years, while the regular anesthesiology residency requires 1 year of preliminary training as an intern followed by 3 years of dedicated anesthesiology training. Categorical anesthesiology residents usually complete a preliminary year in either internal medicine or general surgery before beginning their specialized anesthesiology training as a second-year resident; in an EM/anesthesiology combined program, intern year as part of the categorical EM class replaces this requirement before trainees begin anesthesiology rotations in their second year.

The fields of emergency medicine and anesthesiology share considerable overlap. Both specialties focus on advanced airway management, a range of procedures, and resuscitation of the critically ill patient. Both emergency physicians and anesthesiologists are trained to care for adult, pregnant, and pediatric patients and manage both medical and traumatic illnesses. Emergency medicine and anesthesiology training both offer pathways to further fellowship training in critical care. Dual certified physicians would have a broad range of skills and a wide range of potential career options practicing in either or both fields, from academic medical centers to community private practice. Combining expertise in administering anesthesia with the broader ability to treat a wide range of more common disease processes could be especially useful in remote, austere settings or for individuals interested in international relief work or military medicine.

Part II
Choosing a Career in Emergency Medicine: Pursuing a Fellowship and Additional Training

Chapter 8
Addiction Medicine

Eleanor Dunham

A Brief History of Addiction Medicine

Addiction Medicine has its roots starting from the time that alcoholism was recognized as a disease. The formation of the New York City Medical Society on Alcoholism in 1954 by Dr. Ruth Fox was considered the start of modern addiction medicine. Ruth Fox, MD, is considered the founder of the American Society of Addiction Medicine [1]. Addiction is defined as a treatable, chronic medical disease involving complex interactions among brain circuits, genetics, the environment, and an individual's life experiences [2].

The drug revolution in the 1960s was the beginning of many physicians' journey and learning more about addiction as a brain disease. Over the years, increased research with drug addiction helped demonstrate that addiction is a disease as real and devastating as diabetes or hypertension. Eventually, more state local chapters and national societies began to form to develop health policies, educate and treat the disease of addiction. Previously, those that used to treat addiction were either in psychiatry or toxicology. This made sense as those trained in toxicology have a lot of the same education, training, and overlap as addiction medicine. Addiction medicine has come into its own as its own subspecialty recognized as such by the American Board of Medical Specialties (ABMS) [3]. A landmark study done in Emergency Medicine (EM) demonstrated that starting OUD patients on buprenorphine/naloxone in the ED vs referral or brief intervention were still engaged in addiction treatment compared to the other two treatment modalities [4]. These patients on buprenorphine/naloxone were also reporting less illicit drug use as well as less use of inpatient treatment centers. This was the beginning of the wave for

E. Dunham (✉)
Department of Emergency Medicine, Penn State Hershey Medical Center, Hershey, PA, USA
e-mail: edunham@pennstatehealth.psu.edu

R. P. Olympia et al. (eds.), *An Emergency Physician's Path*,
https://doi.org/10.1007/978-3-031-47873-4_8

MOUD to be started in the ED. Even today in the 2020s, there is still much stigma that needs to be overcome, but there is a more recognized need and increasing dedicated clinics, outpatient treatment centers, and resources both statewide and nationwide to treat addiction and the consequences that come from this disease.

Why Choose Addiction Medicine?

There is such a need at this time for addiction physicians currently with a national crisis that has only increased during and after the pandemic. The US has hit over 100,000 deaths from drug abuse in 2021. Most of these overdose deaths were from synthetic opioids, mainly fentanyl, as well as methamphetamines. This is the highest overdose deaths in the country that we have seen to date [5]. The need for individuals who can treat this disease is greatly in demand. There are so many options and possibilities that open doors should you choose addiction medicine. Here are some examples of possibilities that may come your way.

(a) Outpatient based treatment centers—one would treat patients that needed Medication for their Opioid Use Disorder (MOUD). This is very rewarding area where you can take your time with patients (not as rushed as in the ED), you develop a rapport with patients, and you do get the satisfaction of seeing good outcomes at times and seeing patients progress in a positive direction. You have a set schedule (most of the times) and for the most part, you know what to expect. Also, these patients choose to be here. Unlike the ED, you do not have to convince these patients as fervently to start or stay on MOUD. They are choosing to be there in your clinic and they are *usually* not there as acutely as they present to the ED.
(b) Inpatient consultant for Addiction Consults—this is an option if you are board-certified in addiction medicine to split your time between the ED and the inpatient consultations. Just as you would expect, you would see the admitted patients to treat them and give advice for treatment of their addiction.
(c) Consulting as a free-lance Opioid medical consultant (OMC)— this is probably the best of all worlds in that you could be hired to give your expertise for an independent agency, your Department of Health (DOH) or any entity that might need your expertise in addiction medicine. This is very lucrative in that you can command a salary equivalent to what one what get paid moonlighting with much less stress and acuity involved. You also can bill for time spend on these projects similar to how a lawyer would bill.
(d) There may be other options not yet discovered as this field is still very new and considered still "the wild west and an open frontier." A majority of us that choose EM is because we like to fight and work for "the underdog." The homeless, the poor, the vulnerable, and truly sick people are our "peeps" in EM. With addiction medicine, not only are you helping many that are marginalized in society, but you are truly helping those with serious disease.

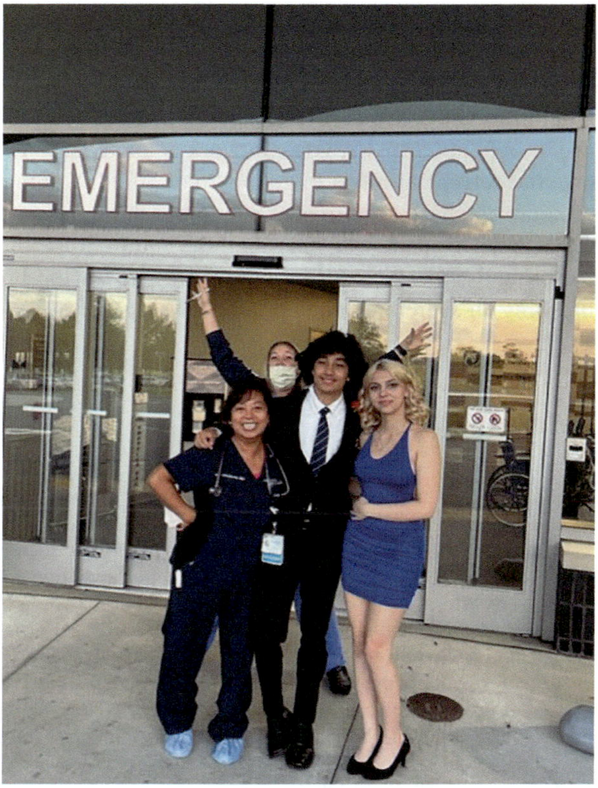

Fig. 8.1 Homecoming Fall 2022 comes to the Emergency Department, Penn State Hershey Medical Center

(e) Another important aspect for addiction medicine is the positive contribution to your over-all wellness and wellbeing. If you are tired of the shift work, the weekends, and holidays, then addiction medicine does have the potential of increasing a more "normal" lifestyle in terms of the hours you would work. If you are looking to increase your longevity in EM as well as another outlet for growth both personally and professionally, also increasing your sustainability in the house of medicine and increasing your financial income, then addiction medicine is most definitely a wonderful option! (Fig. 8.1).

Addiction Medicine Board Certification

Currently there are two paths for Addiction Medicine Board of Certifications. As long as one has board certification through the American Board of Medical Specialties (ABMS), you can get board-certified in Addiction Medicine. The American Board of Preventative Medicine (ABPM) is the society to get board certified and the American Board of Addiction Medicine (ABAM) is the society to maintain the certification. There are two paths to qualify for Addiction Medicine. You can do a 1-year fellowship through an ACGME accredited program. There are 55 approved addiction medicine fellowships in 55 states and the District of Columbia at the time of this publication. After fellowship you would apply for the exam certification to get board certified. The number of fellowships continues to grow as it grows in popularity. Or, you can work at an addiction clinic learning on the job and take the certification test to get board certified. You must have the required number of hours and have seen/treated enough of these patients to be able to qualify to take the exam. This path lasts only until the end of 2024. Starting 2025, this path will be closed and you will only be allowed to sit for the board certification exam after finishing an accredited addiction fellowship.

References

1. Smith DE. The evolution of addiction medicine as a medical specialty. Virtual Mentor. 2011;13(12):900–5. AMA Journal of Ethics.
2. Medicine ASoA. Definition of addiction. American Society of Addiction Medicine; 2019. https://www.asam.org/quality-care/definition-of-addiction.
3. Kunz K, Wiegand T. Addiction medicine: current status of certification, maintenance of certification, training, and practice. J Med Toxicol. 2016;12(1):76–8.
4. D'Onofrio G, O'Connor PG, Pantalon MV, Chawarski MC, Busch SH, Owens PH, et al. Emergency department-initiated buprenorphine/naloxone treatment for opioid dependence: a randomized clinical trial. JAMA. 2015;313(16):1636–44.
5. McPhillips D. In 2021, US drug overdose deaths hit highest level on record, CDC data shows: CNN Health; 2022. https://www.cdc.gov/nchs/pressroom/nchs_press_releases/2021/20211117.htm.

Chapter 9
Administration and ED Operations

Michael Mesisca

Why Administration?

It was a Monday night. The Emergency Department was busting at the seams. Patients were lining up against the dry-wall peeling walls. People everywhere, lying in gurneys and seated in chairs all over. They were coughing, vomiting, and moaning. It was a mess and it was dangerous. Over 120 patients in a 40-bed department and 40-plus patients checked in and not seen yet and waiting for hours. Patients, nurses, and doctors were all frustrated and all concerned. This was my recruitment tour to my current site 5 years ago when I decided to join them as their medical director. I knew based on the willingness and dedication of this passionate team to embrace change that we could do better for our patients and for the team. Together, partnering with physicians, nursing, and administration, we put many small and large changes in place and removed many barriers to improve how care was delivered. This site is currently often the only facility with capacity to accept higher level transfers in the region, has now won multiple awards for care quality and throughput, and leads the region in multiple quality and performance measures. We collectively take tremendous pride in providing efficient, quality care to nearly 100,000 patients a year that visit our department. If you have a desire to serve others by leading a team to make operational changes, you too can impact an entire system of healthcare delivery.

M. Mesisca (✉)
Department of Emergency Medicine, Riverside University Health System, Moreno Valley, CA, USA
e-mail: m.mesisca@ruhealth.org

R. P. Olympia et al. (eds.), *An Emergency Physician's Path*,
https://doi.org/10.1007/978-3-031-47873-4_9

What Is Emergency Medicine Administration and Operations?

Emergency Medicine is a team sport of elite, highly skilled, professional players that demands leaders of an equal caliber to guide success. Great patient care requires an entire team working synergistically to consistently provide multiple, simultaneous, time-sensitive actions. Often, this must be done with limited space and resources. The healthcare team includes Emergency Medical Services (EMS) that encompasses law enforcement and paramedics, nursing, support staff, EMTs, laboratory, radiology, pharmacy, admitting physicians, house supervisors, and specialty support. Effective healthcare leaders can motivate team to work well together, breaking down departmental agendas to achieve the common goal of high-quality, patient-centered care.

In Emergency Departments, efficient operations are usually accomplished by a site management team with strong physician leadership and engagement. Management teams seek to remove as many barriers as possible, so the medical team can focus on clinical work. Well-designed operations function in the background to support those efforts. Leaders create operational efficiencies that foster a culture of excellence making the provision of medical care less frustrating and more engaging for the patient and the treatment team. Effective operational management allows doctors to focus on making medical decisions, nurses to focus on the provision of care, and helps patients feel like they are at the center of focus of the entire care team.

Operational Leadership Structure

Emergency Departments have varying structures, depending on their community or academic focus. Most departments have one or more physician leaders with specific responsibilities. Most commonly they have a Chairperson and Vice Chairperson (some sites use the titles Chief of Service or Medical Director). Many departments, usually higher volume sites, will have more physician leaders that are often assigned as directors over each of the specific areas of ED administration listed below (e.g., Quality Director, Finance Director, etc.). Physician leaders may choose to assume oversight of only one or more administrative areas based on the department need, their personal interest, and the amount of work each role entails.

Emergency Department administration often includes the following responsibilities:

1. **Establishing the team culture and vision**: physician leaders set the tone for the team and take responsibility. A strong leader believes "there are no bad teams, only bad leaders" and "that leadership is the single greatest factor in any teams performance" [1]. Transformational leaders invest heavily into their team and

development of their team members. They identify the strengths and weaknesses of each team member and help them grow. They view their role as one of service to the team. They set a vision and a standard of excellence for their team and help the team understand the why and the how to creating a well-run Emergency Department.

2. **Building the team:** Medical Directors/Chairs are often responsible for the recruitment, hiring, and mentoring of the physician team. At many sites, the physician lead is also responsible for hiring and developing the physician assistant and/or nurse practitioner team. This can be one of the most rewarding aspects of being a leader. Building a strong team with an array of expertise that works cohesively is the best way to positively impact Emergency Department operations. Mentoring other physicians can also be the most challenging and most critical. "The culture of any organization is shaped by the worst behavior the leader is willing to tolerate" and, as such, effective physician leaders will need to have open, direct, and honest communication with members of the team to ensure attitude and effort is consistent with the departmental goals and vision [2].
3. **Quality**: Oversight of cases with opportunities for improvement (through a process called peer review). This includes operations that support specific programs like stroke, sepsis, STEMI, and inter-facility transfers. Quality programs involve peer reviews, legal case reviews from lawsuits or potential lawsuits, and responding to patient grievances. Quality directors provide feedback to physicians on their care and, at times, initiate a performance improvement plan or even disciplinary action.
4. **Operations and Throughput**: Responsible for how things in the department flow. The underlying systems that support where and how care is delivered in the department.
5. **Service Agreements**: Working with admitting teams and specialty services to establish agreed upon workflows that help streamline care and avoid conflict and delays (e.g., creating a hip fracture pathway so Orthopedics, Internal Medicine, and Anesthesia are consulted at time of diagnosis and establishing a clear pathway delineating who will admit the patient right away, expediting operative care).
6. **Support Services**: Site management leaders work with hospital administration and nursing leadership to build support teams that improve patient throughput and care. This can include Case Managers, Social Services, Child Life Specialists, Hospice and Palliative Care, Substance Use Navigators, Behavioral Health Response Teams, Physical Therapy, and others.
7. **Finances**: Many physician groups have a model where the Medical Director or Assistant Medical Director track and share physician-specific performance, such as patients seen per hour and amount of revenue billed and collected per hour, with the physicians. This helps the team identify their strengths and opportunities to capture more revenue for the work they are providing. Physician leaders may also have oversight or input on contracts with the hospital and insurance carriers. Having physicians with an interest and experience in finance can be very valuable to the site management team.

8. **Patient Experience**: Site operations includes a coordinated plan to improve how patients perceive and experience care delivery. Patient experience champions help the care team understand and improve how patients experience and receive care in the department. This teams helps reduce risk and improve patient communication.

Clearly, it can take an entire team with a broad range of experience to create a strong framework to support excellent and efficient patient care. Emergency Medicine Administration can be an incredibly rewarding way to participate and lead a team that is making patient care and outcomes better.

Emergency Department Throughput

There is solid evidence that delays in Emergency Room care contribute to poor patient outcomes [3–5]. Patients that wait longer to see an emergency physician and/or stay longer in the ED after admission (particularly ICU patients) have increased complication and mortality rates [6]. Successful EM site management teams work to improve patient care by creating systems that expedite triage, treatment, and disposition with the goal of reducing patient harm and creating an environment that fosters physician wellbeing. To that end, metrics are used as a guide to measure and sustain operational improvements. The metrics are NOT the goal; they a surrogate for the goal. The goal, and the motivation, is to help improve patient outcomes.

ED Operational Metrics and Why They Matter

Here are a few key Emergency Medicine metrics and why they matter:

1. **Triage time:** time from patient arrival to nursing triage. Obtaining vital signs and assigning an Emergency Severity Index (ESI) score on patient arrival helps identify the sickest patients first and documents an accurate arrival time to the ER. This is typically when the patient's information is logged into the health record.
2. **Time to provider (TTP):** time it takes for a patient to be seen by a physician, PA, or NP once they present to the ED by ambulance or private vehicle. Most Emergency Rooms have a medical screening exam (MSE) process to provide rapid patient assessment within 10–20 min of patient arrival. There is a mantra in Emergency Medicine: "the sickest patient is the one we haven't seen yet." Delays in patient assessment can miss the identification of critical patients and lead to serious injury or even death.

3. **Left without being seen (LWBS):** patients that leave after arrival that are not seen by a physician. Most sites have a goal of <1%. Some patients who leave the ED without being seen are actually suffering from serious illnesses and, without being seen, will go on to experience serious complications.
4. **Ambulance off-load times**: regional and state EMS agencies have different names and goals here but most Emergency Departments track how long it takes to receive care from an ambulance and get the ambulance back into service. Prolonged ambulance offload times can reduce the number of ambulances in service in the community and cause patient harm (e.g., no ambulance to respond to a 911 call for a heart attack because they are all holding in Emergency Departments).
5. **Turnaround time to discharge (TAT-D):** a measure of time from arrival to discharge for patients going home from the ED. This is influenced by triage, TTP, lab and radiology, and discharge processes. As TAT-D increases, the entire department can fill up with patients. The impact is additive. Consider an ER with 100 patients per day. If each patients stays 10 min longer than needed due to delays in operations that is 1000 min of additional time patients are holding in the ED. This creates more congestion, reduced bed/chair availability, more patients requiring nursing support, and increases the potential for error and patient harm.
6. **Turnaround time to admission:** a measure of time from arrival to patients arriving to an inpatient bed. This is impacted by all the same things that impact TAT-D as well as consultant times for writing admission orders and hospital-wide operations that include how quickly beds are cleaned and available, how beds are assigned, inpatient length of stay. Influencing this metric requires great teamwork and support from the entire hospital and support services.
7. **Transfers:** having streamlined ED operations can support the entire region. When tertiary hospitals (facilities that have specialty care services readily available on-call) are at capacity and cannot receive higher level care transfers from outside hospitals, patients can suffer life-threatening delays in care. Operational leaders at sending facilities should establish transfer agreements to help expedite and coordinate patient transfers out to specialty centers. Likewise, physician leaders at receiving facilities should work to maintain operational efficiencies, even during times of surge, to maintain capacity for higher-level care transfers to ensure patient access to time sensitive care. If all the tertiary centers are at capacity, delays in some regions can lead to poor patient outcomes. Watching a patient decompensate that requires specialty care and not being able to get them transferred for definitive care be one most disheartening aspects of the job for a community emergency physician. Leaders should work hard to prevent this from ever happening.
8. **Physician Wellness:** EM leaders need to consider how every decision they make impacts physician well-being. Engage the front-line team in decision making.

Keys to Being a Successful Leader

1. **Understanding that leadership influence**: the goal of an operational physician leader is to try to positively improve every aspect of care in the department. Successful leaders find ways to improve things beyond their direct control and oversight, they expand their influence [7]. There is nothing that impacts EM care that is "not my problem."
2. **Lead with character**: being a servant leader, leading by example, and creating a culture that cares for and supports the care team. "No one cares how much you know, until they know how much you care" [7]. The healthcare team must be heard, valued, and supported.
3. **Working well with others:** being able to collaborate with primary care, specialty care, and hospital administration are essential. There's an old African proverb: "If you want to go fast go alone. If you want to go far, go together." Success requires the ability to find mutual success throughout the entire health system.
4. **Competence**: strong leaders must have the respect from the healthcare team. As a physician, this comes from clinical excellence and strong communication skills. The length of a CV or the caliber of school attended is far less important than how a leader performs and interacts in the department and in meetings.
5. **Start small:** begin by taking on a single project or participating in a single project. Do not assume more responsibility than you can handle. Find some success and learn on the job. Focus less on having a title and more on assuming responsibility and supporting the team to the best of your ability.

Pathway to Operational Leadership

1. **Find the right mentor**: Connecting with a respected physician leader, discussing their role, and gaining feedback about your interests and their experience is incredibly helpful to defining your pathway forward. Ask for honest feedback on your strengths and areas needing improvement.
2. **Experience is a great teacher, find a place to serve**: Ask to participate/lead an operational improvement project. Most sites have a site operations/throughput committee, try to start there to get an understanding of the department operations and challenges. Try to attend a hospital committee and assume responsibility over a project in a given area (e.g., sepsis or stroke champion). Work to identify one project that has a measurable goal that can be used to guide success. Participating in a hospital-wide committee is incredibly helpful in providing knowledge on house-wide operations and building relationships.
3. **Invest in yourself as a leader**: There are many resources available for physician leaders. These include books, online lectures, healthcare management certificate

programs from major universities, MBA programs (not required but can be helpful), medical director courses provided by professional societies, and administrative fellowships. Gain an understanding of organizational leadership, finance and capital investment, negotiations, lean methodology, and kaizen events, amongst others. Develop a plan that works for you and your schedule and make leadership growth a scheduled and ongoing part of your professional and personal development.

4. **Dream Big**: Have a goal for 5–10 years. Do you want to be a quality director, department chair, hospital CMO, or CEO? Developing your leadership skills early and daily, having a mentor who is currently in the role you desire, and gradually expanding your knowledge base, leadership skills, relationships, and communication skills can all help you get there.

Emergency Medicine Leadership's Impact on Me

As an Emergency Department Chair for a public safety-net hospital seeing close to 100,000 patients a year, I strive to be a transformational leader that helps physicians at all stages of their career to grow and develop as leaders. All emergency physicians are in a leadership role every time they are on shift and the amount of positive influence they exert on their team is variable. I believe understanding, embracing, and excelling in that leadership role fosters excellent patient care as well as personal wellness and longevity. I truly enjoy the challenges of my job, as I work every day to empower a team of exceptional physicians to be successful in providing great patient care. Emergency Department leadership comes with tremendous responsibility, and Emergency Medicine needs great, servant-leaders to support our healthcare teams into the future as the practice of medicine becomes more challenging and more complex!

References

1. Willink J, Babin L. Extreme ownership: how U.S. navy seals lead and win. Macmillan; 2018.
2. Gruenert S, Whitaker T. School culture recharged: strategies to energize your staff and culture. ASCD; 2017.
3. Emergency department crowding: high impact solutions. (ACEP Emergency Medicine Practice Committee). https://www.acep.org/globalassets/sites/acep/media/crowding/empc_crowding-ip_092016.pdf. Accessed 5 Sept 2022.
4. Guttmann A, Schill MU, Vermeulen MJ, Stukel TA. Association between waiting times and short term mortality and hospital admission after departure from the Emergency Department: population based cohort study from Ontario, Canada. BMJ. 2011;342:d2983. https://doi.org/10.1136/bmj.d2983.

5. Morley C, Unwin M, Peterson GM, Stankovich J, Kinsman L. Emergency department crowding: a systematic review of causes, consequences and solutions. PLoS One. 2018;13(8):e0203316. https://doi.org/10.1371/journal.pone.0203316.
6. Cowan RM, Trzeciak S. Emergency department overcrowding and the potential impact on the critically ill. Crit Care. 2005;9(3):291. https://doi.org/10.1186/cc2981.
7. Maxwell J. 21 Irrefutable laws of leadership: follow them and people will follow you. Harper Collins; 2022.

Chapter 10
Child Abuse Pediatrics

H. Michelle Greene and Kathryn McCans

Why Child Abuse Pediatrics?

At some point in the general emergency department (ED), you will encounter child abuse—it isn't a question of *if*, but *when*. Families will come ED in crisis after their child discloses sexual assault, either because they don't know what else to do, or because they were referred there by a teacher, police officer, or another medical provider. Infants and toddlers might have subtle or minor injuries from abuse that might go unnoticed if you don't recognize them. Teenagers could be experiencing sex trafficking and come to your ED multiple times for sexually transmitted infections. Children experiencing obvious neglect might come through your doors. What will you do in these situations? At minimum, an emergency medicine (EM) doctor should know how to identify and acutely manage maltreatment allegations or abusive trauma, but this patient population shouldn't cause you to be nervous or want to turn a blind eye. On the contrary, you have a unique opportunity to advocate for these children when there might not be anyone else who can.

As an EM physician, you can frame a family's initial experience with the process of child abuse evaluation and investigation. You can detect injuries that represent abuse, and your medical findings might be the only thing that leads to a child being removed from a life-threatening abusive environment. You can set a teen's mind at ease after an assault. You can provide evidence for law enforcement or give court testimony for attorneys to help prosecute perpetrators. You can also connect a

H. M. Greene
Nationwide Children's Hospital, Columbus, OH, USA
e-mail: Michelle.greene@nationwidechildrens.org

K. McCans (✉)
Penn State Hershey Medical Center, Hershey, PA, USA
e-mail: kmccans@pennstatehealth.psu.edu

R. P. Olympia et al. (eds.), *An Emergency Physician's Path*,
https://doi.org/10.1007/978-3-031-47873-4_10

patient to resources that will help them heal after a devastating experience. Additional CAP training can help you do all of this more effectively and teach others to do the same.

In some ways, when dealing with complicated patient situations involving law enforcement or attorneys, a CAP job can feel a little like Law & Order: Special Victims Unit. However, while the dramatic stories in the CAP world rival television, there are admittedly fewer famous actors encountered on the job.

History of Child Abuse Pediatrics and Pediatric Emergency Medicine

The nineteenth century French forensic pathologist, Ambroise Tardieu, published works describing what would come to be recognized as child abuse 100 years later. In 1946, John Caffey, an American pediatric radiologist, published a paper describing children who had fractures and subdural hematomas and ascribed the cause to trauma. Prior to this such traumatic injuries were attributed to accidents or unknown cause or infections, etc. The medical literature regarding child abuse began to increase. However, it was not until "The Battered Child Syndrome" by Henry Kempe was published in 1962 that child abuse began to be recognized as a medical problem. It was not until 1977 that child sexual abuse was recognized as a medical concern with the publication of Kempe's "Sexual Abuse, Another Hidden Pediatric Problem." Over time more physicians became formally involved in child abuse pediatrics. In 1996, Dr. Stephen Ludwig, professor of Pediatrics at Children's Hospital of Philadelphia and a PEM boarded physician, brought together a group of pediatricians to discuss developing a new specialty in pediatrics dedicated to the evaluation and care of abused children. The first national gathering of the child abuse pediatricians occurred in 1997 in Philadelphia, the inaugural Ray E. Helfer Society meeting.

Child Abuse Pediatrics was recognized as a distinct sub-specialty by the American Board of Pediatrics in 2006, with the first board examination in 2010. It was possible to "grandfather" into the specialty until 2013 by meeting defined practice parameters. After 2013, formal fellowship training was required to become a board-certified Child Abuse Pediatrician (CAP). The recognition of CAP as a pediatric sub-specialty was a culmination of decades of work by dozens of professionals from many fields including pediatrics, emergency medicine, psychiatry, pathology, and other fields.

Pediatric Emergency Medicine (PEM) and CAP specialties have significant overlap regarding injured children. PEM is a relatively young specialty. In the 1970s pediatricians began to dedicate time to working in emergency departments. In the 1980s both the American College of Emergency Physicians and the American Academy of Pediatrics developed sections dedicated to PEM. By the late 1980s, the PEM subspecialty was proposed to the American Board of Medical Specialties. As a result, the first board examination for PEM was offered in 1992. PEM fellowships were accredited in 1998, and graduates of both emergency medicine and general pediatric residencies were eligible to participate. The field has expanded since its inception in academic centers to increasingly community emergency departments.

CAP Fellowship Experience and CAP Attending Role

CAP is a boarded pediatric specialty that requires a 3-year fellowship, usually after a residency in pediatrics. Child abuse pediatricians evaluate pediatric patients with suspected maltreatment, including physical abuse, sexual abuse, human trafficking, neglect, failure to thrive, drug endangerment, and medical child abuse ("Munchausen syndrome by proxy"). Some may be a primary care provider for children in foster care since they have knowledge of the child protection system and long-term psychologic and medical consequences of maltreatment. There are also cases where abuse is *not* to blame—hereditary bleeding disorders, dermatologic conditions, or normal variants sometimes look concerning, but additional CAP training helps diagnose rare or unusual diseases instead!

Child abuse pediatricians might do consults on inpatient cases, work in an outpatient clinic, conduct acute sexual assault examinations, or oversee nurses who complete these evaluations. Often, they work on a multidisciplinary team with social workers, child protective agencies, law enforcement, or forensic interviewers. Forensic interviewers speak to children with possible abuse to obtain specific facts to help with an investigation—child abuse specialists usually do not do these interviews, but they can use the same techniques to gather a medical history from a child. Depending on the practice type, a CAP physician might offer telephone consultation rather than in-person assessments.

CAP fellows usually spend time with the medical examiner or coroner system for child fatalities. A fellowship also gives a physician experience with testimony in court cases of abuse. The child abuse subspecialty is unique in its close interactions with the legal system, and CAPs are often the "translators" between medical providers and attorneys.

Court testimony for child abuse cases can vary based on the location and legal system—some courts utilize CAP experts frequently, and others do not. Child abuse pediatricians might be hired as an expert witness outside of the cases they personally evaluated, and this can be a lucrative career choice depending on the volume and types of cases.

There are a multitude of educational opportunities in child abuse pediatrics, if teaching is a passion of yours. Medical trainees, Emergency Medical Services, lawyers, child protective services, and nurses all can benefit from training in the medical management of child maltreatment. Research is typically a requirement in CAP fellowship, although this might be waived if a fellow has previously demonstrated academic or scholastic achievement such as with previous research experience or an advanced degree (master's or PhD).

Gaining Experience in CAP as an EM Provider

Emergency Medicine physicians can pursue additional experience with the child abuse specialists in their area as part of an elective or clinical focus/track during their residency. Emergency Medicine physicians are not typically eligible for board certification in child abuse pediatrics. A small number of combined PEM-CAP fellowships exist and have been completed by physicians who completed pediatric residency. Combined PEM/CAP fellowships are generally 4 years instead of 3 years for a PEM fellowship and 3 years for a CAP fellowship. Individuals in EM with a specific interest in CAP, particularly in academic research surrounding child abuse pediatrics, might be able to create a fellowship program at an institution if they have support from existing CAP, PEM, and EM faculty.

For those that might not want to pursue a full fellowship, clinical rotations with a CAP are an option. Even spending a few days with a CAP can improve your communication about abuse and neglect with patients, families, and outside agencies (law enforcement, legal workers, CPS). You can also learn trauma-informed approaches to asking questions to children and performing physical or anogenital examinations. CAPs can teach you about local legal statutes surrounding mandated reporting and maltreatment, which are vital to know in a general ED.

The Ray E. Helfer Society (https://www.helfersociety.org/) is made of child abuse specialists, and their website offers information regarding fellowships and practice locations of child abuse pediatricians in the United States. Hospitals and healthcare systems that offer child abuse fellowships would likely offer rotations or clinical clerkships to EM residents, and most child abuse pediatricians would be delighted to have learners from other specialties (Fig. 10.1).

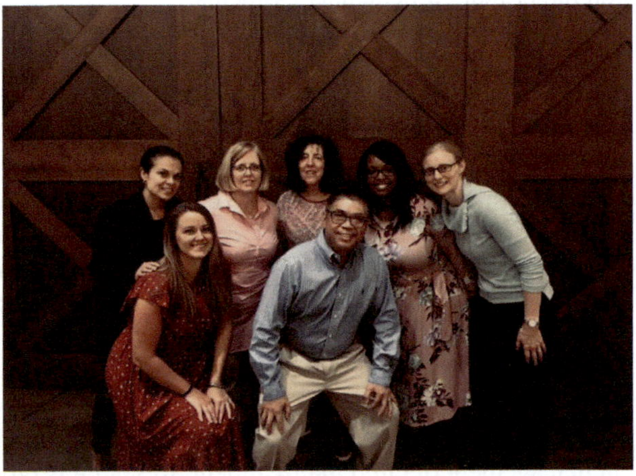

Fig. 10.1 PEM, EM-PEM, PEM-CAP, PEM-pediatric hospitalist, and APP. Photo is from private collection of Dr. Robert Olympia

Implementing CAP Knowledge in an EM Career

In terms of administrative and clinical leadership, EM physicians are vital in creating protocols for their institutions, including immediate management and referral to appropriate specialists. Physical abuse recognition and evaluation can be nuanced, but clinical guidelines can help simplify the approach in a busy ED. Acute sexual assault patients need immediate medical attention including evidence collection ("rape kits"), labs, medications, and examinations—another area for protocols to streamline ED care. For adults, there are sexual assault nurse examiners (SANEs), and general EM physicians can oversee their clinical work if this is an area of interest. Pediatric SANEs (or PSANEs) have separate training in pediatric sexual abuse. EM physicians could oversee these clinicians as well and expand services for pediatric patients needing acute care after a sexual assault.

EM physicians can provide court testimony in wide variety of cases. You might see abused patients whose cases go to trial and communicating effectively with the legal system is an invaluable skill. Providing expert witness testimony for child abuse cases is possible for an EM provider as well, but should be grounded in additional CAP training (either clinical rotations with a CAP or a CAP fellowship).

CAP is a rich area for academic research. There is growing literature in the field, but there is a wealth of topics that have not been explored. Since CAP is a relatively small field, finding mentors and talking with leaders in research is more feasible than other subspecialties. Even without a CAP fellowship, EM providers can easily focus their research on child maltreatment. EM doctors can also lead efforts in quality improvement for child abuse management in their hospital or practice location.

Considerations for an EM/CAP Career

Should you choose to spend clinical, academic, legal, or administrative time with CAP (or any other subspecialty outside of EM), balancing your time and efforts is key. There is a significant need for child abuse providers, and you will find that there is more work in CAP than any one person can do. It is ok to say no to some projects, and you should firmly delineate your expected hours and duties for CAP. Unfortunately, CAP generally pays much less than EM and requires additional training, which should factor into a career decision.

Emotionally, the child abuse subspecialty can be taxing. Overall, the job is fulfilling and can feel like you are addressing/fixing the anguish in the world instead of letting it go unnoticed. One philosophy I have heard is that by the time someone has called me as a child abuse pediatrician, someone has cared enough to advocate for that child. However, it is important to have solid strategies for unwinding after work and be able to recognize when you need to decompress or talk to someone about your experiences. This is especially true when EM can also be a draining career field. If possible, find a practice location where you have colleagues in EM and CAP (even if those colleagues are not combined EM/CAP physicians) where you can debrief or ask questions from someone who understands the specifics of the job.

One benefit of CAP is the close-knit national community of child abuse subspecialists. The Ray E. Helfer Society mentioned above consists of several hundred CAP providers, who offer an annual conference as well as an email Listserv. Child abuse pediatricians ask near-daily questions about child maltreatment literature, difficult cases, or practice variations.

Workforce

Both PEM and CAP workforce are under served. The following data is from the American Board of Pediatrics Pediatric Physician Workforce Data Book 2020–2021 [1]. Of pediatric diplomats ever certified since January 31, 1934, there are 2823 PEM and 394 CAP diplomats. Twenty-four diplomats are dual-certified in PEM and CAP. There are 3.5 PEM and 0.5 CAP physicians (ever board certified nationally) per 100,000 children. By state the range is 0–21 PEM and 0–1.8 CAP per 100,000 children. There are three states, Wyoming, Montana, and North Dakota, that have no PEM or CAP. A different evaluation of the 2020 PEM workforce in the United States used the American Medical Association Physician Masterfile database linked to the American Board of Medical Specialty board certification [2]. This database identified 2403 active pediatric emergency physicians (pEP). Of the pEP population, 71% had emergency medicine training, 27% had pediatric training, 68% were board certified in PEM, and 99% of the pEP worked in an urban setting. The same three states noted above had no pEP's. Three states—Alaska, New Mexico, and North Dakota—had pEP's working in only one county. Based on these demographics and statistics, there will be career security for any physician who chooses the PEM/CAP path.

Organizations Supporting Child Abuse Pediatricians

- Section of Child Abuse and Neglect, AAP https://www.aap.org/en/community/aap-councils/child-abuse-and-neglect/
- The Ray E. Helfer Society https://www.helfersociety.org/
- The International Society to Prevent Child Abuse and Neglect https://www.ispcan.org/

Conclusions

EM providers can advocate for abused and neglected children as part of their clinical shifts, but there are many ways to extend this work outside of the emergency department. When discussing the role of a CAP, people often ask how someone can work in such an emotionally taxing career. The better way to think of a CAP job is that you are empowered to **do something** to stop child abuse and the suffering it causes.

As an EM physician, you will treat children who have been abused and often it is difficult to see the positive effects of your efforts to help the child and family once they leave your ED. When you are involved in the greater child protection system as a CAP, you benefit from getting the "inside scoop" and witnessing the help that is provided to the child and family. The issue of child abuse is massive, but there are concrete ways to help after you've specialized in CAP. Your research could help other clinicians identify abuse or provide resources to victims of maltreatment. By working with abused children and their families, you might be able to prevent a child from being abused, or even save a child's life.

References

1. American Board of Pediatrics. Pediatric physicians workforce data book, 2020–2021. Chapel Hill, NC: American Board of Pediatrics; 2021. https://www.abp.org/sites/public/files/pdf/workforcedata2020-2021.
2. Bennett CL, et al. Evaluation of the 2020 pediatric emergency medicine physician workforce in the US. JAMA Netw Open. 2021;4(5):e2110084. https://doi.org/10.1001/jamanetworkopen.2021.10084.

Chapter 11
Critical Care Medicine

Jordan B. Schooler

A Brief History of Critical Care Medicine (CCM)

Critical care medicine is a specialty devoted to the care of the sickest patients, those at immediate risk of death, or requiring artificial support for organ failure. Like emergency medicine, and in contrast to many medical specialties that focus on a particular organ system, critical care is organized around both a spectrum of illness, and a setting of care, in which there is extensive physiological monitoring, more intensive nursing care, and the ability to provide therapies including mechanical ventilation, vasopressors, inotropes, and often other forms of support including continuous renal replacement therapy and mechanical circulatory support [1, 2]. Some trace the beginning of critical care back to the 1850s, when Florence Nightingale cohorted the sickest patients close to the nurses in battlefield aid stations [3]. In 1923, Walter Dandy launched a three-bed unit at Johns Hopkins for postoperative neurosurgical patients, perhaps the first ICU in the United States. It was during the polio epidemic of the 1940s that mechanical ventilation became widespread. In 1958, Peter Safar created the first modern intensive care unit at Baltimore City Hospital. A giant in resuscitation, Dr. Safar also contributed to one of the first textbooks of emergency medicine, founded one of the first organized urban prehospital emergency medical services in 1967, and pioneered both closed chest cardiopulmonary resuscitation and rapid sequence induction [3]. He wrote that critical care was a continuum that began with prehospital care and continued in the ED and finally the ICU. Critical care medicine was approved by the American Board of Medical Specialties in 1980 (as a subspecialty of anesthesiology, internal medicine, pediatrics, and surgery), only 1 year later than emergency medicine.

J. B. Schooler (✉)
Department of Emergency Medicine and Heart and Vascular Institute, Penn State Health Hershey Medical Center, Hershey, PA, USA
e-mail: jschooler@pennstatehealth.psu.edu

R. P. Olympia et al. (eds.), *An Emergency Physician's Path*,
https://doi.org/10.1007/978-3-031-47873-4_11

Given the overlap in patient population and skill sets, there had been interest in critical care training and board certification among some emergency physicians since the beginning of both specialties. However, this was vigorously opposed by other medical specialties, and in 1989 emergency medicine was finally approved as a primary board, only after agreeing not to pursue the ability to issue a Certificate of Additional Qualification in CCM [4]. Nevertheless, a number of emergency physicians (EPs) did pursue critical care training, with a survey in 2010 finding over 100 EPs in or having completed CCM fellowships [5]. Of note, 42% of those were at the University of Maryland's Shock Trauma Center and the University of Pittsburgh, institutions with a long history of training EPs. In 2011, an agreement was finally reached between the American Board of Emergency Medicine (ABEM) and the American Board of internal Medicine (ABIM) to allow EM graduates to sit for the ABIM CCM boards after completing an IM based CCM fellowship. Similar agreements were made in 2012 with the American Boards of Anesthesiology and Surgery.

Why Critical Care?

Interest in critical care among emergency medicine trainees has steadily grown over the years for many reasons. Many are drawn to emergency medicine in part for the challenge and reward of working with critically ill patients, and critical care medicine offers the opportunity to work exclusively with this population. Because these patients are at great risk of death, there can be the opportunity to have a large impact. Both assessments and treatments are often closely linked to applied physiology. Effects of interventions tend to be seen more rapidly, for better or worse. Critically ill patients more commonly require procedures such as for invasive monitoring, vasoactive medication administration, hemodialysis, or airway access. Intensivists routinely place arterial catheters, central venous catheters, and may also perform bronchoscopy, place chest tubes, intubate, and even do tracheostomies and extracorporeal membrane oxygenation (ECMO) cannulation in some systems. This opportunity to expand the scope of practice is somewhat unique among emergency medicine fellowships, most of which are focused on administration, education, or research regarding focused areas of the emergency medicine core curriculum. CCM also affords longer and deeper patient and family interactions, and the ability to observe and influence the clinical course over days to weeks, rather than the few hours typical in the emergency department.

However, CCM is not ideal for everyone. It can be stressful. Many critically ill patients will die despite optimal care. The increased exposure to death can lead to frustration, burnout, and depression. The desire by family members or patients for what is perceived as futile care is another common stressor in the ICU. Other difficulties of the generalist may be intensified as well: more political demands given interaction with numerous specialty consulting services, lack of respect from subspecialists or hospital administration, and turf battles for procedures. It is not unusual to be trained in a procedure during fellowship only to find that a subsequent hospital requires consultation of another service for that procedure. The work flow is slower, more deliberate, and more detail oriented. Many EM residents may joke about hating rounding and repletion of electrolytes, but these are fundamental activities in critical care. There may also be a misperception of the nature of the care: treatment of the critically ill patient in the ED generally involves the initial resuscitation, with a fast pace and larger share of procedures. But this is only a small part of critical care, much of which involves trying to restore normal function slowly over days while avoiding iatrogenic harm. Extubation is often a greater focus than intubation. Nutrition and physical therapy are of paramount importance, although topics rarely encountered in the ED. It is also worth considering, as with any fellowship, that sub-specialization will narrow one's job prospects. There are far more openings for emergency physicians than intensivists, and as related below, not every intensivist position would consider an EM graduate.

What Are the Options for Fellowship?

There are four pathways to adult critical care board certification in the United States, all potentially open to emergency medicine graduates. They are sponsored by internal medicine, surgery, anesthesiology, and neurology. Emergency medicine does not itself have any way to accredit fellowships leading to critical care board eligibility, although there are programs focused on resuscitation, typically of 1 year duration [4]. Each training pathway will address the core issues of organ support and coordination of care, but they are defined by different patient populations, monitoring, and interventions.

Internal medicine sponsored critical care fellowships have produced the largest number of intensivists in the United States. These programs are 2 years in length, but are frequently combined with pulmonology or other IM subspecialties into 3 year programs. However, those subspecialties are not available to EM graduates, so only the 2 year stand-alone programs may be pursued by emergency physicians. Internal medicine based CCM programs typically spend the majority of their time in the medical intensive care unit, which in academic centers will typically be the default unit for the critically ill patient who does not obviously require care in another specialized ICU. This patient population will often include respiratory failure requiring mechanical ventilation, septic shock requiring vasopressors, or the post cardiac arrest patient.

Surgical critical care (SCC) has perhaps the longest tradition of training emergency physicians, particularly at the R. Adams Cowley Shock Trauma Center in Baltimore, Maryland [4]. The care of the trauma patient is at the very center of surgical critical care, and indeed there is no board certification in "trauma surgery" but trauma surgeons are those who have trained in critical care. This is a 1-year fellowship for the surgeon, but requires 2 years for emergency physicians. The additional year, called the "advanced prelim year," precedes the critical care year, and comprises rotations in various surgical subspecialities in order to learn the medical management of the surgical patient. While emergency physicians will not learn to do surgery in SCC fellowships, they will often become facile in placement and management of chest tubes, tracheostomies, and percutaneous endoscopic gastrostomies (PEGs). Acute resuscitation and ongoing management of the trauma patient as well as many other postoperative populations are heavily emphasized.

Anesthesiology trains many intensivists, and similarly to SCC programs these typically have a focus on the surgical patient. Again, these are 1-year fellowships for the anesthesiologist, but a second year is required for the emergency physician. In contrast to the narrowly prescribed surgical advanced prelim year, this additional content is largely left to the discretion of each fellowship, and will vary widely, but may include elective time or training in advanced airway management, ultrasound, or other procedures.

Neurocritical care is the newest training pathway, accredited not by the Accreditation Council for Graduate Medical Education (ACGME) but the United Council of Neurologic Subspecialties (UCNS). These programs share the core competencies of managing mechanical ventilation, hemodynamic support, nutrition, and other classic critical care topics, but have a focus on the patient with primarily neurological issues, such as stroke, intracranial hemorrhage, status epilepticus, brain or spinal cord injury, CNS infection, or other neurological conditions such as Guillain-Barre. Their graduates will often practice in dedicated neuro ICUs. Their competencies will include both medical management of these conditions as well as specialized monitoring such as electroencephalography (EEG), neuroimaging, and intracranial pressure monitoring. They may additionally be trained in the placement of intracranial pressure monitors or external ventricular drains [6].

There are also critical care units specializing in patients with cardiac issues, both medical and surgical. These are more commonly found in larger or academic hospitals, and may be combined or may be split into a cardiac or coronary ICU (CCU) and a cardiac or cardiothoracic surgical ICU (CTSICU). Cardiac ICUs are typically focused on the care of the sickest cardiology patient, such as those who have undergone emergent catheterization for myocardial infarction, those with unstable arrhythmias such as ventricular tachycardia or complete heart block, or those with severe heart failure requiring inotropic medication. The CTSICU will manage postop cardiac surgery patients, and in many cases, those requiring mechanical circulatory support devices such as ECMO or Impella. Both types of units will be facile in management of inotropic medications, hemodynamic monitoring such as the pulmonary artery catheter, and use of echocardiography. Despite these specialized patient populations and interventions, there are no currently accredited, formal training programs dedicated to cardiac critical care, and these units have a variety of staffing models. Many cardiac ICUs are managed by cardiologists, sometimes in collaboration with medically trained intensivists. CTSICUs are often staffed by anesthesiologists with subspecialty training in critical care, cardiac anesthesiology, or both. However, there are a number of critical care trained emergency physicians who work in these types of units, including the author of this chapter. This may be the next frontier of CCM specialization (Fig. 11.1).

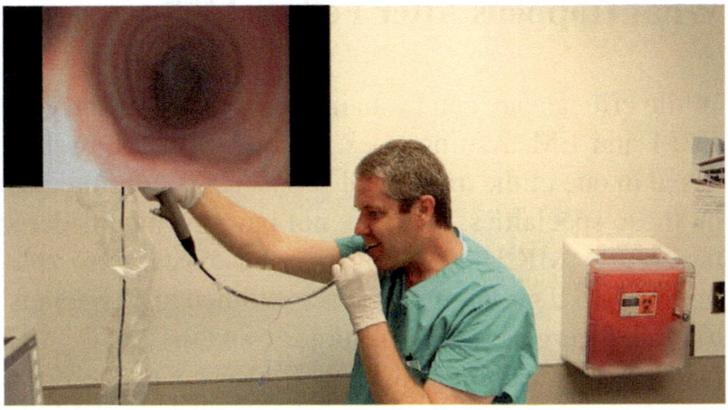

Fig. 11.1 Dr. Schooler performing a self bronchoscopy under local anesthesia during his emergency medicine residency, in order to obtain deeper insight into airway procedures

What Is Important in Fellowship Application?

Given the multiple training pathways across specialties, it is difficult to make any general statements about the competitiveness of critical care fellowships for emergency physicians. However, because there are no accredited critical care fellowships solely for EM graduates, there will usually be fewer spots available for EM compared to the sponsoring specialty. Critical care is a bit more competitive than the average IM fellowship, and a bit less than the average surgical fellowship, but these comparisons mean little to an EM applicant [7]. At present there is no reliable database of which fellowships are even willing to consider EM applicants. It is therefore imperative that the prospective EM-CCM applicant both find a mentor in the field to help navigate this confusing landscape, and also be self-motivated and willing to reach out and investigate programs of interest.

The ideal applicant will have a curriculum vitae (CV) that demonstrates a genuine interest in critical care and documents ongoing involvement in the field. The prospective applicant should have a clear sense of what life will be like in critical care, and where they may fit in. Letters of recommendation from intensivists are important for a successful application, and are particularly helpful if the authors are known to the recipients. Involvement in related hospital committees or academic societies such as the Society of Critical Care Medicine, Eastern Association for the Surgery of Trauma, or the American College of Chest Physicians can both strengthen knowledge and facilitate networking. An SCC candidate could demonstrate interest and provide service by becoming an instructor for Advanced Trauma Life Support (ATLS). Research is not required for a successful application, but will be very helpful in distinguishing an applicant, particularly to academic programs.

Some applicants may find they wish to apply to programs across more than one sponsoring board, which can add complexity to the process. Internal medicine and surgical CCM fellowships use the National Residency Matching Program, while anesthesiology and neurocritical care currently go through the San Francisco match. Since the San Francisco match is earlier, if an applicant matched in anesthesiology critical care, for example, they would have to withdraw any applications in surgical critical care or IM CCM.

What Happens After Fellowship?

While critical care can be an immensely rewarding career, the complexity of joining CCM and EM training does not end with fellowship. Most critical care jobs are based in one of the traditional sponsoring departments, will have expectations based on those specialties, and may not have even considered an emergency physician in the role. A MICU attending may be expected to split time with pulmonology. A trauma/SICU group might be accustomed to physicians able to rotate freely between trauma, emergency general surgery, and the SICU. An anesthesia critical care group may prefer a candidate who will also cover the operating room. These obstacles may become less frequent as the number of EM-CCM graduates increases and awareness rises, but this remains a challenge.

Most EM-CCM physicians will want to split time between their two fields, at least initially, and this can also pose difficulty from an administrative perspective. Academic institutions will usually be more able to accommodate such arrangements, but in a community setting where separate private groups staff the ED and ICU, this may require considerable negotiation. On the other hand, a community ICU may be more flexible about hiring across disciplines, for example an SCC graduate to work in a MICU. Academic institutions often have more specialized units, sicker patient populations, and more advanced interventions. However, they may have more of a bias toward subspecialists, with less autonomy and fewer procedural opportunities. For every such generalization, there will be countless exceptions.

One unique opportunity for the EM-CCM graduate lies in the "ED ICU." This is an area within an ED that is designed to provide some level of critical care services, usually staffed at the physician level either by intensivists or emergency physicians with some additional training. There are multiple models for the ED ICU [8]. Some attempt to fill the gap in care needed for patients who are critically ill and boarding in the ED due to lack of availability of traditional ICU beds. Others are designed as the critical care analog to an observation unit, intending to serve patients requiring critical care services for a short time before stabilizing to go to an intermediate care unit.

References

1. Weil MH, Tang W. From intensive care to critical care medicine: a historical perspective. Am J Respir Crit Care Med. 2011;183(11):1451–3. https://doi.org/10.1164/rccm.201008-1341OE. Epub 2011 Jan 21. PMID: 21257788.
2. Kelly FE, Fong K, Hirsch N, Nolan JP. Intensive care medicine is 60 years old: the history and future of the intensive care unit. Clin Med (Lond). 2014;14(4):376–9. https://doi.org/10.7861/clinmedicine.14-4-376. PMID: 25099838; PMCID: PMC4952830.
3. Weil MH, Shoemaker WC. Pioneering contributions of Peter Safar to intensive care and the founding of the Society of Critical Care Medicine. Crit Care Med. 2004;32(2 Suppl):S8–10. https://doi.org/10.1097/01.ccm.0000110742.81376.fa. PMID: 15043226.

4. Huang DT, Osborn TM, Gunnerson KJ, Gunn SR, Trzeciak S, Kimball E, Fink MP, Angus DC, Dellinger RP, Rivers EP, Society of Critical Care Medicine, American College of Emergency Physicians, Society of Academic Emergency Medicine, Council of Emergency Medicine Residency Directors, Emergency Medicine Residents Association. Critical care medicine training and certification for emergency physicians. Ann Emerg Med. 2005;46(3):217–23. https://doi.org/10.1016/j.annemergmed.2005.04.011. PMID: 16126127.
5. Mayglothling JA, Gunnerson KJ, Huang DT. Current practice, demographics, and trends of critical care trained emergency physicians in the United States. Acad Emerg Med. 2010;17(3):325–9. https://doi.org/10.1111/j.1553-2712.2010.00683.x. PMID: 20370766.
6. Dhar R, Rajajee V, Finley Caulfield A, Maas MB, James ML, Kumar AB, Figueroa SA, McDonagh D, Ardelt A. The state of neurocritical care fellowship training and attitudes toward accreditation and certification: a survey of neurocritical care fellowship program directors. Front Neurol. 2017;8:548. https://doi.org/10.3389/fneur.2017.00548. PMID: 29163327; PMCID: PMC5668669.
7. National Resident Matching Program. Results and data: specialties matching service 2022 appointment year. Washington, DC: National Resident Matching Program; 2022. https://www.nrmp.org/wp-content/uploads/2022/03/2022-SMS-Results-Data-FINAL.pdf. Accessed 2023/02/06.
8. Wessman BT, Mohr NM. Emergency department ICUs add value. Crit Care Med. 2022;50(8):1265–7. https://doi.org/10.1097/CCM.0000000000004708. Epub 2022 Oct 26. PMID: 33105149.

Chapter 12
Disaster Medicine

Daniel Johnson and Avram Flamm

What Is a Disaster?

A disaster is an event that causes a disruption to a community in which the needs surpass available resources [1]. A hurricane, for example, may result in a large number of human casualties, cause damage to existing infrastructure, and require the response of regional and/or federal resources to care for those in need and allow the community to recover. Systems are in place on the local, regional, and federal level to assist citizens and communities respond to disasters. These resources and the role of Disaster Medicine physicians will be described throughout this chapter.

What Is Disaster Medicine and What Makes It a Unique Medical Specialty?

Disaster Medicine is a specialty that has evolved since the mid-1980s. Since the development of the specialty of Emergency Medicine, aspects of Disaster Medicine have been incorporated in the residency curriculum for Emergency Medicine trainees. Indeed, upon graduation from Emergency Medicine residency, emergency physicians will understand some basics of disaster management. This includes medical

D. Johnson
Department of Emergency Medicine, Penn State College of Medicine, Hershey, PA, USA
e-mail: djohnson18@pennstatehealth.psu.edu

A. Flamm (✉)
Department of Emergency Medicine and Public Health Science, Penn State College of Medicine, Hershey, PA, USA
e-mail: aflamm1@pennstatehealth.psu.edu; aflamm@wellspan.org

R. P. Olympia et al. (eds.), *An Emergency Physician's Path*,
https://doi.org/10.1007/978-3-031-47873-4_12

knowledge and skills that are particular useful when dealing with mass casualty incidents (MCIs) and pathologies common to disaster situations. However, the subspecialty of Disaster Medicine involves the in-depth knowledge of not only the medical response to disasters but concepts of emergency management and a deep understanding of local, regional, and federal disaster response frameworks [2]. The response to a disaster is often described by the disaster cycle: mitigation/prevention, preparation, response, and recovery [1]. Disaster Medicine physicians are involved in each phase of the disaster cycle on various levels and this provides the basis for a career in Disaster Medicine.

What Might a Career in Disaster Medicine Look Like?

As mentioned, the disaster cycle encompasses all aspects of disaster response from preparedness to recovery which provides ample opportunity for Disaster Medicine physician involvement. Disaster Medicine physicians may serve on hospital disaster planning committees and participate in the development of health system operational plans for the response to local events. They may also serve as a liaison between the local health system and local or regional government for the purposes of disaster planning. Additionally, in communities that tend to host mass gatherings (sporting events, festivals, concerts, conventions, political activities, etc.), Disaster Medicine physicians will likely play a role in planning for these events, which carry a potential to overwhelm local resources.

The response to disasters is an area where Disaster Medicine physicians may provide a "boots on the ground" approach to Disaster Medicine. The Federal Emergency Management Agency (FEMA) maintains a National Urban Search and Rescue (USAR) response system which includes 28 teams located throughout the United States [3]. Select teams also respond to disasters internationally. Emergency and Disaster Medicine physicians provide medical expertise and oversight to the team and are deployed with the unit to the scene of a disaster. Disaster Medical Assistance Teams (DMAT) are units that are supported by the federal government and also respond to disasters. Their primary role is to provide expanded capacity for medical treatment in areas where local capacity is exceeded or infrastructure damage limits the ability to care for patients. There are 55 teams nationally and they consist of medical providers, including emergency and Disaster Medicine physicians, who may be called upon to support medical operations [4]. There are also various federal programs whose goal is to create a registry of medical professionals who are available to assist in the setting of a disaster. The Medical Reserve Core (MRC) is a federally sponsored registry of over 200,000 volunteer healthcare personnel who can augment local resources in the setting of a disaster [5]. The Emergency System for Advance Registration of Volunteer Health Professionals (ESAR-VHM) is sponsored by the Department of Health and Human Services and maintains a registration of those who are able and willing to volunteer in the setting of disaster or public health emergencies [6]. These organizations also exist on state levels such as the State Emergency Registry of Volunteers in Pennsylvania (SERVPA) program in the Commonwealth of Pennsylvania [7]. The benefit of these programs includes credentialing and vetting of personnel in advance of a disaster so that barriers to care, such as licensing, can be circumvented in a time of need.

Academic positions in Disaster Medicine also exist, generally in conjunction with Emergency Medicine residencies, Disaster Medicine, or Emergency Medical Services (EMS) fellowship training programs. As a relatively new medical specialty, research and scholarship opportunities in Disaster Medicine are ample. As unfortunate as disasters can be, they provide valuable information and feedback to the disaster cycle. However, there are also many challenges when it comes to research in Disaster Medicine since it is challenging to conduct prospective studies. Scholarly work surrounding disaster response, including lessons learned, generally follows large incidents and tends to be retrospective in nature. Other forms of scholarly work include expert consensus on Disaster Medicine topics. As evidenced by the COVID-19 pandemic, dissemination of best practices and cutting-edge knowledge is crucial to the response.

How Do You Pursue Additional Training in Disaster Medicine?

Certain aspects of Disaster Medicine are incorporated in general Emergency Medicine training. Indeed, in smaller community settings, emergency physicians may be called upon as the "experts" in Disaster Medicine in the absence of those formally trained in the subspecialty. However, specialty training programs do exist in the form of Disaster Medicine fellowships. These training programs are generally 1–2 years in length and follow Emergency Medicine residency training. More information on these specific training programs can be found through the American College of Emergency Physicians' section on Disaster Medicine [8]. Clinical aspects of Disaster Medicine training include in-depth knowledge of disease pathology and treatment that are commonly encountered during disasters. Some examples include mass casualty triage, response to chemical/biologic/radiologic/nuclear exposure, blast injuries, treatment of the entrapped patient, and many others. From an emergency management standpoint, education includes aspects of disaster response on the local, state, and federal level and their responsibilities during a disaster. Response to disasters involves the coordination of many agencies, often across state lines, and requires continuous integration to be successful. This requires a national framework for disaster response and all must be well versed in the "language" of Disaster Medicine in order to function together seamlessly at a moment's notice. Many Disaster Medicine programs have certain niche areas of expertise. Some of these may include international response to disasters, government and special operations, and public health preparedness, amongst others. While EMS fellowships cover a broad range of Disaster Medicine topics and provide an avenue to board certification, currently there is no ACGME accreditation or ABEM board certification for Disaster Medicine fellowships.

For those interested in Disaster Medicine but not able to complete a formal fellowship, additional training opportunities do exist to expand the knowledge base of the general Emergency Medicine physician. Courses offered through the National Disaster Life Support Foundation, such as Basic and Advanced Disaster Life Support, are available and cover Disaster Medicine topics over 1–2 days [9]. There are also courses sponsored by FEMA that cover aspects of the Incident Command System (ICS) and the National Incident Management Systemic (NIMS) in various levels of detail. Many of these are available online and at no charge [10].

Combined Programs in Disaster Medicine

Disaster Medicine naturally lends itself to multidisciplinary collaboration. Accordingly, there are combination programs which may combine Disaster Medicine training with a fellowship in Emergency Medical Services, two specialties with natural overlap. The mitigation, response, and recovery from disasters is closely tied with public health and preparedness efforts and several programs also have opportunities to obtain advanced degrees such as a Masters in Public Health (MPH) [11].

Creating an Application for Disaster Medicine Fellowship

At the point of applying for fellowship, Emergency Medicine trainees are well-versed in the key concepts of applying for training programs; applying for fellowship is no different. A general interest in Disaster Medicine should be stablished throughout medical school and residency training. There may be opportunity to serve on hospital emergency management committees as a resident which would certainly bolster the application. Experience in prehospital care is also closely tied to Disaster Medicine, and EMS electives are often available in residency training and may be tailored to focus on Disaster Medicine. Scholarly work in Disaster Medicine would also be of benefit. With the popularity of free, open-access medical education, there are many opportunities to create scholarly content without as much time and resources traditionally dedicated to conventional research. Certainly, partnering with faculty or creating original research during residency would demonstrate the applicant's dedication to the field. When selecting a program, it is important to thoroughly examine the experiences provided by each program. As mentioned, the field of Disaster Medicine has many niches and programs may be most apt at providing education in a field of particular interest to individual applicants.

Conclusion

Disaster Medicine is a developing field of Emergency Medicine which provides a unique and interesting avenue for emergency physicians to diversify their practice and expand out from the traditional hospital setting. Fellowship training in Disaster Medicine provides a formal post graduate Disaster Medicine training and positions graduates of such programs well equipped to prepare for and respond to disasters. Many of these programs can be combined with additional training in Emergency Medical Services, Public Health, and international Emergency Medicine. Applying for Disaster Medicine fellowship follows many of the same principles as any other specialty training program and educational opportunities outside of traditional fellowship training do exist. Unfortunately, disasters will continue to impact communities, which leaves Disaster Medicine physicians with opportunity to serve their communities in new and innovative ways (Table 12.1).

Table 12.1 Summary of disaster response agencies/systems, common acronyms, and roles in disaster preparedness and response

Federal Emergency Management Agency	FEMA	Coordinate federal response to disasters
Disaster Medical Assistance Team	DMAT	Supported by the federal government—provides support and supplements local health care resources during a disaster
Urban Search and Rescue	USAR	Multidisciplinary teams deployed to disaster scenes to assist with search and rescue operations
Medical Reserve Corps	MRC	Registry of health care providers able to assist during a disaster
Emergency System for Advance Registration of Volunteer Health Personnel	ESAR-VHM	Registry of those willing to volunteer during a disaster
State Emergency Registry of Volunteers in Pennsylvania	SERVPA	Similar to ESAR-VHM but on a state level
Incident Command System	ICS	Provides a leadership and management structure for large scale incidents and disasters. Several online courses introducing the ICS are available through FEMA
National Incident Management System	NIMS	Framework for national disaster response. Courses outlining the NIMS are also available through FEMA

References

1. Ciottone GR. Introduction to disaster medicine. In: Ciottone's disaster medicine. 2016. p. 2–5.
2. Lennquist S. Education and training in disaster medicine. Scand J Surg. 2005;94(4):300–10.
3. Urban Search and Rescue. November 4, 2020 [cited 2022 September 6]. https://www.fema.gov/emergency-managers/national-preparedness/frameworks/urban-search-rescue.
4. Disaster Medical Assistance Teams. 2021 [cited 2022 9/6/2022]. https://www.phe.gov/Preparedness/responders/ndms/ndms-teams/Pages/dmat.aspx.
5. The Medical Reserve Corps. 2022 [cited 2022 9/6/2022]. https://aspr.hhs.gov/MRC/Pages/index.aspx.
6. The Emergency System for Advance Registration of Volunteer Health Professionals [cited 2022 9/6/2022]. https://www.phe.gov/esarvhp/pages/about.aspx#:~:text=Main%20Content-,The%20Emergency%20System%20for%20Advance%20Registration%20of%20Volunteer%20Health%20Professionals,public%20health%20and%20medical%20emergencies.
7. State Emergency Registry of Volunteers in Pennsylvania [cited 2022 9/6/2022]. https://serv.pa.gov/.
8. Disaster Medicine Fellowships and Other Training Programs. 2021 [cited 2022 9/6/2022]. https://www.acep.org/disastermedicine/resources/disaster-medicine-fellowships-and-other-training-programs/.
9. All Courses [cited 2022 9/6/2022]. https://www.ndlsf.org/all-courses.
10. National Incident Management System. 2015 [cited 2022 9/6/2022]. https://training.fema.gov/nims/.
11. Shafer K, York P. EMRA fellowship guide 2018. Emergency Medicine Residents' Association; 2016.

Chapter 13
EMS/Prehospital Care Medicine

Monica Corsetti and Jeffrey S. Lubin

A Brief History of Emergency Medical Services (EMS)

Emergency Medical Services (EMS) is a branch of medicine dealing with the emergency treatment and transport of patients in the out-of-hospital setting. EMS involves multiple levels of professionals—from emergency medical technicians to paramedics to dispatchers—and may respond to everything from joint pain to a biological weapon attack. The beauty of EMS is that it is truly a vast specialty dealing with everything in the realm of out-of-hospital medical emergencies. When thinking of EMS, most people envision an ambulance. However, EMS encompasses a variety of topics: air ambulances, tactical medicine, wilderness care, event medicine, and much more.

EMS, in its modern form, is a surprisingly recent development. It was envisioned to reduce morbidity and mortality for conditions that occur outside of a clinical environment and are amenable to treatment before arriving at a hospital. The 1966 *Accidental Death and Disability: The Neglected Disease of Modern Society* report from the National Academy of Sciences envisioned a system of prehospital care, but it was not until 1970 that the National Highway Traffic Safety Administration was founded and started to develop EMS systems. EMS and Emergency Medicine (EM) itself have grown together; the first EM residency program opened in 1972, around the same era that organized EMS systems were emerging. However, it was not until

M. Corsetti
Department of Emergency Medicine, Penn State Health, Harrisburg, PA, USA
e-mail: mcorsetti1@pennstatehealth.psu.edu

J. S. Lubin (✉)
Departments of Emergency Medicine and Public Health Sciences, Penn State Health Milton S. Hershey Medical Center, Hershey, PA, USA
e-mail: jlubin@pennstatehealth.psu.edu

R. P. Olympia et al. (eds.), *An Emergency Physician's Path*,
https://doi.org/10.1007/978-3-031-47873-4_13

2010 that EMS was recognized as a subspecialty of EM by the American Board of Medical Specialties (ABMS).

EMS has evolved into an academic specialty with representation at national assemblies and organizations including the American College of Emergency Physicians (ACEP) EMS-Prehospital Care Section and the National Association of EMS Physicians (NAEMSP). EMS topics are covered in prominent medical journals, including the *New England Journal of Medicine* and the *Annals of Emergency Medicine*. EMS also has developed its own dedicated medical journals including NAEMSP's *Prehospital Emergency Care*, which published its first issue in 1997. Improvements in prehospital care have been extensively studied in many high-acuity conditions such as cardiac arrest, stroke, acute coronary syndrome, and trauma. Data registries developed by EMS professionals have been instrumental in research, such as the Cardiac Arrest Registry to Enhance Survival (CARES) and the National EMS Information System (NEMSIS). EMS has also branched out to include multiple topics including tactical medicine, disaster medicine, critical care, aeromedical transport, and ground transport.

Why Would You Choose EMS?

1. **Multiple Topics and Areas of Medicine.** Emergency Medicine is already a field spanning varied areas of medicine. Additional training via an EMS fellowship presents an opportunity to add areas such as tactical medicine, disaster medicine, wilderness medicine, aeromedical transport, ground transport, and confined space rescue to a physician's practice.
2. **Varied work and workplace.** In EM, our workplace lies primarily in the emergency department (ED). However, EMS provides emergency physicians opportunities to work beyond our typical environment. During an EMS fellowship, emergency physicians can work in ambulances, including air ambulances, and at events such as concerts, rallies, and sporting events, and at the scene of medical and traumatic events: everywhere from roadsides to patients' homes. The ability to work anywhere and everywhere makes EMS simultaneously exciting and challenging; it can be a great way to "mix up" the EM experience from the typical ED setting. EMS physicians may also work as prehospital physicians, treating patients in these non-hospital environments and driving emergency vehicles.
3. **Opportunities for Additional Income.** For those who look for opportunities to supplement their income in EM, EMS might provide an additional source of income. Sometimes, although not always, physicians who provide medical direction for EMS companies are offered compensation for their activities. Contracted employees may obtain protected time from their employer for EMS oversight including medical direction, education of EMS professionals, and even prehospital physician duties.
4. **Working with a Diverse Team.** Perhaps no subspecialty provides the opportunity to work with such a diverse number of professionals as EMS. In addition to

working with emergency medical technicians (EMTs), paramedics, prehospital nurses, respiratory therapists, and other physicians, EMS physicians also can work with dispatchers, firefighters, police officers, and community leaders. EMS has the potential to reach members of the community that few other specialties can. In addition, EMS brings physicians together across medical and hospital groups. Running a successful EMS service means knowing local resources and EMS companies. Thus, meeting with other EMS physicians in your area to discuss regional issues, regulations, disease outbreaks, events, and more becomes a must. Working on regional committees and working with your local EMS federation may help to forge lifelong working relationships and friendships with these colleagues.

5. **Community Outreach.** An EMS fellowship often provides the opportunity to participate in community outreach. Because law enforcement, fire departments, and EMS companies are often staples of the community, an EMS fellowship may include a chance to provide education during community events or gatherings. This can be anything from showing your vehicle at a community picnic while talking to the public about the roles of local EMS, performing wellness checks for community members, or providing first aid at charity events. A fellowship in EMS can be a great way to reach out and serve your local community.
6. **Teaching Opportunities.** For those interested in education, EMS can be particularly rewarding. As mentioned above, EMS has established itself as an ACGME-accredited subspecialty within EM. Being board-certified in EMS may open the doors to practicing in an academic setting for those physicians who desire to teach at a residency program, or perhaps even start an EMS fellowship of their own. In addition, the field of EMS is one of perpetual learning. Paramedics, EMTs, and other first responders are life-long adult learners. As an EMS physician, the responsibility and privilege of teaching these professionals can be extremely rewarding. As a medical director for an EMS company, or even simply an EMS physician, you may provide lectures, hands-on simulations, demonstrations, and knowledge assessments. So, if you enjoy teaching and helping prehospital workers improve the care they deliver to patients, an EMS fellowship may provide a way to step into the role of educator.
7. **Academics.** EM's vast and growing body of research has expanded in recent decades to include research in prehospital care. EMS research is still a relatively young field, but publications in major medical journals, dedicated EMS journals such as *Prehospital Emergency Care*, and an ever-increasing database of prehospital statistics make this field an exciting one in which to pursue a career rich in scholarly activity. Studies on everything from efficacy of epinephrine in cardiac arrest to optimal airway devices in the out-of-hospital environment have been hot topics both in EM and EMS and are being explored in journals such as the *New England Journal of Medicine* and *Journal of the American Medical Association*. If your goal is to build a research reputation or contribute to the field with new findings, EMS can help you reach those goals.

The Fellowship Experience

While training in EMS, fellows participate in emergency response, various subsets of EMS, and have teaching and EM patient care responsibilities. EMS fellows provide field response to medical emergencies as an ACGME requirement, and most fellows can use a physician response vehicle, allowing fellows to drive directly to the scene of an emergency. EMS fellows may also respond to emergencies or transport patients with air ambulances, as many fellows are afforded the opportunity to provide care via helicopter. Commonly, programs provide education for fellows regarding critical care transport and offer the opportunity to participate directly in the transport of critical patients. As part of their training, fellows also engage in disaster planning activities, with most programs offering experiences with hospital systems or EMS agencies. EMS fellows often create medical plans for and provide coverage for mass gathering events, most commonly marathons, concerts, or sporting events. Furthermore, most programs offer some participation in special operations experiences, with the most common being tactical EMS, fireground, and HAZMAT experiences. Some programs also offer wilderness medicine, urban search and rescue, military medicine, and other experiences. One of the great things about EMS is that applicants can pick a fellowship that has resources that best align with their interests, while simultaneously receiving all of the core training required to become board certified in EMS.

In addition to EMS duties, fellows continue to shape their practice in EM, as all fellows in a national survey continued to treat patients in the ED during their fellowship. EMS fellows can expect to have ample opportunity to participate in education, with most fellows participating in training EMS providers and in the education of EM residents.

Applying to Fellowship

Becoming an EMS physician is an arduous but rewarding journey through residency, fellowship, and multiple board certification exams. However, before starting your application process, there is perhaps a more critical step in this path: determining what type of EMS physician you want to become. Because the field of EMS is so broad, no two EMS physician jobs are the same. This extends to fellowship training; no two programs are alike. It may be helpful to reflect on your own interests and experiences before beginning your application and choosing a program. Do you especially enjoy wilderness medicine and working in austere outdoor environments? Do you enjoy a more urban experience? Or perhaps you have always wanted to work with an air ambulance service and are interested in critical care and air medical transport?. For many applicants, time spent as an EMT or paramedic before medical school may give you an idea of where your interests lie. If you are unsure about your goals, consider spending some time working, volunteering, or shadowing with an EMS agency. If you have an interest in a particular field, find a way to obtain some experience prior to your fellowship application. EMS has many niche subject areas. Like medicine itself, having some experience in a topic before entering EMS training will help you to determine whether this is the specialty interest for you long-term.

Because EMS is a subspecialty, to become EMS board-certified, you must first become certified in emergency medicine or another ABMS specialty. This means that, for an emergency physician, securing an EM residency spot is the first step towards EMS. When making your EM residency rank list, it may be advantageous to consider programs with attached EMS fellowships or at least significant EMS exposure and learning opportunities. Not only will this provide opportunities for EMS research, but it may give you additional ability to rotate with EMS services as part of your residency experience. Review program websites and speak to physicians at the program to determine if their faculty's interests align with your own.

It is important to build your CV and network during residency, so continue to seek out EMS-related experiences. In addition to riding with local EMS services, consider volunteering in a medical capacity at local mass gathering events such as races or concerts to gain EMS experience. Collaborating with EMS professionals, including physicians and paramedics, on research projects is another great way to get started in the world of EMS and can often serve to meet residency research requirements for graduation. Consider turning your research into a poster or peer-reviewed journal abstract; national conferences with groups such as the American College of Emergency Physicians, Society for Academic Emergency Medicine, the National Association of EMS Physicians, and others frequently feature research conducted by residents and can be a great way to start your national EMS reputation. Find opportunities to teach and present to EMS professionals, such as grand rounds presentations. Regardless of what kind of experiences you pursue during residency, allow your CV to reflect your own interests and passions.

As you approach the last year of your residency, begin your fellowship application. Remember to tailor your choice of fellowships to the experiences you are seeking. You should also consider the quality and resources of the fellowship. Many programs offer a physician response vehicle for their fellows, which allows them to respond to emergencies independently and can be a valuable learning experience. Many fellowships also provide funding to attend conferences and medical direction courses. Finally, consider other factors such as protected conference time, direct medical oversight opportunities, and EMS faculty qualifications. The National Association of EMS Physicians provides valuable resources for those looking to apply and typically maintains a list of accredited fellowships on its website. It also offers a fellowship guide for applicants that details each program including the program director information, whether the program participates in the match, salary, faculty roles, typical conference/course attendance, response vehicle availability and more. It is important to familiarize yourself with these resources to help select the fellowship that is right for you (Fig. 13.1).

Once you have created a list of preferred programs, be sure to meet all application deadlines. Most fellowship positions are offered within the National Residency

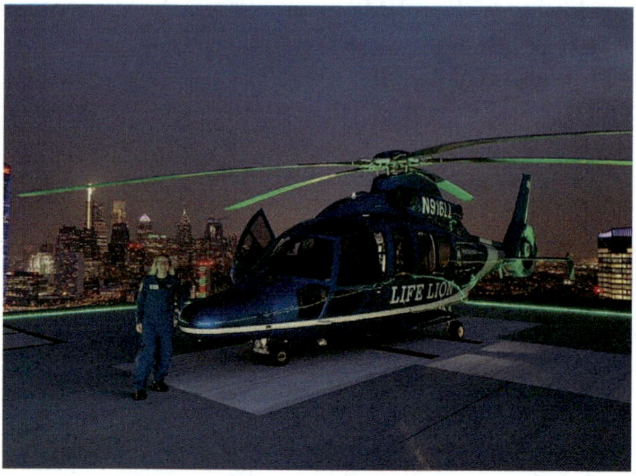

Fig. 13.1 Many EMS fellowships offer in-depth training in the clinical practice and operations of air medical services as part of their curriculum

Match Program (NRMP). In 2021, the Match had 111 certified positions within 70 programs, most programs being 1 year in duration. The match typically occurs in the fall, and NRMP keeps a calendar on their website for aspiring applicants. Most programs require several letters of recommendation; programs vary and you should ensure you are meeting the requirements, but three is typical. Ensure that your letter writers can speak to both your professional capabilities such as your enthusiasm and experience in EMS and your clinical performance as well as your personal attributes like your work ethic, positive demeanor, and so on. Letters from your residency program director, EMS faculty, or a local EMS medical director are all good options. Ensure that you review the match deadlines to give your letter writers ample time to write and submit your recommendation. A personal statement is also typically required and can be a great time to let an EMS program know what makes you a competitive applicant. Do not be afraid to let your special interests shine through in your statement and convey your passion and experiences thus far in EMS.

Applying to EMS fellowship can seem daunting, but to a physician with a passion for EMS, and a well-organized application calendar, the rewards can be enormous and result in a career and a passion lasting a lifetime. The variety of experiences, topics, professional collaboration, and opportunities for research and teaching make EMS an unparalleled sub-specialty within the world of emergency medicine.

Further Reading

50 years of modern EMS. Ems.gov, https://www.ems.gov/OEMShistory.html.

ABMS recognizes EMS as subspecialty. EMS World; 26 Sept. 2010. https://www.hmpgloballearningnetwork.com/site/emsworld/news/10336918/abms-recognizes-ems-subspecialty.

ACGME Program Requirements for Graduate Medical Education in Emergency Medical Services. ACGME; 1 July 2020. https://www.acgme.org/globalassets/pfassets/programrequirements/112_emergencymedicalservices_2020.pdf.

Flamm A, Burch K, Lubin J, Mencl F. Characteristics of EMS fellowships in the United States. Prehosp Emerg Care. 2023;27(1):84–9. https://doi.org/10.1080/10903127.2021.2015023.

Bucher J, Zaidi HQ. A brief history of emergency medical services in the United States. EMRA; 2021. https://www.emra.org/about-emra/history/ems-history/.

Cardiac Arrest Registry to Enhance Survival (CARES). Cardiac Arrest Registry to Enhance Survival (CARES)—healthy people 2030. US Department of Health and Human Services. https://health.gov/healthypeople/objectives-and-data/data-sources-and-methods/data-sources/cardiac-arrest-registry-enhance-survival-cares.

Emergency medical services eligibility criteria for certification. American Board of Emergency Medicine; Feb 2020. https://www.abem.org/public/docs/default-source/default-document-library/eligibility-criteria-ems_rev02242017final.pdf?sfvrsn=ae20c8f4_10.

Emergency Medicine Match Calendar. NRMP; 2022. https://www.nrmp.org/fellowship/emergency-medicine/.

EMS fellowship guide. National Association of EMS Physicians Council of EMS Fellowship Directors; 2021. https://naemsp.org/NAEMSP/media/NAEMSP-Documents/2021-Supp_List.pdf.

Fellowship Programs, National Association of EMS Physicians. https://naemsp.org/career-development/fellowship-programs/.

Match results statistics. NRMP; Nov 2021. https://www.nrmp.org/wp-content/uploads/2021/11/2022-MTOX-Match-Statistics-Results.pdf.

National Association of EMS Physicians. Prehospital Emergency Care. https://naemsp.org/resources/prehospital-emergency-care-journal/.

National EMS Information System (NEMSIS). 9 Jan 2023. https://nemsis.org/.

Perkins GD, Ji C, Deakin CD, Quinn T, Nolan JP, Scomparin C, Regan S, Long J, Slowther A, Pocock H, Black JJM, Moore F, Fothergill RT, Rees N, O'Shea L, Docherty M, Gunson I, Han K, Charlton K, Finn J, Petrou S, Stallard N, Gates S, Lall R, PARAMEDIC2 Collaborators. A randomized trial of epinephrine in out-of-hospital cardiac arrest. N Engl J Med. 2018;379(8):711–21. https://doi.org/10.1056/NEJMoa1806842. Epub 2018 Jul 18.

The history of the national registry and EMS in the United States. National Registry of Emergency Medical Technicians; 2021. https://www.nremt.org/about/history.

Wang HE, Schmicker RH, Daya MR, et al. Effect of a strategy of initial laryngeal tube insertion vs endotracheal intubation on 72-hour survival in adults with out-of-hospital cardiac arrest: a randomized clinical trial. JAMA. 2018;320(8):769–78. https://doi.org/10.1001/jama.2018.7044.

Chapter 14
Geriatric Emergency Medicine

Katherine Selman and Christine Binkley

Abbreviations

ACEP	American College of Emergency Physicians
ACGME	Accreditation Council for Graduate Medical Education
AGS	American Geriatrics Society
ED	Emergency Department
EM	Emergency Medicine
ENA	Emergency Nurses Association
GED	Geriatric Emergency Department
GEM	Geriatric Emergency Medicine
SAEM	Society of Academic Emergency Medicine

History of Geriatric Emergency Medicine

The population of older adults in the United States is growing at a rapid rate, and older patient ED utilization is increasing out of proportion to population growth [1, 2]. Older adults are more likely to require more resources overall including hospital admission, imaging, critical care services, and social considerations [2]. Older adults experience unique geriatric syndromes, such as falls and atypical presentations of disease. Despite this, many EM physicians feel less comfortable with older

K. Selman (✉)
Department of Emergency Medicine, Cooper University Healthcare, Camden, NJ, USA
e-mail: selman-katherine@cooperhealth.edu

C. Binkley
Department of Emergency Medicine, Northwestern Medicine, Kishwaukee Hospital, DeKalb, IL, USA

R. P. Olympia et al. (eds.), *An Emergency Physician's Path*, https://doi.org/10.1007/978-3-031-47873-4_14

patients who often have nonspecific chief complaints such as dizziness. The ED typically approaches patients as having one problem; however, older patients are more likely to have chronic issues, multiple problems, and social factors that impact their visits [3].

Geriatric Emergency Medicine (GEM) evolved to investigate and to address the needs of this population and to improve their care while being evaluated in the ED. The first recognized Geriatric ED opened in 2008 at St. Joseph's Regional Medical Center in New Jersey, and the first GEM fellowships started at Beaumont Hospital, Royal Oak and New York-Presbyterian Hospital in 2005. Since then, leaders in GEM have developed different models of delivering high-quality geriatric care in the ED and GEM research has increased exponentially in the past decade [4]. In 2009, competencies for EM residents related to the care of older patients were published and incorporated into residency training [5]. The identified core domains in GEM in which residents are expected to be proficient include:

- Atypical presentation of disease
- Trauma including falls
- Cognitive and behavioral disorders
- Emergency intervention modifications
- Medication management
- Transitions of care
- Effect of comorbid conditions

In 2013, the first GED guidelines were published as a collaboration between American College of Emergency Physicians (ACEP), Society of Academic Emergency Medicine (SAEM), Emergency Nurses Association (ENA), and the American Geriatrics Society (AGS) and outlined best practices and recommendations for high-quality geriatric care in the ED setting. In 2018, ACEP started the GED Accreditation Program and defined standardized criteria for an ED to be considered a GED based on these guidelines. Since 2018, over 300 EDs nationwide have been accredited as GEDs.

GEM is represented as a section within ACEP and an academy within SAEM. Research within GEM is published widely across many journals, including a dedicated *Journal of Geriatric Emergency Medicine*, and on a variety of topics such as polypharmacy, improved communication with care facilities, delirium identification, and fall prevention.

Why Choose a Career in Geriatric Emergency Medicine?

An EM physician's average patient census can be at least one-third older adults on any given shift. By 2040, the population of older adults is projected to increase by over 25 million, and this trend will be naturally reflected in our practice [1]. GEM champions can assist with this transition in population change. We will continue to see large numbers of older adults both from the community and long-term care facilities, so it is imperative that we become adept at meeting their needs.

In this way, GEM is applicable to EDs anywhere, and you can create a niche specialty that medical directors will want to recruit and hire. ACEP has recognized hundreds of GEDs, and accreditation is now a goal for many hospitals and healthcare systems. The hope is that these recommendations will one day become a standard for every ED. As this is an emerging field, there are relatively few EM doctors who specialize in geriatrics, and you can expect to be in high demand in any region.

GEM offers a huge diversity in career opportunities. You can focus on research, clinical practice, medical education, administration, or a mix of all. There is a lot of emerging research in GEM but it is still a new field with many gaps in the literature about best care practices for older adults from the EM perspective. Hot topics in the research domain include how GEDs can reduce future repeat visits, avoid unnecessary admissions, and decrease overall healthcare spending; the role of the ED in preventing falls and delirium; and practical implementation of interventions in the ED. Medical education in GEM can be directed to medical students and residents, but good geriatric care requires significant engagement of nursing and ancillary staff, so you can incorporate teaching even at non-academic centers for multiple levels of learners. If you are interested in administration, GEDs develop specific policies and initiatives for geriatric patients, which requires interfacing with ED leadership, hospital administration, ancillary services, and many hospitals are interested in quality improvement and metrics related to older adults.

Whether academic or community, big city or rural area, GEM will be relevant to your future.

GEM Fellowship: Next Steps

Next step is the completion of a 1–2 year fellowship for EM residency graduates, which includes completion of a research and quality improvement requirement, with opportunities to obtain a concurrent master's degree at some programs. There are currently five GEM fellowships in the United States and one in Toronto, Canada. Alternatively, you may consider other fellowships such as Research, Medical Education, Simulation, or Administration and still maintain a focus on geriatrics through these fellowships. While GEM fellowships are approved by SAEM, they are not currently ACGME accredited. GEM fellows are not currently eligible for Geriatric Medicine board certification, which is presently only available to Internal Medicine or Family Medicine trained physicians.

In addition to ED shifts, fellows may rotate through geriatric inpatient units, geriatric outpatient clinics, skilled nursing facilities, geriatric consult services, and subspecialty services such as palliative care, hospice, hip fracture services, and rehabilitation. The didactic curriculum covers geriatric syndromes and core domains of GEM including falls, cognitive impairment, atypical presentation of disease, end of life care, medication management, and transitions of care. Fellows are expected to participate in at least one scholarly project during their fellowship. This may be a quality improvement initiative, a research project, or an educational process, depending on the fellow's areas of interest.

Typically, there are between 2 and 5 fellows per year nationwide. While it is not necessarily competitive, program directors are looking for self-directed, passionate individuals. It is helpful to familiarize yourself with common topics and the core domains in GEM beforehand and have an idea of areas within GEM in which you would like to concentrate. The GEM community is supportive and valuable in terms of resources and mentorship. Since GEM physicians are not a standard at every institution, getting involved with SAEM or ACEP is a great way to connect with mentors nationally and even internationally.

A key tenet of Geriatric medicine is to focus on what matters most. Apply this to your career as well, and it will serve you well!

References

1. Centers for Disease Control and Prevention. Atlanta, GA. 2022. https://data.cdc.gov. Accessed 15 Aug 2022.
2. Pines JM, Mullins PM, Cooper JK, Feng LB, Roth KE. National trends in emergency department use, care patterns, and quality of care of older adults in the United States. J Am Geriatr Soc. 2013;61(1):12–7. https://doi.org/10.1111/jgs.12072.
3. Ringer T, Dougherty M, McQuown C, Melady D, Ouchi K, Southerland LT, et al. White Paper-Geriatric Emergency Medicine education: current state, challenges, and recommendations to enhance the emergency care of older adults. AEM Educ Train. 2018;2(Suppl 1):S5–16. https://doi.org/10.1002/aet2.10205.
4. Southerland LT, Lo AX, Biese K, Arendts G, Banerjee J, Hwang U, et al. Concepts in practice: geriatric emergency departments. Ann Emerg Med. 2020;75(2):162–70. https://doi.org/10.1016/j.annemergmed.2019.08.430.
5. Hogan TM, Losman ED, Carpenter CR, Sauvigne K, Irmiter C, Emanuel L, et al. Development of geriatric competencies for emergency medicine residents using an expert consensus process. Acad Emerg Med. 2010;17(3):316–24. https://doi.org/10.1111/j.1553-2712.2010.00684.x.

Chapter 15
Health Policy

Aaron R. Kuzel and Philippa Soskin

A Brief History of Health Policy in Medicine

This issues of access to health care and health care reform have long dominated American politics. At the heart of this a complex history is the relationship between government and private industry; consequently, rather than having a cohesive health care system, this has led to an amalgamation of systems including employer-based, private insurance, and government funded. For the first half of the twentieth century, there was not much demand for health insurance and most was bought privately. World War II triggered a major change when, in response to labor shortages and an attempt to reduce inflation, businesses were prohibited from increasing their wages to attract employees. Employers instead started offering benefits including health insurance to compete for workers. In 1943, employer-based health insurance became exempt from taxation making it an even more affordable benefit for employers to offer. Government took on a much larger role in health insurance coverage in 1965 when President Lyndon B. Johnson signed the Medicaid and Medicare Act establishing are health insurance program for the elderly and those with limited income. Over the years there have been many attempts to reform the U.S health care system and improve health insurance coverage. President Barack Obama signed the Patient Protection and Affordable Care Act in 2010 to increase coverage for the uninsured and broaden the health insurance market [1].

A. R. Kuzel
Department of Emergency Medicine, University of Louisville School of Medicine, Louisville, KY, USA
e-mail: Aaron.kuzel@louisville.edu

P. Soskin (✉)
Department of Emergency Medicine, MedStar Georgetown University Hospital and Washington Hospital Center, Washington, DC, USA
e-mail: Philippa.Soskin@medstar.net

R. P. Olympia et al. (eds.), *An Emergency Physician's Path*,
https://doi.org/10.1007/978-3-031-47873-4_15

Emergency medicine is particularly affected by changes in health care policy and access to care. As the safety net specialty, emergency medicine cares for all people who come through the door; a concept that became federal law in 1986 with the passage of the Emergency Medical Treatment and Labor Act (EMTALA). Patient volumes, workforce issues, quality of care, prescription drug policy, and access to primary care and specialty services are just a few of the many policy issues that impact our practice and patients. The American Medical Association (AMA) includes advocacy in its Declaration of Professional Responsibility [2]. Given our direct experience with patients' demographics, needs, and challenges navigating the health care system, emergency physicians are uniquely positioned to serve as advocates, create and advise policy, and implement change.

How Can You Incorporate Health Policy in Your Career?

There are many ways to use health policy knowledge and training in your career. Some choose to develop their niche within their hospital and alongside their clinical responsibilities. Some take advantage of the flexibility of emergency medicine to work part time clinically and part time on their policy work while others may transition fully to a non-clinical job in health policy.

Academic medicine. You may choose to work as an academic emergency physician with healthy policy as your niche. This may involve health services research, and/or educating and mentoring medical students, residents, fellows, and other faculty and staff in health policy.

Hospital leadership. An in-depth understanding of health policy and the health care system are valuable skills for service on hospital committees as well as within hospital leadership and administration.

Advocacy. Physicians are important advocates for the needs of their patients as well as for their fellow doctors and the specialty of emergency medicine. This may involve lobbying your local, state, or federal representatives on a specific bill or issue. You may choose to advocate through organized medicine by joining the leadership of one of the medical or emergency medicine specialty societies such as the AMA, the American College of Emergency Physicians (ACEP), or the American Academy of Emergency Medicine (AAEM). You can use your voice through writing on policy topics, contributing op-eds, and through radio, podcast, social, and television media.

Government and non-profits. You may advise a government representative or policy committee. Physicians over the years have run for office themselves in all areas of government including congress. You may work for a non-profit or serve on their advisory board.

Pursuing a Health Policy Fellowship in Emergency Medicine

Health policy fellowships are designed to provide additional academic, professional, and clinical training and experience so that fellows gain the tools to successfully integrate health policy into their careers and affect positive change for patients and the practice of emergency medicine. When selecting a fellowship, it is important to consider what is of value to you and your career goals; these may include location, research opportunities, teaching responsibilities, advanced degree options, moonlighting availability, and internship sites. This is a personal decision based on one's passions and interests and future personal and professional goals. Most emergency medicine health policy fellowships consist of three main components: policy education, policy experience, and clinical work.

Currently, healthy policy fellowships in emergency medicine do not yield an additional board certification and are not accredited by the Accreditation Council for Graduate Medical Education (ACGME). Many fellowships do offer formal credentials through master's level training such as a Master of Public Policy or Master of Public Health. There are benefits to being a non-accredited fellowship such as flexibility for moonlighting, potential for higher salary, and less restrictions to duty hours for fellow education and opportunities.

One of the major benefits of a health policy fellowship is the professional experience gained through internships. Most fellowships offer at least one if not multiple internship opportunities for fellows to gain high level real world professional experience in their area of interest. Examples of internship placements include local, state, and federal government entities such the Center for Medicare and Medicaid Innovation, the Department of Health and Human Services, the Agency for Healthcare Research and Quality, departments of public health, and working on health care issues for a specific member of congress or legislative committee. Opportunities also include non-governmental entities such as the National Quality Forum, Environmental Defense Fund, and many other non-profit and advocacy organizations working on a wide range of health care issues. Often one of the challenges of finding employment in health policy is not having prior work experience and a health policy fellowship can provide a structured opportunity to gain this experience and build a professional network (Fig. 15.1).

Location. Is the fellowship located somewhere you feel you will be happy to work and practice for one to two years? Does the location provide a rich breath of professional opportunities in your areas of interest for your internship placements? Will the network you will gain assist you in your future career? For example, if you are committed to living in a specific city or state, you may consider a program that will allow you to build a network in that area or provide national contacts that are transferrable.

Length of training. There are both one-year and two-year health policy fellowship options. Two-year fellowships are more likely to offer a formal master's program as part of their curriculum. Some may offer a one-year option for those not seeking an additional advanced degree or who already hold a relevant master's

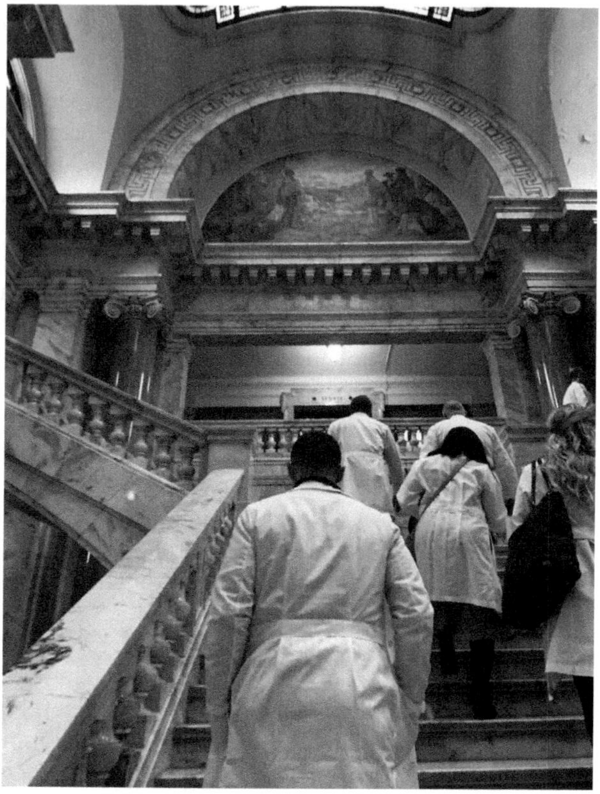

Fig. 15.1 Physicians from the Greater Louisville Medical Society attend Physician's Day at the Capitol in Frankfort, Kentucky, to discuss with legislators regarding issues affecting the practice of medicine

degree. One-year programs may be more limited in the amount of education and professional experience there is time to offer but there is also a personal cost-benefit analysis one must do in terms of considering an additional year of training and the opportunity cost that comes with this in terms of time and salary.

Formal education and degree programs. Health policy fellowships differ widely in how much classroom education they provide and in what format. Some offer a series of lectures from their own faculty while others may have their fellows take classes through the program's affiliated university resulting in a "Certificate in Health Policy" or similar credential. Others offer a formal advanced degree such as a Master of Public Policy, Master of Public Health, or Master of Policy Management. These differ in the focus of their core curriculum. For example, the core curriculum in public health often focuses on epidemiology and statistics whereas public policy programs often favor economics and organizational management. Look carefully at the core curriculum and elective offerings for the programs you are considering to be sure they align with your interests and goals.

Clinical responsibilities. As a health policy fellow, you are also spending time clinically as an attending physician in emergency medicine. If you are starting your fellowship directly following residency, this may be your first experience as an attending. Consider the clinical practice sites offered by the fellowship. Are these sites where you want to practice? Do they offer the experience you want whether that be community practice, academics and teaching opportunities, or some combination of both? You will likely be working less clinically than the average full time attending due to your fellow responsibilities. Does the program offer the right balance of dedicated fellowship time but also allow you to gain the clinical experience you need as a new attending?

Salary and benefits. Some fellowship salaries will follow the post-graduate year (PGY) structure and you will be paid as a PGY-4 or PGY-5 depending on the length of your residency training. Some will offer higher salaries and/or supplement your salary with moonlighting hours. Also consider the value and expense of a master's degree which is generally included in the salary agreement. You may receive other benefits such as continuing medical education (CME) dollars and reimbursement for board exams.

Applying for a Health Policy Fellowship

So you have decided to apply for a health policy fellowship. What makes a strong applicant and what are the next steps? Fellowship programs are looking for applicants with a strong level of interest and a desire to gain additional training with a goal to incorporate health policy in their careers. First and foremost a candidate should demonstrate an enthusiasm and interest in the field of health policy. There are many ways to demonstrate this interest such as involvement in advocacy days, health policy interest groups, health policy electives, and involvement in research. There are many opportunities to be involved in health policy sections or committees within emergency medicine and beyond through organizations such as ACEP, AAEM, SAEM, EMRA, AMA, ACP, and AOA. Interested applicants can also attend special rotations or "min-fellowships" in health policy offered by non-profit entities and through EMRA and AAEM.

While this chapter is focused on emergency medicine heath policy fellowships, you may also consider more general fellowship training including but not limited to the Robert Wood Johnson Heath Policy Fellows Program, the National Academy of Medicine Fellowships for Health Science Scholars, and the White House Fellows Program. An internet search will help you locate fellowship programs and their contact information. The exact number of fellowships and fellowship positions is fluid from year to year; currently there are approximately twelve emergency medicine health policy fellowships and most offer one to two positions per year. Most emergency medicine fellowships are listed on fellowship information sites through EMRA and SAEM and some will be represented at fellowship fairs through ACEP, SAEM, and AAEM. Your program director is also a good resource as they may receive recruitment information from individual programs.

Programs generally require a curriculum vitae (CV), letter of intent or personal statement, and typically two to three letters of recommendation. Based on the program's review of these initial materials, you may be invited for an interview. There may be a separate or additional application process if there is a master's degree involved. There is no match process or universal deadline for health policy fellowships and each program differs in their process, requirements, and deadlines. Applicants should review the program's website and reach out to the program director and/or coordinator to determine the exact application requirements and deadlines for each program.

References

1. Kaiser Family Foundation. Timeline: history of health reform in the U.S. Kaiser Family Foundation Website. https://www.kff.org/wp-content/uploads/2011/03/5-02-13-history-of-health-reform.pdf. Accessed 2 Aug 2022.
2. American Medical Association. AMA declaration of professional responsibility. American Medical Association Website; 4 Dec 2021. https://www.ama-assn.org/delivering-care/public-health/ama-declaration-professional-responsibility. Accessed 25 Aug 2022.

Chapter 16
International Emergency Medicine

C. James (Jim) Holliman

A Brief History of International Emergency Medicine (IEM)

The sub-specialty of IEM (also now termed "Global Emergency Medicine") started in the early 1990s when a relatively small number of academic emergency physicians in the U.S.A. looked around and realized that the specialty of Emergency Medicine (EM) was not officially recognized and in fact did not even exist in most of the countries around the world. So they decided collectively to try to fix this situation and develop the field of IEM as a recognized EM sub-specialty. Early on they faced opposition and ridicule from some of the U.S. national leaders in EM who thought IEM was just an excuse for "medical tourism" (which in fact many of these leaders practiced when going to other countries). So the early founders of IEM started an Interest Group for IEM within the Society for Academic Emergency Medicine (SAEM), and published a series of journal articles to provide academic legitimacy for the sub-specialty of IEM [1–9]. SAEM's leaders then recognized the potential value of IEM and upgraded the Interest Group to an SAEM Committee, which then later morphed to the Global Health Academy under SAEM.

At about the same time, the leaders of the American College of Emergency Physicians (ACEP) became interested in IEM, and ACEP started its IEM Section, which quickly became the largest dues paying membership section in ACEP. The IEM section achieved a number of accomplishments, including starting the ACEP IEM Ambassador Program, the IEM Scholarship Program, facilitating international members of ACEP, sponsoring IEM conferences, maintaining web based resources

C. James (Jim) Holliman (✉)
Emergency Medicine and Public Health Sciences, Pennsylvania State University M. S. Hershey Medical Center, Hershey, PA, USA

Military and Emergency Medicine, Uniformed Services University of the Health Sciences, Bethesda, MD, USA
e-mail: cholliman@pennstatehealth.psu.edu

R. P. Olympia et al. (eds.), *An Emergency Physician's Path*, https://doi.org/10.1007/978-3-031-47873-4_16

for IEM, and publishing additional articles on IEM in the Annals of Emergency Medicine.

Early on the leaders in IEM recognized the importance of providing post-residency training in IEM to develop future leaders in this field, and so the first IEM Fellowship programs were started in a number of academic Emergency Medicine (EM) departments. Because of the burgeoning interest in Global Health issues by both medical students and EM residents, the number of IEM fellowship programs rapidly increased and now numbers over 40 in the U.S.A. The IEM Fellowship Consortium (now renamed the Global EM Fellowship Consortium) was started to link activities between the many IEM fellowship programs, and developed an on-line application process and web site to coordinate and standardize applications from residents for the IEM fellowship programs.

So Why Should You Choose a Career in IEM?

Why is there such a recent increase in interest in IEM? I think a number of things have contributed to this, including the recent awakening by many countries that they should develop better EM for their patients. EM in the U.S.A. has fully matured as a specialty and is looked upon as a role model by other countries. The collapse of Communism has opened up multiple countries to people and new ideas from the outside, and EM is a relatively new idea for many countries. Multiple international EM conferences have just gotten started in the past 20 years and many of these have been very successful, and there is expanding interest in participating in these in the future. Within individual other countries, a number of factors have also contributed to the increasing interest in developing EM. There has been overall medical system development improvement in most countries. Most countries, even the ones with poor economies classed as "developing," are undergoing rapid urbanization. This has resulted in a "demographic transition" with increasing frequency of cases of trauma from motor vehicle crashes and of cardiorespiratory illnesses. These have now assumed greater public health importance in most urbanized areas than were the previous prominent problems of infectious and parasitic diseases. Hospital-based EM is well-suited to manage these problems of trauma and cardiorespiratory illnesses [10]. Also, in most countries there are increasing outpatient visits and also an increasing percentage of elderly patients who require emergency services at a greater frequency than younger patients. In addition, the demonstrated success of EM in the U.S.A. has resulted in increased public expectations in other countries for improvement of the quality and availability of emergency health care services. This has also been promoted by international exposure of the previous very popular television programs "ER" and "Rescue 911." Increased international travel has also promoted awareness of the need for improved EM in many countries.

What general benefits does international EM experience offer U.S. EM physicians? I think one of the most important benefits for U.S. EM physicians is the potential for exposure to, and interaction with, other cultures. EM physicians can learn more of the historical background of other cultures and can better understand how culture can influence compliance with medical care. Also, this cultural experience might enable EM physicians to better deal with emergency department (ED) patients in the U.S.A. who are from other cultures. There is also the possibility of the EM physician discovering new foods and/or crafts which he or she could continue to enjoy into the future. Another important benefit is that EM physicians can learn novel approaches to common clinical problems. Most urban EDs in other countries see a very similar case distribution as do U.S. ED's. This includes (as noted above) trauma from motor vehicle crashes, acute coronary syndromes, acute respiratory emergencies such as tuberculosis and pneumonia, and simple fractures and lacerations. Many practicing EM physicians in other countries have extensive experience in dealing with these same medical problems that we have here in the U.S.A. and often can show us different effective ways to deal with these same medical problems. Also, in some other countries, there may be some pharmaceuticals that are not available in the U.S.A. and physicians can learn about the benefits of these. Overcrowding is unfortunately also a common problem in ED's in other countries, and there is the potential to take some lessons from management of this problem in other countries back to the U.S.A. In contrast, another potential benefit of international EM work is the opportunity (which is obviously dependent upon the locale) to see clinical problems that are not common in the U.S.A. These can include malaria, arborviral fevers, parasitic diseases, cutaneous and systemic mycoses, tetanus, rabies, and neurotoxic snake bites (Fig. 16.1).

Another benefit of international work is the personal satisfaction in having deeply appreciative patients. ED patients in other countries in general appear to be more appreciative of the care given them by physicians than are patients here in the U.S.A. It is very common for even very economically disadvantaged patients in

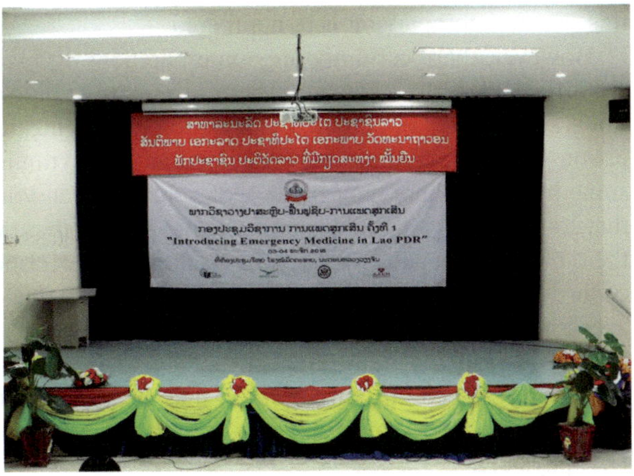

Fig. 16.1 Emergency Medicine extending worldwide (photo courtesy of Dr. James Holliman)

other countries to give thank-you gifts to emergency physicians for care they have received. In addition, there can be the personal satisfaction of having deeply appreciative emergency physician colleagues from other countries. Most of these physicians are very "hungry" for interaction and teaching. Most also enjoy maintaining long-term correspondence links with U.S. physicians.

Another potential benefit of international EM work is the opportunity as a single individual to have a very big impact on influencing development of EM on a national basis. This can include helping to train EM faculty, organizing EM residencies, recommending ED facility design features, coordinating prehospital and ED care, and obtaining government support for EM development. Statements by visiting U.S. EM physicians may have very big influential impact on both government officials and hospital administrators in assisting with EM development.

International EM work may also provide the opportunity for U.S. physicians to perform procedures which may often be done (or argued as to who is going to do the procedure) by other specialties in U.S. ED's. These can include thoracotomy, placing thoracostomy tubes, doing peritoneal lavage, performing peritoneal dialysis, doing complex facial and hand laceration repairs, performing closed fracture reductions, performing emergent amputations, and endoscopy. There is also the possibility in some countries to act as or assist surgeons in the performance of major surgical procedures that would not normally be done by emergency physicians in the U.S.A.

Another common reported benefit of U.S. physicians doing international work is to experience the fun of clinical practice without the excessive U.S. paperwork and worry about malpractice suits. There is also the possibility for physicians to learn how to practice without excessive reliance on diagnostic testing, because of the resource limitations in some other countries' ED's. However, despite all of the current U.S. health care system problems, most U.S. physicians returning from international work experiences report that this has enabled them to appreciate how good the U.S. system is by comparison to all other national health care systems. This can make getting back to day-to-day work in the U.S. somewhat more enjoyable when this sense of comparison is remembered.

However, there certainly are some potential disadvantages of international EM work for U.S. EM physicians. There can be frustration due to local resource limitations, such as lack of certain lab or radiology diagnostic tests. Some effective medications (such as certain antibiotics and anti-arrhythmics) may not be available. In some hospitals there may be lack of ventilators and/or intensive care unit beds so that some patients may die simply due to lack of these resources. In some hospitals there may also be lack of specialty backup for performance of certain surgical procedures. In some countries it can be frustrating to deal with the lack of guaranteed access to emergency or inpatient care unless the patient or family is able to pay for their care. Language differences may also inhibit patient or staff interactions. However, it is certainly my opinion that these potential disadvantages are far outweighed by the many advantages and rewards of international work for U.S. physicians.

IEM Fellowship: The Next Steps

IEM has not yet been certified by the American Board of Emergency Medicine (ABEM) as an officially ABEM recognized sub-specialty so it does not have a standardized sub-certification exam. There also is not a standardized structure for the various IEM fellowship programs. Most programs are involved with EM residency development and support in other countries, and the IEM fellows in most programs provide bedside and didactic teaching and direct patient care. Some IEM programs are focused on disaster management, refugee aid, mass casualty management, leadership development, faculty development, public health programs, and/or EM research. Some of the programs are focused just on one country, and others have multiple country connections. Some are directly affiliated with international organizations such as the International Medical Corps or Doctors Without Borders. Many of the programs offer completion of a Masters of Public Health Degree (having this degree as part of your pedigree can be very helpful in dealing with stodgy elderly physicians in other countries who may be reluctant to take advice from younger physicians). So when considering applying for an IEM fellowship, look carefully at each program's web site to see if the program's activities and foci are in line with your career interests.

Most of the IEM fellowships require completion of a Canadian or U.S. EM residency, but some are open to graduates of other specialty residencies. Once you have done a careful check of program web sites (and considered making site visits to selected programs), send in your application(s) through the online system operated by the Global EM Fellowship Consortium. Not all the programs require an on-site interview, and many have gone to having online interviews as part of the application process.

References

1. Holliman CJ, VanRooyen MJ, Green GB, et al. Planning recommendations for international emergency medicine and out of hospital care system development. Acad Emerg Med. 2000;7(8):911–7.
2. Kirsch TD, Holliman CJ, Hirshon JM, et al. The development of international emergency medicine: the role of United States emergency physicians and organizations. Acad Emerg Med. 1997;4(10):996–1001.
3. Holliman CJ, Kirsch TD, Green GB, et al. Guidelines for evaluation of international emergency medicine assistance and development projects. Ann Emerg Med. 1997;30(6):811–5.
4. Arnold JL. International emergency medicine and the recent development of emergency medicine worldwide. Ann Emerg Med. 1999;33:97–103.
5. VanRooyen MJ, Thomas TL, Clem KJ. International emergency medicine services: assessment of developing prehospital systems abroad. J Emerg Med. 1999;17(4):691–6.
6. Shayne P, Holliman CJ, Wang E, Parrillo SJ. International emergency medicine reference list. J Emerg Med. 1999;17(1):159–61.
7. Keyes LE, Holliman CJ. Reference listing of international emergency medicine journals and web sites. Ann Emerg Med. 1999;34(6):786–9.

8. Holliman CJ, Green G, VanRooyen MJ, et al. Proposed curriculum for an "observational" international emergency medicine fellowship program. Acad Emerg Med. 2000;7(4):359–64.
9. VanRooyen MJ, Clem KJ, Holliman CJ, et al. Proposed fellowship training program in international emergency medicine. Acad Emerg Med. 1999;6(2):145–9.
10. Holliman CJ, et al. The efficacy and value of emergency medicine: a supportive literature review. Int J Emerg Med. 2011;4(1):44. https://doi.org/10.1186/1865-1380-4-44.

Chapter 17
Medical Education

Joshua Ginsburg

Do You Want a Career in Academic Medicine?

To answer the first question, consider one study by the Association of American Medical Colleges (AAMC), in which three overarching themes were identified as reasons physicians chose academic medicine [1]:

1. Educating the next generation of physicians
2. Conducting research
3. Providing high-quality patient care

Additionally, the most frequently cited work-related values among academic physicians pursuing the above themes were the following:

1. *Variety.* Physicians in academic medicine can pursue any combination of clinical, research, teaching, service, and leadership opportunities.
2. *Intellectual stimulation.* Academic medicine allows one to work with residents and/or students, which leads to daily learning opportunities and motivates academic physicians to stay up to date and increase their knowledge base. Academic emergency departments tend to see sick and medically complex patients as well.
3. *Service.* Many academic institutions are safety net hospitals that care for the underserved.
4. *Fulfilling relationships.* Academic physicians have the opportunity to form valuable relationships with residents, students, faculty colleagues, patients, and the community.

J. Ginsburg (✉)
Department of Emergency Medicine, UT Southwestern Medical Center, Dallas, TX, USA
e-mail: Joshua.Ginsburg@UTSouthwestern.edu

R. P. Olympia et al. (eds.), *An Emergency Physician's Path*,
https://doi.org/10.1007/978-3-031-47873-4_17

If these appeal to you, you may want to consider a career in academic medicine. Personally, I pursued academics as I felt that the above factors were essential for a long and satisfying career. It is absolutely worth noting that these characteristics can be found in some community medicine careers as well. Indeed, many community doctors are responsible for vital resident and student education. However, as will be described further, medical education fellowships tend to focus on topics that are more valuable to physicians who plan to be heavily involved in academic medicine rather than teaching in community hospitals.

Additionally, note that many academic physicians have completed fellowships in subspecialties other than medical education, such as Ultrasound or Emergency Medical Services (EMS), and others have gone directly into academics without completing a fellowship. This brings us to the second question of whether it is necessary or beneficial to pursue a fellowship in medical education prior to pursuing an academic career.

Is It Necessary or Beneficial to Receive Fellowship Training in Medical Education in Order to Have a Successful Career in Academic Medicine?

In other fields, completion of a fellowship has been associated with increased research productivity and academic rank. For example, family medicine physicians who completed fellowships were more likely to achieve senior rank than their colleagues who did not complete fellowships [2]. In a study of emergency medicine physicians specifically, although not compared to non-fellowship-trained colleagues, graduates of medical education fellowships generally went on to be academically productive and take on leadership positions. Nearly 90% of graduates subsequently worked in academic settings, nearly 70% served on national medical education committees, and graduates on average had written more than three book chapters and authored five peer-reviewed medical education papers [3]. It can reasonably be said that while completion of a medical education fellowship neither guarantees future work in an academic institution nor is a prerequisite for academic success, historically it is associated with both.

For the motivated fellow, medical education fellowships also provide mentorship and networking opportunities that can make the job hunt and early career advancement easier. Medical education fellowship graduates often take positions as assistant residency program directors, clerkship directors, core faculty, or other leaders in education [4]. This is, however, not the only path. For example, I went straight from fellowship into community emergency medicine to gain more clinical experience prior to returning to academics. After 2 years, I returned to academics with a desire to use my background in medical education to teach residents how to practice in less resource-rich environments.

What Do I Need to Know About Medical Education Fellowships?

The first medical education fellowships were started in the 1970s, with rapid expansion in the number of programs in the 1990s and 2000s that continues to this day [5]. At the time of this writing, there are about 30 medical education fellowships under departments of emergency medicine alone. These fellowships take either 1 or 2 years to complete, and some programs offer both 1-year and 2-year options. Typically, 2-year fellowships encourage or require pursuit of an additional advanced degree, such as a Master's in Education. Additionally, fellowships require clinical work as an attending physician in the emergency department [6].

Although there is no uniform curriculum for a medical education fellowship, most fellowships focus to varying degrees on the themes of career development, learning theory, clinical teaching methods, education research/scholarship, and educational program administration [7, 8]. Although medical education fellowships are not accredited by the Accreditation College for Graduate Medical Education (ACGME), the Society for Academic Emergency Medicine (SAEM) does have an approval process to be considered an Educational Scholarship Fellowship, which ensures that a program will address certain curricular elements. Of course, programs that choose not to go through this approval process certainly may address the same topics. By attending the Council of Residency Directors (CORD) and American College of Emergency Physicians (ACEP) annual conferences, in addition to exploring program websites, you can learn much more about the individual fellowships, their curricula, and their particular focus.

The Next Steps

Program Factors to Consider

1. Perhaps the most obvious distinguishing factor between fellowships is whether they are 1 or 2 years in length. Many people choose to do a 2-year program specifically so that they can simultaneously pursue a Master's degree, as this allows them to learn more about educational theory and practice and to leave their fellowship training with more formal education credentials. Consider whether you want an advanced degree and, if so, which degree (Master's in Education, Master's in Health Professions Education, etc.) and in what learning format (remote, on-site, or a combination of the two).
2. Consider the amount of time you need to accomplish your fellowship goals. With a 1-year fellowship, I found that it was time to start the job search within a few months of starting my fellowship. While this worked well for me and may work well for you, you also may find that you have not yet fully explored your niche or made sufficient progress on your scholarly work by this time. Two-year

fellowships provide additional time to explore one's interests, complete scholarly projects, and explore the job market.
3. Some fellowships have a certain focus, such as undergraduate medical education, graduate medical education, research, simulation, or innovation depending on the fellowship director and the particular department within which the fellowship exists. By networking and exploring the fellowship's website, you can learn more about which program caters best to your interests.

When to Apply

Many final offers come in early November. With that date in mind, it is reasonable to target June for writing your personal statement, finalizing your curriculum vitae (CV), identifying writers for your letters of recommendation, and preparing for your interviews. I recommend getting your CV to programs that interest you by early August.

The Interview

Interviews often occur in September and October, many at the ACEP Scientific Assembly. Although nobody expects you to have your career fully planned or your niche fully defined, be able to state your general interests and goals and identify how that program can help you achieve those goals.

Although I am still early in my career, I know that academics was the correct path for me; however, I am not sure that I would have felt prepared to pursue academics or gotten the job I wanted were it not for excellent fellowship training and mentorship. I hope that this chapter has helped you with your decision, and I wish you a long and satisfying career whatever that decision may be.

References

1. Bunton SA, Dandar VM. AAMC analysis: in brief. Sept 2017.
2. Taylor JS, Friedman RH, Speckman JL, Ash AS, Moskowitz MA, Carr PL. Fellowship training and career outcomes for primary care physician–faculty. Acad Med. 2001;76(4):366–72. https://doi.org/10.1097/00001888-200104000-00015.
3. Jordan J, Ahn J, Diller D, et al. Outcome assessment of medical education fellowships in emergency medicine. AEM Educ Train. 2021;5(4):e10650. https://doi.org/10.1002/aet2.10650.
4. Reyes M, Dimeo S, Carmelli G, Shamoon M. Why you should do a MedEd fellowship. [online] Emra.org. 2019. https://www.emra.org/about-emra/publications/emra-cast/MedEd-fellowships/. Accessed 8 July 2022.

5. Thompson BM, Searle NS, Gruppen LD, Hatem CJ, Nelson EA. A national survey of medical education fellowships. Med Educ Online. 2011;16:10.3402/meo.v16i0.5642. https://doi.org/10.3402/meo.v16i0.5642. Published 2011 Apr 4.
6. Coates WC, Lin M, Clarke S, et al. Defining a core curriculum for education scholarship fellowships in emergency medicine. Acad Emerg Med. 2012;19(12):1411–8. https://doi.org/10.1111/acem.12036.
7. Cataldi M, Yarris LM, Coates WC, Lin M, et al. A suggested core content for education scholarship fellowships in emergency medicine. Acad Emerg Med. 2012;19(12):1425–33. https://doi.org/10.1111/acem.12032.
8. Cataldi ML, Kelly-Hedrick M, Nanavati J, Chisolm MS, Anne LW. Post-residency medical education fellowships: a scoping review. Med Educ Online. 2021;26(1):1920084. https://doi.org/10.1080/10872981.2021.1920084.

Chapter 18
Pain Management

Samuel Wood

My Story

At age 16, while most of my friends were playing on varsity teams and contemplating steps towards college, I was crouched on my bedroom floor, staring at my swollen and immobile hands. One year earlier, I was diagnosed with lupus thanks to a suspicious-looking butterfly rash, and diffuse rheumatoid arthritis had left me nearly incapacitated. Each morning was spent kneading out my inflamed joints until I could finally get up and start my day. The experience was terrifying but instilled a deep respect and curiosity towards the power of pain.

Even at that young age, I vividly recall asking the same fundamental questions people suffering from chronic pain ask themselves every day. "How is this possible?" "Will it ever get better?" And perhaps most challenging, "Why me?" While the physical pain was a brutal adversary, I found an even more formidable foe in the battles within the mind. Pain cast a shadow on all aspects of my life, and I fought daily to maintain hope that relief would someday come. My struggles with lupus continued into the following year, until finally receiving the treatments I needed to enter full remission, which I have remained in without complication for the past 15 years.

The impact of my personal relationship with pain remained with me throughout medical school and residency. During my rotations, I discovered a love for emergency medicine due to the diversity of patient presentations, procedural components, and emphasis on a broad scope of medical knowledge. At that time, I had no knowledge or understanding that pain medicine was a specialty, but pain was all around me, accounting for nearly 80% of all emergency department visits

S. Wood (✉)
Department of Pain Management and Rehabilitation, University of Minnesota, Minneapolis, MN, USA

R. P. Olympia et al. (eds.), *An Emergency Physician's Path*, https://doi.org/10.1007/978-3-031-47873-4_18

nationally. I saw much of my own struggles in these patients and began feeling discouraged by my inability to offer long-term and sustainable options for treatment outside of the ED.

It was as this time that a close friend and mentor happened to mention that he was pursuing a fellowship in pain medicine after graduating from his EM residency program. I was shocked, and it hadn't occurred to me that this option was available. Some quick research revealed that while it is rare, programs were becoming more and more open to EM applicants, so I decided to give it a shot. Thankfully, after a lot of work and extremely helpful mentors, I matched and will be completing my pain fellowship in 2023.

The Job

The EMRA Fellowship Guide describes the specialty of pain medicine as follows: "A pain medicine physician treats all pain disorders, ranging from pain as a symptom of a disease to pain as a primary disease. A specialist in this field utilizes various levels of care such as evaluating complex pain problems, prescribing and managing pain relieving medications, acting as an integral component in a multidisciplinary team, and dispatching skills to perform interventional procedures such as nerve blocks and spinal injections." The specialty can be traced back to the International Association for the Study of Pain (IASP), founded in 1973, whose goals were "to foster and encourage research on pain and improve the management of patients." This agency did not accredit pain medicine clinicians, thus in 1983, the American Academy of Pain Medicine (AAPM) was formed for this purpose. Traditionally, pain medicine fellows graduate from Anesthesia or PM&R programs, however Psychology, Radiology, and Neurology are often listed as acceptable. Emergency medicine is new to the arena, having been formally approved to sit for the pain medicine boards in 2014.

Why Pain?

There are multiple reasons to apply for a pain medicine fellowship, particularly coming from emergency medicine.

1. **Relevance to the ED**: Pain is the most common complaint in the ED, and further training in this field can provide more tools in the toolbox for your patients. The training also provides deeper insight into the psychology, pathology, and treatment of chronic pain, addiction, and withdrawal.
2. **Career Flexibility**: Pain medicine is one of the few fellowships that offers career options outside of the ED. An individual can pursue countless different paths including interventional procedures, outpatient clinic, addiction medicine, medi-

cal floor consultation, acute pain management, academia, entrepreneurialism, etc. This provides a powerful ability to diversify one's career, especially when combined with the flexibility of shift work in the ED.

3. **Continuity of Care**: While it is true many EM providers do not feel the need to have regular follow-up with patients, the opportunity to form long-term relationships in clinic can be both refreshing and fulfilling.
4. **Academic Opportunities**: Being dual board-certified in emergency medicine and pain medicine is unique and undoubtedly adds a competitive edge to applicants looking to enter educational or academic careers.
5. **Hours**: In general, pain physicians work Monday through Friday with minimal call and most holidays off. This is, of course, a generalization and can vary, but a regular schedule without nights is a clear advantage to the field.
6. **Salary**: Both emergency medicine and pain medicine physicians make good money. According to The Medical Group Management Association (MGMA) data from 2018, the median total compensation of a pain physician was $453,128. It is critical to view this in perspective however, as it also includes private practices before overhead costs. According to Medscape's annual report, the average EM salary is $354,000/year. The income potential for pain is wide and dependent upon multiple factors including hospital-employed vs private practice, RVU models, location, bonuses/incentives, etc. When taking these variables into account, there is significant potential for income in a pain management practice.

What About the Downsides?

Every job has its downsides, and it's important to consider these before applying to a pain fellowship.

1. **Not as flexible as shiftwork:** Many of us went into EM because of the flexible schedule and ability to swap shifts, request days off, go to Disney on a random Tuesday afternoon, etc. With the "banker's hours" of pain management comes the sacrifice of losing much of this flexibility.
2. **Home calls:** EM offers the ability to leave work at the hospital. While this can certainly be true in a pain practice, you are generally still operating an outpatient clinic that requires attention even when you are "off shift."
3. **Insurance battles:** Unfortunately, words like "prior authorization" are well known in the pain community, and discussions with insurance companies regarding prescriptions and procedures are common.
4. **Patient population:** Chronic pain patients can be extremely challenging to manage every day. This can be especially frustrating when combined with issues of addiction, manipulation, treatment non-compliance, and treatment failures.
5. **Extra Training:** As with any fellowship, you are sacrificing a year of an attending salary to pursue further education.

Application Timeline

The vast majority of ACMGE-accredited pain fellowships use the Electronic Residency Application Service (ERAS). It is important to note that pain medicine participates in a December cycle through the Anesthesiology subspecialty match, which is in contrast to most other fellowships which operate on a July cycle. This means that if you are participating in a 3-year EM program, your application will need to be submitted between November and January of your second year, with an ERAS final deadline for submission in April. Interviews are extended anytime between the submission of your application to the summer of the application year. Match day generally falls mid-October of the subsequent year. Please note these dates are just for reference and subject to change, so refer to the appropriate calendar for your application year.

Doing the math, this timeline leads to a lot of waiting. Consider the fact that my application was submitted November 1st, 2020, during my second year of residency. January to July of 2021 was spent patiently and anxiously awaiting interviews, and Match Day occurred October 14th, 2021, just 2 weeks shy of an entire year. Considering these factors is critically important, especially when many of your colleagues are functioning on a July application cycle which does not pertain to the Anesthesiology match. I harp on this point because I almost made the fatal error of thinking I had nearly a year to gather my materials, when in fact the application cycle began far earlier.

Application Contents

The application contents are much like applying to residency again and will be familiar to anyone who has used ERAS before. Generally they include the following:

- Personal Statement
- Curriculum Vitae (CV)
- Copy of Formal Transcripts
- Official Test Scores (United States Medical Licensing Exam/Comprehensive Osteopathic Medical Licensing Examination)
- Letters of Recommendation (at least two, one of which should be from your Program Director)
- In-training Exam Scores (this is less common, but happens)

It is important to leave plenty of time to complete these items. As stated above, the application timeline starts midway through your second year if you are in a 3-year program, so you'll ideally be acquiring the necessary documents early (especially letters of recommendation) as not to be rushed. Other time-consuming items to consider include your personal statement and revised CV.

A Word on Elective Rotations/Audition Rotations

As of this writing, COVID has made auditioning exceptionally difficult. Further, many programs don't offer elective time early enough to take advantage. Despite these hurdles, I would fight hard to acquire experiences in the field. Like any application, you need to prove your interest, and this is especially true if you are applying from a "non traditional" track like EM. Start at your local institution. Ask to shadow the pain medicine docs, observe fluoroscopy and interventional procedures, and inquire about any research opportunities you can participate in. In my experience, most of these individuals were more than happy to assist and are often intrigued by the notion of EM residents taking an interest in pain management. Further, your application should have a letter from at least one pain physician for obvious reasons, so it's best to form these relationships early.

Research

As above, you need to "sell" your interest in the field, and an application with no pain-related research would be a red flag. Poster presentations and attending conferences are great ways to network and bolster your application. Even a presentation of a pain-related ED case is better than nothing.

Interviews

It's safe to assume all readers who are considering a fellowship are well versed in interviews, so I won't focus on them here. However, I will mention the question of "Why do you want to do pain medicine coming from emergency medicine?" should be clearly answered throughout your essay, application, and interview.

Conclusion

Pain accounts for a significant proportion of emergency medicine visits. A pain medicine fellowship offers a unique opportunity to expand and diversify an emergency physician's career, while simultaneously providing a broader scope of treatments and interventions for these patients. More and more emergency medicine graduates are applying for, and being accepted to these fellowship programs, and that trend is likely to continue. I hope you have found the information in this chapter helpful, and please feel free to connect with me via email at any point.

Further Reading

https://www.ncbi.nlm.nih.gov/pmc/articles/PMC3027428/#:~:text=The%20reported%20prevalence%20of%20any,patients%20who%20presented%20with%20pain.
https://www.ncbi.nlm.nih.gov/pmc/articles/PMC6548151/.

ERAS Application Timeline

https://students-residents.aamc.org/eras-tools-and-worksheets-fellowship-applicants/eras-2023-fellowship-application-timeline.

Anesthesiology Fellowship Match

https://www.nrmp.org/fellowship-applicants/participating-fellowships/anesthesiology-match-fellowship/.

EMRA Fellowship Guide, Pain

https://www.emra.org/books/fellowship-guide-book/18-pain-management/.

2021 Match Results

https://www.nrmp.org/wp-content/uploads/2021/11/2021-Anesthesiology-Match-Results-Statistics.pdf.

2021 Match Calendar

Abdolrazaghnejad A, Banaie M, Tavakoli N, Safdari M, Rajabpour-Sanati A. Pain management in the emergency department: a review article on options and methods. Adv J Emerg Med [Internet]. 2018;2(4):e45. https://www.ncbi.nlm.nih.gov/pmc/articles/PMC6548151/
Anesthesiology [Internet]. NRMP. 2021 [cited 2023 Jan 23]. https://www.nrmp.org/fellowship/anesthesiology/.
Anesthesiology Fellowship Match [Internet]. NRMP. [cited 2023 Jan 23]. https://www.nrmp.org/fellowship-applicants/participating-fellowships/anesthesiology-match-fellowship/.
ERAS® 2023 Fellowship Application Timeline [Internet]. Students & Residents. [cited 2023 Jan 23]. https://students-residents.aamc.org/eras-tools-and-worksheets-fellowship-applicants/eras-2023-fellowship-application-timeline.
https://www.nrmp.org/fellowship/anesthesiology/.

Match Results Statistics [Internet]. [cited 2023 Jan 23]. https://www.nrmp.org/wp-content/uploads/2021/11/2021-Anesthesiology-Match-Results-Statistics.pdf.

Medscape.com. 2023 [cited 2023 Jan 23]. https://www.medscape.com/slideshow/2021-compensation-emergency-medicine-6013847?icd=login_success_email_match_norm.

Pain Management Fellowships [Internet]. www.emra.org. [cited 2023 Jan 23]. https://www.emra.org/books/fellowship-guide-book/18-pain-management/.

Todd KH, Cowan P, Kelly N, Homel P. Chronic or recurrent pain in the emergency department: national telephone survey of patient experience. West J Emerg Med [Internet]. 2010;11(5):408–15. [cited 2023 Jan 23]. https://www.ncbi.nlm.nih.gov/pmc/articles/PMC3027428/#:~:text=The%20reported%20prevalence%20of%20any.

Updated MGMA? [Internet]. Student Doctor Network. [cited 2023 Jan 23]. https://forums.student-doctor.net/threads/updated-mgma.1378790/.

Chapter 19
Palliative Care

Callie Schnitker

Palliative Care: What Is It?

Palliative care is a medical model that focuses on optimizing quality of life through the assessment, management and when possible, prevention of physical, psychological, and spiritual suffering faced by patients and their families with serious, complex, and terminal illnesses. The physicians who subspecialize in HPM are distinguished from other specialists by their expertise in symptom control interventions, knowledge and skill around the topics of death and dying, bereavement, a dedication to an interdisciplinary team approach, and their focus on the patient as a whole.

A Brief History of Modern Hospice and Palliative Medicine

While medical practice related to symptom management is as old as medicine itself, the concept of providing specialized care for the dying and seriously ill did not formally take off until the nineteenth and twentieth centuries. From Herbert Snow's development of the Brompton Cocktail, to Howard Barrett's discovery regarding the benefits of providing scheduled morphine to the dying, and more recently Dame Cicely Saunders who is credited with founding the modern hospice movement, modern training in HPM is the culmination of a multitude of innovative physicians who shared a passion for alleviating the suffering of the seriously ill and dying

C. Schnitker (✉)
University of Minnesota, Minneapolis, MN, USA

Department of Emergency Medicine and Hospice and Palliative Care, Regions Hospital, Saint Paul, MN, USA
e-mail: Callie.k.schnitker@healthpartners.com

R. P. Olympia et al. (eds.), *An Emergency Physician's Path*,
https://doi.org/10.1007/978-3-031-47873-4_19

[1–3]. While the term hospice has been in use since the fourth century, and hospice homes having existed abroad since the 1800s, it wasn't until 1974 that the first hospice facility opened in the United States (U.S.). There are now more than 3600 hospices in the U.S., serving more than one million patients annually [4]. In contrast, the concept of palliative care is relatively new. The term "palliative care" was not officially coined until 1974, and it was not until 1990 that the World Health Organization recognized palliative care as a distinct specialty. While palliative care was initially limited in its scope and was delivered predominantly through hospice, it is now found throughout the spectrum of medical practice locations, and no longer limited to only end-of-life disease states. Among its many benefits, palliative care results in improved quality of life, better quality of medical care, less aggressive end-of-life care, and less emotional distress for the patient, their families, and medical practitioners [5–11]. In turn, palliative care has become one of the most rapidly growing fields in health care in the U.S. in the last two decades [11]. In recognition of its growing impact, the American Board of Medical Specialties in 2006 approved the creation of hospice and palliative medicine as a subspecialty of ten participating boards, including EM. Since 2014, in order to be eligible to take the certification examination, all physicians are required to complete a 12-month, accredited HPM fellowship.

Why You Should Choose a Career in Hospice and Palliative Medicine

1. Schedule – The majority of palliative care jobs (inpatient consult service and ambulatory clinic) involve regular, day-time hours with minimal or no requirements for being on-call after hours. Depending on the practice, there may be no weekends involved either – some inpatient consult services only work weekdays, while others provide seven-days-per-week coverage. For those who are employed by a hospice agency, on-call times may be more involved but the degree and frequency depends heavily on the group structure with some being very heavily Advanced Practice Provider-run and algorithm-driven.
2. Job security – Jobs within EM are projected to become significantly more competitive. An alarming workforce study published in 2021 predicted a surplus of 7845 emergency physicians in 2030 [12]. While subsequent analysis supports a surplus but not quite as dire a situation as initially predicted, employment within EM is nevertheless on track to become increasingly competitive [13]. For those physicians who desire greater job security, academic employment, or to practice in a competitive location, sub specialization within HPM is likely to aid in attaining employment that achieves these goals. HPM remains a rare subspecialty within EM; in 2019 there were only 176 boarded EM/HPM physicians [14]. Sub-specialization in a unique field like HPM will enable an applicant to stand out compared with their peers. For those physicians who split time between EM

and palliative care or hospice, employers in either field may have greater flexibility with hiring for positions which individually are part-time, but when combined within a healthcare system, may equate to a full-time position. Hiring someone who works in both EM and HPM may also be desirable to EM groups who wish to have a greater reach or collaboration within the hospital system.

3. "Work-work" balance – EM/HPM provides physicians with a unique work balance. EM is fast-paced and exhilarating. In turn it can be exhausting, both physically and mentally. Patient interactions are often brief and without continuity. HPM, on the other hand, is measured and renowned for its emotional connectedness. While they seem like two divergent fields, they share a surprising amount in common. Physicians in both fields are skilled at acute symptom management, high stakes communications, and death. For physicians practicing in both areas, HPM and EM offer a buffer for one another. When you find yourself drained from the drug use and traumas of EM, the deep patient interactions and slower pace of HPM are rejuvenating. Similarly, when you find yourself drained from being present in times of grief and serious illness, the blood and chaos of the ED offers an escape. Burnout is a significant issue for EM physicians [15], while HPM suffers from their own significant burnout [16], the complimentary and divergent nature of the two fields may offer some degree of career longevity.
4. Rewarding/life fulfilling – Helping someone die peacefully, or cope with difficult news about their health, or improving debilitating symptoms are just a few of the incredible effects HPM physicians can have on a daily basis. Several studies have shown that HPM physicians report high levels of job satisfaction [17–19].

HPM Fellowship: The Next Steps/How to Prepare Yourself for Applying for a Fellowship and What to Expect

The majority of programs participate in the Electronic Residency Application Service (ERAS) July application cycle: with the application process opening in June, interviews in early fall, and the Match occurring in December with programs starting the following July 1st. In general, the application includes the ERAS standard application which involves a list of work and education experiences, three letters of recommendation, and a personal statement. Average board scores, experiences, and publication numbers for successful applicants can be found on the NRMP website.

While not a requirement, it would be wise for applicants to obtain experience within hospice and palliative medicine prior to applying, not only to obtain worthwhile letters of recommendation, but also to ensure that this is a field for you. For a small group of EM residencies, a hospice and palliative medicine rotation is included in their residency curriculum [20]. For the vast majority, residents will need to explore completing a rotation within HPM during another part of residency, likely the elective rotation. In order to obtain meaningful letters of recommendation, any such rotations are ideally completed in the second year of residency. For applicants who have completed residency or cannot allocate time for a whole rotation block, options exist for rotations with faculty in HPM clinics (involving a single or handful of days a week), weekly hospice interdisciplinary team rounds, or shadowing hospice medical directors on home visits. It has been my experience that HPM physicians are more than happy to have learners join them, especially if they are interested in exploring the field.

The HPM fellowship is a 12-month experience. Training must include clinical education in a minimum of four educational locations, including inpatient acute care, long-term care, home visits, and ambulatory practice settings. While training typically occurs concurrently, a very limited number of programs may allow for training to occur over a longer period of time, with blocks of training staggered between periods of working within a fellow's primary specialty. Some degree of call is typically involved within the fellowship but hours are generally daytime with occasional weekends, and vary by program. Moonlighting is generally permitted and feasible as long it does not affect your fellowship performance.

Following fellowship, physicians will sit for the HPM certification exam. For allopathic physicians this is administered by the American Board of Internal Medicine every 2 years (even numbered years). In order to qualify for the certifying exam, physicians must be board certified and in good standing with the American Board of Emergency Medicine (ABEM). For recent residency graduates, depending on the year, this may mean sitting for the ABEM written and oral boards during fellowship training, especially if the goal is to take HPM boards as soon after fellowship graduation as possible. For osteopathic physicians, the process is relatively similar; the hospice and palliative medicine subspecialty certification exam is administered by the Hospice and Palliative Medicine Conjoint Committee. Unlike allopathic HPM boards, this exam is administered annually. Similarly, in order for osteopathic applicants to qualify for the certifying exam, physicians must be board certified and in good standing with their respective board, the American Osteopathic Board of Emergency Medicine.

What to Expect in Your Career in Hospice and Palliative Medicine

There are many career paths for EM physicians who subspecialize in hospice and palliative medicine. Some physicians continue to work in clinical emergency medicine exclusively, using their newly acquired skills to strengthen their EM clinical practice while also retaining the ability to transition into hospice or palliative medicine practice later in their careers. Others choose to fully transition to careers in hospice and palliative medicine immediately after training. Finally, some choose to split their time between emergency medicine and palliative medicine. The opportunities in this regard are multiple. The flexibility of EM schedules allows physicians to work in virtually any area of palliative medicine. This can include working a set number of inpatient palliative medicine weeks each year – a schedule generally mirroring a hospitalist schedule of 5 or 7 days/week seeing consults in the hospital followed by a number of weeks off when you can work EM shifts. Some physicians work in ambulatory clinic with set days per week or per month in dedicated palliative clinic or entrenched in specialty clinics like oncology, nephrology, or cardiology, and then working their EM shifts during non-clinic days. Others may choose to work as hospice medical directors or running weekly hospice interdisciplinary team meetings.

References

1. Saunders CM, Sykes N. Introduction – history and challenge. In: The management of terminal malignant disease. Essay, E. Arnold; 1993.
2. Saunders C. The evolution of palliative care. Patient Educ Couns. 2000 Aug;41(1):7–13.
3. Clark D, Graham F. Morphine, cocaine, and 19th century cancer care. Lancet Oncol. 2008;9(10):1018.
4. National Association for Home Care & Hospice. Home care and hospice facts and stats. 2009.
5. Higginson IJ, Finlay I, Goodwin DM, Cook AM, Hood K, Edwards AG, Douglas HR, Norman CE. Do hospital-based palliative teams improve care for patients or families at the end of life? Pain Symptom Manage. 2002;23:96–106.
6. Higginson IJ, Finlay IG, Goodwin DM, Hood K, Edwards AG, Cook A, Douglas HR, Normand CE. Is there evidence that palliative care teams alter end-of-life experiences of patients and their caregivers? J Pain Symptom Manag. 2003;25:150–68.
7. Rabow MW, Schanche K, Petersen J, Dibble SL, McPhee SJ. Patient perceptions of an outpatient palliative care intervention: "it had been on my mind before, but I did not know how to start talking about death...". J Pain Symptom Manag. 2003;26:1010–5.
8. Ellershaw JE, Peat SJ, Boys LC. Assessing the effectiveness of a hospital palliative care team. Palliat Med. 1995;9:145–52.
9. Flory J, Yinong YX, Gurol I, Levinsky N, Ash A, Emanuel E. Place of death: U.S. trends since 1980. Health Aff (Millwood). 2004;23:194–200.
10. Jack B, Hillier V, Williams A, Oldham J. Hospital based palliative care teams improve the insight of cancer patients into their disease. Palliat Med. 2004;18:46–52.
11. Hughes MT, Smith TJ. The growth of palliative care in the United States. Annu Rev Public Health. 2014;35:459–75.
12. Marco CA, Courtney DM, Ling LJ, Salsberg E, Reisdorff EJ, Gallahue FE, Suter RE, Muelleman R, Chappell B, Evans DD, Vafaie N, Richwine C. The emergency medicine physician workforce: projections for 2030. Ann Emerg Med. 2021 Dec;78(6):726–37.
13. Gettel CJ, Courtney DM, Janke AT, Rothenberg C, Mills AM, Sun W, Venkatesh AK. The 2013 to 2019 emergency medicine workforce: clinician entry and attrition across the US geography. Ann Emerg Med. 2022 Sep;80(3):260–71.
14. American Academy of Hospice and Palliative Medicine. Workforce data and reports. AAHPM. n.d. Retrieved September 1, 2022, from http://aahpm.org/career/workforce-study#HPMphysicians
15. Dyrbye LN, Burke SE, Hardeman RR, Herrin J, Wittlin NM, Yeazel M, Dovidio JF, Cunningham B, White RO, Phelan SM, Satele DV, Shanafelt TD, van Ryn M. Association of Clinical Specialty with Symptoms of burnout and career choice regret among US resident physicians. JAMA. 2018;320(11):1114–30.

16. Kamal AH, Bull JH, Wolf SP, Swetz KM, Shanafelt TD, Ast K, Kavalieratos D, Sinclair CT. Prevalence and predictors of burnout among hospice and palliative care clinicians in the U.S. J Pain Symptom Manag. 2020;59(5):e6–e13.
17. Lupu D, Salsberg E, Quigley L, Wu X. The 2015 class of hospice and palliative medicine fellows-from training to practice: implications for HPM workforce supply. J Pain Symptom Manag. 2017;53(5):944–51.
18. Yoon JD, Hunt NB, Ravella KC, Jun CS, Curlin FA. Physician burnout and the calling to care for the dying: a national survey. Am J Hosp Palliat Care. 2017;34(10):931–7.
19. Granek L, Buchman S. Improving physician Well-being: lessons from palliative care. CMAGranek L, Buchman S. Improving physician Well-being: lessons from palliative care. CMAJ. 2019;191(14):E380–1.
20. Kraus CK, Greenberg MR, Ray DE, Dy SM. Palliative care education in emergency medicine residency training: a survey of program directors, associate program directors, and assistant program directors. J Pain Symptom Manag. 2016;51(5):898–906.

Chapter 20
Pediatric Emergency Medicine

Lilia B. Reyes and Angel L. Schuster

Introduction to Pediatric Emergency Medicine (PEM)

A. ***A brief introduction to PEM*** The field of PEM originated in the 1970s, when discussions regarding the optimization of care for critically ill and injured infants and children began amongst general pediatricians. [1, 2] The goal of PEM was to improve and ensure the quality of patient care, teaching, and research in this new field of pediatric medicine [1, 2]. In the 1980s, sections of PEM were established in the American Academy of Pediatrics (AAP) and American College of Emergency Physicians (ACEP) [1, 2]. The 1980s also introduced specialized certification for the management of critically ill and injured infants and children, including Pediatric Advanced Life Support (PALS), a module for injured children in Advanced Trauma Life Support (ATLS), and Advanced Pediatric Life Support (APLS), and the first PEM-dedicated journal, *Pediatric Emergency Care* [2].

B. The first pediatric trauma center in the country was established in 1975 in Maryland [1]. Currently 70% of pediatric emergency departments (PEDs) are located in large urban areas affiliated with or located within university teaching hospitals, with 50% of the PEDs population under the age of 3 years and the greatest pediatric volume presenting to the PED between 3 p.m. and midnight. While most PEDs are prepared to manage the acutely injured infant or child they also care for acutely ill pediatric patients presenting with respiratory distress, abnormal mental status, abnormal rhythm or perfusion, ingestions/poisonings, and acute surgical conditions. The most common PEDs diagnoses seen in

L. B. Reyes (✉) · A. L. Schuster
Department of Emergency Medicine & Pediatrics, Penn State Children's Hospital, Hershey, PA, USA
e-mail: lreyes@pennstatehealth.psu.edu; aschuster@pennstatehealth.psu.edu

R. P. Olympia et al. (eds.), *An Emergency Physician's Path*,
https://doi.org/10.1007/978-3-031-47873-4_20

are acute febrile illness, acute respiratory illness, otitis media, viral infection, and asthma exacerbation, and the most common diagnoses in adolescents are acute headache, non-specific abdominal pain, and psychiatric-related complaints [3, 4].

C. Board-certification in PEM requires the completion of a three-year fellowship for pediatric residency graduates and a two or three-year fellowship for emergency medicine residency graduates. During fellowship, in addition to completing the curriculum guided by ACGME requirements, the physician will also complete a scholarly project [7]. Scholarly projects may include traditional research, quality improvement projects, or other opportunities. Upon the completion of fellowship, the physician is "board eligible" in PEM and must pass the certifying examination through the American Board of Pediatrics (ABP) to become "board certified." Currently the PEM certification exam is available biannually only.
D. The dissemination of PEM research is well represented at both regional and national scientific assemblies, including the AAP National Conference & Exhibition, Pediatric Academic Societies (PAS) meeting, ACEP Scientific Assembly, and Society for Academic Emergency Medicine (SAEM) meeting. Research in the field of PEM is often published in high impact factor journals, most recently including topics such as pain management, asthma, procedural sedation, bronchiolitis management, ultrasound, resuscitation, and simulation [3, 4].

So Why Should You Choose a Career in PEM?

A. **Salary.** Let's get right to the compensation of a PEM physician. While salary continues to be lower on the list of motivators/factors for becoming a physician and being a satisfied physician, it is still important to know how your career choice will provide income stability [5, 6]. Currently, the mean annual salary for a non-specialized EM physician is $354,000/year. The mean annual salary for a general (non-specialized) pediatrician is $221,000. The mean annual salary for a PEM physician is $280,000 [6]. While these are averages and actual salary depends on many factors such as training, location, practice setting, and years of practice, it can be generally stated that PEM physicians make more than a general pediatrician and less than a non-specialized EM physician. For a pediatric residency-trained physician, a career in PEM offers a salary bump. However, this must be weighed against the additional costs of subspecialty applications, the additional 3 years of training, subspecialty board certification maintenance of certification, and any interest accrued on student loans during training. If a physician is EM trained and plans to pursue a career made solely of PEM (versus doing both EM and PEM), the PEM salary may not be a check mark under the "pros" column.

B. ***How a fellowship trained PEM physician is different from other physicians.***

(a) In terms of pursuing a PEM fellowship as an EM residency graduate, one could argue that there are limited benefits. EM physicians are expected to care for pediatric patients, they are skilled in emergent and urgent procedures, and the very nature of EM lends to physicians who will jump to care for whoever walks through the door, regardless of age. However, there are benefits to a PEM fellowship if a candidate is EM-trained. PEM fellowship allows for continued learning of pediatric medicine. When a five-day-old, ill-appearing, cyanotic infant arrives at the ED, an EM physician will likely initiate the ABCs based on PALS algorithms. While this neonate presenting in extremis is being resuscitated using PALS, a pediatric subspecialist thinks more broadly on the "what is next?" and the special considerations based on this patient's age. For example, How is this five-day-old's physiology different from a 5-month-old infant? What routine interventions may be harmful for this five-day-old that may not be an issue for an older infant or child? In addition to advanced training in pediatric medicine, PEM fellowship provides opportunities that allow for training in pediatric emergency guidelines, clinical tools, protocols, and provides the opportunity for introduction into scholarly activities for those that are academically-bound.

(b) For pediatric residency graduates, who may also work in an emergency department without being fellowship-trained, it is a bit different. While a pediatrician spends at least 3 years learning the medicine in residency, PEM fellowship will help train a physician in management of patient flow in the ED, as well as emergent procedures needed in children. In addition, just like EM graduates, pediatric graduates will benefit from fellowship by learning pediatric emergency guidelines, clinical decision tools, protocols, and provides the opportunity for an introduction into scholarly activities for those that are academically-bound. Finally, as mentioned above, the mean salary for a fellowship-trained PEM physician is likely to be higher than a general pediatrician, even if the general pediatrician is practicing in an ED without fellowship training (this can happen in various ED settings, such as in the community, in rural settings or other resource-limited settings, and in resource-rich locations where urgent care physicians are needed).

(c) Both EM and pediatrics-trained PEM physicians have opportunities to expand their career with leadership positions in the Pediatric Emergency Department. Though non-fellowship-trained emergency and pediatric specialists can work in a PED, it is less likely that they will hold a position of PED Director, Division Chief, or higher.

C. ***What are special considerations to keep in mind when applying to PEM fellowships***? So you have decided that a career in PEM is the way to go and you want to apply for a fellowship position. There are currently 86 PEM fellowship programs in the United States, which is not enough. For the 2022 fellowship match, there were 214 open PEM fellowship positions for 310 applicants. This means that 96 applicants did not match equaling a match rate of 69.0%. Compare this to other pediatric subspecialties such as Critical Care, Gastroenterology, Infectious Disease and Nephrology with match rates greater than 80% and Cardiology, Endocrinology, Hematology/Oncology and Rheumatology whose match rates were all above 90%. In fact, the highest match rate for PEM fellowship between 2018 and 2022 was 77.1% (in 2020), making PEM one of the most competitive pediatric fellowships [8]. Although these numbers may seem daunting, do not let these statistics deter you from your desire to pursue a career in PEM. With strategic planning, one can work to create a competitive application. Here are things to think about when preparing to apply:

(a) Paramount to the PEM application process is building your curriculum vitae (CV). Search for opportunities that mirror your professional interests (what areas of PEM are you really passionate about?): (1) Seek out educational opportunities with medical student, within your residency, or even outside your institution (other non-pediatric residency programs, Grand Rounds at other institutions, or with community outreach programs). Turn every lecture into a review article or book chapter. (2) Get involved in research and quality improvement opportunities, but choose projects that you can complete during the first 2 years of residency, usually during less stressful rotations. Consider taking research electives to collect and analyze data, and write up abstracts and manuscripts. Retrospective studies and case reports work well within your time constraints. Turn every research and quality improvement project into a lecture, an abstract to present at a regional or national scientific assembly, and/or a peer-reviewed journal manuscript submission. (3) Participate in committees within your residency program, your hospital and institution, your medical school, your profession (such as AAP, PAS, ACEP, or SAEM), and your community. This will benefit you by demonstrating leadership and the ability to work within a team structure.

(b) Another important requirement for the PEM application are letters of recommendation (LOR). Similar to medical school, you want to find LOR writers who know you well [professionally (i.e. can comment on your clinical acumen, research and teaching abilities, service) and personally, if possible] and can write a strong letter on your behalf. Most PEM fellowships require three to four LORs, typically one from your residency program director, at least one from a PEM attending physician, and at least one from a pediatric critical care attending. LOR writers who have connections to your top PEM choices will may improve your chances of success. If you are fortunate to be able to do an away PEM elective, attempt to obtain a LOR from a senior attending who can accumulate the comments from the physicians with whom you worked.

(c) The final step to a well-rounded PEM fellowship application includes a personal statement. Trying to describe yourself in words can be very difficult. As it is a personal statement, each individual's story will be unique. PEM physicians already appreciate the field of PEM so we recommend that you avoid listing out all of the awesome things PEM has to offer. Focus on the background and traits that make you a unique candidate. Highlight things in your CV that you are truly passionate about. Describe what the PEM fellowship program should expect from you during fellowship and what you can contribute to the PEM field after fellowship. Sell yourself, be honest, and let your words shine through.

(d) As you begin to put your application together, it is also important to begin considering the programs to which you will apply. On average, most applicants apply to approximately ten programs; however, this may vary by applicant circumstance [5]. When selecting programs, consider what is important to you: location, fellowship size, research opportunities, teaching/supervisory responsibilities, advanced degree opportunities, moonlighting opportunities, etc. The American Academy of Medical Colleges (AAMC) website provides resources on applying for fellowship, a list of fellowships, and links to the Electronic Residency Application Service (ERAS) with deadlines for applications. Undertaking the process of applying to a PEM fellowship can be confusing and overwhelming at times. Remember to reach out to your mentors regularly throughout residency to help guide and encourage you along your pathway to success.

D. The things we love about being PEM physicians:

(a) ***Organized chaos***. Pediatric emergency medicine can be fast paced, with a variety of ages and chief complaints making every presentation different, providing for an exciting career. If you dislike the monotony of rounding, then PEM is perfect for you. PEM physicians are frontline diagnosticians, under time restraints to solve each undifferentiated patient that comes through the door. We are the frontlines for providing healthcare during a pandemic when outpatient offices and urgent care offices are closed.

(b) ***Flexibility***. Often you can choose how many shifts you work per month, days or nights, weekdays, or weekends. On average, PEM physicians work 10.6 shifts a month that are 8.9 hours in duration. When looking at the total hours per week, PEM physicians work 26.7 hours fulfilling clinical duties and 42.7 hours when accounting for all clinical and non-clinical responsibilities [3]. If you consolidate your ED shifts up it makes for an instant vacation afterwards. The PEM world is so versatile that you have options to purely work clinical ED shifts, add research, add education, and/or add administration to your responsibilities. Adding research, education or administrative duties can allow for buy down of clinical shifts to allow more time for those duties.

(c) ***Location, location, location***. In the past, most PEM attending positions were located in urban areas affiliated with academic institutions. Currently, many community hospitals and academic institutions are opting to have PEDs staffed by board-certified specialists, PEM physicians now have more options on where to establish their careers.

(d) ***A career of scholarship.*** The volume of patients, the variety of disease processes, new technologies, and innovations in the field of PEM, such as simulation, ultrasound, and point-of-care diagnostic testing, allow the PEM physician a multitude of opportunities to perform research and quality improvement projects, with the goal of academic promotion while simultaneously improving the care of children.

(e) ***The jack of all trades***. One minute, you are running a traumatic resuscitation and placing a chest tube, and the next minute you are intubating a post-operative congenital heart infant. Procedural sedations, fracture reductions and casting, lumbar punctures, complex laceration repairs, and central venous lines are some of the procedures we routinely perform. Complex patients, critically ill, and injured medical or surgical patients are the mainstay of whom we provide care. The variety of patients and procedures is exhilarating and mind stimulating.

(f) ***The ultimate team sport.*** Whether it is a cardio-respiratory arrest or a traumatic resuscitation, status epilepticus or septic shock, or a non-urgent chief complaints, the success of your patients depends on shared mental model approach working as a synchronous unit with the PEM attending as the coach of the team. Resident physicians and medical students, PED nurses and technicians, registration and environmental services, diagnostic and laboratory technicians, social workers, chaplains, transport, child life, and subspecialty services all need to work hand-in-hand.

(g) ***Get out in the community and serve.*** Whether it's injury prevention, school-based health, emergency and disaster pediatric preparedness, or community education on immunizations, gun violence, teen distracted driving, substance use disorders, suicide prevention or bullying, PEM physicians feel an innate desire to impart knowledge to the communities they serve. Community service allows the PEM team to be more entrenched in the needs and lives of the children of their surrounding community.

(h) ***Gaining trust is our challenge.*** Parents bring their children to the PED, usually stressed, fearful, and vulnerable. They are often unfamiliar with those who will make, at times, life-saving decisions on behalf of their loved ones. We must listen attentively, communicate clearly, and gain their trust unconditionally in a short time span. It is a challenge that we as PEM physicians accept willingly.

(i) ***The PEM family is tight.*** Whether it's scanning the medical literature, running into PEM colleagues at conferences and scientific assemblies, or listening to social media podcasts or webcasts, PEM physicians are well represented. We are a small, tight knit community, where everyone knows your name. We work hard and play hard, and we have fun working as a united front for the health and wellness of infants and children.

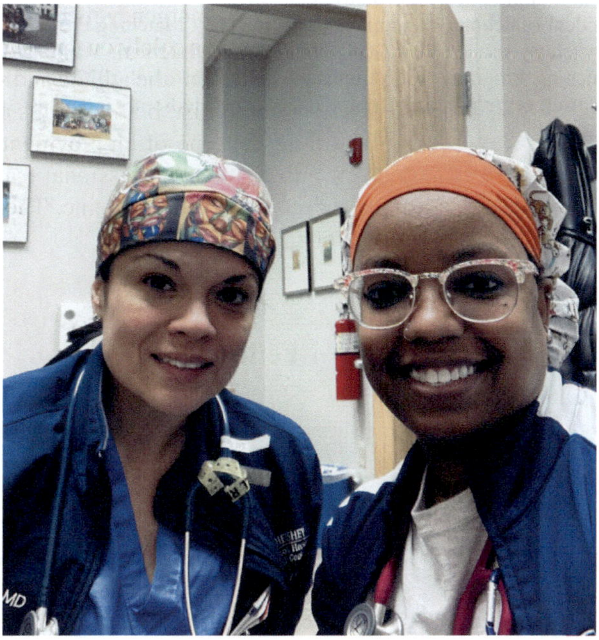

Caption for the Photo: Wonder Woman Work Sisters

Acknowledgements We would like to thank Lauren McNickle, MD, for her invaluable assistance in preparing this chapter.

References

1. Institute of Medicine. Emergency care for children: growing pains. Washington, DC: The National Academies Press; 2007. https://doi.org/10.17226/11655.
2. Pena M, Snyder B. Pediatric emergency medicine the history of a growing discipline. Emerg Med Clin. 1995;3(2):235–53.
3. Spurkeland N, Rixe J, Glick J, Lehman E, Olympia RP. Publishing trends in the field of Pediatric emergency medicine from 2004–2013. Pediatr Emerg Care. 2016;32(12):840–5.
4. Alpern ER, Stanley RM, Gorelick MH, Donaldson A, Knight S, Teach SJ, Singh T, Mahajan P, Goepp JG, Kuppermann N, Dean JM, Chamberlain JM. Pediatric emergency care applied research network (PECARN). Epidemiology of a pediatric emergency medicine research network: the PECARN Core data project. Pediatr Emerg Care. 2006;22(10):689–99.

5. Gorelick MH, Schremmer R, Ruch-Ross C, Radabaugh C, Selbst S. Current workforce characteristics and burnout in pediatric emergency medicine. Acad Emerg Med. 2016;23(1):48–54.
6. Katzowitz, J. How much do doctors maker? The white coat Ivenstor [Internent]; 2022. Available from: https://www.whitecoatinvestor.com/how-much-do-doctors-make/
7. Wall J, Ford CJ. Pediatric emergency medicine [Internet]. Irving, TX: Emergency Medicine Residents' Association; 2018. [Cited 2020 Jun 9]. Available from: https://www.emra.org/books/fellowship-guide-book/19-pediatric-em/
8. National Resident Matching Program. National Resident Matching Program, results and data: specialties matching service 2022 appointment year. [Internet]. Washington, DC: National Resident Matching Program; 2022. [updated 2022 Feb; cited 2022 Jun 6] Available from: https://www.nrmp.org/wp-content/uploads/2022/11/Medicine-and-Peds-Specialties-MRS-Report.pdf

Chapter 21
Population Health and Social Emergency Medicine

Philippa Soskin

Introduction

As emergency physicians we have a front row seat to the social factors influencing our patients' lives and health. The uninsured patient who struggles to access specialty care or obtain their medications. The man with chronic wounds who is living on the street. The young woman who triggers your concern as a possible victim of trafficking. The patient who is receiving his third head CT of the week after being brought in intoxicated with a head injury. The child who lacks access to healthy food and a safe neighborhood. We know that the medical care we provide in the Emergency Department (ED) is only a very small piece of what influences our patients' health and ability to access care. If you are interested in further exploring the social, racial, cultural, and historical forces that shape health and strategizing to address these upstream factors, further specialization in population health and social emergency medicine may be for you.

A Brief History of Social Emergency Medicine

Emergency medicine is unique as a specialty in that it developed out of a need to address access to care and serve the poor and underserved. ED visits tripled between 1940 and 1960 in response to care provided in EDs regardless of insurance or ability to pay as well a growing shortage of primary care doctors. At this time EDs were staffed by an assortment of physicians from different specialties with none solely

P. Soskin (✉)
Department of Emergency Medicine, MedStar Georgetown University Hospital & Washington Hospital Center, Washington, DC, USA
e-mail: Philippa.Soskin@medstar.net

R. P. Olympia et al. (eds.), *An Emergency Physician's Path*,
https://doi.org/10.1007/978-3-031-47873-4_21

devoted to ED care. In 1961, Dr. James Mills Jr. and three internist colleagues entered into a contract with Alexandria Hospital in Alexandria, Virginia, to provide ED coverage. Around the same time, 23 community physicians worked part time to cover the ED at Pontiac General Hospital in Michigan. Dr. Mills was a champion for social justice and found that his work in the ED allowed him to focus on providing care for those with social and financial needs. In the late 1960s, riots were occurring in cities around the United States in response to civil unrest and racial conflict. In Cincinnati poor access to care and concern regarding dysfunction in the ED at Cincinnati General Hospital were particular issues behind the riots in this area. In response, Cincinnati city officials and hospital leadership committed to improving emergency care which lead to the first university emergency medicine residency program at the University of Cincinnati in 1970 [1]. From its inception, emergency medicine has operated as a medical and social safety net. This concept became federal law in 1986 with the passage of the Emergency Medical Treatment and Labor Act (EMTALA).

While the premise of social emergency medicine is as old as emergency medicine itself, the term "social emergency medicine" was coined by Dr. Harrison Alter and Dr. Barry Simon of Highland Hospital in Oakland in 2009 with the formation of the Andrew Levitt Center for Social Emergency Medicine [2]. The first social emergency medicine fellowship was founded in 2010 at Highland Hospital in Oakland. Over the next decade, the American Academy of Emergency Medicine (AAEM), American College of Emergency Physicians (ACEP), and Society for Academic Emergency Medicine (SAEM) all established social emergency medicine sections or interest groups [3]. In 2016, the American Board of Emergency Medicine (ABEM) updated their Model of the Clinical Practice of Emergency Medicine to include the understanding of health care disparities as a core competency within the practice of emergency medicine [4].

The Terminology

While Dr. Alter and his colleagues have worked to define the concept and specialty of social emergency medicine, educational programming and fellowships have taken on a variety of phrases. We seek to define a few here:

- **Social emergency medicine** can be defined as the "interplay between social forces and the emergency care system as they together influence the health of individuals and their communities, with the goal of improving population health while decreasing system costs." [5].
- **Population health** can be defined as "health outcomes of a group of individuals, including the distribution of such outcomes within the group." [6].
- The Center for Disease Control (CDC) defines the **social determinants of health** as "conditions in the places where people live, learn, work, and play that affect a wide range of health and quality-of life-risks and outcomes." [7].

- The CDC defines **health disparities** as "preventable differences in the burden of disease, injury, violence, or in opportunities to achieve optimal health experienced by socially disadvantaged racial, ethnic, and other population groups, and communities." [8].
- The CDC defines **health equity** as "achieved when every person has the opportunity to attain his or her full health potential and no one is disadvantaged from achieving this potential because of social position or other socially determined circumstances." [9].

How Can You Incorporate Social Emergency Medicine into Your Career?

Understanding the social influences on your patients' health and ability to access care will make you better able to provide compassionate and patient-focused care to all your patients. You can work with your department and hospital to develop strategies to address social determinants and reduce health disparities such as employing social determinants screenings and advocating for programs such as community health advocates, community violence intervention programs, drug/alcohol harm reduction programs, and medical-legal partnerships. You can participate in research and develop educational programming for staff, faculty, residents, students, and fellows. You can partner with community organizations to improve access to care in particular neighborhoods in need and provide additional resources to your patients. Emergency physicians suffer from high rates of burnout compared to physicians in other specialties in part due to the moral injury of being unable to provide adequate care due to constraints that are beyond our control. Developing interventions and solutions to the social challenges facing our patients may provide the agency and empowerment to improve burnout and job satisfaction [10].

Pursuing Fellowship Training in Social Medicine

Fellowships in social medicine and population health are designed to provide additional academic, professional, and clinical training and experience for fellows looking to gain a greater understanding of the social, cultural, and historical forces affecting individual and population health with an aim to improve their individual practice, departmental strategies, and broader outreach. In 2021 there were at least ten fellowships available [11]. The terminology is not standardized throughout the specialty and fellowships come under different names including social medicine, population health, minority health, street medicine, health disparities, and health equity. When selecting a fellowship, it is important to consider what is important to you and your career goals. Considerations include location, research opportunities, teaching responsibilities, advanced degree options, moonlighting availability, and partner organizations/internship sites. This is a personal decision based on one's passions and interests and future personal and professional goals.

Currently, social emergency medicine and population health fellowships do not yield an additional board certification and are not accredited by the Accreditation Council for Graduate Medical Education (ACGME). Some fellowships do offer formal credentials through including masters level training such as a Master of Public Health. There are benefits to being a non-accredited fellowship such as flexibility for moonlighting, potential for higher salary, and less restrictions to duty hours for fellow education and opportunities.

Location. Is the fellowship located somewhere you feel you will be happy to work and practice for 1–2 years? Does the location provide a rich breath of professional opportunities in your areas of interest for your internship placements? Will the network you will gain assist you in your future career? For example, if you are committed to living in a specific city or state, you may consider a program that will allow you to build a network in that area or provide national contacts that are transferrable.

Length of training. There are both one-year and two-year fellowship options. Two-year fellowships are more likely to offer a formal master's program as part of their curriculum. Some may offer a one-year option for those not seeking an additional advanced degree or who already hold a relevant master's degree. One-year programs may be more limited in the amount of education and professional experience there is time to offer but there is also a personal cost-benefit analysis one must do in terms of considering an additional year of training and the opportunity cost that comes with this in terms of time and salary.

Formal education and degree programs. Several fellowships offer a masters level degree through their affiliated university. For social emergency medicine and population health, the most common degree offered is the Master of Public Health but other examples include a Master of Health Science Research and a Master in Policy Administration. Look carefully at the core curriculum and elective offerings for the programs you are considering to be sure they align with your interests and goals.

Clinical responsibilities. As a fellow, you are also spending time clinically as an attending physician in emergency medicine. If you are starting your fellowship directly following residency, this may be your first experience as an attending. Consider the clinical practice sites offered by the fellowship. Are these sites where you want to practice? Do they offer the experience you want whether that be community practice, academics and teaching opportunities, or some combination of both? You will likely be working less clinically than the average full time attending due to your fellow responsibilities. Does the program offer the right balance of dedicated fellowship time but also allow you to gain the clinical experience you need as a new attending?

Salary and benefits. Some fellowship salaries will follow the post-graduate year (PGY) structure and you will be paid as a PGY-4 or PGY-5 depending on the length of your residency training. Some will offer higher salaries and/or supplement your salary with moonlighting hours. Also consider the value and expense of a master's degree which is generally included in the salary agreement. You may receive other benefits such as continuing medical education (CME) dollars and reimbursement for board exams.

Applying for a Population Health and Social Medicine Fellowship

So you have decided to apply for a population health and social medicine fellowship. What makes a strong applicant and what are the next steps? First and foremost a candidate should demonstrate interest and experience in social medicine. Many residencies offer a social medicine or related concentration or track for further education beyond the core curriculum. Faculty in your department or in another specialty may be doing heath disparities research that you can join. Some residencies have their own social medicine interest groups and you can also join interest groups and committees within the specialty societies including AAEM, ACEP, SAEM, and EMRA. Consider volunteering at a free clinic or with a local community organization or non-profit. The exact number of fellowships offered is fluid from year to year but appears to be growing. An internet search will help you locate fellowship programs and their contact information. Remember that fellowships go by different names so include social emergency medicine, population health, health disparities, and health equity in your search. Most emergency medicine fellowships are listed on fellowship information sites through EMRA and SAEM and some will be represented at fellowship fairs through ACEP, SAEM, and AAEM. Your program director is also a good resource as they may receive recruitment information from individual programs.

Programs generally require a curriculum vitae (CV), letter of intent or personal statement, and typically two to three letters of recommendation. Based on the program's review of these initial materials, you may be invited for an interview. There may be a separate or additional application process if there is a master's degree involved. There is no match process or universal deadline for social emergency medicine fellowships and each program differs in their process, requirements, and deadlines. Applicants should review the program's website and reach out to the program director and/or coordinator to determine the exact application requirements and deadlines for each program.

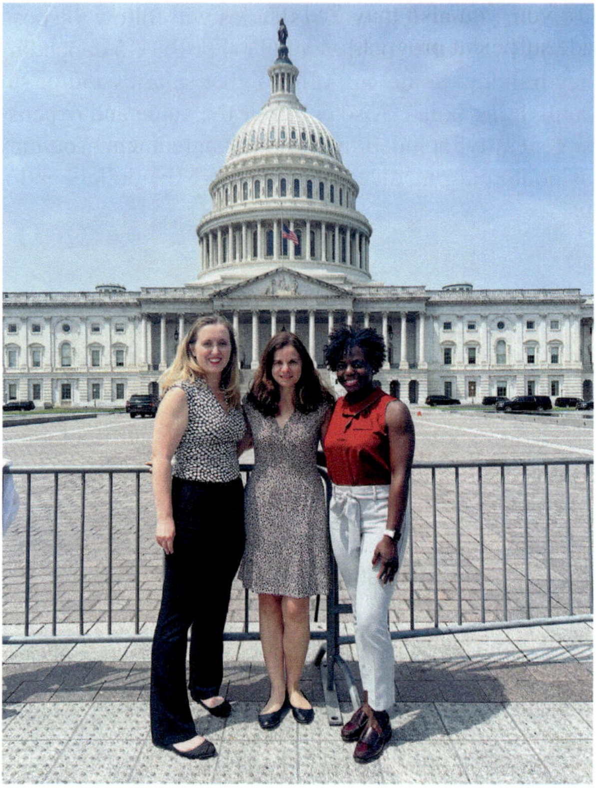

Caption for the Photo – “Emergency physicians advocate on Capitol Hill for workplace violence prevention”

References

1. Zink BJ. Social justice, egalitarianism, and the history of emergency medicine. Virtual Mentor. 2010;12(6):492–4.
2. Alter HJ. Foreword to conference proceedings, inventing social emergency medicine. Ann Emerg Med. 2019;74(5S):S1–2.
3. Fahimi J, Goldfrank L. Principles of social emergency medicine. Ann Emerg Med. 2019;74(5S):S6–S10.
4. American Board of Emergency Medicine. 2016 Model of the clinical practice of emergency medicine. American Board of Emergency Medicine Website. https://www.abem.org/public/docs/default-source/default-document-library/2016-em-model-website-document.pdf?sfvrsn=8b98c9f4_6. Accessed 2 Aug 2022.
5. Anderson ES, Hsieh D, Alter HJ. Social emergency medicine: embracing the dual role of the emergency department in acute care and population health. Ann Emerg Med. 2016;68:21–5.

6. Lewis N. Populations, population health, and the evolution of population management: making sense of the terminology in US health care today. Institute of Healthcare Improvement Website; 2014. https://www.ihi.org/communities/blogs/population-health-population-management-terminology-in-us-health-care. Accessed 4 Aug 2022.
7. Centers for Disease Control and Prevention. Social determinants of health; know what affects health. Centers for Disease Control and Prevention Website. Updated September 30, 2021. https://www.cdc.gov/socialdeterminants/index.htm. Accessed 4 Aug 2022.
8. Centers for Disease Control and Prevention. Health disparities. Centers for Disease Control and Prevention Website. Updated January 31, 2017. https://www.cdc.gov/aging/disparities/index.htm. Accessed 4 Aug 2022.
9. Centers for Disease Control and Prevention. Health equity. Centers for Disease Control and Prevention Website. Updated March 3, 2022. https://www.cdc.gov/chronicdisease/healthequity/index.htm. Accessed 4 Aug 2022.
10. Anderson E, Bernstein E, Xuan Z, Alter HJ. Inventing social emergency medicine: summary of common and critical research themes using a modified Haddon matrix. Ann Emerg Med. 2019;74(5S):S74–7. https://doi.org/10.1016/j.annemergmed.2019.08.464.
11. Goldberg L, Urquhart S, DesCamp R, Cisneros V. Training future leaders: social emergency medicine fellowships. Common Sense. 2021. https://www.aaem.org/UserFiles/SocialPopulationJulyAugust2021.pdf. Accessed 8 Aug 2022.

Chapter 22
Sex and Gender Medicine

Angela F. Jarman and Alyson J. McGregor

Section I: The History of Sex and Gender Based Medicine

Originally, the notion of "women's health" was synonymous with reproductive issues: childbearing, breast health, and menopause. It was thought that men and women were similar in all conditions except the reproductive system. This created a foundation for medical research to be performed only on men, and for those results to be applied to women. We now know that women are different than men in many more ways than just their reproductive system and sex hormones.

Sex- and gender-based medicine (SGBM) embraces the influences that sex (a biological construct) and gender (a sociocultural construct) have on the etiology, diagnosis, progression, outcomes, treatment, and prevention of many conditions that affect both women and men. A decade ago, women walked into emergency departments and could expect that the medical care they received would be based upon research performed on men. We can now clearly see how women are different than men in the ways in which they have heart attacks, strokes, lung diseases, psychiatric disorders, autoimmune conditions, traumatic injuries, and responses to medications and treatment regimens. It is incumbent upon emergency physicians to take patient sex and gender into account when interpreting clinical manifestations of disease, potential limitations in diagnostic imaging, sex-specific thresholds for biomarkers and laboratory value references, and medication dosing – not to mention mitigating potential and often unconscious gender bias. Emergency medicine (EM) today has a unique opportunity to embrace these differences that have major impacts on improving patient care in every aspect of human health and disease.

A. F. Jarman (✉)
University of California-Davis, Sacramento, CA, USA
e-mail: afjarman@ucdavis.edu

A. J. McGregor
University of South Carolina, Greenville, SC, USA

R. P. Olympia et al. (eds.), *An Emergency Physician's Path*,
https://doi.org/10.1007/978-3-031-47873-4_22

Section II: Careers in Sex and Gender

The goal of a SGBM fellowship is to develop physician-leaders with the specialized knowledge and skills for clinical care, education, research, and advocacy in SGBM. Emergency medicine is an influential and ever-growing specialty. The National Institutes of Health also recently initiated a requirement [NOT-OD-15-102] that all research design, analysis, reporting, and generalizability take into account the role of sex as a biological variable in vertebrate and human studies, which has unleashed an exponentially growing quantity of new evidence that must now be incorporated into clinical practice. Thus, it is a great time to get involved, as there is a compelling need both to discover new knowledge as a primary researcher, train residents, students, and peers as a medical educator, incorporate this knowledge in health systems as an administrator, and influence policy-level changes that support health equity.

Completing advanced training in SGBM opens the doors to a number of varied career paths. Rather than describe these in detail here, we have selected several Emergency Physicians who work in SGBM to highlight both the breadth and depth of their work and the ways in which SGBM informs it.

Tracy Madsen, MD, PhD, FAHA, FACEP

Associate Professor, Departments of Emergency Medicine and Epidemiology
Vice Chair of Research, Brown Emergency Medicine
Co-Director, Rhode Island Hospital/The Miriam Hospital Stroke Centers
Alpert Medical School of Brown University/ Brown University School of Public Health

Education and Training

MD: Boston University
EM Residency: Brown University
Sex and Gender Fellowship: Alpert Medical School of Brown University
PhD (Epidemiology), ScM (Clinical/Translational Research): Brown University School of Public Health

Professional Interests

Sex differences in neurologic emergencies, stroke epidemiology/prevention, gender disparities in the academic medicine workforce, acute stroke care.

Impact

SGBM has been critical to my career as a physician scientist. I have a long-held interest in women's health and improving the care of women, and sex- and gender-based medicine allowed me to integrate my passion for women's health into my career as an emergency medicine physician. Through the field of sex and gender, I was able to begin exploring key differences in stroke, ranging from prevention and epidemiology to acute care. Sex and gender became the foundation for my research career, with a focus on topics including cerebrovascular disease, health equity, and workforce disparities.

Rebecca Barron MD, MPH

Assistant Professor of Emergency Medicine, University of Massachusetts Chan Medical School-Baystate.

Education and Training

MD, MPH: Tufts University School of Medicine
EM Residency: Alpert Medical School of Brown University
Sex and Gender Fellowship: Alpert Medical School of Brown University
Post-Master's Certificate in Evidence-Based Teaching in the Health Professions: Johns Hopkins University

Professional Interests

Medical Education, Sexual Assault, Intimate Partner Violence, Women's Health, Reproductive Health, Professional Development.

Impact

The fellowship in Sex and Gender in Emergency Medicine enabled me to develop my preexisting interests; gain expertise in a novel, unique, and widely applicable area of medicine; meet and collaborate with world-renowned leaders in this area; and help others appreciate the relevance of this field.

Kimi Chernoby, MD, JD, MA

Clinical Instructor, George Washington University Department of Emergency Medicine

Attending Physician, Commonwealth Emergency Physicians Mount Vernon (Community practice)

Counsel for Reproductive Rights and Health, National Women's Law Center

Education and Training

MA (Bioethics): New York University

MD/JD: University of Florida

EM Residency: Indiana University

Health Policy Fellowship: George Washington University

Professional Interests

Reproductive Justice, Health Policy, Advocacy

Impact

Studying sex and gender in Emergency Medicine has allowed me to focus my policy and legal work in the area of reproductive health. By combining clinical practice and law, I have been able to affect policy at the state and federal level that has benefited patients far greater in number than my clinical practice alone. Maintaining the practice of medicine gives me the clinical relevance needed for my policy work, and community practice in particular has allowed me the flexibility to pursue this career path.

Despite their varied expertise and day to day activities, these physicians all utilize sex and gender principles in their daily practices in research, education, administration, and policy and represent only a portion of the careers available to individuals with advanced training in SGBM.

Section III: Applying to Sex and Gender Fellowship

The most important aspect in preparing to apply to a sex and gender program is familiarizing oneself with careers in SGBM and establishing alignment with one's professional goals. Given the relative flexibility of many programs, it is likely possible to tailor advanced educational opportunities to one's particular interests, but this should be discussed well in advance of application deadlines with pertinent program faculty and leadership. Within the fellowship at Brown University, for example, candidates can choose a concentration, with a focus on either education or research. Within that concentration, then, come different curricular requirements. Candidates focused on research may be required to apply for a grant, or submit a manuscript, while educational candidates may design a course curriculum for example.

To increase one's chances of success in applying for fellowship, the typical academic advice applies here as in other subspecialties; this includes performing well on rotations, standardized tests, and having strong letters of recommendation, preferably from other sex and gender scholars. In addition, demonstrated interest and commitment to SGBM can be beneficial for any application. This can come in a variety of forms, including experience in educational programming, research projects, volunteerism; any scholarly activity in the area will show program directors that you are dedicated to a career in SGBM.

If your medical school or residency program does not have a program in SGBM, do not despair, there are several national organizations and resources to help you get and stay involved. Principle among these is the Sex and Gender Interest Group of the Society for Academic Emergency Medicine (SAEM). This group, started in 2015, has a robust membership with strong representation across the organization, so no matter your specific interest, you can be matched with an appropriate mentor. The group has free and open membership to all SAEM members, an active listserv, and innumerable mentorship and authorship opportunities available to interested learners. The group holds regular and open meetings and presents multiple didactics at the SAEM annual meeting, so there are ample opportunities to identify mentors at other institutions. This group also publishes a sex and gender column in every SAEM Pulse newsletter, creating many authorship opportunities as well.

The Sex and Gender Women's Health Collaborative (SGWHC), while not specific to EM, is a tremendous repository for all things related to SGBM. Affiliated with the American Medical Women's Association, this group also has a robust interdisciplinary membership with strong representation of students and residents; there are numerous opportunities for learners to become involved with educational efforts and publishing opportunities. The SGWHC also sponsors a recurring Sex and Gender Health Education Summit, which is another great opportunity for learners to gain exposure and experience in SGBM. Lastly, this organization sponsors a number of web-based educational materials, including case-based modules to augment the sex and gender education learners may be receiving at their home institutions.

SGBM transcends specialties, and at this point is present in some form at nearly every medical school and university, so we would also encourage potential applicants to seek out mentors from other specialties if they are not readily available in EM. Cardiology and Internal Medicine tend to have sex and gender scholars and if your university has a Building Interdisciplinary Research Careers in Women's Health (BIRCWH) program, you can likely find a number of interdisciplinary mentors.

There are several other national organizations that can be helpful, including the National Institute of Health's Office of Research in Women's Health, which holds regular web-based seminars and sponsors the BIRCWH program. The NIH and the Canadian Institute of Gender and Health publish a number of resources, including several free online learning modules. When completed, these award a certificate – which is beneficial to include on your application and curriculum vitae.

While we expect new programs to develop, likely by the time this book is published, there are several well-established programs worth familiarizing yourself with. The Department of Emergency Medicine at Warren Alpert Medical School of Brown University established the first of its kind Division of Sex and Gender in Emergency Medicine (SGEM), dedicated to conducting the research needed to discover differences in men and women in emergent conditions as well as designing educational programs that teach this new knowledge. Brown hosts the most storied fellowship in SGEM and has trained several of the faculty profiled in Sect. II. A number of other programs are now in development at The University of California-Davis, the University of South Carolina, and the University of Alabama. There is also an interdisciplinary Global Women's Health Fellowship housed at Brigham and Women's Hospital for those that are interested in the intersection of SGBM and global health.

Careers in sex and gender are varied, flexible, and incredibly rewarding. As the authors of this chapter, and content experts in sex and gender, we illustrate this variety and flexibility. Dr. Jarman, who completed the fellowship at Brown, is a physician-scientist, currently working on a BIRCWH grant at her institution to study sex differences in pulmonary embolism and venous thromboembolism. After founding and leading the SGEM division and fellowship at Brown for many years, Dr. McGregor is now an Associate Dean for Clinical Faculty Affairs and Development at the University of South Carolina School of Medicine, in addition to her ongoing SGBM scholarship. Your interest and your career are infinitely malleable and we encourage you to reach out to leaders in SGBM if you are interested in joining this increasingly recognized and essential field.

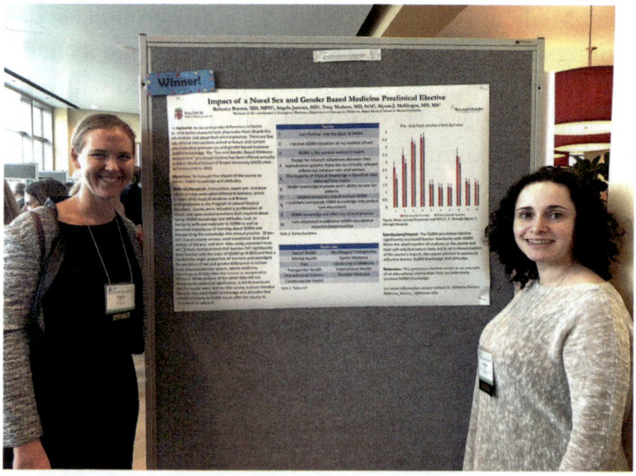

Caption for the photo – "Drs. Barron and Jarman presenting an award-winning poster at the 2018 International Sex and Gender Health Education Summit in Salt Lake City, Utah."

Selected Readings

1. McGregor A, Choo E, Becker B, editors. Sex and gender in acute care medicine. Cambridge University Press; 2016.
2. Jenkins M, Newman C, editors. How sex and gender impact clinical practice: an evidence-based guide to patient care. Elsevier Academic Press; 2021.
3. Legato M, editor. Principles of gender-specific medicine. 3rd ed. Academic Press; 2017.
4. Global Women's Health Fellowship. Boston: Brigham & Women's Hospital. https://connorscenter.bwh.harvard.edu/fellowships/
5. Sex & Gender in Emergency Medicine Fellowship. , Providence: Alpert Medical School of Brown University. https://www.lifespan.org/centers-services/sex-and-gender-emergency-medicine-sgem/sgem-fellowship-and-elective-education
6. Canadian Institute of Gender and Health. https://cihr-irsc.gc.ca/e/8673.html
7. Learning modules. https://cihr-irsc.gc.ca/e/49347.html
8. NIH Office of Research in Women's Health. https://orwh.od.nih.gov/
9. Building Interdisciplinary Research Careers in Women's Health (BIRCWH). https://orwh.od.nih.gov/career-development-education/building-interdisciplinary-research-careers-in-womens-health-bircwh
10. Sex & Gender Women's Health Collaborative. https://www.sexandgenderhealth.org/resources.html
11. SAEM Sex & Gender Interest Group. https://community.saem.org/communities/community-home?CommunityKey=ab6db66f-c94b-4ebf-a9a7-5025b69d606c&tab=groupdetails

Chapter 23
Simulation

Diana V. Labrada

Prior to residency, I had only thought about completing a Simulation fellowship once. I was interviewing at an institution where they advertised their Simulation fellowship using images of physician teachers demonstrating procedures and activities that, on a very basic level, looked fun. There were mannequins covered in fake blood, pork ribs as chest tube task trainers, and pictures of smiling residents learning how to perform procedures. I had always known I wanted to go into academic medicine, but this was the first time I envisioned teaching in a way other than lectures and PowerPoints. It was not until a few months into my third year of residency that I decided to commit to a Simulation fellowship at the same institution I was completing my residency. The biggest challenge? I would be the first fellow of our Simulation program.

History

"To Err is Human" was a shocking paper released in 1999 that identified medical errors as a source of morbidity and mortality in patients. This led to the idea that procedural proficiency is equally important as medical knowledge for patient care [1]. Although many of us only heard of this paper in medical school, it affected the way we train and continue to teach medicine. When I think back to my own medical school experience, simulation was a huge part of my training, although I did not think of it at the time. Every standardized patient encounter I had, every clinical skills lab, every procedure lab that taught me how to be a doctor was simulation based.

D. V. Labrada (✉)
University of Kentucky, Lexington, KY, USA
e-mail: DLA258@uky.edu

R. P. Olympia et al. (eds.), *An Emergency Physician's Path*,
https://doi.org/10.1007/978-3-031-47873-4_23

Per the Society of Academic Emergency Medicine, there are currently 45 Simulation fellowships in the United States [2]. Since this is not an ACGME-accredited fellowship, several differences exist among programs, including length of training. Per review of fellowship lists, most programs are 1–2 years after a 3–4 year Emergency Medicine residency program. There is no board certification in simulation; however, there are certifications available through different programs including The Center for Medical Simulation Instructor Certificate Series and Harvard Macy Institute's Program for Educators in the Health Professions. This lack of consistency and structure may seem daunting, but in true Emergency Medicine fashion, allows for improvisation, adaptation, and improvement.

In 2016, Frallicciardi et al. surveyed Simulation fellowships throughout the country to determine core content that could be used as a guide to tailor each program's simulation curriculum while also allowing for individual variation [3]. Core components include curriculum development, technical operations and techniques, simulation directorship/administrative, simulation research, Simulation fellowship teaching and education, and simulation theory.

Simulation includes everything from practicing ultrasound-guided IVs to lumbar punctures, codes to polytrauma, as well as standardized patient encounters. It has become a major teaching method in medical school and residency.

Why Should You Choose Simulation?

1. **Utility in Medical Education**

   My main reason for choosing simulation was that it fulfilled my desire to teach in a way that was not behind a podium. I often get stage fright giving lectures, but all of that goes away when I get to explain a procedure, debrief a simulation case, or teach interns how to run a code or trauma resuscitation. If you want to be a physician teacher and prefer hands-on activities, this may be a way for you to achieve that. In my experience, we have used simulation with learners of all levels and learners across multiple disciplines. Medical students have used simulation to learn how to manage sepsis and perform ACLS. I have used simulation to teach interns how to perform a primary and secondary survey on trauma patients. Upper level residents have participated in simulation cases to learn how to perform rare, but vital, procedures like pericardiocentesis, lateral canthotomy, and a resuscitative hysterotomy.

2. **Creative Outlet**

   Writing simulation cases is a perfect opportunity to create clinical scenarios you infrequently encounter (massive GI bleed requiring Minnesota tube placement), cases you are scared to have (resuscitative hysterotomy), and common cases presented in a variety of ways (pediatric status epilepticus, polytrauma, massive pulmonary embolus). Creating a simulation case requires using all tools available to you to try and make the simulation as high fidelity as possible. This includes creating models out of household objects to teach critical procedures.

At my institution, for example, we have used toilet paper rolls attached to a child size doll to simulate performing percutaneous transtracheal jet ventilation.

Additionally, simulation requires adding moulage onto the mannequin or leaving clues to help learners identify key points of the case. For example, during my fellowship we ran a simulation case based on significant trauma after a motor vehicle collision. The patient had an unstable pelvis, left sided chest wall crepitus, and seatbelt sign. As such, our mannequin had purple makeup across his chest and abdomen to demonstrate a positive seatbelt sign along with plastic bags tucked underneath the mannequin skin to simulate crepitus. This same case required a chest tube task trainer during the simulation.

3. **Technological Advancements**

   Simulation has greatly advanced over the last several decades. As such, there is a wide array of mannequins and models and even new programs rooted in virtual reality that can be used. There are mannequins that have breath sounds, lung sounds, voices, and pupillary changes. Similarly, there are models that simulate a positive FAST exam to help learners identify free fluid in the abdomen and pelvis. New virtual reality programs could be used to teach new learners how to make therapeutic decisions and decide the next step in management [4].

4. **Patient Safety**

   If practice makes perfect, it makes intuitive sense that the more times a physician performs a procedure, the better they will be at the procedure. However, simulation extends far beyond technical skills. A quick search pulls up thousands of articles relating simulation and patient safety across multiple specialties and disciplines. One study in particular published in the *Journal of Public Safety* outlines expert consensus on ways simulation can improve patient safety [5]. Besides technical skills, this expert consensus agreed simulation can improve physician readiness assessments, handoff, team training, interpersonal skill training, use of new technology, and improvement of debriefing skills.

5. **Teach Non-procedural Skills**

   Simulation is obviously important for teaching and assessing procedural competencies and medical management; however, simulation also offers the opportunity to have learners practice difficult conversations. This includes goals of care discussions, breaking bad news, how to take a history in a transgender patient, and more. Additionally, mannequins are now being created in different skin colors to further promote diversity and inclusion in medicine, allowing for broader conversations to be held about health equity. A March 2021 study investigated medical students' self-reported knowledge of social determinants of health and confidence treating underserved populations through the use of a new curriculum that utilized simulation. This study describes how students take on the role of a member of the community experiencing a barrier to healthcare and discuss what they learn [6].

If these points have convinced you to consider a fellowship in simulation, you may be wondering what to do next.

1. Complete ACGME Emergency Medicine residency program.
2. Simulation is, as of the writing of this chapter, not an ACGME-accredited fellowship, and therefore has no official match. Apply directly to programs with their specific criteria and requirements.
3. Choosing a program: There are several programs to pick from all over the country. Therefore, pick a program that lines up with how involved you want to be with medical students and/or residents. Inquire about what resources you would have and what your role in education will be. Will you be participating in monthly resident didactics? What deliverables are you expected to have by the end of your fellowship? Conversely, see what educational opportunities are available to you, as some programs offer Master's degrees in health professional education while others offer opportunities to complete American College of Emergency Physician Teaching Fellowship or other certificates. As is necessary when choosing the next step in your career, pick a city that you would enjoy living in as well as a program that matches how long you would like to continue training (1 or 2 years).

What to Expect

To complete my story, I was able to outline what I wanted from my fellowship: completion of the ACEP teaching fellowship, creation of new simulation cases, and more involvement with simulation with our medical students. Over my year-long fellowship, I gained skills that have translated to several new opportunities and projects, allowing me to create a niche for myself in academic medicine. I have had the opportunity to create a trauma simulation case for a graduating medical student course. I have developed a multidisciplinary simulation program to improve how my institution performs trauma resuscitations. I continue to participate and create simulation cases for medical students and Emergency Medicine residents. This has been incredibly fulfilling to me, but the residents and medical students I have worked with seem to enjoy it (and learn from it!) too.

Although I am very happy with my choice, Simulation is not currently an ACGME-accredited fellowship, meaning that it will only be as involved as the program you choose. As previously mentioned, this lack of standardization can create great opportunities with appropriate support or unfortunately could lead to disappointment. As such, it is important to have an idea of what each simulation program can offer you and what your trajectory will look like.

In closing, a Simulation fellowship is a wonderful way to receive further training and develop more skills to be an effective medical educator. It has several applications ranging from medical student education to multidisciplinary team building. If you are interested in being a medical educator but dislike the thought of having to create lectures or do not like speaking behind a podium, simulation allows a new way to teach the same information in a more involved manner. If this is the path you choose, I hope you find it as fulfilling and rewarding as I do.

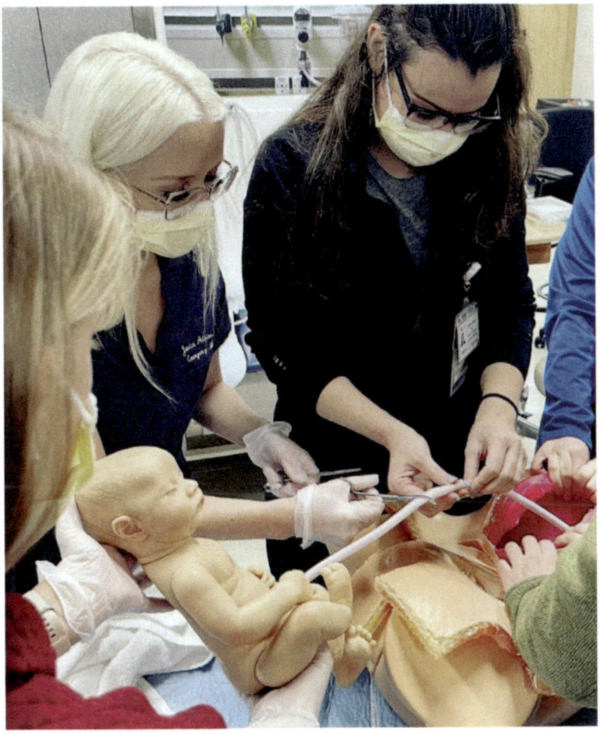

Caption for photo – "University of Kentucky Emergency Medicine residents Dr. Jessica Adkins Murphy and Dr. J.E. Robyn Hanna simulating a resuscitative hysterotomy"

Resources

1. Al-Elq AH. Simulation-based medical teaching and learning. J Family Community Med. 2010;17(1):35–40. https://doi.org/10.4103/1319-1683.68787. https://www.ncbi.nlm.nih.gov/pmc/articles/PMC3195067/
2. Advanced Solutions International, I. Fellowship directory. Fellowship directory – list view. n.d. Retrieved November 27, 2021, from https://member.saem.org/SAEMIMIS/SAEM_Directories/Fellowship_Directory/SAEM_Directories/P/FellowshipList.aspx
3. Frallicciardi A, Vora S, Bentley S, Nadir N-A, Cassara M, Hart D, Park C, Cheng A, Aghera A, Moadel T, Dobiesz V. Development of an emergency medicine simulation fellowship consensus curriculum: initiative of the Society for Academic Emergency Medicine Simulation Academy. Acad Emerg Med. 2016;23(9):1054–60. https://doi.org/10.1111/acem.13019. https://onlinelibrary.wiley.com/doi/epdf/10.1111/acem.13019
4. McGrath JL, Taekman JM, Dev P, Danforth DR, Mohan D, Kman N, Won K. Using virtual reality simulation environments to assess competence for emergency medicine learners. Acad Emerg Med. 2018;25(2):186–95.

5. Sollid S, Dieckman P, Aase K, Søreide E, Ringsted C, Østergaard D. Five topics health care simulation can address to improve patient safety: results from a consensus process. J Patient Safety. 2019;15(2):111–20. https://doi.org/10.1097/PTS.0000000000000254.
6. Denizard-Thompson N, Palakshappa D, Vallevand A, et al. Association of a health equity curriculum with medical students' knowledge of social determinants of health and confidence in working with underserved populations. JAMA Netw Open. 2021;4(3):e210297. https://doi.org/10.1001/jamanetworkopen.2021.0297.

Chapter 24
Sports Medicine

Joseph Andrie and Matthew Silvis

Background of the Specialty

There continues to be growing interest in pursuing additional training in primary care sports medicine among all specialties, but particularly within emergency medicine. As of the 2022 match [1], there were a total of 11 PCSM fellowship programs accredited through the American Board of Emergency Medicine (ABEM). However, 75 programs specifically mention emergency medicine as being an acceptable background for their fellowship applicants.

A fellowship in sports medicine was initially born out of emergency medicine, when, in 1992, the American Board of Medical Specialties approved sports medicine as a subspecialty through ABEM. Shortly after that, the American College of Emergency Physicians created a sports medicine special interest group in 1993 [2]. Since then, the number of emergency medicine physicians who have completed a fellowship in sports medicine has continued to climb steadily. In fact, within the last 10 years, over 150 certificates of added qualification (CAQ) in sports medicine have been awarded to emergency medicine physicians [3].

Why Choose Additional Training in PCSM?

In reality, physicians who are trained in sports medicine have greatly expanded their scope of practice beyond the athletic field and beyond a population of elite athletes. Primary care sports medicine trained physicians are well-versed to address the

J. Andrie · M. Silvis (✉)
Departments of Family and Community Medicine and Orthopedics and Rehabilitation, Penn State Milton S. Hershey Medical Center, Hershey, PA, USA
e-mail: jandrie@pennstatehealth.psu.edu; msilvis@pennstatehealth.psu.edu

R. P. Olympia et al. (eds.), *An Emergency Physician's Path*,
https://doi.org/10.1007/978-3-031-47873-4_24

medical and orthopedic needs of a variety of individuals from youth athletes to weekend warriors to Olympic level athletes. According to the American Society for Sports Medicine, sports medicine physicians are specialized in both the treatment and prevention of illness and injury to help each individual achieve a healthier lifestyle and maximize their athletic performance [4].

A trainee in primary care sports medicine should be interested in more than just athletics, because, quite frankly, attending sporting events becomes another day in the office. Generally, sports medicine physicians have a drive to help their patients reach their goals, rehab their injuries, and prevent re-injury. The ability to communicate with the rest of the team and a genuine love for interacting with those around you, building relationships, and making connections are the cornerstone of sports medicine practice.

Career Options Within PCSM

Career options for an emergency medicine-trained sports medicine physicians are numerous. Often times, by completing extra training in sports medicine, trainees are seeking to enhance their knowledge of musculoskeletal care and procedures, so they can improve patient care within the emergency department setting. Others may use the extra training to seek part-time employment through an orthopedic office or primary care office as a way to supplement their emergency medicine practice. Still others might see the extra training as a way to focus solely on sports medicine, possibly even at the university setting through the care of the athlete and student health. In reality, a variety of different practice options exist, both in terms of the logistics of the weekly schedule, but also regarding the type of employment organization, whether academic, private practice, or university or professional team-based. This is perhaps one of the most exciting aspects of sports medicine. The extra training can either define a career or supplement an existing practice.

What to Expect Out of a PCSM Fellowship

Regardless of where the training occurs – it is sure to be a busy year (or years)! All sports medicine fellowships are either 1 or 2 years depending on the program. It will be a year full of hands-on learning, adapting to unique settings to practice medicine, and shifting the framework of treatment plans to address nuanced aspects of return to play for athletes. According to the 2017 American Medical Society for Sports Medicine recommendations for a primary care sports medicine fellowship [5], each program will contain the following at their core:

1. Longitudinal experiences

Longitudinal experiences will occur across a variety of settings including sports medicine clinic, the emergency department setting, and the athletic training room setting.

2. Event coverage opportunities

   Coverage of a variety of sporting events at all levels is perhaps one of the things that truly sets apart the educational experience of a sports medicine fellow. A large proportion of training and time occurs at athletic events, which enhances the ability to care for acute injuries on the field or facility. The type of events covered varies based on the program, but will include a mix of different sports and also a mass coverage opportunity such as a marathon or a large tournament.

3. Training in the use of ultrasound

   In today's practice, ultrasound is an essential tool for the sports medicine physician, both for diagnostics, but also for treatment through ultrasound-guided procedures. Each program is required to provide this training to their applicants through didactic programming as well as in the clinical setting. Some programs may have dedicated ultrasound clinics whereas others may incorporate the ultrasound training into everyday practice.

4. Monthly rotations

   Similar to most residency programs, each fellowship program is structured around monthly rotations for the fellow. These rotations will focus almost exclusively on orthopedic specialties and subspecialties to enhance the knowledge of the care and recovery of orthopedic injuries. Many fellowship programs will also have rotations in student health or concussion clinics.

5. Sports Medicine specific procedures and skills

   (a) In addition to ultrasound-guided procedures, each sports medicine fellow will be trained in other specific procedures to include compartment testing, orthobiologic procedures such as platelet-rich plasma injections, creating exercise prescriptions, casting and splinting, exercise treadmill testing, and care of the concussed athlete.

Lifestyle and Compensation

As with most fields of medicine, the career of a sports medicine physician can often be a demanding one but also incredibly rewarding. There are often additional hours outside of what may be considered traditional clinic hours. In particular, coverage of sporting events, which often occur in the evening or on weekends, will often be a part of your practice. Additionally, some job descriptions include the athletic training room clinic as part of the weekly schedule, which often happens outside of normal office hours. Furthermore, communication with athletic trainers often will occur outside of normal office hours as well. The exact schedule and lifestyle will vary based on the position, but is sure to expand beyond normal outpatient hours.

Compensation levels can vary widely and depend on a number of factors including years in the field, practice-setting and geographic location. However, in 2022, the average salary for a sports medicine physician was $247,066 [6]. Typically, in addition to salary, benefit packages will be included as well, but vary widely depending on employer.

Primary Care Sports Medicine Fellowship (PCSM): Next Steps

Preparing To Be an Applicant

PCSM is a competitive fellowship option for the following resident types: emergency medicine, family medicine, internal medicine, osteopathic neuromuscular medicine, pediatrics, and physical medicine and rehabilitation. Based on data from the National Resident Matching Program (NRMP), there were a total of 222 certified programs in the match with 353 certified positions. 81.1% of applicants matched into a PCSM fellowship (18.9% unmatched) [1].

The American Medical Society for Sports Medicine (AMSSM) provides a pdf application check sheet as a guide to exemplify what program directors expect in qualified candidates [7]. Building your curriculum vitae is critical to your success at becoming a qualified applicant for the PCSM fellowship match. Search for opportunities throughout your residency to experience PCSM across mission areas: clinical, education, research, and community service. Many residency programs have curriculum dedicated to musculoskeletal and sports medicine with published suggested content [8]. If your program has an area of concentration in PCSM or a sports medicine track, that is a great way to begin building experiences that not only prepare you for fellowship but also help to solidify your interest in the field. Share you interest in PCSM as early in residency as you can so you begin to accumulate experiences. Sports medicine coverage is particularly valuable for your development and should demonstrate both a breadth of experiences and depth with continuity (i.e., covering high school football at the same school throughout residency). Engaging in musculoskeletal rotations whenever possible throughout residency and adding in special elective experiences if possible is also helpful, including procedural electives such as musculoskeletal ultrasound. Whether or not you complete an away rotation is a difficult decision but could be a good idea to get to know programs of interest to you.

Strongly consider engaging in scholarly work during your residency. For instance, you may choose to begin a research or quality improvement project early in residency with a focus on completing your project in the first 2 years of residency, usually during less stressful rotations. . Retrospective studies, along with case reports and series, are particularly well suited to the timeframe that you may have to take an idea and see it result in a scholarly work. Presentations at the local, regional, and national level are important for a competitive PCSM fellowship application. Attendance at annual sports medicine meetings [for example: AMSSM, American

College of Sports Medicine (ACSM), American Osteopathic Academy of Sports Medicine (AOASM)] creates an opportunity to meet program directors and get involved in AMSSM to set yourself apart from other applicants. A recent publication focused on scholarly activity during PCSM fellowship is a great resource to consider during residency as well [9].

Application Content

Similar to medical school and residency applications, all applicants to a PCSM fellowship should think carefully about who they ask to complete a letter of recommendation (LOR). Letter writes should know you well professionally and be able to comment on your clinical acumen, research and teaching abilities, and community service activities. Specific stories or examples highlighting your accomplishments and not just a rewrite of your curriculum vitae are ideal. They should also be able to comment on you personally, including attributes that set you apart from others with a focus on how your characteristics are likely to lead to future success as a PCSM physician. Most PCSM fellowships require three to four LORs, often one from your residency program director with other LORs written by PCSM faculty members with whom you have worked. If you choose to complete an away PCSM elective, attempt to obtain a LOR from a PCSM physician from that elective location.

Your personal statement is another key aspect of your PCSM application. Trying to describe yourself and sharing your story can be very difficult. Some applicants try too hard to differentiate themselves by being creative in a way that is unnatural for them (i.e., injecting humor into a personal statement). Every applicant's story will be unique. PCSM faculty members already appreciate the field so your focus should be on traits that make you a unique applicant, highlighting specific accomplishments or experiences from your curriculum vitae that you are truly passionate about. You should also consider closing your personal statement with what you are looking for in a PCSM fellowship and future career. Remember to be true to yourself!

Process of Applying

Based on data from the National Resident Matching Program [1], PCSM is considered one of the more competitive fellowship options for emergency medicine physicians. For applicants in the 2021–2022 fellowship season, 11 programs offered a total of 17 positions in PCSM. 26.7% of the applicants did not match. As a PCSM fellowship applicant, you should focus your search on accredited fellowships to ensure you can sit for the certificate of added qualification (CAQ) in PCSM – essential for many aspects of your career, including sports medicine credentialing and how you are viewed by insurance carriers.

As you begin your application process, it is important to consider the programs to which you will apply. On average, most applicants apply to approximately 15–25 programs; however, this may vary based upon applicant circumstances. When considering programs, the following questions are important to consider: What area of the country are you most interested in pursuing your education? Do you prefer a community or hospital setting? What sport coverage experiences are included in the fellowship? Are there research opportunities available for you? What are the clinical, educational, and research interests of the faculty members? The AMSSM website provides resources for applying to fellowships including a list of all accredited PCSM fellowships with associated website links.

Applicants apply for PCSM fellowship positions after registering in the Electronic Residency Application Service (ERAS). Applicants are encouraged to register in ERAS the June prior to the interview season to begin work on their application. On July first, applicants can officially begin work on their PCSM fellowship application. Programs begin to review their applicant pool on July 15th with application deadlines ranging from September through November depending on the program. In September, the NRMP match opens for registration. The NRMP rank list deadline is in December, with match officially occurring in early January each year.

References

1. National Residency Matching Program. National residency matching program, math results statistics, sports medicine – 2022. [Internet]. Washington, DC: National Residency Matching Program; 2022. [updated December 17th, 2021; cited August 30th, 2022].
2. Henehan MJ, Cappellari AM, Stromwall AE, Donaldson NG. Sports medicine training and practice opportunities for emergency physicians. J Emerg Med. 2013;45(4):619–23.
3. American Board of Medical Specialties. [Internet, cited August 28th, 2022]. http://www.abms.org/board-certification/abms-board-certification-report/
4. American Medical Society for Sports Medicine. [Internet, cited August 28th, 2022]. http://www.amssm.org/MemberFiles/PatientBrochure.pdf
5. Asif I, et al. Primary care sports medicine fellowship: AMSSM proposed standards of excellence. Clin J Sports Med. 2018;27(3):231–44.
6. Salary.com. [Internet, cited August 29th, 2022]. http://www.salary.com/research/salary/benchmark/sports-medicine-physician-salary
7. American Medical Society for Sports Medicine. [Internet, cited August 30th, 2022]. http://www.amssm.org/Content/pdf%20files/ERAS_APP_Worksheet.pdf
8. Chow Y, et al. Recommended musculoskeletal and sports medicine model curriculum for emergency medicine residency training. Curr Sports Med Rep. 2021;20(1):30–46.
9. Rao A, et al. Recommended sports medicine fellowship scholarly activity curriculum. Curr Sports Med Rep. 2022;21(2):63–9.

Chapter 25
Tactical Medicine

Scott Goldstein

History of Tactical EMS

Tactical Emergency Medicine came to fruition after the Vietnam War when wartime medics came back to the United States. They returned with a vast knowledge of how to care for the severely wounded to a place that was not optimally managing severely injured people, as outlined in the paper "Accidental Death and Disability: The Neglected Disease of Modern Society" [1]. These newly returned veterans wanted to take the knowledge they obtained during wartime back to the community to make life back as safe as possible. At about the same time, the need for specialized police forces, like Specialized Weapons and Tactics (SWAT) teams, was being introduced during the period of civil unrest in the 1960s [6]. After these "higher fire powered" teams were created, the need for medical support followed. This was due to different ballistic injuries and blunt injuries that were occurring with the different weapons the police were using on these specialized teams. This medical follow-through took almost 20 years, but when it came, it was warmly welcomed and needed. This was first written about in *Military Medicine* by Captain Frank Butler in 1996 [2]. It was the first time the general public was exposed to what Special Operations providers did during wartime and explained how certain principles could be translated into current policing to provide emergency medical care to providers. The inception of the National Tactical Officers Association occurred in the early 1980s and it took until 1994 to have understanding and need to endorse the concept of TEMS [3].

Soon after, many specialty associations put out consensus statements endorsing this new specialty of tactical EMS and the importance of this life-saving service, for the police and civilians. Some of the colleges that were for TEMS were ACEP,

S. Goldstein (✉)
Temple University Hospital, Department of Emergency Medicine' Chief,
EMS and Disaster Medicine, Philadelphia, PA, USA
e-mail: scott.goldstein@tuhs.temple.edu

R. P. Olympia et al. (eds.), *An Emergency Physician's Path*,
https://doi.org/10.1007/978-3-031-47873-4_25

NAEMSP, SOMA, and ACOS along with the Hartford Consensus 2, which continued to emphasize the need for this type of service [4]. Since then, the implementation of EMS within police forces has increased and TEMS are now embedded in most police and SWAT units around the world.

What Does It Take to Become a Tactical Emergency Medical Service Provider?

To become a tactical EMS provider, all you need to have is a primary interest and drive to help law enforcement, with the understanding you will be helping the community also. You do not need to be a paramedic or EMT prior to embarking on this specialty, but having that knowledge would be helpful to understand how the prehospital environment functions. Whether you have prehospital experience prior to involvement, or not, once you become a TEMS provider, you will get this exposure regardless of what you did in a prior career. The prehospital TEMS environment is different from the expected "usual" prehospital environment. Most pre-hospital providers are taught to make sure a scene is safe prior to rendering any type of aid. The primary difference in TEMS is that the scene is inherently not safe, and therefore requires a specially trained medical provider. Any type of medical provider can be a tactical medical provider; there are specialists in Emergency Medicine, Surgery, Anesthesia, and Family Medicine who are tactical medical providers. Once you have the basic medical knowledge, taking courses and classes on tactical medicine is what is needed. Tactical EMS is a different mindset and way of thinking compared to how medical routine/civilian providers are trained to think and act. There are numerous courses across the county, but the main course that others have modeled after is Counter Narcotics and Terrorism Operational Medical Support (CONTOMS) [5]. They offer basic tactical medical courses, along with advanced and medical director's courses. This course is the archetype, because after the 5-day intensive course, you have an EMT-Tactical certificate, which is well known in the police and medical community. Completing this course then allows you to take advanced courses and gives a great footing to start off on, along with the added knowledge of how to provide basic tactical medicine. Any course should provide the basic knowledge of tactical medical training along with how to handle non-emergent conditions that may affect the outcome of a mission.

I am Trained, Now What?

Once you have received the basic tactical EMS training, it is time to put it to good use. Like most specialties there are numerous organizations that are always looking for members who want to be involved, locally and nationally. The need for group and political involvement is paramount. Joining these groups helps them provide the support and policy recognition to the politicians that usually provide the financial backing. These groups can shape political viewpoints and reimbursement for tactical providers, which can lead to better services to the community and allow providers to devote the time needed. Depending on your location/hospital affiliation, this may be done as a volunteer or you may get payment for non-clinical time.

Providing TEMS for agencies can be more political than you might think. Wanting to help the police is a noble cause, but if the service is run by an elected official, like sheriffs, there may be outside pressures that may make it difficult to pursue. The want to provide TEMS for an organization is the easy part, the not-so-easy part is the understanding on the other side. There are other viewpoints and interests that need to be taken into consideration and might actually not be seen that feel like you are being hindered. If a team is not interested, it is most likely because of unseen reasoning and not because they don't want the medical care.

You cannot just "be on a team." These teams train and work together for years to become a tight-knit group. It takes time to be trusted along with being considered a fellow provider, let alone trusted with their lives. The time put in going to police functions, trainings, and non-work related events to gain their trust is worth it and will be paid back tenfold!

First, you need to know your geography. Are you moving somewhere to get on a team or are you moving somewhere (clinical job, family, etc.) and then will look into getting on a team? This may seem like a nuance, but location is more a predictor of acceptance than you might expect. If you are moving to find a team, the south and west of the United States would be your best options, as they are more readily accepting of non-law enforcement providers on their teams. Some federal teams may utilize outside physicians for TEMS, but for the most part, most use internal medical providers that are cross trained to maintain operational security. Some of these teams even deputize their physicians to make legal and medical malpractice coverage easier but can lead to "role confusion" and the need for additional proficiencies (firearm training, etc.). Some hospital systems are well aware of the nuances, while others are not, and educating your administration on the pros/cons of this scenario might work out the best, especially if they do not have to cover malpractice.

If you are looking more in the north and northeast, joining a team is more of a political nature and may require years of offering didactics, training, and availability before being invited to be on a team. Some ways to ingratiate yourself is to put the time in by offering to give presentations and hands on demonstrations that are helpful to the law enforcement teams (e.g., Stop the Bleed, basic first aid, etc.). This will show your worth as an educator and provider. Make sure you are available for advice to the agency members and provide contact information so they can reach out.

Another way to show your worth and interest is to become an "assistant" or "associate" Medical Director to the current Medical Director for the team, if they have one. Different Medical Directors have different interests and abilities. The current Medical Director might just support first aid aspects and not tactical aspects, which could be your niche.

A third way is to volunteer to be a tactical physician, which has its own inherent risk necessitating a conversation about medical malpractice and life insurance with your employer. As EMS has blossomed as a specialty, we try not to "work for free" as our services and time are worth money, but depending on your yearning and financial status, volunteering may be a way to show your value. This only works if your clinical place of employment or you personally find medical malpractice coverage for your actions while involved in a tactical event.

A final way is to solicit. There are benefits to tactical medicine for the county and the insurance stance of the municipality. There are benefits to morale, decreased attrition, immediate illness treatment, and "clearing for incarceration," instead of waiting in Emergency Rooms for this to happen. Make a brochure or one page of "why" tactical EMS is beneficial and approach local teams and District Attorneys. (See Fig. 25.1).

You can take a combination of above approaches to try and solidify a team. At the end of the day, you need to feel connected and willing to help everyone, so make sure you feel that connection. The best part of being a tactical physician is the close connections you make with officers and their families. They will look at you as a

Tactical Emergency Medical Support (TEMS)

What is Tactical Emergency Medicine Support (TEMS)?

- Nonmilitary EMS that has been modified for the tactical environment
- A spectrum of services necessary to establish and maintain the health, welfare and safety of Law Enforcement Providers
- Unit Commander's "Medical Conscience"

What is the Value of TEMS?

- Operational Security
- Train team members on individual medical care
- Increased performance
  - Conditioning, Training
- Preventive maintenance
  - Hydration, injury prevention
- Treatment of medical emergencies/urgencies
  - Heat/cold illness, penetrating and blunt injury
  - 24 hour availability for any medical reason
- Medical Records/History and advocacy

Why is TEMS needed? (How will this benefit the team?)

- Conventional EMS is inadequate (delay in care, no preplan, opsec)
- Immediate Life-saving interventions
  - 21% of fatally wounded can be saved with immediate care
  - 80% die within 30 min without treatment
    - *25% die within 5 min without treatment*

How will this benefit the logistics/legal aspect?

- Improve agencies liability posture
- Decrease injury and lost work time of specialized officers
- Cleared for confinement from scene
  - Eliminates need for long ED travel and stay

Fig. 25.1 TEMS

Will this save money?

- Eliminates need to have EMS/Fire on 'standby'
- Decrease workers compensation claims
- Decrease need to train more officers (if less are hurt)
- Increase liability posture (possible insurance discount)
- Decreases officer hours (no ED transport and stay)

How will this benefit the community?

- Eliminates unnecessary travel with a prisoner to a public area (emergency department)
- Eliminates taking 2 (or more) officers out of the field (to transport and guard)
- Treat bystanders if needed
- Community outreach teaching

What is my training?

- EMT-Tactical (CONTOMS)
- Pre hospital Physician for the Commonwealth of PA
- Emergency physician for over 17 years
- EVOC/HazMatOps/FEMA IS course
- Tactical medical Director/Operator for Dauphin County Crisis Response Team for 2 years

What Special Skills/Attributes does a tactical physician provide?

- Teaching of medical care to the team (self/buddy aid)
- Specialized zones of care and equipment
- Preventive Medicine
- Medical Threat Assessment
- Remote Assessment
- 24 hour team care
- Physician Response

Fig. 25.1 (continued)

fellow provider and reach out to you with questions, day or night. These questions may be related to them or their family, but this shows the trust they have in you. It is exhilarating to help the team and go on calls, knowing you are making a difference in the community to both officers and civilians. That said, one of the negatives is possibly being on call essentially 24/7. As mentioned above, phone calls can come at any time (vacation, dinner, etc.). Call outs are not planned too far in advance and some are literally unknown. How does that fit with your clinical and non-clinical schedule? How does this fit with your personal life? Sometimes the days are long, especially training days, which can be physically grueling. But it's all to make you a better provider!

What do you need to be a good or great tactical provider? It depends on your geographic location and distance from definitive care. For example, in the northeast United States, you do not have to worry about poisonous snakes on outdoor operations, but may need to be more vigilant about ticks.

Location may also alter what medication you decide to carry on your person. Everything you carry adds weight and weight is the main enemy for all operations. At minimum you will be wearing a uniform, ballistic vest (with or without a ceramic plate, which can add 30 lbs. at minimum), along with what you have in your medical back and what you carry on your persons. Intravenous fluids are heavy and not necessarily needed, but airway management and tourniquets are worth the weight. These decisions will vary based on the operations, time of year, location, and expected needs. This can be best figured out by a preoperative evaluation of needs, also called a "medical threat assessment." (Fig. 25.2).

Operational Information						
Date:		Location:				Latitude:
Time:						Longitude:
Operation type	Warrant (#):	Barricaded Suspect (#):	Hostage (#):	Dig. Protection (#):	Training (#):	Active Shooter: (#):
LEO/Medical	Tactical:	EMS:	Supervisors:	Patrol:	K9:	Other: (#):
Perpetrators	Male(#):	Female(#):	Ages:	Weapons: o handgun o automatic o knife o shotgun o other:		
Innocents	Children(#):	Ages:	Elderly(#):	Bystanders(#):		

Hospital Facilities	Type	Address	Distance	ED Contact No.
1				( ) -
2				( ) -
3				
4				

Transport Plan			
HELICOPTER	Contact no: ( ) -	Company:	
Landing Zone	Address:	Latitude:	Longitude:
	LZ Type:	Obstructions / Debris:	
Ground	Contact no: ( ) -	Company:	
ALS/ BLS	Staging: crossroads:	Latitude:	Longitude:

Weather								
Temp Hi:	Precip (%):	Heat Index:						
Temp Lo:	Sunrise :	Cold Risk? Yes / No	Wet Bulb Temp	<60	60-78	78-82	82-85	85-88
Wind (mph):	Sunset :	Uniform Adjustments? Yes / No	H20 Qt/hr	0.5	0.5	0.5	0.75	1.0
Humidity (%):	Night Ops Yes / No	Recs:	Rest min/hr	0	0	0	10	15

Animal Threats				
Domestic Animals	Yes / No /Unknown	#:	Types:	Animal Control: ( ) -
Poisonous Snakes	Yes / No/Unknown	#:	Types:	

Plant Threats			
Poisonous plant exposure likely?	Yes / No	Types:	Poison Control: 1-(800) 222-1222
Uniform Adjustments needed?	Yes / No	Recommendations:	

Hazardous Materials				
Ignition risk	Yes / No/Unknown	Types: flashbang,smoke,	Recommendations	HazMat Team: ( ) -
Clandestine Lab	Yes / No/Unknown	Types:petrol liquids,fumes,traps,	Nomex? Yes / No	
Industrial chemicals	Yes / No/Unknown	Types: ammonia,chlorine,	Other special PPE? Yes / No	Chemetrec 1-(800) 424-9300
Other HazMats	Yes / No/Unkown	Types: **Appendix B**	Plackards:	

Public Works				
Street Closings	Yes / No	Location:	Crossroad:	Reason:
( ) -		Alternate route:	Crossroad:	
Road Hazards	Yes / No	Location:	Crossroad:	Reason:
Misc.				

Medical Threat Assessment

Extended Operations					
Work cycles determined	Yes / No				
Nutrition	Yes / No	List:	Sleep area determined:	Yes / No	
Water potable	Yes/No	List	Food Safety	Yes/No	

Fig. 25.2 Medical threat assessment

Like most things that are glorified, the one hour of adrenaline rush during a mission does not show the hours of behind the scenes work that you will be doing. There are tasks that need to be done to make sure the team is "mission ready" at a moment's notice. These range from training and didactics to medication reconciliation and stocking. When these all come together, the team can work knowing their medical needs are met and they can focus on the mission at hand.

References

1. National Academy of Sciences (US) and National Research Council (US) Committee on Trauma, National Academy of Sciences (US) and National Research Council (US) Committee on Shock. Accidental death and disability: The neglected disease of modern society. Washington, DC: National Academies Press; 1966. https://www.ncbi.nlm.nih.gov/books/NBK222962/. https://doi.org/10.17226/9978.
2. Butler FK Jr, Hagmann J, Butler EG. Tactical combat casualty care in special operations. Mil Med. 1996;161(Suppl):3–16. https://doi.org/10.1007/978-3-319-56780-8_1. PMID: 8772308
3. https://www.ntoa.org/sections/tems/tems-position-statement/
4. Joint Committee to Create a National Policy to Enhance Survivability from Mass-Casualty Shooting Events, Jacobs LM, Rotondo M, McSwain N, Wade DS, Fabbri WP, Eastman A, Butler FK, Sinclair J, Burns K, Brinsfield K, Carmona R, Serino R, Conn A, Kamin R. Active shooter and intentional mass-casualty events: the Hartford consensus II. Bull Am Coll Surg. 2013 Sep;98(9):18–22.
5. https://contoms.chepinc.org/
6. https://www.lapdonline.org/office-of-the-chief-of-police/office-of-special-operations/metropolitan-division/swat/

Chapter 26
Toxicology

Laura J. Fil

The History of the Medical Toxicology Fellowship

Although there is evidence that effects of xenobiotics on humans were first recognized thousands of years ago, the formal study of toxicology was only developed within the past 75 years [1]. Poisons were initially used as weapons such as an arrow dipped in a poison, an accelerant of death, or used as a method of murder. One of the first scientists to study the dose-response effect of xenobiotics was Paracelsus. He is best known for saying "What is there that is not poison? All things are poison and nothing without poison. Solely, the dose determines that a thing is not a poison." [2]

So how did we get from this cursory understanding of xenobiotics to the modern study of toxicology?

In the beginning of the twentieth century, the United States government created many regulatory acts to help protect the public from unsafe foods and medications. One of the better known acts in this era was the Federal Food, Drug and Cosmetic Act of 1938. This Act empowered the already existing Food and Drug Administration to have legal authority over the marketing of drugs based on safety [3].

After World War II, a combination of increased production of new medications, increase in deaths due to suicide using medications, and an increase in children with exploratory exposures made it apparent that increased support for how to manage the poisoned patient was needed, and thus the first poison control center opened in 1953 [7].

L. J. Fil (✉)
Department of Emergency Medicine, Vassar Brother's Medical Center, Poughkeepsie, NY, USA
e-mail: Laura.Fil@nuvancehealth.org

R. P. Olympia et al. (eds.), *An Emergency Physician's Path*,
https://doi.org/10.1007/978-3-031-47873-4_26

The development of poison control centers led to further expansion of the field of medical toxicology. Additional poison prevention legislation was passed, societies were developed, and scientific assemblies were held. One society that was created was the American Academy of Clinical Toxicology in 1968 [4]. Their work led to the development of the American Board of Medical Toxicology [5]. Subsequently, the first medical toxicology board exam was administered in 1994. In 1999, the Accreditation Council of Graduate Medical Education (ACGME) in the United States officially accepted medical toxicology as a subspecialty [6]. This led to the growth of 28 medical toxicology programs as of 2022.

Why Do a Medical Toxicology Fellowship?

As a trainee in an emergency medicine residency, our first exposure to toxicology is may be a dedicated medical toxicology rotation, which is typically reserved for second year or higher classes. Of course, we have seen and managed cases in the emergency department by the time we do this rotation, but this rotation is special because it is usually about two to four weeks of non-stop lectures, cases, and breaking down the mechanisms of action, pharmacokinetics, and toxicokinetics surrounding xenobiotic exposures. It is through this rotation that many residents become initially interested in toxicology. Here are a few, but not all, major reasons many people become a toxicologist.

1. ***You are still a nerd at heart.***

   Some toxicologists are intrigued by the interesting ways ordinary pharmaceuticals act in an overdose situation, some are intrigued by all the rare xenobiotic exposures that can occur. For others, we trained as scientists in college, continuing many of those basic science classes in medical school such as biochemistry, and as we delve further and further into clinical medicine, we are not using our basic sciences as often - and we miss the basics. Studying medical toxicology gives us a reason to still discuss biology and chemistry at the cellular and molecular levels.
2. ***You like the magic of an antidote.***

   For me, few things in medicine are as satisfying and as exciting as administering an antidote. Nothing makes you feel more like David Copperfield than giving someone who appears blue, administering methylene blue as an antidote, and watching them turn pink. Another antidote that usually draws a crowd is physostigmine. To watch an anticholinergic patient that is hallucinating, unable to even phonate because their mouth is so dry receive physostigmine and suddenly become alert and oriented and tell you a coherent story, feels nothing short of a chemical card trick. If closing QRS intervals with bicarbonate and using antidotes interests you, then this may be the field for you.
3. ***You want to be an "expert" in something.***

   As an emergency physician, we are experts in knowing a great deal of information about a multitude of medicine. We are experts in many areas including resuscitation. However, our main focus is knowing the emergencies of each specialty. Doing a toxicology fellowship gives one the opportunity to truly delve into an area of medicine and become the specialist in that field.

4. ***Academics.***

   There will be a plethora of opportunities to be involved in academics as a toxicologist. Many residency programs will welcome a toxicologist to their core faculty as you are fellowship trained. During a toxicology fellowship, you will learn how to critically review journal articles and studies, write case reports, develop and perform original research, write letters to editors, submit abstracts, and so much more. These skills are not only highly sought after, but help to diversify your practice of medicine and make it more enjoyable.

5. ***Outlet for other ways to practice medicine.***

   The field of medical toxicology is dominated by emergency medicine trained physicians, with the majority still working full time in the emergency department. Many toxicologists have concurrent toxicology services in their hospitals and have some protected and subsidized time from the emergency department to run their services.

The path of a toxicologist after fellowship can also follow many routes. There are medical toxicologists who have their own toxicology practices/clinics, addiction medicine clinics, work as medical directors of poison control centers, fellowship directors, expert witnesses, work in pharmaceutical fields overseeing regulatory compliance and product safety, and forensic toxicology.

If any of what I have described to you thus far is resonating with you, then I would try to get exposure in the field as early as possible in your training.

How to Get Exposure to the Field and Build Your Toxicology Resume

Whether you know you want to be a toxicologist or want to gather more information to see if this is the specialty for you, there are many ways to get involved.

During residency, if your residency does not require a toxicology rotation, do one as an elective, and if you are interested in fellowship, do a toxicology elective where there is a fellowship established. Many fellowship programs welcome "drop-in" learners as well, as long as you give them a heads up. There is usually one day they review all of the most interesting and complex cases of the week, and that would likely be the best day to attend.

If you have an interesting toxicologic patient case, write it up! Submit it to a conference or a journal. Even if you are not accepted the first time, it is a great learning experience.

Another great way to familiarize yourself with the field is to attend conferences. The two largest conferences are the North American Congress of Clinical Toxicology (NACCT) which is held in the fall, and the American College of Medical

Toxicologists (ACMT) which is held in the spring. At these conferences you can listen to lectures, review case posters, and meet many toxicologists from various hospitals and fellowship programs. ACMT even has a dedicated resident/student membership section.

Another way to become involved with a fellowship program while you are in residency is to reach out to a program and ask if they have any research with which they need help, or possibly come to them with a research idea with which you can combine forces to accomplish.

Choosing the Type of Toxicology Fellowship for You

Just as there are many different factors that go into which emergency medicine residencies you rank, there are also many different characteristics of a toxicology fellowship that should be considered.

First, different fellowships have different areas of focus. There are some fellowships that are primarily clinically based. These fellowships involve a large amount of bedside consults and usually management of a toxicology service in a hospital or health system. There are some fellowships that are based at hospitals with poison center affiliations. In these fellowships, fellows receive calls from throughout a particular area or state and manage many of these patients over the phone. These fellowships are still based at a hospital so there are still bedside cases to be seen. There are some fellowships where the focus is on research. Again, there are still the opportunities to see plenty of patients, but a heavy emphasis is on conducting research in the field. There are also fellowships that focus more on public health as it relates to toxicology. All fellowships have some exposure to all of these factors, but it is important to consider the particular areas of focus for a given fellowship.

Second, consider what types of cases you would be interested in seeing. If you aspire to run a snake bite center one day, then you may want to choose a fellowship in the southwest. If you are interested in body packers, you may want to choose one near a major city and airport. The list can go on and on. The idea is to consider the toxins and areas of toxicology that excite you and to choose a location where you will likely see those cases.

Finally, be sure to ask about the schedule as a fellow. What is the call schedule and weekly schedule like? Make sure the schedule is something that allows you to successfully balance both your work, family, and social life. As emergency physicians we are used to shift work, and any other type of schedule can feel foreign to us.

Final Thoughts

If you are considering a toxicology fellowship, please reach out to a toxicologist. Any of us would be happy to tell you how we navigated our journeys as toxicologists.

References

1. Mann RH. Murder, magic, and medicine. New York: Oxford University Press; 1992.
2. Deichmann WB, et al. What is there that is not poison? A study of the third defense by Paracelsus. Arch Toxicol. 1986;58:207–13. [PubMed: 3521542].
3. Wax PM. Elixirs, diluents, and the passage of the 1938 Federal Food, drug and cosmetic act. Ann Intern Med. 1995;122:456–61. [PubMed: 7856995].
4. Comstock EG. Roots and circles in medical toxicology: a personal reminiscence. J Toxicol Clin Toxicol. 1998;36:401–7. [PubMed: 9734269].
5. Anonymous. American board of medical toxicology. Vet Hum Toxicol. 1987;29:510.
6. Nelson LS, Howland M, Lewin NA, Smith SW, Goldfrank LR, Hoffman RS. Goldfrank's Toxicologic emergencies. 11ed. McGraw Hill; 2019.
7. Press E, Mellins RB. A poisoning control program. Am J Public Health Nations Health. 1954;44:1515–25.

and help them appreciate the

History

The Florida Human

errors as a source of morbidity and mortality

procedural proficiency is equally important as

[1]. Although many of us only heard of this

Chapter 27
Ultrasound

Nicholas W. Macklin

History of Point-of-Care Ultrasound in Emergency Medicine

Completing a fellowship in Advanced Emergency Ultrasound opens many doors for the emergency physician. Similar to other fellowships available to Emergency Medicine, it allows for the carving out of one's niche in the professional world – both in the academic and community setting. However, again similar to other fellowships, investing one year of your early earning potential is a decision to be considered with great care. This is not to say that this fellowship is not a valuable endeavor, but that one should understand the expected return on investment in terms of professional opportunities and personal fulfillment.

Point-of-care ultrasound (POCUS) developed as a field out of necessity, and therein lies its promise as an ongoing subspecialty. In the 1990s, the role of ultrasound became an area of interest as bedside diagnostics such as the FAST exam and procedural applications such as dynamic needle guidance emerged. The initial role, privileging, and scope of non-radiologist physicians performing ultrasound were not well-defined. One of the first landmarks in the inception of this field was the policy statement by the American Medical Association (Privileging for Ultrasound Imaging H-230.960) in 1999 which affirmed the use of ultrasound for any appropriately trained physician. The language was broad, but a crucial section of this statement recommended that ultrasound training standards be developed by the individual specialties. This notion was most eagerly embraced by national Emergency Medicine leadership as evidenced by the American College of Emergency Physicians (ACEP) policy statement "Emergency Ultrasound Guidelines" in 2001. As early adopters, Emergency Medicine has developed much of the point-of-care standards widely in use throughout the United States today, and we continue to be leaders in the field.

N. W. Macklin (✉)
Department of Emergency Medicine, Wake Forest University School of Medicine, Winston-Salem, NC, USA
e-mail: nmacklin@wakehealth.edu

R. P. Olympia et al. (eds.), *An Emergency Physician's Path*,
https://doi.org/10.1007/978-3-031-47873-4_27

Point-of-care ultrasound has grown at a steady rate since its start but has remained true to its core tenets: augmenting clinical practice with bedside sonographic techniques and supplementing gaps in available diagnostic imaging. Some benefits of POCUS are obvious, such as dynamic needle guidance in both central and peripheral vascular access, arthrocentesis, pericardiocentesis, and regional anesthesia. Others are more situationally dependent. Some emergency physicians raise valid questions regarding the utility of performing one's own diagnostic sonographic examinations, such as for biliary pathology or deep vein thrombosis, as opposed to ordering a study to be performed by the Radiology Department. Depending on the setting and resources available in one's practice, it may indeed be more efficient to order a study rather than perform it oneself. However, many emergency departments to this day do not have 24/7 access to some or all ultrasound applications, particularly in a timely fashion. This holds true both in community and academic settings. POCUS offers the emergency physician the means to better evaluate and care for their patients regardless of time or location.

The nomenclature regarding this training has evolved, with many fellowships and organizations using the titles "emergency ultrasound" and "clinical ultrasound." Most recently, ACEP and ABEM (American Board of Emergency Medicine) have chosen the designation Advanced Emergency Ultrasound, abbreviated AEMUS, for fellowship training. However, many organizations continue to use the original titles with which they were started. POCUS is a commonly used and appropriate term to describe bedside ultrasound performed by the clinician and is not limited to Emergency Medicine.

As we recognized and protocolized a growing number of POCUS applications, a need for dedicated leadership formed organically and the position of "ultrasound director" was developed. Early on, such positions were often held by those with experience and training obtained after residency through workshops or mentorship. Ultrasound fellowship programs were developed throughout the 1990s and 2000s which provided training in both the clinical aspects of ultrasound and the leadership of its implementation. As the body of fellowship-trained emergency physicians has grown, so has the expectation for directors of ultrasound to have fellowship training. However, not all who pursue fellowship do so in order to lead, and may instead seek to fulfill personal practice goals or carve out their niche in an educational or research space.

Reasons for Pursuing Ultrasound Fellowship

1. *Leadership.* Ultrasound fellowship will provide you with the training to create, maintain, and advance an ultrasound program, both in a community practice or an educational site. Even in a community setting, if members of your group are using POCUS in their clinical practice, some degree of oversight is needed. Quality assurance should be performed periodically, documentation and billing

need to be managed, and machines will need to be maintained. Your colleagues will come to you with questions. Often you will have physicians, physician assistants, or nurse practitioners seek additional training either from you or your recommendations. Fellowship will give you the foundational knowledge to succeed in such a position, which is key to a group or institution supporting your time financially.

2. *Education.* Ultrasound lends itself well to enjoyable teaching. Learners of ultrasound are often enthusiastic about learning a new skill or honing what they have practiced. Bedside teaching provides a pleasant reprieve from the routine of working clinically or spending time in the office. Didactics in ultrasound tend to be more engaging, with lectures having more multimedia, fewer words, and increased interactivity. Further, ultrasound education can often be done in a simulation lab where you spend less time talking and more time guiding excited learners. The most challenging aspect of ultrasound education is finding ways to convey concepts of three-dimensional spatial reasoning through words or screens, but this comes with training and practice.
3. *Scholarship.* If you are seeking an academic career, scholarship will be a necessary component of your professional life. Ultrasound has a strong advantage here in being a ripe venue for scholarship. There are many areas within emergency ultrasound and POCUS supported only by sparse or low-level evidence where one can always find a question yet to be answered. Further, there exists a desire among many to shift from technique-oriented studies to those evaluating large-scale outcomes wherein many investigators will be needed. Publication in educational journals is common among ultrasound educators as unique challenges to developing spatial comprehension are addressed.
4. *Procedural expertise.* Perhaps one of the most attractive aspects of AEMUS fellowship training is the expertise garnered in ultrasound-guided procedures. These include more traditional applications such as vascular access and paracentesis as well as more advanced techniques such as ultrasound-guided lumbar puncture, regional anesthesia, and arthrocentesis. Fellowship training provides an understanding of the technical aspects of ultrasound physics and mechanics, which lends itself not only to expertise in these advanced applications but also to a higher standard for more routine procedures such as arterial and central venous catheterization. The ability to perform and teach these skills makes you a valuable member of any group.
5. *Diagnostic expertise.* AEMUS training also affords the opportunity to explore ultrasound applications that might be less commonly performed by an emergency physician. These applications include bowel pathologies such as pyloric stenosis, intussusception, appendicitis, and bowel obstruction; advanced echocardiography including transesophageal echocardiography, right heart evaluation, and diastolic evaluation; musculoskeletal ultrasound, and transcranial ultrasound. Further, a broadened knowledge base of sonographic findings in commonly performed applications will allow you to be a resource to your colleagues when coming across less common findings.

6. *Practice setting.* As fellowships in the Emergency Medicine subspecialties have become more common, competition for faculty teaching positions at university hospitals has increased significantly. A young physician must distinguish themself to gain such a position. A fellowship in AEMUS will be of value if your goal is to work in an academic setting. If you are geographically flexible, finding an ultrasound director or assistant director position out of fellowship is certainly possible. However, many of the most desirable locations have a well-staffed ultrasound section or division.
7. *Industry.* Beginning in fellowship and continuing throughout your career, you will interface with various personnel from the ultrasound industry. Most commonly, these will be sales representatives when you need a new probe, accessory, or ultrasound machine. However, as you develop professional relationships with the major corporations in this field, you will have opportunities of varying magnitude to contribute your expertise to technology research, development, and implementation. Your opportunities may lead to compensated consulting work, and some physicians have even successfully pivoted their careers into the private sector. Ultrasound is uniquely positioned for this career trajectory, if so desired.
8. *Immediate gratification.* Emergency Medicine, in general, tends to draw those who enjoy being able to answer their questions immediately. Unlike hospital and outpatient medicine, we rarely have to wait hours, days, or weeks to get the results of the tests we ordered. POCUS amplifies this sense of immediate gratification. Experienced clinicians may take their ultrasound machine in the room when they first evaluate a patient to perform their diagnostic study. In this way, you can have a sonographic diagnosis (or exclude a differential) before leaving the room. It is incredibly satisfying to introduce yourself to a patient and, within minutes, show the patient their culprit disease process, such as cholelithiasis, hydronephrosis, pneumonia, or systolic dysfunction. If you find satisfaction in continually improving your capabilities, you can always improve your image acquisition and interpretation proficiency. There is no skill ceiling for emergency ultrasonography. Finally, if unsure of your findings, you can compare your images with that of a different modality or a radiology-performed ultrasound for immediate feedback.
9. *Technophilia.* The small world of AEMUS tends to appeal to those who enjoy technology and gadgetry. If you maintain any position of ultrasound leadership, you will be invited to demonstrations of new equipment. Pushing new buttons, learning new features, and seeing the latest in image quality can be quite enjoyable. You may be given charge of making recommendations for ultrasound equipment purchasing. With handheld ultrasound devices and increasingly modern cart-based platforms, there is no shortage of equipment to test and learn.
10. *Interdepartmental networking.* POCUS has always been open to other specialties but with varying levels of interest. In recent years, other specialties such as Internal Medicine, Anesthesiology, Neurology, Family Medicine, and others have become more involved in advancing their capabilities. These specialties are often navigating similar obstacles to what we, as a specialty, have encoun-

tered. This provides ready networking opportunities for interdepartmental collaboration and support. The benefits of such relationships are mutual and, while often intangible initially, ultimately worthwhile. Interdepartmental scholarship, educational initiatives, and reciprocal teaching are just a few benefits of having friends in diverse places within the hospital.

11. *Fulfillment.* Finally, while not unique to ultrasound, the decision to pursue a fellowship should first be considered in the context of your fulfillment with the general practice of Emergency Medicine. We have a hard job, but we are well compensated, we get to leave our job at the end of our shift, and we can work in nearly every part of this country. While there are many benefits of fellowship training, you are giving another year of your youth and earning potential for it. If enough satisfaction can be maintained by enjoying your personal life and practicing Emergency Medicine, a fellowship may not be needed to reach your goals. Unlike many other subspecialties, ultrasound is unlikely to increase your annual compensation. Your time should be supported by your institution for your ultrasound leadership whereby you work fewer clinical shifts for the same base pay, but this is not guaranteed in the community setting. You must consider if the fulfillment in a more diverse scope of day-to-day work including teaching, scanning, research, and administrating is worth the initial investment of time and delayed income.

What to Expect in Fellowship

Advanced emergency ultrasound fellowships require the completion of an Emergency Medicine residency, including the ultrasound requirements of one's program. Most fellowships last one year and include a research project, bedside teaching as both a learner and instructor, image review for quality assurance, and didactic education. Depending on the program, much of the time will be spent developing your ability to provide ultrasound education and manage an ultrasound program. Finally, and most importantly, a fellow spends many hours *scanning* – performing, acquiring, and interpreting ultrasound images. All of these activities prepare a fellowship-trained physician to sit for the focused practice designation examination offered by ABEM to formally recognize expertise in this field.

Residents considering an AEMUS fellowship commonly want to know how much exposure they will have to non-core examinations – that is, applications beyond those they practiced in residency. This is particularly true for those who feel they received a robust ultrasound education during their training. The answer is unsatisfying in that it varies greatly both by program and the initiative of the fellow. These opportunities depend on having fellowship faculty with experience in such applications or instruction from external departments such as Radiology, Cardiology, or Anesthesia. Such external instruction requires an ongoing relationship between these departments and that of Emergency Medicine, which is not the case in all hospitals.

A common misconception is that an AEMUS fellowship is ideal for those who did not get enough ultrasound training in residency. While a fellowship will enhance your ability to perform the core ultrasound applications of Emergency Medicine, it is not an efficient means of accomplishing this goal. An AEMUS fellowship has only one year to provide a large body of information and develop the expertise needed to independently lead in the field of Emergency Medicine. This valuable time is best spent building upon skills and interests developed during residency.

AEMUS fellowships are not ACGME-certified, and therefore receive no graduate medical education funding. These programs are typically funded internally via clinical shifts worked by the fellow. This arrangement has its benefits and drawbacks. A significant benefit is that the transition from supervised resident to independent attending is somewhat more gradual, as you will not have a full clinical load. Conversely, the expected salary is not standardized and varies widely among institutions — a potential drawback. Salaries can range from a typical house officer pay scale to a partial attending salary roughly commensurate with your clinical hours. These are important factors to consider when evaluating potential programs.

Preparing to Apply

As noted above, you can prepare yourself for fellowship by maximizing your exposure to ultrasound during residency. This should include completing and logging a robust number of ultrasound examinations, ideally at least 100 per year of residency. Depending on what is available at your program, consider taking an elective in ultrasound as early as possible to spend additional time with ultrasound faculty and learn how their non-clinical time is utilized. Look into assisting with the instruction in ultrasound for junior residents, such as during resident conferences or orientations. If there is a medical school associated with your program that has ultrasound integrated into its curriculum, consider reaching out to assist with instruction. Identify a mentor to guide and encourage along your path of ultrasound excellence. By developing a strong foundation of the core applications and concepts in residency, you will be poised to successfully transition to fellowship and harness the opportunities available to you.

The application cycle is similar to that for residency. Applications are submitted to programs through an organization known as SCUF (Society for Clinical Ultrasound Fellowships), and fellowship programs now participate in the National Resident Matching Program. Even if you apply to one program, you will still need to go through the match. You will need letters of recommendation, a personal statement, and good standing in your residency program. As you begin to research programs you are interested in applying to, the plethora of abbreviated terms can be confusing. A table is provided below which summarizes some of the more common abbreviations and their relevance.

ABEM	American Board of Emergency Medicine	Offers the FPD examination and certification to fellowship-trained emergency physician
AEMUS	Advanced emergency ultrasound	Current designation endorsed by ABEM and ACEP for fellowship training in ultrasound by emergency medicine physicians
CUS/ EUS	Clinical ultrasound / Emergency ultrasound	Commonly used terms for the field of ultrasound in emergency medicine and associated fellowships
FPD	Focused practice designation	The certification offered by ABEM to designate expertise. You cannot sit for this until you have passed both written and oral board examinations – No need to consider until after fellowship
EUFAC	Emergency ultrasound fellowship accreditation council	Accredits ultrasound fellowship programs as of 2020. Accreditation will eventually be required of programs to qualify graduates for the FPD, so accreditation status may be of interest to an applicant
NRMP	National Resident Matching Program	Matches applicants with fellowship programs. Of note, the NRMP uses the term "clinical ultrasound" for matching purposes
POCUS	Point-of-care ultrasound	General term for ultrasound performed at bedside by the treating clinician (performed at the "point of care")
SCUF	Society of Clinical Ultrasound Fellowships	Primary national organization for ultrasound fellowships. Formerly known as EUS fellowships. *This is where you will submit your application to fellowship programs.*

Chapter 28
Undersea and Hyperbaric Medicine

Kelly Johnson-Arbor

Introduction

Undersea and Hyperbaric Medicine (UHM) is a medical subspecialty dedicated to the diagnosis, prevention, and treatment of conditions associated with exposure to environments with increased ambient pressures such as SCUBA diving, as well as the diagnosis and treatment of conditions with hyperbaric oxygenation [1]. The American Board of Medical Specialties recognizes UHM as a subspecialty of both the American Board of Emergency Medicine (ABEM) and the American Board of Preventive Medicine (ABPM). As of 2022, physicians may become board-certified in UHM by completing an ACGME-accredited one-year fellowship in UHM and by passing the written board certification examination. Although a practice pathway to board certification was previously available, it is no longer an option for board certification in UHM as of 2022. Board-certified UHM physicians must complete regular recertification requirements through their primary medical specialty board (ABEM or ABPM).

There are limited UHM fellowship programs available in the United States, and, for unclear reasons, UHM has historically not been a popular subspecialty in Emergency Medicine. The Undersea and Hyperbaric Medical Society (UHMS) (www.uhms.org) maintains a list of UHM fellowship programs on their website (https://www.uhms.org/resources/credentialing/fellowship-programs.html). Both civilian and military UHM fellowship programs are available. UHM fellowship programs are located in various areas of the United States.

The clinical practice of UHM varies based on facility type and geographic location. UHM programs that are located in coastal areas may concentrate primarily on the diagnosis and treatment of diving-related injuries, while other programs may

K. Johnson-Arbor (✉)
MedStar Georgetown University Hospital, Washington, DC, USA

R. P. Olympia et al. (eds.), *An Emergency Physician's Path*,
https://doi.org/10.1007/978-3-031-47873-4_28

focus more on clinical hyperbaric medicine, including wound care. There is no "typical" hyperbaric medicine practice: UHM physicians can practice hyperbaric medicine, undersea medicine, or a combination of both.

Undersea Medicine

While clinical hyperbaric medicine is an important facet of the subspecialty, undersea medicine is also a primary aspect. Undersea medicine, often described as diving medicine, encompasses the prevention, diagnosis, and management of diving-related injuries. Physicians who practice undersea medicine care for various types of SCUBA divers, including recreational, technical, scientific, and commercial divers. Because of this, a simple interest in recreational SCUBA diving generally does not provide medical professionals with enough undersea medicine experience to treat all SCUBA divers, and highlights the importance of specialized UHM training when managing the diving population. Medical standards for recreational, scientific, and commercial divers may differ, and there are varying guidelines for returning to diving after sustaining an injury such as decompression illness, based on the diver's classification. Because of the complexity of diving medicine, there are additional courses and certifications that are available for physicians who have an interest in diving medicine in addition to completion of the UHM fellowship. These courses allow physicians to achieve advanced level certification as a "Diving Medical Examiner" or a "Diving Medical Physician" by the UHMS. Physicians who obtain and maintain these certifications can partner with the Divers Alert Network (DAN), a non-profit organization dedicated to diving safety, to provide medical care to divers of all ages. Becoming a DAN-affiliated physician allows you to treat divers of all ages and classifications, from children who are interested in participating in SCUBA diving activities at summer camp to elderly recreational or technical divers. DAN-affiliated physicians typically evaluate and treat divers in a medical clinic environment. Depending on the diver's condition and medical needs, the DAN-affiliated physician may refer the diver for laboratory tests, cardiac evaluation, pulmonary assessment, or other subspecialty testing. These medical visits and associated tests may be paid by the diver out-of-pocket, billed to the diver's health insurance, or reimbursed by the diver's employer (in the case of commercial divers). The medical evaluation of divers is typically a pleasant experience, as most divers are generally healthy and motivated to maintain their physical condition so that they can engage in safe diving practices. It is not uncommon for divers to keep in touch with their physicians over time and send them pictures of their diving excursions. Additionally, because there are a limited number of physicians in the United States who specialize in diving medicine, patients may travel from long distances for appointments with their dive medicine physician. For certain dive medicine patients, telehealth appointments may be an option, although many patients require a physical examination that can only be performed in a face-to-face, in-person setting.

The clinical practice of diving medicine differs from the practice of Emergency Medicine or other medical-based specialties. When evaluating a SCUBA diver, it is important to remember that conditions that may be associated with morbidity on land may be fatal if they occur during underwater submersion. For example, seizures, loss of consciousness, or hypoglycemia that occurs underwater can result in fatality, as an intact level of consciousness is required to breathe through a SCUBA regulator. Divers who have asthma or other lung disease may experience difficulties in breathing through a regulator, due to the dense nature of the compressed breathing gases used during diving as well as the increased resistance associated with breathing through a regulator. Individuals who have uncontrolled or poorly controlled psychiatric conditions, such as panic disorder, may expel their regulator during unexpected conditions that may occur during diving. Finally, although diving is perceived by many as being a low-risk recreational activity, it can be exertional at times, as divers may have to swim against currents, climb on and off of boats while carrying heavy gear, or even evade hazardous marine life. Individuals who engage in recreational diving as teenagers or young adults often do not have the same exertional tolerance when they become older, and each year there are diving-related deaths reported due to undertreated or undiagnosed coronary artery disease. For this reason, one of the main focuses of the diving medicine physician is to ensure that divers have adequate cardiac endurance.

In addition to preventive diving medicine evaluations, some divers are referred to UHM physicians for treatment of diving-related injuries such as immersion pulmonary edema (IPE), pulmonary or otic barotrauma, or decompression illness (DCI). Patients who are referred for treatment of adverse events that occur as a consequence of SCUBA diving require a thorough assessment by the diving medicine physician to investigate potential predisposing factors and discuss ways to mitigate diving-associated risks in the future. While many divers are able to return to diving after they experience adverse events, some divers are advised to cease diving due to an unacceptable risk of recurrent or future events.

Hyperbaric Medicine

UHM physicians often supervise clinical hyperbaric treatments in hospitals or outpatient clinical settings. There are more than 1300 hyperbaric facilities in the United States, and many hospitals have hyperbaric chambers located within outpatient wound centers [2]. There are two types of hyperbaric chambers used in clinical medicine: class A, or multiplace chambers, hold more than one person, while class B, or monoplace chambers, are designed for single-person occupancy. Multiplace hyperbaric chambers are pressurized with air, and patients breathe oxygen through hoods or masks. These chambers are typically large and can accommodate patients who are intubated and require invasive monitoring, medication administration, or telemetry during their treatments. Multiplace hyperbaric chambers are often utilized as emergency hyperbaric facilities and may be open and able to accept and treat patients 24 hours a day. Multiplace hyperbaric chambers are also more costly to maintain and staff compared with monoplace chambers, and for that reason, they are infrequently found in the United States. Most clinical hyperbaric medicine facilities found within hospitals are monoplace chambers. Monoplace hyperbaric chambers are designed to hold a single patient. These chambers are pressurized with 100% oxygen. Most monoplace chambers are not configured to allow invasive monitoring or telemetry, so the UHM physician must ensure the patient's clinical stability prior to recommending the patient for hyperbaric medicine administration. Hyperbaric chambers are typically operated by nurses or respiratory therapists who are specially trained as hyperbaric technicians. While the UHM physician does not generally operate the hyperbaric chamber, he or she is responsible for the clinical supervision of each hyperbaric treatment and also can work in conjunction with the hyperbaric facility's safety director to ensure that the facility is engaged in the safe practice of hyperbaric medicine.

Clinical hyperbaric medicine practice can vary by location. In hyperbaric facilities that are located within outpatient wound centers, UHM physicians may supervise hyperbaric treatments while practicing wound care. Since some wound center patients may have indications for treatment with hyperbaric medicine, the UHM physician can evaluate those patients for hyperbaric medicine candidacy within the wound center as well. In some outpatient wound centers, the UHM physician is also responsible for performing inpatient hyperbaric medicine consultations and treatments, while other hospitals may not offer hyperbaric medicine treatments to inpatients due to financial or logistical concerns.

There are a limited number of clinical indications for the use of hyperbaric medicine. As of 2022, the UHMS has approved 14 conditions for use of hyperbaric medicine. These conditions include selected problem wounds (typically severe diabetic lower extremity ulcerations that have associated osteomyelitis, abscess, tendonitis, or gangrene and that have failed to heal despite use of standard conservative therapies), sudden sensorineural hearing loss, compromised skin grafts and flaps, decompression illness, carbon monoxide poisoning, and severe anemia with inability to accept blood transfusion due to religious or medical constraints. The UHM physician must be familiar with the approved indications for hyperbaric medicine, as well as the rationale for the use of hyperbaric oxygen therapy to treat these conditions. As the insurance coverage for hyperbaric oxygen therapy can vary geographically by carrier and hyperbaric indication, it is also the responsibility of the UHM physician to maintain a working knowledge of the hyperbaric medicine-related medical policies of insurance carriers in his or her region. For example, as of 2022, Medicare does not consider hyperbaric oxygen therapy to be medically necessary for the treatment of severe anemia in patients who are unable to receive blood transfusion, and the Blue Cross Blue Shield Federal Employee Program does not consider hyperbaric oxygen therapy to be medically necessary for the treatment of compromised skin grafts or flaps [3, 4]. It is important to ensure insurance coverage for hyperbaric treatments due to the costly nature of outpatient hyperbaric treatments. The hospital facility fee associated with a single outpatient hyperbaric treatment may exceed several thousand dollars. Due to these high costs, the use of hyperbaric oxygen therapy for experimental or "off-label" conditions is limited in the United States, as most patients cannot afford the self-pay costs of hyperbaric treatments that are administered in hospital settings. For this reason, hyperbaric oxygen therapy is typically not utilized for experimental conditions such as autism, traumatic brain injury, and Lyme disease in hospital settings. Some UHM physicians may choose to open standalone hyperbaric medicine facilities, not associated with healthcare facilities, to treat these and other experimental conditions. As the use of hyperbaric medicine as a treatment of these conditions is not considered medically necessary by insurance carriers, patients must pay out of pocket for these treatments.

Research and Publication

Given the significant medical expenses associated with the administration of hyperbaric oxygen therapy, it can be difficult to perform undersea and hyperbaric medicine related research due to funding constraints. During the COVID-19 pandemic, hyperbaric oxygenation was studied as a potential therapeutic modality for patients infected with the SARS-CoV-2 virus in a limited number of hyperbaric medicine facilities within the United States and abroad. DAN also performs research and provides grant funding related for studies involving diving safety. There are two main undersea and hyperbaric medicine journals in which clinical research, case reports/studies, and commentaries can be published: *Diving and Hyperbaric Medicine* and *Undersea and Hyperbaric Medicine*. Both journals are peer-reviewed and are indexed in Medline, although they are published quarterly instead of monthly.

Summary

A career in Undersea and Hyperbaric Medicine involves the evaluation and treatment of divers as well as hyperbaric medicine patients. The daily activities of an Undersea and Hyperbaric Medicine physician vary widely and may include supervision of hyperbaric oxygen treatments, outpatient routine medical evaluation of divers, inpatient hyperbaric medicine consultations, teaching, and research. While hyperbaric medicine facilities are found in hospitals throughout the United States, there are relatively few physicians who undergo subspecialty training in this field, and board certification can only be achieved by completing a one-year fellowship. Considering that the need for board-certified Undersea and Hyperbaric Medicine physicians will likely increase in future years as the number of clinical hyperbaric medicine facilities continues to expand across the United States, Emergency Medicine trainees should strongly consider this training pathway as a potentially viable career option.

References

1. American Board of Emergency Medicine. Undersea and Hyperbaric Medicine. https://www.abem.org/public/become-certified/subspecialties/undersea-and-hyperbaric-medicine. Accessed 30 Aug 2022.
2. Johnson-Arbor K, Verstraete R. No bad blood-surviving severe anemia without transfusion. JAMA Intern Med. 2021;181(1):7–8.
3. Centers for Medicare and Medicaid Services. National coverage determination: hyperbaric oxygen therapy. https://www.cms.gov/medicare-coverage-database/view/ncd.aspx?ncdid=12. Accessed 30 Aug 2022.
4. Blue Cross Blue Shield Federal Employment Program. FEP 2.01.04 Hyperbaric Oxygen Therapy. https://www.fepblue.org/-/media/PDFs/Medical%20Policies/3-18-2022/Medical_Policies/20104%20Hyperbaric%20Oxygen%20Therapy.pdf. Accessed 30 Aug 2022.

Chapter 29
Wilderness Medicine

Hillary E. Davis and Martin Musi

So you Want to be Involved in Wilderness Medicine?

Wilderness Medicine is the multidisciplinary practice of implementing techniques for healing or preventing injury in resource-poor, natural environments where definitive care is not immediately available. Emergency Medicine is particularly applicable to wilderness settings due to its breadth of training in acute-care scenarios. Core tenants of Wilderness Medicine are the improvisation with supplies at hand, dissemination of solutions, teamwork, and ensuring participants remain healthy and safe; this is not dissimilar to being active in an emergency department (ED). However, unlike working in the ED—participants are usually outside, exposed to the same objective risk that created the initial injury, and usually on "epic" adventures!

The field of Wilderness Medicine is continuously in flux as new specialties are added to its scope [1]. Although traditionally thought of as "mountain medicine," this is now viewed as a subclassification; wilderness physicians are involved in care in both hypobaric and hyperbaric environments, and every extreme in-between. While not all-inclusive, Table 29.1 lists several recognized categories of Wilderness Medicine.

Physicians can serve in wilderness roles as three entities: advisors, caregivers, or participants [2]. As advisors, physicians may be board members or provide medical direction for corporations involved in space flight, commercial travel, or media

H. E. Davis (✉)
Department of Emergency Medicine, University of Tennessee Medical Center, Knoxville, TN, USA
e-mail: Hedavis1@utmck.edu

M. Musi
Department of Emergency Medicine, University of Colorado, Boulder, CO, USA
e-mail: martin.musi@cuanschutz.edu

R. P. Olympia et al. (eds.), *An Emergency Physician's Path*, https://doi.org/10.1007/978-3-031-47873-4_29

Table 29.1 Common subfields in Wilderness Medicine

Topics in Wilderness Medicine		
Altitude and Mountaineering Medicine	Diving and Hyperbaric Medicine	Tropical and Travel Medicine
Expedition Medicine	Tactical Combat and Casualty Care	Aerospace Medicine
Polar and Desert Medicine	Sports Medicine and Physiology	Disaster Medicine
Climate and Health Sciences	Rescue and Evacuation	Survival Medicine and Bushcraft
Toxicology	Preventative Medicine and Field Sanitation	Event and Endurance Medicine
Trauma Management	Female Health Considerations	Diversity and Inclusion

ventures. They can also work for government entities, including the National Park Service (NPS), the National Aeronautics and Space Administration (NASA), the Department of Defense (DOD), or even the National Science Foundation (NSF). Non-profits, such as the National Outdoor Leadership School (NOLS), seek out wilderness physicians to help develop or teach curricula. Further, wilderness physicians have established themselves in academia by being part of fellowship programs and developing wilderness tracts in both medical and residency training.

As caregivers, wilderness physicians may work in stationary and remote locations providing treatment for injured patients. There are roles for wilderness physicians in polar stations, high altitude clinics, and clinics in tropical locations encountering sea and jungle-related illnesses. These physicians are not only proficient in diagnostics related to their surroundings, which may not have been emphasized during their Emergency Medicine residency, but are also comfortable with making decisions regarding field treatment versus evacuation. Patient care can also occur in technically challenging circumstances, such as being a medical officer during an expedition or participating in complex search and rescue operations. Wilderness physicians can administer onsite care, but to fill this roll competently, additional rescue training is often necessary.

Lastly, wilderness physicians have an enthusiasm for partaking in wilderness activities themselves, either for recreational or lifestyle objectives. Possessing supplementary knowledge of how their own physiology adapts to certain exposures prevents unintended consequences and allows for unique experiences that were previously unobtainable. When in groups, they can transform into caregiver roles should an injury or illness occur, providing a most welcome resource for all involved.

Wilderness physicians have exceptional opportunities to entwine their passion for the outdoors and their profession. However, competency in this field requires a mastery of knowledge, procedural skills, and the development of an improvisational mindset not typically emphasized in Emergency Medicine residencies. To ensure proficient wilderness medical care, additional education by Emergency Medicine physicians is often warranted.

Pre-Fellowship Wilderness Medicine Educational Opportunities

There are many Wilderness Medicine training options available, exclusive of an Accreditation Council for Graduate Medical Education (GME) fellowship. Some Wilderness Medicine fellowship program directors might even consider involvement with a few of these opportunities as necessary precursors before applying for a formal Wilderness Medicine fellowship. The following are a few that are accessible in the United States:

1. ***The Wilderness Medical Society (WMS)***: conceived by three pillars of the American Wilderness Medicine community, Drs. Auerbach, Geehr, and Kizer founded this non-profit society in 1983 to further wilderness-related healthcare, research, and education [3]. Today, the WMS is largely considered the leading Wilderness Medicine organization and offers its own research journal (*Wilderness and Environmental Medicine*), magazine, clinical practice guidelines, and library of wilderness presentations, along with the following selected activities:

   (a) *Conferences:* hosted twice a year, these gatherings bring together past and present leaders of Wilderness Medicine to educate, present research, and discuss areas of advocacy. Meetings are held in picturesque locations and can be an informal way to meet future fellowship directors.
   (b) *The Fellowship in the Academy of Wilderness Medicine (FAWM)*: this is an educational program that is separate from GME wilderness fellowships designed to demonstrate exemplary education, leadership, and service in the field. Resident physicians are eligible for this designation and upon paying the initial fee, have 5 years to complete the curriculum (or pay a renewal fee).

2. **Wilderness Medicine Electives/Away Rotations**: there are many formal medical student rotations in Wilderness Medicine hosted by both academic institutions and the WMS. These courses are often open to Emergency Medicine residents using elective time to assist in teaching. Further, there are several resident-only Wilderness Medicine rotations available that involve working in austere locations or being involved in wilderness emergency medical system (EMS) activities. Comprehensive lists of these opportunities can be found online on the predominant Emergency Medicine association pages.
3. **Additional Certifications**: these are not only an easily digestible way to consume didactic education on wilderness topics, but they also offer tangible skills and serve as a means to meet future colleagues.

   (a) *Advanced Wilderness Life Support (AWLS or WLS:MP designations), Wilderness Advanced Life Support (WALS) or Advanced Wilderness and Expedition Provider (AWEP):* usually 3–4-day courses that cover patient assessment, stabilization, and evacuation. Courses are hosted by either academic institutions, the WMS, or commercial medical adventure companies.

(b) *Diploma in Mountain Medicine (DiMM):* this course combines both didactic and practical education to provide rescue skills to students in mountain-wilderness settings. The foundational course is at least 120 hours of education with follow-up specialty courses ranging anywhere from 42 to 53 hours of dedicated teaching time. In the United States, at the time of this publication, there are three foundational courses offered (WMS, the University of New Mexico, and the Uniformed Services University—open to military only) and one expedition specialty course (University of Colorado).

(c) *Diploma in Dive and Marine Medicine (DiDMM):* this program is geared to train participants to care for patients in marine environments. This certification is currently only offered by the WMS and is completed in blocks over a two- or three-year period.

4. **Memberships:** besides for the WMS, there are several Wilderness Medicine-oriented groups within the larger Emergency Medicine assemblies, including the Emergency Medicine Resident's Association (EMRA), the American College of Emergency Physicians (ACEP), and the Society for Academic Emergency Medicine (SAEM).
5. ***Medical* Wilderness Adventure Races (MedWARs):** a competition-style event where students, residents, physicians, or other healthcare professionals race using various modalities (foot, bike, canoe, etc.) and complete stations involving Wilderness Medicine tasks.
6. ***Practical* Experience**: albeit difficult to arrange during Emergency Medicine residencies due to scheduling limitations, but if possible, participating in search-and-rescue teams or ski patrols provides practical experience and demonstrates to potential fellowship directors the ability for teamwork in extreme environments.
7. ***Wilderness* Medicine Research**: a career in Wilderness Medicine includes advancing the knowledge associated with the field. To ensure project completion, the best course is to identify a principal investigator and project locally. The WMS does have several grants available for Wilderness Medicine research.

Why Do a GME Wilderness Medicine Fellowship?

The finances of being a GME fellow can be complicated. Wilderness Medicine fellowships are located throughout the United States and moving expenses are not covered. Fellows are still required to work several clinical shifts (on average, eight per month) as an attending physician and salaries are much lower than non-fellow clinical earnings. There is no additional board certification that is associated with the fellowship despite one or two additional years of post-residency training and consequently, graduates of these programs do not generally earn higher pay. Why then are there still so many applicants?

1. ***Focused Teaching.*** There is no substitute for having direct access to world-class faculty that are invested in furthering wilderness knowledge and technical skills. Unlike a wilderness course where there may be many participants, most fellowship programs typically only have one or two fellows at a time.
2. ***Lifetime Mentors and Friends***. Advisors have a sincere interest in seeing their fellows succeed in their wilderness careers as they supply feedback for the program and can further future collaborations. Long after the fellowship is complete, a fellow can often rely on these mentors for job recommendations or to forward wilderness opportunities.
3. ***Exposure to Novel Wilderness Adventures.*** There is an established core content for wilderness fellowships developed by a Wilderness Medicine Fellowship Subcommittee and Taskforce [4]. Most individuals would be hard-pressed to have come across all aspects of this extensive curriculum prior to fellowship training. Further, each individual fellowship program has certain concentrations of the core content; fellowships in California may emphasize Dive Medicine while a fellowship in Colorado is more likely to highlight Altitude and Mountaineering Medicine. Fellows should commit themselves to programs that have strengths in the areas of Wilderness Medicine that they desire more exposure.
4. ***Elements to Build an Academic Career.*** Pursuing a career in academia may not be for everyone, but those who complete a wilderness fellowship may find themselves more desirable to certain institutions. To date, many residency programs do not have wilderness faculty, and many are interested in expanding their residency curriculum by creating a "wilderness track" or developing a medical student wilderness elective. Moreover, several institutions are likely considering adding wilderness fellowship programs of their own.
5. ***Community.*** The fellowship-trained Wilderness Medicine group provides an endless supply of friends willing at moment's notice to partake on any (well or poorly) conceived wilderness escapade. By being a member of this collection of special people, fellows are privy to exclusive opportunities advertised in email chains or social chat groups.
6. ***Opportunity to Expand Worldview:*** Most wilderness fellowships have protected travel-time built into the curriculum to explore other communities or countries. Fellows are typically sent to destinations not usually frequented by tourists. Oftentimes these are wonderful opportunities for personal reflection and to explore the interplay of health, environment, and culture.

Ultimately, graduates of Wilderness Medicine GME fellowships are satisfied with their decisions to obtain this additional wilderness training [5]. Certainly, Wilderness Medicine fellowship provides an unforgettable experience.

History and Background of Fellowship Programs

The first GME Wilderness Medicine fellowship was established in 2003 at Stanford. Since initiation there have been more than twenty programs established, including a military fellowship. In recent years, the WMS has offered a peer-review process of the curriculum of programs via the Wilderness Medicine Fellowship Certification Process; to date, 18 fellowships have been certified.

Wilderness Medicine Fellowship: The Next Steps

Interested applicants should decide on which fellowships they are interested in applying to based on the type of supplementary training, mentorship, and location desired. Applicants must be board-eligible or board-certified, as they will eventually need to pass a credentialing process for clinical privileges. Some programs require applicants to graduate from a four-year Emergency Medicine residency or have an additional year of post-graduate training to ensure that they can appropriately supervise senior residents during clinical shifts. Program directors often advise interested parties to be in contact as early as possible either via email or by introduction at meetings as there may be opportunities to be involved in the program's activities during residency.

GME Wilderness Medicine fellowships are not involved in the national resident matching program (NRMP) specialties matching service (SMS) but instead fill positions using an agreed upon offer date set by the fellowship directors, usually in the beginning of November [6]. Each program requires different application materials, which can be viewed on their individual websites, but typically consist of a personal statement, curriculum vitae, and letters of recommendation. Applicants should apply as early as possible to leave time for site visits and interviews. Generally, most programs do not cover interview costs (flights, hotel) so applicants should be wary of this additional expense. However, recently many programs have established virtual interviews.

In previous years, fellows would receive a phone call from fellowship programs on the agreed upon offer date and either accept or deny a position. Fellowship Directors would subsequently continue calling applicants based on their program ranking until their program opening was filled. In 2022, the WMS is organizing a GME internal match in which both applicants and program directors submit rank lists. Competitiveness for fellowship varies by year and program. Applicants should bear in mind that the entire application process is a small inconvenience for potentially securing an incredible year full of wilderness adventure and establishing friends and mentors for a lifetime.

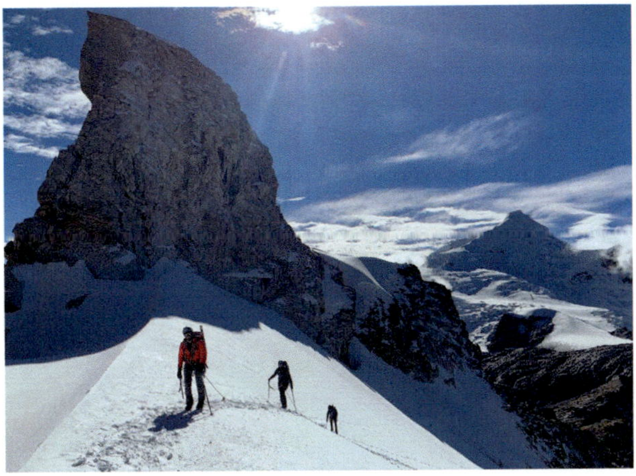

The University of Colorado Wilderness Medicine Fellow of 2018 follows her program director up a mountain in Peru's Cordillera Blanca region while learning invaluable lessons in glacier travel and friendship

References

1. McIntosh SE, Cushing TA, Keyes LE, Pollock NW. What is wilderness medicine? Wilderness Environ Med. 2015;26:1.
2. Bowman WD. Perspectives on being a wilderness physician: is wilderness medicine more than a special body of knowledge? Wilderness Environ Med. 2001;12:165–7.
3. Sward DG, Bennett BL. Wilderness medicine. World J Emerg Med. 2014;5:5–15.
4. Lipman GS, et al. Core content for wilderness medicine fellowship training of emergency medicine graduates. Acad Emerg Med. 2014;21:204–7.
5. Dove AJ, Castaneda R, Spano SJ. Professional outcomes and satisfaction among graduate medical education wilderness medicine fellowship alumni in the United States. Wilderness Environ Med. 2022;33:154–61.
6. Spano SJ. Is it time for wilderness medicine fellowships to join the National Resident Matching Program Specialties Matching Service? Wilderness Environ Med. 2021;32:12–8.

Chapter 30
Additional Degrees to Supplement Your Professional Career

Jeffrey S. Lubin

In the past, physicians who pursued advanced degrees in business, healthcare administration, public health, education, or another field generally did so only to attain leadership roles. Most physicians were generally able to acquire skills in healthcare administration, education, and business through passive observation of peers and mentors. However, these role models were sometimes inconsistent in their behavior, leaving growth in these areas largely to anecdote and trial-and-error.

This has changed as patient demographics, advances in medical science, the development of new technologies, and the growth of new business trends have started to challenge healthcare providers to expand their knowledge base and skill sets. Many physicians, therefore, choose to pursue additional training to complement their existing clinical and research competencies and interests. The choice to pursue an advanced degree should not be made lightly; degree programs can be costly and time-consuming, even overwhelming, for the typical overstretched physician. Therefore, before pursuing an additional advanced degree, you should take the time to do a careful and thorough assessment of your motivation for pursuing more credentials.

Which Physicians Pursue Additional Advanced Degrees

There is scant literature about the impact of additional advanced degrees on the careers of the physicians who obtain them. In one survey of 568 physician members of the American College of Physician Executives (ACPE), 90% of respondents who

J. S. Lubin (✉)
Departments of Emergency Medicine and Public Health Sciences, Penn State College of Medicine, Hershey, PA, USA
e-mail: jlubin@pennstatehealth.psu.edu

R. P. Olympia et al. (eds.), *An Emergency Physician's Path*,
https://doi.org/10.1007/978-3-031-47873-4_30

had advanced management degrees reported that their investment in the additional education was worthwhile. They found that some physicians, particularly primary care physicians, stood to gain more money and satisfaction relative to specialists. Physicians equipped with additional advanced degrees appear to be better equipped to face the challenge of the dynamically evolving healthcare landscape, and, like almost everyone else in the nation's increasingly sophisticated workforce, doctors who have the longest string of degrees or titles after their name tend to earn the highest salaries.

If there is only limited data available about the number of overall physicians who pursue additional advanced degrees after training, there is even less information about Emergency Physicians who choose to pursue this additional education. Similar to other specialties, obtaining additional credentials can focus or shift an Emergency Physician's academic development and career trajectory. It allows for increased networking by interacting with classmates in other medical specialties and professions. For those interested in academics, research, or administration, it may provide additional knowledge and training in skills that are not well covered in a typical Emergency Medicine residency.

Why (and Why Not) to Pursue an Additional Advanced Degree

Knowing your motivation for pursuing this kind of training is critically important as you consider further formal coursework toward a degree. You should consider this investment in the same way you consider investing in stock or real estate: it comes at a price, requires time and energy, and carries opportunity cost. Although some programs may be offered fully or partially online, graduate degrees require participation in classes and a considerable amount of time completing coursework. This means less time to see patients, less time for other scholarly work, and less free time to spend with family or pursuing non-medical interests.

In looking through the medical literature and experiences posted on blogs related to physicians who have pursued these degrees, the following arguments are often made:

- An additional advanced degree can improve a doctor's practice management knowledge and skills.
- Getting an additional advanced degree can aid doctors in advancing their careers.
- An additional advanced degree can help doctors better understand health care policy and how it affects them.

Conversely, the following counter-arguments are often made:

- Additional advanced degree programs often do not teach doctors the specific skills they need to manage a clinical practice.

- Physicians can learn a lot of the health care-related business through several other avenues that do not have to include another degree.
- Additional advanced degrees can create the potential for conflict with office managers, practice administrators, and others.
- If a physician is feeling burned out, pursuing additional coursework may make things worse instead of better; they should not add more to their plate until they have addressed the original burnout.
- A physician's time is best spent treating patients and generating revenue instead of performing administrative or management tasks.

Still, forgoing that additional degree may come at a cost in today's increasingly complex and competitive healthcare environment. The decision a physician makes about additional education comes down to the available program options and to what extent the experience, knowledge, and skills gained in any one program can be applied to a healthcare practice.

With those things in mind, you should have a clear understanding of the outcome and impact you desire. You may find it helpful to have conversations with trusted colleagues who have completed similar training; they may help you explore options and become more aware of your own blind spots. Speak with others about what they hoped to gain from their coursework and whether they actually achieved those gains. Articulate what you expect to achieve given the cost, effort, and attention required and ask if your expectations are realistic. Discuss what kinds of support they accessed to be able to earn their degree. Most importantly, listen generously and consider what they say.

In summary, commit to obtaining an additional advanced degree only after you have an unambiguous understanding of:

- What your motivation is for training toward an additional advanced degree
- What you hope to gain from the additional degree
- What sources of support (financial, professional, and personal) you will need to successfully complete the degree

Which Program to Choose

If you believe your motivation to pursue a degree is sound, the timing is right, and you have the necessary resources, you should explore options. When evaluating a specific degree program, remember that the skills obtained from an advanced degree are more important than the degree itself. For example, students pursuing a Master of Public Health (MPH) take courses in a wide variety of health care fields, while students pursuing a Master of Science (MS) might take courses only in epidemiology and biostatistics. Therefore, an MPH may be a better choice for a physician interested in a career in medical education, but an MS might be more useful for a physician seeking research skills. Having a vision for your career path and the skills you need to get there are the best guide to which coursework or degree you should consider.

Keep in mind that several advanced degree programs have been specifically curated for the needs of physicians and the medical field. Their curriculum is focused toward topics such as the business of healthcare, health policy, and healthcare law. Furthermore, the professional network gained through these programs may be more relevant to physicians than the connections that would be made in a non-physician program. Some allow for a more flexible schedule, and some even offer continuing medical education credits for their courses.

Although there are too many different advanced degrees to list, some of the most commonly pursued are described below:

Master of Business Administration (MBA)

A Master of Business Administration is an internationally-recognized advanced business degree with a history dating to the nineteenth century. An MBA provides practical and theoretical training to better understand the general functions of business management, with a focus on business theory, concepts, and principles. Initial coursework typically covers management functions and the analytical skills required for management. Programs are offered online, in hybrid online/on-campus formats, or as immersive on-campus experiences, and typically last from 1 to 2 years. "Executive MBA" programs are specifically structured for, and targeted towards, corporate executives, and senior professionals who are already in the workforce. Programs often culminate in a comprehensive exit examination, program capstone, and/or dissertation. An MBA is considered a generalist degree, with programs that are designed to broadly apply to a wide variety of industries and professional contexts.

Master of Health Administration (MHA)

A Master of Health Administration is designed to help professionals effectively run the business side of healthcare organizations and manage teams of health care professionals. Topics covered include core business courses such as management, finance, and strategy, as well as health policy, law, and ethics. While an MBA is applicable to many different industries, an MHA degree specifically focuses on management within the healthcare industry. Full-time programs can be completed in as little as 1 year, while part-time programs, which may be ideal for working physicians, can often be completed in two or 3 years and sometimes up to five or six.

Master of Medical Management (MMM)

The Master of Medical Management is designed specifically for physicians, with coursework focused on business, management, and informatics. The key difference between the MMM and other relevant master's degrees is that the MMM is exclusively targeted to physicians, whereas the other degrees are open to a much wider range of healthcare professionals. The MMM also is generally meant for physicians with some post-training experience, typically those who are at least 3 to 5 years out of residency. Programs generally run 12–18 months, and prerequisites might be required. The programs often incorporate online learning and an on-site residential component, in some cases several times annually. Common courses include health policy, organizational management, health economics, operations management, health finance, quality management, and health care law.

Master of Public Health (MPH)

A Master of Public Health is an interdisciplinary graduate degree designed to educate and build skills in a range of areas including epidemiology, environmental health, health policy, biostatistics, program planning, and program evaluation. The degree trains students to protect and improve the health of entire populations, providing insight into issues that affect communities, education on how to work with people across sectors, and ways to educate the public about best health care practices. Some think of an MPH as a healthcare research degree with a sprinkling of health policy and management. That said, there tends to be a lot of flexibility in the courses taken to complete an MPH, with most programs providing avenues for students to concentrate in particular areas of public health. These may include health policy and management, global health, social and behavioral sciences, community health, communicable disease, and public health preparedness. Similar to MBA programs, different programs are offered online, in hybrid online/on-campus formats, or in on-campus formats. Programs typically last from 1 to 2 years. Most programs require some sort of experiential component and/or some sort of capstone or dissertation for completion of the degree.

Master of Education (MEd, MSEd, MSPE)

There are several different graduate degree programs designed for physicians and other professionals interested in further training, expertise, and immersion in educational theory and practice. Most programs focus on theories of teaching and learning, teaching practice, assessment and evaluation, educational research and scholarship, and/or leadership; many are designed specifically to address the education of healthcare providers. Programs are often developed in a way that accommodates students using a combination of on-line and/or on-site learning modalities. Depending on the intensity of the program, coursework may last from 18 months to 5 years.

Master of Science (MS)

Finally, some physicians may want to consider a Master of Science (MS). The main difference between an MS and any of the other master's degrees is that an MS tends to be more focused. It allows the student to emphasize a particular area of specialization. There are countless concentrations for MS degrees, some of which have a heavy emphasis on research. Examples include bioethics, biomedical informatics, biostatistics, business analytics, clinical epidemiology, healthcare management, healthcare quality and safety, organizational behavior, translational research, and many others.

Table 30.1 summarizes these degrees and their scope of study.

You will notice that there is a lot of overlap between degree types. Graduate schools try to set themselves apart, and forming new degree-granting programs is a

Table 30.1 Graduate degree program accreditation and scope of study

Discipline/degree	Scope of study
Master of Business Administration (MBA)	Covers the foundations of general management including courses such as finance, business ethics, leadership, marketing, and operations. Elective courses may include a wide variety of topics such as HR management, nonprofit management, and entrepreneurship.
Master of Health Administration (MHA)	Includes business topics limited in scope to management of health systems and hospitals. Topics covered include core business courses as well as health policy, law, and ethics. Specifically focuses on management within the healthcare industry.
Master of Medical Management (MMM)	Management training designed specifically for physicians, generally several years out of training. Coursework is focused on business and management topics.
Master of Public Health (MPH)	Designed to educate and build skills in a range of areas including epidemiology, environmental health, health policy, biostatistics, program planning, and evaluation. Somewhat more clinical than MBA, MHA, or MMM degrees, but can often be tailored to focus on healthcare leadership and health systems science.
Master of Education (MEd, MSEd, MSPE)	An avenue for physicians interested in further training, expertise and immersion in educational theory and practice. Programs generally focus on theories of teaching and learning, educational research and scholarship, and/or leadership.
Master of Science (MS)	Tends to be more specialized than other masters degree programs, sometimes with a heavy focus on research. Wide variety of concentrations available.

way for them to do this. In truth, there is no single best master's degree for physicians. The degree and program you choose should be based on many factors, most of which should be specific to you and what you hope to achieve by completing this additional training.

Other Avenues to Obtain Skills and Experience

Obtaining a master's degree is not the only way to develop new areas of expertise. Taking coursework in non-degree or certificate programs, even through open online courses, can fill knowledge gaps. Looking for opportunities for hands-on experience can provide a chance to show your work ethic and obtain mentorship. When challenges arise, view them as a chance to take action and prove yourself. Offer to assume more responsibility, even taking on unpaid leadership challenges, as a chance to learn and develop. There will inevitably be opportunities to serve on task forces, committees, and ad hoc initiatives; participate enthusiastically and be vocal about your willingness to lead and serve in these roles. You can even volunteer to take on tasks others avoid like conflict resolution, scheduling, or compliance issues. Depending on your career goals, these real-life opportunities may be the best training of all.

Conclusion

Ultimately, the desire to complete an advanced degree while in practice takes time, advanced planning, and dedication. Be careful to understand your motivation behind pursuing an additional advanced degree and choose a program that will best meet your needs. If you are not ready or able to commit to a full degree program, consider ad hoc elective courses to determine if the curriculum is right for you. There are also plentiful non-degree options to augment your knowledge and skills without the associated cost or timeline. If you have decided that pursuing an additional advanced degree is the right course of action, ensure you have the financial, professional, and personal support you need to be successful.

Suggested Readings

1. Weeks WB, Lazarus A, Wallace AE. Is a management degree worth the investment for physicians? a survey of members of the American College of Physician Executives. J Med Pract Manage. 2008;23(4):232–7.
2. Romano M. Rising by degrees. Management titles, diplomas lead to higher salaries for physicians, survey shows. Mod Healthc. 2003;33(46):16.

3. Turner AD, Stawicki SP, Guo WA. Competitive advantage of MBA for physician executives: a systematic literature review. World J Surg. 2018;42(6):1655–65.
4. Bendix J, Lutton L. Three reasons why doctors should get an MBA degree (and three why they shouldn't) – Medical economics. (2021). https://www.medicaleconomics.com/view/three-reasons-why-doctors-should-get-an-mba-degree-and-three-why-they-shouldn-t-. Accessed 12 Aug 2022.
5. Grigsby RK. Advanced leadership training: pursue an MBA or other advanced degree? Psychiatr Clin North Am. 2019;42(3):439–46.
6. Kossoff L. Why more MDs, Medical residents are choosing to pursue additional academic degrees – ENTtoday. (2019). https://www.enttoday.org/article/why-more-mds-medical-residents-are-choosing-to-pursue-additional-academic-degrees/?singlepage=1&theme=print-friendly. Accessed 01 Aug 2022.

Part III
A Career in Community-Based Emergency Medicine

Chapter 31
Choosing the Job of your Dreams – A Career in Community-Based Emergency Medicine

Ngoc-Anh Nguyen

Just like choosing a partner, there is no dream job that is perfect for all Emergency Physicians (EPs). However, with some searching, you can find a job perfect for you. Community hospitals offer excellent opportunities for emergency physicians to practice true emergency medicine without ready access to consultants, to earn a very competitive salary, and to have more time off to enjoy a work–life balance. To successfully compete for these jobs, organize practice aspirations and research job opportunities to prioritize what is most important to you. In the following, I have provided some major criteria that are paramount in choosing a job. They are broken into Tier 1 and Tier 2 considerations.

Tier 1 considerations consist of the major items that affect your personal life and those of your family members (Table 31.1):

Table 31.1 Tier I Considerations

Tier I Considerations	
Consideration	Rank
Location	
Salary	
Schedule	

N.-A. Nguyen (✉)
Houston Methodist Hospital, Houston, TX, USA

R. P. Olympia et al. (eds.), *An Emergency Physician's Path*, https://doi.org/10.1007/978-3-031-47873-4_31

Location

As a real estate agent would say, the three most important factors in finding a home (and job) are location, location, location. Proximity to family, spousal career considerations, safe neighborhoods, and quality schooling will significantly affect your life outside of work. Urban versus rural healthcare will vary dramatically, and the supply and demand of physicians are always in flux depending on location.

Pro Tip: Locums tenens is an option that could be the dream job for many. Know that you may work in undesirable locations or undesirable hospitals that have trouble finding full-time coverage. You will be compensated handsomely for your time and flexibility [1, 2].

Salary

As doctors and emergency medicine residents, we are given very little training in finances and billing, but these are paramount to practicing in the real world. Identify billing models for each job, whether it be straight salary, salary + RVU bonus, or strictly RVU reimbursement. These are the most common models, but each job will vary slightly. In addition, benefits such as retirement and health insurance will change net pay significantly. Applicants who fail to do their research may end up in a reimbursement model that does not match their practice style, which contributes greatly to burnout. RVU-only reimbursement models may vary widely from month to month due to factors out of the EP's control such as patient volume. This model may work for classically "high producers" but might be a strain on an EP who relies on a steady paycheck each month. Plan for this when budgeting.

Schedule

Aspiring medical students choose EM for its "flexible" schedule and lack of call. However, if you end up in a practice where you work primarily nights, weekends, or holidays as a junior partner, this will significantly negatively affect your life. Night owls might consider nocturnist jobs for higher pay and a more regular schedule, whereas early risers may choose to work more weekends in exchange for a favorable day schedule. Many practices will give schedule priority to directors or senior physicians, so inquire about this when considering job options.

Pro Tip: It is important to understand that a full-time ER job is approximately 120–130 hours a month. This will play out to be approximately 12–13 shifts a month, or 10–11 12-hour shifts. Per diem is another option here, as you can start out by getting your feet wet at different hospitals before committing to a full-time position. Of course, the downside will be that you will not be guaranteed shifts. In addition, for more competitive locations, you can usually get your foot in the door by getting a per diem position. Ideally, with good performance, a familiar friendly face, and up-to-date credentials, the per diem EP can ramp up to full-time as openings become available.

Tier 2 Considerations are the intangibles that can differentiate a miserable work life from a wonderful one (Table 31.2). Once you have a location locked down and a minimum salary you are willing to tolerate, it is time to differentiate jobs by their Tier 2 considerations.

Pro Tip: The most meaningful indicator of a desirable workplace is low turnover. EM physicians are savvy, and if they are happy in a location, very few will leave. If

Table 31.2 Tier II Considerations

Tier II Considerations	
Consideration	Rank
Culture matches Ideally, the hospital's culture and mission statement will align with yours. Happy coworkers and support staff make for a happy work environment. Befriending your colleagues will make for a much more fulfilling life. Make sure you ask about culture regarding signing out patients at the end of shift, and availability for coverage/shift swaps.	
Commute Will you be getting on a train for 1 hour each day, or driving 5 minutes? Is the area surrounding your hospital safe for when you need to leave at 3 a.m. after a swing shift?	
Employer Large private-equity (PE)-backed groups will have more resources but will be a less personable employer. PE-backed firms are less likely to respect seniority and tenure and may have stricter metrics. Democratic physician-owned groups may force you to "buy in" or start out as a junior with lower pay, but you may end up being a partner with equity in the company. Hospital-employed physicians will have benefits directly from the hospital but might carry a lower salary in a tradeoff for more job stability. Hospital employees are usually mandated to attend conferences and meet hospital-set metrics.	
Development/career growth Is it important to you to continue career development as an attending, or would you like to check in and check out and focus on your life outside of work? Are there any EPs in leadership at your hospital or staffing company?	
Mentorship/opportunities for junior attendings As a junior attending, I wish I had sought out more mentorship opportunities. I had the misconception that mentorship ended with residency. To this day, a decade after becoming an attending, I still appreciate advice from senior doctors and leadership. I have since joined committees in the hospital to become more involved in the behind-the-scenes decision-making process.	
Rural versus urban Rural and urban emergency medicine are two entirely different beasts. Your patient population will be different, and your job might have difficult patients particular to that region. You will have to educate and establish rapport with patients with vastly different life experiences from yours. Consider whether the political climate of a region might be something that will significantly affect your practice and mindset.	

(continued)

Table 31.2 (continued)

Tier II Considerations	
Consideration	Rank
Number of consultants Chances are, you have trained at a tertiary care hospital with a multitude of consultants. As you graduate and practice, you take on more independence as an EP. Are you comfortable with less available resources and consultants? In my first job, I had no radiologists reading X-rays after midnight and no vascular ultrasound. MRI was an inpatient procedure only. I reduced my own fractures, established my own pediatric vascular access, and made tough decisions on when to transfer a patient to a higher level of care. Less resources can mean less timely treatment of certain acute conditions, higher morbidity and mortality, and higher EP burnout.	
Throughput Long waits for inpatient beds is a symptom of an overall hospital system issue. However, it causes real morbidity and mortality for ER patients and highly contributes to EP burnout. It also delays critical diagnoses and decreases patient satisfaction [3, 4].	
Patient acuity With expectations of productivity such as patients per hour being tracked closely, what is the patient acuity of the site? Will you be admitting or discharging the majority of patients? At my hospital, I admit 80% + of my patients and call a lot of consults. This can slow an EP significantly who is not able to multi-task. If the majority of the patients are less acute, you can easily see 3+ patients per hour.	
Physician coverage Thin physician coverage can put you at risk of poor patient outcomes in the event of multiple simultaneous emergencies. While some hours of single coverage are expected at all facilities, well-run departments should be staffed with physician hours appropriate for patient safety.	

the majority of physicians in a certain department have tenure time in the order of decades, and leadership is steady, it is a job you will want to take a very serious look at. Many tumultuous EDs will hire directors every few years, turn them over as they get burnt out, or assign them impossible tasks, and the personnel will be unrecognizable after a few years.

One Major Caveat: The emergency medicine landscape is changing rapidly. Our field has operated with an EP shortage in recent memory. Projections state that this will change. All information in this chapter may be moot in several years, and you may be competing with other graduates to even land a job. Reimbursement models and staffing models may change. Many companies have cited their goal to add more advanced practice provider coverage in the ER. It is impossible to know how the future will play out, and the savvy EP should keep abreast of these changes [5, 6].

No job in Emergency Medicine is perfect. However, at the end of the day, it is the field that we chose and love. Pick the downsides that you can tolerate. Having worked at several hospitals, I committed to the one where I was happiest. I do not dread going into work each day, and I do not leave work feeling completely mentally and emotionally drained. Trial and error is perfectly acceptable; with some self-reflection and aggressive application and interviewing, you will be able to find your dream job.

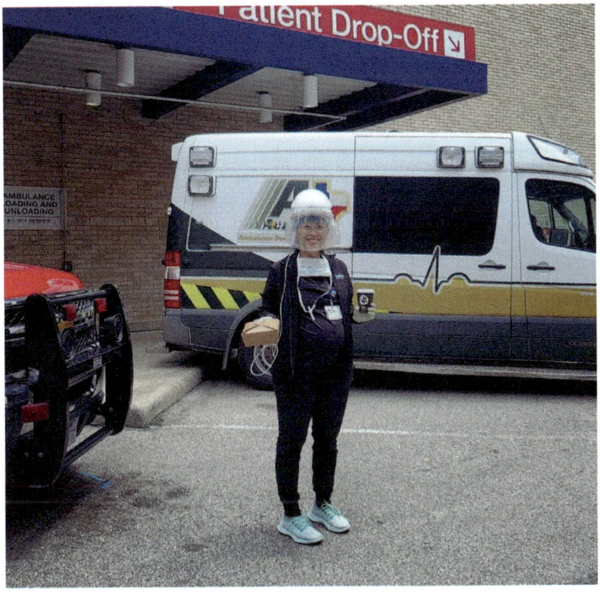

Throughout the pandemic, many physicians had to adjust to a new normal as they scrambled for PPE and learned entirely new workflows. Dr. Nguyen is pictured here at 9 months pregnant on a short coffee break

References

1. Cook TP. After the match: the disappointing match was exactly what EM needed. Emergency Medicine News. 2022;44(6):1–33. https://doi.org/10.1097/01.EEM.0000834092.52542.42.
2. Lucas R, Dandar V, Scott J. Engagement and workplace satisfaction of emergency medicine Faculty in the United States. AEM Educ Train. 2020;5(2):e10474. https://doi.org/10.1002/aet2.10474. PMID: 33842803; PMCID: PMC8019150
3. Goel NN, Durst MS, Vargas-Torres C, Richardson LD, Mathews KS. Predictors of delayed recognition of critical illness in emergency department patients and its effect on morbidity and mortality. J Intensive Care Med. 2022;37(1):52–9. https://doi.org/10.1177/0885066620967901. Epub 2020 Oct 29. PMID: 33118840; PMCID: PMC8081733
4. Patel PB, Combs MA, Vinson DR. Reduction of admit wait times: the effect of a leadership-based program. Acad Emerg Med. 2014;21(3):266–73. https://doi.org/10.1111/acem.12327.
5. Haas MRC, Hopson LR, Zink BJ. Too big too fast? potential implications of the rapid increase in emergency medicine residency positions. AEM Educ Train. 2019;4(Suppl 1):S13–21. https://doi.org/10.1002/aet2.10400. PMID: 32072104; PMCID: PMC7011403
6. Reiter M, Allen BW. The emergency medicine workforce: shortage resolving, future surplus expected. J Emerg Med. 2020;58(2):198–202. https://doi.org/10.1016/j.jemermed.2020.01.004. Epub 2020 Apr 3. PMID: 32253112

Chapter 32
Your First Job – Application and Interviews

Ngoc-Anh Nguyen

The time is finally here! You have been in school and training for over a decade, and you have delayed gratification all for the end goal of becoming an attending. What is the next step? Your first job. You are understandably excited and nervous. To establish a viable job that will provide a runway for the rest of your career, you must decide exactly what you want to accomplish. While this may seem obvious, we interview many applicants who are an obvious mismatch with the prospective department, which is a waste of time for both the interviewee and the employer. Applicants who procrastinate will end up "settling" for a job, and while EM is a fairly flexible field, your first job will be formative in how you practice as an attending and it has the potential to set you up for a long and successful career.

Research Job Opportunities

The first step is identifying a practice model that fits your personality. All hospitals are required to have an emergency department (ED). However, some hospitals view the ED as merely a requirement, whereas others have developed and grown around the department, realizing the value of emergency care as a gateway for new admissions and patients to the hospital system. This culture will vary widely. Evaluate what your strengths are and focus on finding jobs that will emphasize those strengths. For example, a person who is great at procedures may choose to practice in a higher-acuity setting with fewer available consultants. A graduating resident who needs more guidance on reading imaging may need a hospital with 24/7 imaging services

N.-A. Nguyen (✉)
Houston Methodist Hospital, Houston, Texas, Usa

R. P. Olympia et al. (eds.), *An Emergency Physician's Path*,
https://doi.org/10.1007/978-3-031-47873-4_32

and radiologists. Someone who is very good at handling multiple tasks at once may choose a high-volume hospital that reimburses for RVU production. It is your responsibility to research these characteristics unique to each emergency department and evaluate your own strengths and weaknesses [1].

From there, you will need to decide where you want to live. Focus your efforts by location and cast a wide net. For my first job, my spouse and I made a list of cities where we wanted to live, and I began by compiling a list of all the hospitals in each region. Next, use your contacts. Emergency medicine is a small field and your current residency attendings will have some connections to help you. If not, a simple web search will reveal the names of the directors of each department and their contact information. It is important to note who staffs each hospital, whether it be a large staffing company such as Envision or Team Health, or whether the EM physicians are in a democratic group, or hospital employees. Online web forums can also help clarify these differences.

It is perfectly acceptable to send emails with your interest. It is also acceptable (and preferred) to have your program director or attending mentors reach out on your behalf. The director of the department of interest will likely respond to you personally or refer you to a hiring specialist/recruiter. In addition, you may seek out jobs and recruiters on LinkedIn and Doximity. The large staffing companies such as Envision, Team Health, Schumacher, and USACS will all have recruiters by region who can help you assess job availability and set up interviews. Make your list by the end of your penultimate year, and send out cover letters and CV in July of your last year in residency. If the department is hiring, they will send you an application which should be relatively straightforward. Slightly alter your cover letter to fit the hospital you are applying to. Attend conferences such as ACEP and AAEM where there will be large job fairs during your last year of residency. During this process, keep all your important documents and licensure in a safe place to improve your efficiency. In addition, if you know the state you want to practice in, it is recommended you start applying for a license in that state 6 months before graduation.

Despite a recent surge in emergency medicine residency graduates, the job market is still favorable in many areas. Some markets will be completely saturated; if this is your dream location, still make a strong effort but have backup plans at smaller hospitals or surrounding cities. Networking will be important in all instances.

The Interview Process

Preparation is paramount to a successful interview. Formulate a strategy specific to each job opportunity to maximize your outcome. Understand that every potential employer will want to know why you want to work at their institution, and what value you bring to the table. As a graduating resident, you may feel like you lack negotiating power; however, interviews are always a two-way street [2].

It is unlikely you will be asked medical questions or to demonstrate any skills. EM is about reputation and logs of cases, skills, and comfort and confidence level.

Table 32.1 Interview Considerations

Interview Considerations	
Pay	• Estimated workload • Sick call obligations • Patient population/payor mix • Reimbursement model (RVU, salary, and salary + RVU) • Loan forgiveness • Partnership track • Guaranteed shift count and flexibility on shift count • Extended vacation time • Support staff (scribes, schedulers, billers, and practice administrators) • Malpractice/disability insurance coverage • Benefits vs 1099 • CME allowance
Resources	• Coverage (importantly, note single coverage hours) • Consult services and hours of availability • Expectations on transferring patients • Radiology availability • Equipment availability (GlideScope/ultrasound) • Physician extenders (advanced practice providers) • Medical students and resident rotators • Nurse staffing
Intangibles	• Expectations on "undesirables" such as holidays, weekends, and nights • Administrative expectations • Culture • Vacation time/long periods of time off • Maternity or paternity leave • Medical director quality/personality

Tell the interviewer what your strengths are – are you particularly good at procedures? Do you have the capacity to manage multiple sick cases at once? Do you have particularly high patient satisfaction ratings? Are you a pleasure to work with?

Table 32.1 lists topics you should broach in your interview. Research and answer what you can, and ask the rest in your interview either with the recruiter or director. These will all significantly change your quality of life. After the interview, ask to shadow on the floor for a few hours. The medical director of a well-run emergency department will have no qualms about this. If there is hesitation, be extremely cautious about moving forward.

A Note for Graduating Residents

Perhaps something not often discussed about a first job is the fear of practicing alone for the first time. I am here to say that you will make mistakes. You will have cases with bad outcomes and missed diagnoses. You will fail procedures. You will miss radiology findings. Understand this is a universal experience and will happen to all of you. (It has happened to even the most experienced competent attendings who are teaching you now!) Of course, you will get excellent training in residency, but it is impossible to see all cases and be confident in everything that walks through the door. You may suffer devastating patient outcomes, and receive patient complaints that hit close to your heart. Only time and repetitions will improve your confidence level, and this only happens over a period of several years. Knowing this, I wanted a workplace with an empathetic medical director with whom I had a good relationship. During interviews, I made a note of the directors with whom I established a good rapport. I asked myself who I would feel comfortable approaching with a bad patient outcome or with questions about patient care. My first medical director grew to be my mentor and friend throughout the years, and although we are no longer in the same hospital system, I can still always count on him for advice. While learning to be comfortable on your own and figuring out your practice style, it is important to have someone in your corner. It has been shown that mentorship decreases attrition and improves engagement for a long career in emergency medicine [3]. Personally, I knew that my strengths were procedures and speed, and I worked on connecting more with patients during our brief encounters and documenting with more detail. My first director helped me greatly in the areas I was lacking while being understanding as I learned and developed.

At the end of the day, remember that the first job is just that, a first job. It is not your only job or your forever job. It is a place where you will grow in spades. An ideal department will be welcoming, receiving, well-functioning, and not particularly punitive on physicians. Avoid frustration early in your career by understanding that it may take several years for you to feel truly comfortable as an emergency physician and to develop your practice. Organize and define the things that are important to you, and you will be effective at asking for them. Constantly reassess what is going well and what is not, and if necessary, redefine your search for your second job.

References

1. Osborne AG. Finding your first job in a community hospital. J Orthop Trauma. 2011;25(Suppl 3):S108–10. https://doi.org/10.1097/BOT.0b013e318237bcea.
2. Ziran BH, Bray TJ. How to negotiate with your hospital. J Orthop Trauma. 2012;26(Suppl 1):S14–7. https://doi.org/10.1097/BOT.0b013e3182644fcc.
3. Lucas RH, Dandar V. Importance of mentoring on workplace engagement of emergency medicine faculty: a multi-institutional study. West J Emerg Med. 2021;22(3):653–9. https://doi.org/10.5811/westjem.2020.11.48510. PMID: 34125042; PMCID: PMC8203009

Chapter 33
Understanding and Negotiating your Contract – A Career in Community-Based Emergency Medicine

Michael LeWitt

Community or Military Hospital?

This is a personal choice and sometimes may override other decisions. Military medicine is different from community or academic medicine, both in patient population and reporting relationships. One can practice as a civilian physician in a military setting or enlist (with a suitable ranking, generally O-3 or higher) with good benefits, job security, and a generally appreciative population. The salary, however, may be somewhat lower than that of the surrounding community.

The most important advice I can provide is to have your contract(s) reviewed by an experienced attorney, ideally one familiar with both healthcare law and contracts. Too often, this is overlooked by even the most experienced of physicians; the relatively small cost of this service will be outweighed by the reduction in stress, misunderstandings, and, ultimately, long-term financial costs associated with potential traps within a contract. Physicians are not trained in the law (generally) and what may seem minor or even trivial can be a minefield. I will provide one personal example. One potential employer presented me with a lengthy contract that contained the phrase "This document is a mutually agreed upon contract written by both parties." Seems harmless, right? However, when I tried to change one part of it, an especially egregious demand written in (in small type), I was told that "no changes to the contract are permitted." This removes the presumption that the drafting parties are deemed equally responsible for the document and removes any leverage you might have. This is a red flag warning and one of many reasons why I did not sign the contract. Caveat Emptor (let the buyer beware). Everything, and I mean everything, is negotiable. If it is not, that is, in itself, a red flag, and you should walk, I mean run, away.

M. LeWitt (✉)
Berwyn, PA, USA

R. P. Olympia et al. (eds.), *An Emergency Physician's Path*,
https://doi.org/10.1007/978-3-031-47873-4_33

Google or otherwise search the reputation and stability of the hospital/system. Nowadays, little can be hidden on the Internet. Is the hospital likely to be closed or sold in the foreseeable future? Will there be reductions in staffing or replacement of physicians by non-physicians? If there is a new owner will that entity assume previous liabilities (especially pension programs and malpractice tails)? Will it retain previous employees, especially if a contract management group (CMG) takes over? What EHR (electronic health record) is being used (if that is important to you)? Will new ownership change the EHR (remember, these are often more billing records than health records)? Why are you looking to fill this position (retirement, disability, death, and expansion of services)? What other people are you looking to add? Why? How can my hiring help you to meet your goals? What needs will I be providing?

It Is Not Just the Dollars, but it Is Also the Sense

As you will see, in reading through the contract, it is not just the amount you are being compensated. It is not just a simple sale, but rather something with impact on your professional career and personal life. Do not hesitate to ask for more compensation, especially if you are being offered less than other physicians in your area (much less non-physicians) or less than the "going rate" in your catchment area. You are not just a commodity, but you do have additional worth, so do not sell yourself short. Do you get a signing bonus (negotiable) and a relocation amount (negotiable)? Do you have to repay some or all of these if you leave before some specified time (all negotiable), whether it is because you are leaving for health or personal reasons, are fired, transfer jobs (within or outside the system), or the health system is taken over?

Will you be compensated by a straight salary or hourly rate, partial salary and partial RVU, or all RVU? Is there a guarantee? If so, for how long? Bonuses? What criteria? Each compensation scheme has some advantages and disadvantages. With full RVU, you may be at the mercy of a slow period of time. With a straight salary, you may be working in a crowded emergency department (ED) with high acuity and not get additional compensation despite working more than anticipated.

What benefits are offered? What do you need? What type of malpractice coverage is offered (occurrence, claims made, or incident)? Who pays the annual premium, the tail? What choices doe you have for health insurance coverage? Who is covered? (just you, you and spouse, you and significant other, children, other family members)? Are there co-pays? Are you covered for a work-related injury or illness (worker's compensation pays a small amount of your hourly rate) in part or at your normal salary? Disability insurance is important; you are three times as likely to be disabled as to die before age 65, so I suggest getting it when you are the youngest and healthiest. Is there an individual or group policy? Is it portable if you change jobs? I strongly recommend buying your own policy to the maximum amount you can get, for your own specialty (not just medical practice). How long do you have to work before you can take time off for an illness or injury, whether work-related or not?

Life insurance is important to cover expenses of education, and if you die, for a family. Term insurance is the better buy, especially if you have the discipline to make the payments, and save the difference between the cost of a term and whole life policy. You will likely never be in better health, so get the longest term you can afford (15–20 years, if possible). Some employers offer a small policy, generally up to the amount of 1 year's earnings. I recommend that you get your own policy, at least $1,000,000 in coverage. It does not go as far as it used to.

Does your employer offer dental or vision insurance? These generally are expensive, do not cover much (unless, perhaps, your kids might need braces), and are usually not worth getting on your own. Are you offered a medical savings account? This helps you put away pre-tax dollars for non-covered expenses (e.g., glasses, hearing aids, dental care, medications, optional surgery or treatments, etc.). Is there a pension plan? Is it matched, contributory, or non-contributory? Who supervises and manages the plan? How long until you vest (usually 5 years)?

Are you entitled to vacation days, personal time off days, or CME days? Compensated or not? Are you given money for CME, for state licenses, and DEA licenses? Are you given a bonus for board certification? Do you have paid holidays? Is there parental leave? Are you an employee (employer withholds taxes, pays half of FICA, Social Security/Medicare) or an independent contractor (1099 employee, figure 40% of your compensation for taxes and benefits)? All of these issues are negotiable.

Are there restrictions on your employment? Is there a restrictive covenant (this is pointless for an emergency physician, and generally unenforceable in many states)? If so, try to get this taken out of the contract. It is potentially harmful to you and offers no benefit. Are you allowed outside employment? Do you need to get permission from your employer to work on your own, personal time? Your malpractice coverage will generally not extend to other jobs, including locums tenens. Can you independently do telemedicine, consultation, malpractice review, supervise EMS, own a medspa, work as a hospitalist/intensivist, own a cosmetic practice, or an opioid clinic, or have other employment? Are your other professional earnings your own, such as writing, lecturing, consulting, and surveys? All of these issues are negotiable.

Location, Location, Location

This is the mantra of real estate professionals everywhere. If the perfect (house, job, school, etc.) is not where you are, how much are you willing to compromise for the inconvenience of relocating? Most jobs have one of three "hooks" to attract people – great location, great opportunity, great compensation and benefits. You rarely get all three, sometimes not even two in any job. Make a chart and give points to each aspect. I strongly recommend not buying a home for your first 6–12 months in a community. Rent, get a feel for the community (and schools if that is, or will be, important) and the job. Be assured of some stability in the work environment. before you buy. Physicians are notoriously bad at business decisions, and buying a home is usually the second most expensive decision you will make, after educational expenses.

It Is Not Just you!

Do you have a spouse or significant other? Will he/she/they be accepted in the community? Do you have children and/or other family considerations (relatives and friends)? What are the schools like? Are there job opportunities for spouse or significant other? Are there cultural and social activities consistent with your interests? What is important in a community to you and yours, and is it available within that community? Even if you are uncommitted in a relationship now, you might not be in the future, and you may want to give consideration as to whether you would have an opportunity to meet someone in the community under consideration.

What Do you Have to Do?

Likely, you will be expected to see patients, but do you have other responsibilities and duties? Do you have to supervise midlevel practitioners, sign their charts, see patients with them, and supervise and/or teach med students, other students, residents, and fellows, other medical people? Are you expected to participate in hospital committees, do EMS or toxicology work, occupational medicine, worker's compensation, telemedicine? Do you want to? Can you? Do you have other responsibilities within the hospital (responding to codes outside the emergency department)? What happens if you leave the ED to attend an emergency elsewhere? What if you are in a single coverage situation? Are you expected to do/help with deliveries, intubations, and central line placement?

What is the staffing of the ED? How many physicians, nurses, NPs, PAs, and clerical people? What is the response when there are (physician) call-outs? How are sign-outs handled? If you are in a resource or tertiary care hospital, what are your responsibilities in accepting or refusing patients? If you are in an academic environment, will you be given protected time for teaching, research, publication, lecturing, and other academic pursuits? If so, how much will you be allocated and compensated for this?

What are the minimum hours you must work? How do you get compensated above the minimum? Are days/nights/holidays/weekends discussed in the contract? How are they distributed? If you are the newest, is the distribution equitable? Most contracts specify a minimum number of hours, often 1680 per annum. Is this the total number, or just clinical hours? Are you compensated for chart completion, meetings, and other duties outside of clinical hours? How are personal time-offs, sick leaves, and CME compensated?

Who does the schedule? How flexible is it? How are call-outs handled and compensated? Do you have input to your work schedule?

Who do you report to? Who does that person report to? Who are you working for (the hospital, the group, a CMG, a private equity group, the federal/state/local government, or the military)? It is becoming more difficult to find a job with an independent group, or even an independent hospital/system, as CMGs and private equity groups are, well, metastasizing in many desirable areas and even opening residencies to provide feeders for their jobs. I suggest reading the position papers of the two major EM societies (ACEP and AAEM), and also the SAEM, to educate yourself. It is pretty discouraging how the field has gone from an anticipated shortage of EM physicians of some 25,000 a few years ago to an expected glut due to midlevel practitioners assuming positions originally staffed by physicians. It is increasingly unusual for the top administrators in a hospital to be physicians, with the exception (generally) of the chief medical officer (CMO), so anticipate that issues will be resolved with an administrative spin more than a medical one.

What Are the Job Requirements?

Do you have them, or will you in a reasonable length of time? Does the job require board certification (ABEM/AOBEM)? Will it accept an alternative board, or another specialty (IM, FM, pediatrics, surgery, etc.)? Does it matter if you have a different degree from an MD or DO (i.e., MB BS), or were trained in another country? Is completion of a residency (in EM or another specialty) required? Years ago, I applied to a hospital for a job but was turned down because I had not done a residency in EM (despite the fact that there were only a handful available when I graduated, and I "grandfathered" into EM and maintained certification), but this is no longer an issue as those of us of a certain age are, generally, retired. Would it matter if you have practiced EM for years without board certification? Are you able to be hired if you finished a residency but have not (yet) completed certification? Do you get a bonus when you do get board certification? If you get subspecialty certification (EMS, toxicology, ultrasound, critical care, pediatric EM, occupational medicine, etc.), do you get additional compensation? How long does credentialing take? Are you allowed to work before every last document is completed?

What Can you Be Fired/Suspended for?

One serves many masters in the fishbowl that is Emergency Medicine, so reviewing the contract closely is important. Most contracts have a morals clause, meaning if you are convicted of a felony (or, in some cases, even a misdemeanor), have a substance abuse problem, a sexual or other abuse offense, or anything that might jeopardize your medical or DEA license, board certification, or even driver's license, might be reported to the National Practitioner's Data Bank (lawsuits, suspension of privileges, etc.), and cause you to lose your job. Sometimes, a patient complaint or comment on social media, and even something appearing innocuous, can create huge problems. Talk with an attorney. Most EM physicians do not have due process; you can ask for it in a contract, but you may not get it. Consider whether or not you want it to be a deal breaker.

Are you Looking for your Forever Job, or Is this a Stepping Stone?

It is easy when you have the equivalence of a huge mortgage in school debt to choose the job that pays the most. Remember, though, that there is often a reason why they are offering a lot of compensation. It is the rare physician who maintains significant longevity (i.e., 20 years or longer) at the same place, though many of us start with hopes that the job will be long-term. Lately, there has been a great deal of unexpected downsizing, often when hospitals suddenly close, reduce their services, consolidate, or hire midlevel practitioners to replace physicians. A non-physician-run ED is an increasingly common entity, frightening to many. One should try to plan at least 5 years into the future, anticipate needs and gaps in employment (health issues, educational opportunities, family issues, environmental issues, etc.), and act accordingly.

Termination? Your terms, Their terms, or an amalgam?

Can you be fired at will? For cause? If so, what causes? These should be spelled out in the contract. Are you entitled to due process? This is often a deal breaker for employers, and you might not be successful in trying to negotiate it. If you are fired, you generally lose medical staff privileges (and this is reported to the National Practitioner's Data Bank). How much notice would you need to give to leave employment (1–3 months is reasonable)? How onerous would it be to walk away if you're really unhappy? Are you able to survive a few months without income from this employer (try to put away 6 months of expenses if possible)?

This monograph is meant to be a guide to physicians who are signing a contract; it is not meant to be legal advice, nor should it be used without consulting a qualified legal professional. Thanks to my wife, who is an attorney, who has reviewed all my contracts, and taught me most of what I have shared here.

Chapter 34
Billing and Insurances

Jonathan Ken

Billing and coding in Emergency Medicine has historically been a poorly understood topic, one that is usually not taught in depth during medical or residency training. We are often focusing our efforts on refining our medical skills and knowledge, that we often forget the importance of the business and reimbursement side of our specialty. We are innately selfless as emergency physicians, but we should also be paid appropriately for the unique services we provide. It is important not to undervalue the cognitive and physical work that you have put into patient care. Your practice group and hospital's financial viability often depends on it. If your income structure takes into account your individual productivity and generated revenue, then your own financial viability may also depend on it. At a previous institution, my individual productivity accounted for 80% of my take-home pay. You can imagine how closely I paid attention to my own billing and coding.

The billing process has traditionally been driven by documentation, where a medical coder will assign Current Procedural Terminology (CPT) codes for the services and procedures provided to the patient and subsequently billed out to the payer (e.g., Medicare, Managed Care, and Private Payers). Patient visits to the emergency department (ED) are assigned an Evaluation and Management (E/M) level, a specific CPT code that quantifies the complexity of work performed by the physician or medical provider. These E/M CPT codes are 99281–99285, which are often referred to as levels 1–5, respectively. Higher levels represent greater complexity of patient care, thus greater reimbursement. Separately billable procedures, such as endotracheal intubation, central venous catheter placement, thoracostomy tubes, and even EKG interpretation, all have their own CPT codes for billing, in addition to the E/M code for the ED encounter.

J. Ken (✉)
Department of Emergency Medicine, Penn State Hershey Medical Center, Hershey, PA, USA
e-mail: jken@pennstatehealth.psu.edu

R. P. Olympia et al. (eds.), *An Emergency Physician's Path*,
https://doi.org/10.1007/978-3-031-47873-4_34

Previous documentation guidelines required you to complete a minimum number of elements within the history of present illness (HPI), physical examination (PE), review of systems (ROS), and past medical/family/social history (PFSH) in addition to medical decision-making (MDM) in order for you to reach a certain level of billing. However, starting in 2023, the American Medical Association (AMA) published new CPT documentation guidelines which are based solely on MDM and eliminate the "check box" requirements of hitting a combination of elements in your history and physical exam [1]. That being said, your documented history and physical should include enough detail to appropriately support the risk and complexity of the ED visit. Medical coders, who often do not have clinical backgrounds, translate your charts into billable CPT codes, which is why it is important to clearly convey the level of services that you provide.

Sloppy charting will lead to "downcoding," where the documentation does not support a higher level of service that was provided and is coded at a lower level. For example, a chart that should be billed at level 5 for a complex patient ends up being billed at level 4 due to missing documentation. Even though the loss of revenue seems like a small amount per chart, this adds up quickly over a short period of time and can equate to hundreds of thousands or even millions of dollars in professional fees for a department, depending on its annual volume. Small changes in your documentation habits will increase the accuracy and reimbursement of your chart. In this challenging environment, where medical reimbursement continues to be threatened by pay cuts year after year, there is no excuse to ignore the importance of billing and coding.

What Are Relative Value Units (RVUs)?

Relative value units (RVUs) are the standard measure used by the Centers for Medicare and Medicaid Services (CMS), and often by private payers, to quantify the amount of work performed by the physician or provider. The RVU itself does not directly translate to a dollar amount but is multiplied by a conversion factor (CF), dollars per RVU, to determine the total payment. The CF for CMS is updated and published each year, but the CFs for private payers are not transparent or they often utilize contracted amounts that can be a percentage of the total fee. At the time of writing, the CMS conversion factor for 2023 is $33.06 per RVU [2]. This is a 4.5% reduction in CF from the previous year. In general, private payers (e.g., UnitedHealth, Anthem, and Aetna) have a higher reimbursement. A study by RAND Corporation found that private health plans paid hospitals on average 224% of what Medicare would have paid during 2020, for both inpatient and outpatient services [3]. This varied by state, ranging from some states with relative prices around 175% of Medicare, while other states were at or above 310% [3].

RVU is made up of three components:

1. Work RVU (wRVU)
2. Practice expense RVU (PE RVU)
3. Malpractice RVU (MP RVU)

Work RVU is the value of the physician's work, while PE RVU reflects the cost of labor and expenses of the practice, and MP RVU reflects the cost of professional liability insurance. Each of these components has variations based on the geographic location, called Geographic Pricing Cost Index (GPCI). The GPCI is multiplied by the RVU as an adjustment factor. For example, the cost differences for practice expense and malpractice insurance may be significantly different in a city like Miami, FL (2023 MP GPCI 2.564), versus the state of Nebraska (2023 MP GPCI 0.269) [2].

The formulas for Total RVU with geographic variation and Total Payment are as follows:

Total RVU = (wRVU × work GPCI) + (PE RVU × PE GPCI) + (MP RVU × MP GPCI)
Total Payment = Total RVU × Conversion Factor

E/M Levels 1–5

Based on 2021 CMS Medicare E/M emergency physician-specific data, 99284 (level 4) and 99285 (level 5) compose greater than 75% of the billed acuity levels (with 21.5% of 99284 and 56.5% of 99285) [4]. This is the latest Medicare data at the time of writing, as a compilation of CMS data usually lags by greater than a year (see Table 34.1 for the rest of the acuity distribution). In addition to levels 1–5, there are also critical care codes (99291 and 99292) based on the amount of time critical care services are provided. A minimum of 30 minutes of critical care services must be provided in order to bill for 99291. AMA defines critical care when "a critical illness or injury acutely impairs one or more vital organ systems such that there is a high probability of imminent or life-threatening deterioration in the patient's condition" [5]. Physician groups will often measure the acuity distribution (99281–99285

Table 34.1 Total Relative Value Units (RVUs), CMS reimbursement, and national distribution per E/M level [2, 4]

E/M Level	Total RVUs (2023 CMS)	Total Reimbursement (2023 CMS RVU × CF)	National EM Physician Acuity (2021 CMS)
99281 (level 1)	0.35	$11.57	0.2%
99282 (level 2)	1.24	$40.99	1.2%
99283 (level 3)	2.13	$70.42	9.3%
99284 (level 4)	3.58	$118.35	21.5%
99285 (level 5)	5.21	$172.24	56.5%
99291 (critical care)	6.31	$208.61	11.3%

and 99291) among their group and compare this against group, state, and national averages to look for outliers and opportunities for improvement in physician billing.

As you can observe from Table 34.1, being downcoded from E/M level 99285 to 99284 would mean an approximate loss in revenue of $53.89 (or 1.63 RVUs) in professional charges per patient. Downcoding to level 99283 from a 99285 would be a greater loss of about $101.82 (or 3.08 RVUs) per patient. If the latter example made up 5% of your charts for a 75,000 annual-visit ED, this would equate to over $380 K in lost revenue in professional charges (based on CMS reimbursement). Again, keep in mind that reimbursement from private payers can range from 175% to 310% of what Medicare would have reimbursed [3]. In addition to the "professional" charges described above, there are separate "facility" charges that reflect the volume and intensity of resources utilized by the facility [6]. Facility billing and coding is beyond the scope of this chapter and based on an institution's own established guidelines instead of centralized AMA or CMS guidelines [6].

Importance of Medical Decision-Making

Starting in 2023, the level of billing will be determined *only* by the medical decision-making (MDM), instead of a combination of history, physical exam, and MDM [1]. The 2023 changes to the AMA CPT documentation guidelines are quite monumental, as E/M guidelines have not significantly changed for almost three decades. In my opinion, the MDM has always been the most important part of the chart, not only does it drive the level of billing, but it also communicates your thought process and reasoning from a patient care and quality aspect and can help mitigate medico-legal risk. This change emphasizes its importance even more.

MDM for billing and coding can be broken down into three categories:

1. **Number and complexity of problem(s) that are addressed during the encounter –** Takes into account the number and severity of acute and/or chronic diseases, conditions, injuries, illnesses, signs, and/or symptoms being addressed.
2. **Amount and/or complexity of data to be reviewed and analyzed –** Data include tests, documents, orders, or independent historian(s); independent interpretation of tests; discussion of management or test interpretation with an external physician or other qualified health care professional.
3. **Risk of complications, morbidity, and/or mortality of patient management decisions made at the visit, associated with the patient's problem(s), the diagnostic procedure(s), and treatment(s) –** High-risk examples include administration of parenteral controlled substances, drug therapy requiring intensive monitoring for toxicity, decisions regarding hospitalization, or escalation of care.

Together, these components determine "high," "moderate," "low," or "straightforward" MDM. New changes in 2023 only require a "low" level of MDM to reach 99283, while you previously needed a "moderate" level of MDM to reach this level

Table 34.2 Changes in MDM complexity per E/M level from 2022 to 2023

E/M Level	2022 MDM	2023 MDM
99281	Straightforward	Not required
99282	Low	Straightforward
99283	Moderate	Low
99284	Moderate	Moderate
99285	High	High

*2023 MDM Changes

of billing (see Table 34.2). In my opinion, this rightward shift assigns greater value to the emergency physician's MDM and cognitive work. Documentation should never be manipulated to falsely increase revenue. Doing so would be fraud! However, including the following key elements in your documentation, if asked or completed, can help accurately and consistently communicate the level of complexity of your MDM to a coder and avoid downcoding: [1].

- Independent interpretation of diagnostic tests (e.g., CT scan, X-ray, EKG, and cardiac tracing).
- Testing *considered*, but not performed (after shared decision-making, clinical decision tools, and risk/benefit analysis) *
- Procedure or treatment *considered*, but not performed (after shared decision-making) *
- Review of prior *external* documentation.
- Obtaining history from an independent historian (e.g., parent, guardian, surrogate, spouse, and witness)*
- Decision or discussion regarding escalation of care/hospitalization*
- Discussion of management or test interpretation with an external physician or other qualified health care professional (e.g., consulting physician or admitting house officer).
- Severity of chronic illness exacerbation.
- Acute or chronic illness/injury that poses a threat to life or bodily function.
- High-risk medication administration (e.g., parenteral controlled substances such as opioids or benzodiazepines and drug therapy requiring intensive monitoring for toxicity).
- Social determinants of health (i.e., economic and social conditions) that may influence or limit diagnosis or treatment*

As emergency physicians, we are great at providing high-quality, timely care to our patients but often ignore the financial value of the services that we provide. Hospitals continue to operate under greater financial constraints and our specialty continues to face increased cuts to reimbursement. Updated CPT E/M guidelines attempt to decrease the administrative burden of documentation by placing focus on our medical decision-making. With little extra effort, paying closer attention to your documentation will prevent undercoding and subsequent loss of revenue. You should never undervalue the importance and difficulty of your work as an emergency physician.

References

1. “CPT Evaluation and Management (E/M) Code and Guideline Changes.” American Medical Association, Aug. 2022. https://www.ama-assn.org/system/files/2023-e-m-descriptors-guidelines.pdf
2. “Physician Fee Schedule.” Centers for Medicare & Medicaid Services, CMS, 2 Nov. 2022. https://www.cms.gov/medicare/medicare-fee-for-service-payment/physicianfeesched
3. Whaley CM. “Private health plans during 2020 paid hospitals 224 percent of what Medicare would pay.” RAND Corporation, 17 May 2022, https://www.rand.org/news/press/2022/05/17.html
4. “Medicare Coding Acuity for Emergency Medicine Groups, by the Numbers in 2021.” Zotec Partners, 22 Sept. 2022. https://zotecpartners.com/resources/medicare-coding-acuity-for-emergency-medicine-groups-by-the-numbers-in-2021/
5. CPT 2023 Professional Edition. 1st ed., American Medical Association, 2022.
6. “ED Facility Level Coding Guidelines.” American College of Emergency Physicians, 2011. https://www.acep.org/administration/reimbursement/ed-facility-level-coding-guidelines/

Chapter 35
Getting Involved in Your Community

Charles Finch

After completing residency in emergency medicine and spending two and a half decades in school, excitement for practicing emergency medicine is often at its highest. Developing a solid foundation of medical education in both basic science and clinical medicine, and expanding that into the field of emergency medicine, is an outstanding achievement and time commitment. Becoming an emergency physician requires ongoing yearly training in new techniques, medications, and delivery of care. In addition to education, delivery of emergency care requires the understanding of engaging community-based resources (housing, behavioral health, toxicology/poison control, and public health) for patients and families. Many physicians believe that, in addition to providing high-quality care in the emergency department, active community involvement is vital for their own medical identity as well.

Research on Service: Gap Between Values and Clinical Practice

Research examining physician volunteerism in their communities is limited and has focused primarily on the provision of charity care services or level of political activity [1]. A recent survey found that 95% of physicians rated community participation, defined as providing health-related expertise to local community organizations, as important [2]. However, just 54% of physicians reported volunteering in this capacity over the prior 3 years. Factors such as limited time, family obligations,

C. Finch (✉)
Department of Integrated Medicine, Midwestern University – Arizona College of Osteopathic Medicine, Glendale, AZ, USA
e-mail: cfinch@midwestern.edu

R. P. Olympia et al. (eds.), *An Emergency Physician's Path*,
https://doi.org/10.1007/978-3-031-47873-4_35

unfamiliar territory, as well as uncertainty with respect to what one should or should not do were associated with getting involved in one's community.

Given the amount of professional time spent in your daily work as an emergency physician, why then is it important to get involved in your community?

Enhance Collegial Partnerships at Work

A majority of emergency medicine group practices, including my own, hire emergency physicians who have interest in their community. Knowing this at the beginning of my career inspired/encouraged me to develop a direct pathway to active community involvement. This also fostered a more collegial relationship between our emergency group, the hospital, and our community. The medical staff was incredibly supportive of our group, as each member of the group was engaged in medical staff committees as well as community-based leadership and events. Given that our hospital was a community hospital, run by a board of local community leaders with a stable administration, this involvement was critical to my individual growth and success within our group. Many colleagues in various groups across the country have told me the same thing: that your emergency department contract is only as good as the working relationship between your ED group, administration, and the hospital board.

Understand and Embody Healthcare and Teamwork

As you begin your career and expand on your knowledge and skills, it is important to continue to foster new opportunities to develop and grow. I reached out to our hospital volunteer department and provided community-based lectures on important topics of interest to the community. Working outside of the emergency department on Friday night high school sporting events, weekend community health fairs, hospital-based community forums, or specialty-related state and national conferences are all ways to gain this growth and development outside of your own specialty. During the school year, I volunteered for a local high school athletic department in need of a physician to be available for their weekly varsity football and basketball games. During the summer, I volunteered with a residential asthma camp, sponsored by an organization on which I also served as a board member. These opportunities allowed me to work together with other specialties – i.e., Family Medicine, Sports Medicine, Orthopedics, General Surgery, Critical Care, and Internal Medicine – which impacted my own ability to better understand the individual needs and what each has to offer.

Establishing these collegial relationships early in your career can help you to start developing a much better understanding of how the entire healthcare team works. For me, it gave me great insight into building referral sources, allowing the ability to “bounce off” questions/concerns/thoughts, as well as work together with others on hospital and community-based committees – all of which helped me to provide better patient care, access resources available within our hospital and community, and share quality referral networking for my patients and families.

Relationships, Meaning, and Impact: A Common Denominator

Through community involvement, you can meet people who share similar interests. These individuals may or may not be involved in the medical profession, which provides growth in your professional and personal networking. Joining a local, state, or national board of directors gives you an avenue to share your knowledge and expertise while learning about other professions, i.e., legal, human resources, sales, and marketing, to name a few. For example, I was out of residency for less than 1 year when I joined a local board of directors for the American Lung Association of Arizona. Over the course of 7 years, I transitioned into several leadership roles, culminating with becoming President of the American Lung Association of the Southwest.

Through involvement in the community, you will meet people with similar as well as diverse interests and purposes. The relationships you develop through service become an important focus as you grow your own professional portfolio. Up to the point of graduating from your residency, many of your professional contacts and relationships surround primarily the field of emergency medicine. While this is certainly good to have, it does not help with many of the obstacles that you will face when dealing with the community. The varied and diverse relationships built over the course of several years provided me with a solid foundation, a sense of purpose, and a tremendous impact on the local, state, and national community.

Learn New Skills

Collaborating with professionals from other disciplines, occupations, and organizations around the country has provided me with skills and talents that I did not learn while in medical school or during residency training. Working with colleagues in the business sector, and learning how important budget reporting and income/expense spreadsheets impact current and future goals, provided me with a heightened awareness of daily business practice. I was also able to identify my own leadership delivery as I transitioned through different positions at both the state and national levels – leading to representing our State Osteopathic Medical Association for two terms. These skills and talents have proven instrumental in my own personal leadership journey. Developing an understanding of how other occupations and organizations function and interact establishes methods to navigate your daily practice smoothly and easily. Networking and developing key relationships are important building blocks in your personal and professional career.

Develop and Sustain Role Models

The benefits that come from active involvement in the community go far beyond what you may realize. I was able to establish key role models from many different communities and professions. The opportunity to learn from several local, regional, and national CEOs of large non-profit organizations established a learning platform that I use today in my practice and organizational structure. Understanding the political nuances that impact healthcare from local and state policy leaders provided me with a means for effective change in the practice of medicine [3]. These role models offered connections and a willingness to serve, which gave me a heightened sense of myself and what I can give back to my own community. Starting early enabled me to identify pathways about which many people are often unaware, and it led to new adventures, opportunities, and resources in the community.

You may be asking at this point "Is getting involved in the community really that important?" Yes! Meeting individuals from diverse backgrounds and sharing experiences, both personally and professionally, provides opportunities for personal and professional growth and development [4]. Through this community involvement, you are likely to identify with more individuals who share similar interests, likes, abilities, and ideals [5]. This serves as reinforcement of your interests, which leads to personal satisfaction and a greater sense of purpose. Early in my career, I developed a local non-profit grief organization, which provided individuals with special resources within their community. The use of key role models enabled me to develop a sustainable non-profit business that delivered high-quality support services for the community. Having the opportunity to share different experiences with others gave me a much more meaningful understanding of how to provide care for my own patients, engage in the community, and gain personal fulfillment.

Looking back, what I would suggest to someone just starting in the field of emergency medicine is to get involved with your community in the beginning. Offer to serve on committees, boards, service networks, and weekend events. Make yourself known. Establishing purpose in what you do – each and every day – becomes more evident the more you engage in the community. Become someone who people can reach out to and get answers. Be there to help others, and you may find you learn far more than what you give. Involvement in the community is not something to "consider" – it is an expectation that comes with practicing in the field of emergency medicine. Take the opportunity and run with it! You will look back and feel proud of the accomplishments you have made.

References

1. Grande D, Asch DA, Armstrong K. Do doctors vote? J Gen Intern Med. 2007;22:585–9.
2. Gruen RL, Campbell EG, Blumenthal D. Public roles of US physicians: community participation, political involvement, and collective advocacy. JAMA. 2006;296:2467–75.
3. Fitzgerald T. Building a democratic independent, Community ED Practice ACEP Now March, 26, 2019; 1–5.
4. Stukas A, Snyder M, Clary G. Understanding and encouraging volunteerism and community involvement. J Soc Psychol. 2016;156(3):243–55.
5. Frank E, Breyan J, Elon LK. Pro bono work and nonmedical volunteerism among US women physicians. J Women's Health. 2003;12:589–98.

Part IV
A Career in Academic-Based Emergency Medicine

Chapter 36
Choosing the Academic Job of Your Dreams

Daniel Freess

Types of Academic Emergency Medicine Jobs

Jobs in academic Emergency Medicine come in all shapes and sizes. If you can envision a niche, you can likely find it or create it within academic Emergency Medicine. To help categorize jobs though, you can start by dividing jobs into two general types or tracks: clinical/teaching and research. While the line between these two tracks is becoming increasingly blurred and almost every academic job is now some type of hybrid between the two, it can be helpful to understand both tracks in order to better understand the roles and expectations within academic Emergency Medicine.

Within the clinical/teaching track, you can expect more "time" requirements and less "production" requirements. You are expected to create educational content, give lectures, act as a mentor to learners and others, provide leadership within the department, residency, or medical school, and attend various teaching and learning activities. You can also expect to spend comparatively more time within the department caring for patients and providing bedside teaching.

Within the research track, you can expect more "production" and publication requirements in exchange for slightly more autonomy and less "time" requirements. For example, while the number of clinical shifts and departmental/local activity may be less, you may be required to have a certain number of articles published in high-impact journals, give a certain amount of national-level lectures, or bring in a certain amount in grants every year. While some find this to be daunting, others enjoy their research time and find great career fulfillment in advancing the science of Emergency Medicine. Of note, if you are interested in a research-type track, it is expected that you will have begun research or proven an interest in academic

D. Freess (✉)
Department of Emergency Medicine, Hartford Hospital, Hartford, CT, USA

Integrated Residency In Emergency Medicine, University of Connecticut, Hartford, USA

R. P. Olympia et al. (eds.), *An Emergency Physician's Path*,
https://doi.org/10.1007/978-3-031-47873-4_36

activity during residency or for at least a few years prior to applying to an academic job. Your CV and application will need to demonstrate a track record of production before hiring.

As mentioned, every role is some hybrid of the two tracks and models, but when considering a job in academics, you must consider your personal goals, your envisioned niche, and how you personally find job satisfaction. Is it by constantly being around learners and applying knowledge at the bedside? Is it by being a mentor and role model for others? Is it by advancing science and knowledge for the whole medical community? Is it by having job flexibility and autonomy to vary your career as you go?

Why Are you Going into Academics?

When I interview medical students for residency and ask about their future vision and goals, about 80% of them state they envision a career in academics of some form. I do not fault them for this as they are applying to learn in an academic environment, are interviewing with academic physicians, and are likely to some extent to have been coached that this is what they are "supposed" to want, but the reality is that only about 20% of emergency physicians end up practicing in an academic environment. So now that you are looking for a job, why do you want to go into academics? It is not what you are "supposed to do" anymore, it has to be what you want to do.

The "benefits" of academics include:

- Working in a collaborative role with colleagues and learners
- Constant learning, education, and an environment of inquiry
- Generally high career satisfaction and lower "burnout"
- Job diversity and flexibility.

The "costs" of academics include:

- Comparatively lower pay and reimbursement
- Despite more time flexibility, greater overall time requirements
- Potential pressures to produce and create/publish

Most physicians go into academics because they feel they have or want to develop a niche within the field, enjoy research and want a supportive platform to complete it, and/or enjoy teaching. All of these things can also be performed in community Emergency Medicine and outside the walls of an academic center but typically can be better explored in an academic environment if you are willing to put in the time and energy required of an academic setting.

Similarly, many residents and physicians speak longingly about earning and receiving "protected time." The issue is that it is generally an empty term as the assignment of "non-clinical time" leaves your time neither protected nor reduced. While it may give you more time flexibility, those in academics will almost universally tell you that any reduction in clinical time leads to a multiple of total hours spent on non-clinical activities. For example, if you are granted 10 hours of "protected time" per month for something like residency teaching or organizing a research collaborative, it is common to spend 20–30 hours per month preparing and performing these duties. On the contrary, if these activities bring you job satisfaction, joy, and fulfillment, they may be more than worth the time tradeoff.

Finding Your Personal Balance of Clinical Practice, Teaching, and Research

Most academic jobs are going to require at least some time in three main areas: clinical medicine, teaching, and research. What percentage of time each accounts for in your ideal job is up to you and needs to be something you maintain control over. While it may be tempting to agree to most everything in order to get your foot in the door or appease your superiors, your happiness in a job depends on finding a good balance of activities that meet your goals and needs. Just in my local region, I know of an academic emergency physician who runs a research lab/institute, works four shifts a month, and gives a lecture or two to learners each year. On the opposite end of the spectrum, I have a member of my group who does almost no research, works nearly a full complement of shifts, and spends 5–10 hours per week in a teaching role. I also know that each of these physicians would hate their job if they were to switch roles/jobs with someone on the other end of the academic spectrum.

Second, while certain physicians and institutions put more "weight" on work and achievements in one or two of the three academic areas, it is important to remember that all three are equally important for a well-functioning department and program. Do not be afraid to justify your time in any one area if you feel that it adds value to the group, the department, or our specialty. Everyone's niche, interests, and role in academics are somewhat unique, and your job should reflect that, not just model that of a colleague or the typical "job description" of an individual department.

Aligning Your Goals with that of the Department

To that extent, every academic department is a little different. Some favor teaching and education, while some are focused on research. As noted, all departments need physicians acting in all roles, and a personal niche can be found in most departments. However, it is important to understand the vibe and priorities of a given department before considering a job. Do your goals, skills, and values, along with your desired job description, match that of the department? For example, if your interest is in medical school and resident education, but a department is only a secondary teaching site and heavily values research production, there may not be value in trying to fit a square peg into a round hole. Similarly, if you are interested in starting your own research lab/group/collaborative, but an academic department does not currently have employed research assistants or many connections to outside grants/funding, it may be too heavy a lift or take more time than you are willing to commit in order to achieve your goals within the stated job setting.

Mentors

When asked to assess the quality of a job, most people point to various objective criteria such as salary, hours, the nature of hours worked, the location, and the facilities, but much more important is the people and the support you receive at a job. Whether it is someone in your niche or just someone supportive to help you through the ups and downs of the academic world, it is critically important to have mentors. Ideally, you should have mentors both older than you and younger than you, both in your field and outside. Second, it is important to have a boss or director who you can trust and who you feel can advocate for you both within the department and the hospital/university system. If you can find this within an academic department or group, many of the above factors leading to what makes a job your dream job become more apparent and attainable.

Making a Decision

As has hopefully been made clear, when finally deciding which job to take or whether to take an individual job, many factors come into play. While many of us like to make lists and compare pros and cons, it can be incredibly difficult to compare jobs head-to-head or even in concept. Overall, it comes down to where you feel you will be supported, where there is the infrastructure to allow you to succeed, and where you will enjoy working, even on a bad day.

Along the same lines, while this chapter has focused on many of the unique aspects of academic medicine and medicine in general, you must not also forget to consider the factors that weigh into evaluating any job. Is it in a location where you and your family want to live? If you take the job, will you be able to live in an area near your job or will there be a long commute? How does the pay compare to other similar jobs? Are there unique benefits that make one job more valuable than another (for example, free tuition for children, convenient child care, or "state-employee" health benefits at some academic sites)?

Finally, when it comes to making a decision, take your time. Never be rushed into making a decision or taking on an overly defined role. While there may be a limited number of jobs or spots available in a given academic department, it is about creating a unique role, not filling an empty spot. If possible, visit the department and facilities multiple times and at different times of the day or week. Talk with multiple different faculty members, both new and more veteran (a prior colleague once told me that, when interviewing for any job, ask to speak to the newest hire and the longest-tenured worker). Have detailed discussions with the director and/or administrators about your expected role and do not be afraid to be honest about your goals, desires, and expectations. Finally, have fun and enjoy the process. It is your life and your career. Make the best of it at every step along the way!

Chapter 37
Committee Participation and the Development of Policies and Procedures

Daniel Freess

Why Join Committees?

Ask the average emergency physician if they want to join or serve on a committee, any committee, and you are likely to receive a stern look and possibly an exaggerated eye roll! I get it, we are emergency physicians. We cannot sit still. We like action, quick decisions, and immediate results. We do professional Zoom calls while hiking and biking. However, we also work in an incredibly integrated system and rely on numerous different parties to make our jobs satisfying and rewarding.

On any given day, we interact with and/or rely upon:

- Hospital administrators
- Emergency department (ED) staff
- Non-physician providers
- Payors
- Governmental regulators and policymakers
- Patients
- Law enforcement professionals
- Community resources and officials
- Emergency Medicine colleagues
- Other physicians/consultants
- Our communities

As emergency physicians, we also like being in control. There are famous sayings that "if you aren't at the table, you are on the table" and "if you aren't seated at dinner, you are what's for dinner." In order to advocate for ourselves, we need to be at the table, discussing issues we are having, defining best practices, regulating our

D. Freess (✉)
Department of Emergency Medicine, Hartford Hospital, Hartford, CT, USA

R. P. Olympia et al. (eds.), *An Emergency Physician's Path*,
https://doi.org/10.1007/978-3-031-47873-4_37

jobs and work environments, and defining our practice. This takes time, energy, and persistence; fortunately, we as emergency physicians tend to have all three. Committee and policy work also does not have to be boring. If you have a niche within medicine or take leadership of a project, you will often find that you are valued, are able to make meaningful changes for yourself and your colleagues, and gain job satisfaction knowing you had a role in defining the standards and practices you work and live by.

While you may start out at the end of the table or the low man/woman on the totem pole, you will quickly find that your presence and voice alone make a difference and can have profound long-term effects on your career and workplace. To give an example, when I was the only resident on one of the largest committees within ACEP, sitting next to some of the most prominent names within our specialty, I once raised my hand during a discussion on whether to renew an important ACEP policy. Sheepishly and a bit guiltily, I spoke against the comments of a few prominent individuals who had previously spoken and recommended a major change to the policy. Three minutes and some minor discussion later, the whole committee voted to accept my recommendations, and the policy was modified in what I felt was a meaningful way for myself and my colleagues. This story may sound heroic and self-congratulatory, but after many years of working and serving in this arena, I have come to learn that my story is, in fact, just routine. This is how committees work and typically every person's voice and presence matter.

On the flip side, serving on committees and performing policy work can be just as important defensively as it is offensively. Everyone remembers when they created a new policy or had a breakthrough, but it is just as important to be there to protect your interests against others who do not understand your specialty. As another example, when I was asked to serve on a 16-person statewide committee (composed of doctors, insurance lobbyists, government regulators, and private citizens) reviewing certain aspects of the billing interactions between doctors, patients, and insurance companies, we (myself and my fellow doctors on the committee) got zero of our proposals and recommendations ratified by the entire group but were wildly successful in educating government officials on the unique nature of emergency medicine billing and the financial strains placed on departments. Since then, while we have still never gotten our "dream" billing legislation passed on the state level, in a state known as "the Insurance Capital of the World," where many if not most state healthcare regulators come out of the insurance industry, we have been able to defend against encroachments and inequitable billing proposals by the insurance lobby. Consistently, legislators and regulators have stood up and cited what they learned from us on that committee as reasons to protect doctors and emergency physicians from unfair billing practices by the insurance industry.

What Change Are you Interested in Effecting?

Emergency physicians affect a great amount of change by serving on committees and helping to create policies and procedures, but one physician cannot do everything. In fact, if you try, and overextend yourself, you will likely be less effective and less satisfied with your work and the time spent. Rather, it is important to find a niche or a few areas where you feel you have some knowledge and/or passion to contribute. That knowledge could be from past experiences, from a desire to learn, or even from a single patient where you feel a change in policy could have made a human difference. You also need to define in what arena you wish to contribute. While you can obviously contribute in multiple arenas, you must first decide whether you are interested in local departmental issues, hospital-wide issues, state-wide issues, national issues, or even issues slightly outside medicine (homelessness, community resources, and mentorship).

The following are all areas where committee and policy work can make a meaningful difference:

- Intra-Departmental Committees
  - Quality, Scheduling, Billing, Patient Experience, and Education
- Inter-Departmental
  - Trauma, Neurology, Hospitalist, Cardiology, and Transfer Protocols
- Hospital.
  - Medical Staff, Quality Review, Physician Executive, Diversity Equity and Inclusion, Wellness, Credentialing, Finance, Legal/Risk Management, and Ethics
- Local
  - Town/Hospital Relations, Philanthropy, Community Engagement, and Public Education
- State-wide
  - Legislative, Regulatory, Medical Board, and State Medical Societies/Colleges
- National
  - Legislative, Regulatory, and National Medical Societies/Colleges

Local vs. Regional vs. National

As mentioned above, there are various levels on which you can serve and make a difference. Like running for office, you must decide on what level you wish to make a difference. Do you want to fix the admission process at your local ED, or do you want to create admission standards for the nation? Both are necessary and both can be fulfilling. Do you want to work on the state level to improve the local malpractice and/or medical billing environment, or do you want to try to set insurance and coverage standards for the nation? While the easy answer is to work on both, both take significant time, dedication, and advocacy. On the local front, changes and improvements can often be made quicker and with more efficiency. You see them and live them on a daily basis. Changes on the regional and national levels typically take more time and patience but can be more long-lasting and influential.

How to Get Involved?

It is said that 90% of success is showing up. When I was a young and eager second-year resident, I carved out time in my schedule to attend the ACEP Leadership and Advocacy Conference. There I ended up at a state dinner sitting at a table with multiple members of the ACEP Board of Directors. I did not know exactly how or if I wanted to "get involved," but in conversation, I mentioned some of my personal interests and experiences to one of the board members. Three days later, I was the EMRA Representative to one of the largest committees within ACEP. Fast forward a decade, I am now finishing my third year as Chair of that very same committee. I relate this not as a message of personal accomplishment, but rather as a statement of inclusion. Leaders are always looking for interested individuals to assist and serve. All you have to do is ask and/or show interest. While there are rare committees that have a waitlist or hurdles to get involved, in most situations, a willing participant will always be accepted and even promoted if they show effort and dedication.

With this in mind, a long-time ED department director once lectured that he requested all his junior faculty pick an "unpopular" hospital committee on which to serve. This may sound like a punishment or counterproductive to getting engaged, but he explained that, on these committees, even the smallest amount of effort and interest can make a monumental difference, gain notice from hospital administrators and colleagues, and quickly lead to leadership roles within the committee and the hospital. In other words, if you show interest and are willing to work/give of your time, you will be rewarded both in professional advancement and career fulfillment.

Roles Stemming from Committee Participation and Involvement

Emergency physicians are uniquely qualified to hold administrative and leadership positions within healthcare. We have a broad base of medical knowledge, deal with the entire healthcare landscape on a daily basis, interact with physicians of all specialties, and have an insider perspective on the needs of our communities. We have the ability to analyze data and information quickly in order to make rapid decisions and we feel comfortable being the person or people to make decisions. Additionally, depending on the position or role, we tend to have more flexible schedules than many other physicians. The one main qualification emergency physicians often lack in terms of leadership credentials (besides a willingness to get dressed up "fancy" for work) is experience with committees and collaborative meetings. Hence, if you can gain experience and even better find professional satisfaction within this realm, endless opportunities are available.

As with involvement, positions can be held both locally and nationally. While certainly not an exhaustive list, some examples of positions for which emergency physicians are often qualified are:

Locally
- Department Chair or Administration
- Quality Director
- Wellness Director
- Medical Staff Board of Directors or Physician Executive Committee
- CMO/CEO/Vice President of Medical Affairs
- Town or Local Elected Office

Regionally
- Board of Directors of State ACEP Chapter
- Committee Chair of State ACEP Chapter
- Leadership in other State Medical Societies
- CMO or similar for Private Medical Companies

Nationally
- Elected or Appointed Positions within ACEP
- Elected or Appointed Positions within other National Medical Societies
- National Elected Office

In conclusion, we can all make a difference in our departments and communities if we take the time to share our knowledge, experiences, and expertise. Whether that is through joining a committee within your department, creating practice standards through your national professional organization, becoming CEO of your hospital system, or running for public office, emergency physicians are uniquely qualified to lead. Beyond recognition and the benefit to the community, working on committees and taking on leadership roles improves job satisfaction, diversifies one's career, and often opens up opportunities that might not otherwise be available. However, it takes raising your hand, volunteering your time, and starting somewhere! What change can you make if you put your mind to it?

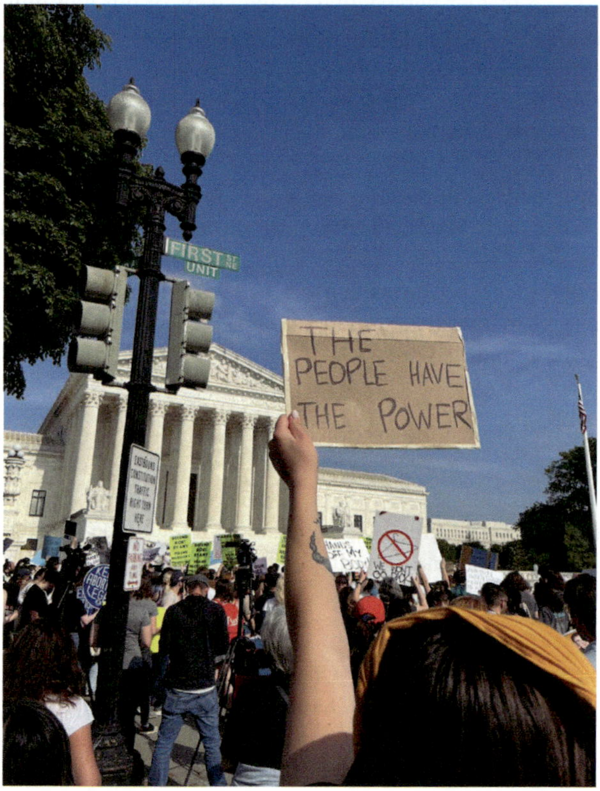

The scene outside the U.S. Supreme Court while in Washington DC for committee and policy work on the date the "Dobbs" decision was leaked

Chapter 38
Understanding and Negotiating Your Contract: A Career in Academic-Based Emergency Medicine

Michael LeWitt

Have Your Contract Reviewed by an Attorney

Ideally, this should be a counselor who is familiar with health law, medical practice, and contract law. This individual is your defense against signing something that is not in your best interest. As you are familiar with medical practice, an attorney is familiar with legal practice and contract law and can help you avoid a minefield that could impact severely your job, financial future, and even your career.

This is probably the most important piece of advice in this article, and one too often overlooked by new and even experienced physicians. We are not, generally speaking, trained in the law, and the playing field is unfamiliar and tilted for the unwary. A word or phrase, used in an unfamiliar context, may represent more than it appears. I will provide one personal example. One potential employer presented me with a lengthy contract that contained the phrase "This document is a mutually agreed upon contract written by both parties." Seems innocuous, right? However, when I tried to change one part of it, an especially egregious demand written into the contract, I was told "No changes to the contract are permitted." This removes the presumption that the drafting parties (writers of the contract) are deemed responsible for the writing of the document and removes any leverage you might have. This is a red flag warning, and, one of many reasons why I did not sign the contract. Caveat emptor. Everything is negotiable. If it is not, that is also a red flag. You should be prepared to walk, or run, away.

M. LeWitt (✉)
Berwyn, PA, USA

R. P. Olympia et al. (eds.), *An Emergency Physician's Path*,
https://doi.org/10.1007/978-3-031-47873-4_38

Google, or Otherwise Research, the Stability of the Hospital, System, and Program

Is it likely to be closed in the foreseeable future? Has it become embroiled in financial problems and lawsuits, or is it a target for buyout by another system? Have there been reductions in staffing, replacement of key executives, and replacement of physicians by non-physicians either in clinical or administrative settings? If there is a new owner, do you have any guarantees that your contract will be continued or honored? Will a new owner assume previous liabilities? Will it retain current employees and maintain staffing levels the same? If a contract management group (CMG) is coming in, what stability will you have regarding salary, benefits, or hiring? What EHR (electronic health record) is being used (if that is important to you – and it should be)? Will this change if there is new ownership?

It Is Not Just the Dollars, but it Is Also the Sense

As one will see in reading through the items listed, the terms of the contract are far more than just the amount you are being compensated for. It is not just a simple sale, like one that might occur at a store, but rather one with an impact on your professional and personal life. Do not hesitate to ask for more compensation, especially if you are being offered less than other equivalent physicians (much less non-physicians), or less than the comparable rate in your community or catchment area. You are a commodity, it is true, but you have worth, and you should not sell yourself short. Do you get a signing bonus? It is negotiable. If so, how much (it is negotiable)? Do you get a relocation bonus (it is negotiable, as is the amount)? Do you have to repay some or all of any bonuses you receive if you leave before the contracted time (if you are fired, quit, disabled, transfer jobs within the system, or die)?

Location, Location, Location

This is the mantra of real estate professionals everywhere. If the perfect (job, house, school, etc.) is not where you are or might be, to what degree are you willing to compromise for the inconvenience of relocation? Most jobs have one of three hooks to attract people – compensation and benefits, opportunity, and location. Most jobs do not have all three, and many do not even have two. If you have your heart set on practicing in, say, San Diego, San Francisco, Boston, New York, Austin, Pacific Northwest, Atlanta, Washington DC, or other highly desirable locations, consider that these are desirable for others, and you may have to give up something in exchange, and the same is true with regard to opportunity or compensation and benefits. Make a chart, give points to each item in the contract, and compare it with your ideal job.

I strongly recommend that you do not buy a house within your new community for at least 6–12 months. Rent first, and give yourself time to look around for the best location and assurance of stability in the work environment. Physicians are notoriously bad at business decisions, and buying a house is one of the most expensive you will make.

It Is Not Just you

Do you have a significant other or spouse, partner, children, parents, other relatives, or other family considerations? What are the school systems like? Are there job opportunities for others? What are the cultural, sports, and social opportunities in the community? What is important to you and yours, and is this easily accessible nearby? Even if you are uncommitted now, you might not be in the future, and you need to see if a potential partner/significant other would be available in the community under consideration, and how that person might regard the community.

What Are Your Responsibilities?

Are you just seeing patients clinically? In an academic setting, you will likely have teaching responsibilities. Does this include medical students, interns, residents, fellows, and other physicians? Do you have others to teach, such as EMTs, paramedics, EMS students, nurses and nursing students, NPs and students, PAs and students, and pre-medical students? Do you have to supervise any or all of these people, see patients with them, and sign their charts? Do you have any authority or choice over who you might be responsible for, or are you a "liability buffer?" Are you expected or required to serve on hospital committees? Do you want to? Can you? Are you expected/required to do telemedicine?

Do you have other tasks within the hospital, such as responding to codes outside of the emergency department (ED)? What happens if you leave the ED unattended because of a code elsewhere? Are you expected to do deliveries? Are you expected to assist outside of the department (e.g., central lines, intubations, etc.), especially in a single coverage situation?

What is the staffing of the ED? How many physicians (minimum and maximum) and how many pharmacists (if any), mid-levels (PAs and NPs), RNs, LPNs, aides, and clerks? How are sign-outs handled? Are you responsible for signing charts of mid-levels? If you are a receiving hospital, do you have responsibilities in accepting or declining patient transfers (study EMTALA!)?

Will you be given protected time for teaching, research, and other academic pursuits? If so, how much will you be allocated, and compensated, for this?

What are the minimum hours you must work? How do you get compensated above the minimum? Are you the "newbie" with regard to days, nights, holidays, weekends, and CME time, or is there equitable distribution from the beginning?

Most contracts specify a minimum number of hours (often, 1680 per annum), but you must clarify if this is total hours, just clinical hours, or does it include academic time, as well? Do not expect compensated time for chart completion; that is a rarity these days. Do you get PTO, compensated or not? How much CME time are you allowed? What is your CME stipend?

Who does the scheduling? How flexible is it? Who covers gaps? Is this compensated or mandatory? Do you have any meaningful input to your work schedule and time off, or is this done by fiat? In one of my prior jobs, I offered to do the schedule. I did not mind scheduling myself for an extra shift to help balance the load and used a commercially available and inexpensive program (AMION) to do so. I did get compensated for my time in doing the schedule; though some places schedule up to a year in advance, I found 1 month at a time was more manageable. It may be easier to make switches, especially at the last minute, if you are not booked out for the entire year.

Who Is the Boss?

Who do you report to? Who does that person report to? Who are you actually working for (independent group, hospital, or CMG)? It is becoming increasingly uncommon to find a job with an independent group, and even a hospital or hospital system, as CMGs and private equity groups are becoming increasingly prevalent and, in some areas, dominant or exclusive in a region. Choices are becoming limited. Some CMGs have even taken over academic residencies, partially to control the direction of new graduates. I suggest reading the position papers of the major EM groups (ACEP, AAEM), and SAEM on this topic, to educate yourself; it is pretty discouraging. You will generally have an ED director, often but not always on site. I hope it is a physician, though not infrequently it is not. The director generally reports to someone in the C-suite, either the CMO or COO, sometimes the CEO. Only the CMO is (generally) a physician, so do not expect medical issues to have the same import as administrative issues that go up the corporate ladder.

What Do you Need to Do your Job?

Does the job require board certification (generally either ABEM or AOBEM, though some places accept boards in other specialties such as IM, FM, GS, Peds, or even some of the boards not designated by the NBMS)? If not, will you have it within a few years? Do you get a bonus for passing the certification exams, for recertifying? Does it matter if you have a non-traditional medical degree (i.e., not an MD or DO) like MBBS? Do not try passing for a physician if you have a doctorate such as DNP or doctorate in medical sciences (PA), or a PhD. You are not a physician, even if you call yourself one (eg. chiropractor, podiatrist, "cathopathic" physician, etc.).

Is completion of a residency in EM required? This is not much of an issue as board certification is no longer grandfathered, but it was a problem at one time. Can you be hired if you haven't taken/passed the board examinations, assuming you still have eligibility? Do you get a bonus if you have taken training in, or have certification by one or more of the subspecialty boards (EMS, ultrasound, toxicology, Peds EM, Occupational Medicine, and critical care), or have an additional certification (Peds, IM, GS, OB-Gyn, FM, and OccMed)?

How Could you Lose Your Job?

One serves many masters in the fishbowl that is Emergency Medicine. Most contracts have a morals clause, meaning if you are convicted of a felony (and sometimes a misdemeanor), especially if it involves drug dealing, sometimes drug or alcohol use, abuse, sexual crimes, etc., or anything that might jeopardize your state or federal (i.e., DEA) licenses, or, in some instances, your board certification, you may lose your job and/or be reported to the National Practitioner's Data Bank. Sometimes, unfortunately, an innocuous appearing patient complaint (often "I didn't get the medications I wanted") can come back to haunt you, as can (anonymous) complaints on social media (yours or others), from co-workers, a complaint about waiting to be seen or overcrowding, as well as legal action, whether meritorious or not. Most EM physicians do not have due process, and, while you can ask for it in a contract, it should not be a deal breaker if you do not get it (as you likely will not).

Is this a Stepping Stone, or Your "Forever" Job?

It is the rare person who maintains significant longevity (i.e., 20 years or longer) in the same position, though many of us start with high hopes that this will be the case. Lately, there has been a great deal of downsizing of physician jobs in EM, unexpectedly in many cases, as hospitals close or consolidate, reduce services, or, unfortunately, hire mid-levels to do the work of physicians. A non-physician-run ED is an increasingly common entity, though frightening to many. It was not so long along that a shortfall of EM physicians on the order of 25,000 was predicted; now, there may be a glut, as non-physicians have increasingly taken on what were previously exclusively physician responsibilities an practice. One should try to plan at least 5 years in the future and anticipate needs and possible gaps in employment (health issues, educational opportunities, family obligations, environmental issues, etc.) and budget/plan accordingly.

Academia – University, Community, or Military?

This is a personal choice and sometimes must override other decisions. An otherwise perfect job that is/is not (thanks, Schrödinger) academic might be a factor in your signing. Most people in residency can handle an academic environment, but the expectations, and politics, are much different when you are an attending. It is more difficult to get back into academia if you have been away for years, but still possible. Military medicine is quite different, as the politics, reporting relationships, expectations, patient population, and patient needs are often quite different from those in a community hospital. One can practice as a civilian in a military setting, or enlist (generally with the rank of captain or higher in the Army or Air Force, O-3 or Lt. Cmdr. in the Navy), with good benefits, though often a lower salary initially than non-military standards.

Show me the Money

Are you earning a straight salary, partial salary and part RVU, or all RVU? Any guarantees or minimums? Any bonuses? Every compensation plan has benefits and disadvantages. With all RVU, you are at the mercy of a slow week (or longer), though with current volumes, that may be less of an issue. With straight salary, you may feel overwhelmed and under-compensated in the event of a bad week (or year, such as with COVID). See if your research provides you with information about patient volumes over several years, not just the last few (which have been skewed – 2020–2023). Do you have a guaranteed minimum regardless of which plan you have? Do you have to repay?

Benefits! What Is Offered? What Do you Need?

1. Malpractice coverage. Do you pay in part or in whole? What type do you have? Occurrence or Claims Made? Who pays the tail?
2. Health insurance. Do you pay in part or in whole? Who is covered? What is covered? What are the limits of the policy, the deductibles, what are the co-pays?
3. Worker's compensation. Are you covered for a work-related illness or injury, or do you have to use your personal health insurance? Most jobs use a state's worker's compensation schedule for weekly payments, but these amounts are far below what a physician might earn. Do you have to use personal time if you are away from your job? Who determines work relationship?
4. Disability insurance. Who pays in whole or in part? Does it cover long term or just short term? What are the dollar amount and time limits? What is the waiting period (a good reason to have up to 6 months of expenses in savings or liquid assets)? Can you supplement a job policy with your own coverage? Does it cover you for your own specialty or your profession, or is it generic? How long do you have to work before you are entitled to sick days?
5. Life insurance. Type, coverage, or term? Who pays in full or in part?
6. Dental, vision, or medical savings account? Avoid accident (solely) insurance.
7. Pension. Is it contributory or non-contributory? 401 K, 403B, Roth, IRA, military, or annuity? Who supervises and manages? Does your employer match some or all of your contributions? How long until you vest? Is the plan portable if you leave the job?

8. CME. How much time off, how many $ are you allowed? Any limitations? Are you compensated for CME time, for presentations?
9. Licensures. Are you reimbursed for state and DEA licenses, in whole or in part?
10. Board examinations. Reimbursed in whole or in part? Recertification?
11. Vacation and PTO. How much at any one time? Compensated? How far in advance? When are you eligible? Parental leave and FMLA?
12. Are you entitled to have Holidays off? If so, which ones? Are you given compensatory time off if you work all or part? How are they distributed (especially Thanksgiving, December, and New Year's)?
13. Taxes. Are you an employee with (FICA, Social Security, Medicare, State, Local, and Federal) taxes taken out, or an independent contractor (read the IRS rules regarding this carefully), in which case figure at least 40% of your income going to taxes and benefits?

Restrictions

Do you have a restrictive covenant (meaningless for EM physicians, but often written in)? This is typically not enforceable in many states but is often included as a sign of other potential red flags. Are you allowed outside employment? Can you do locum tenens elsewhere, and, if so, do you need to get permission from your employer? Can you independently do telemedicine, consult, own or work at a medical spa or cosmetic practice, work as a hospitalist or intensivist, run an opioid or ketamine clinic (all requiring a separate malpractice policy), practice occupational or worker's compensation medicine, or teach/lecture/write/do surveys?

This Is the End

Your terms, their terms, an amalgam? Can you be fired at will? For cause? If so, for what causes? This should be spelled out in the contract. Are you entitled to any due process (generally no)? If you're fired, do you lose medical staff privileges? This is usual and may be reported to the NPDB. How much notice would you need to give to leave employment (aside from health reasons)? How onerous would it be to walk away if you are really unhappy? Are you able to survive a few months without income from this employer?

The Fine Print

This document is meant to be a guide to physicians who are signing reading and then signing a contract; it is not meant to be legal advice, nor should it be used without consulting a qualified legal professional. Thanks to my wife, who is an attorney, who has reviewed all my contracts, and who has taught me most of what I have shared here.

Chapter 39
Mentorship: Finding and Being a Mentor

Aisha Mirza

Mentorship: Formal and Informal

Mentorship can be formal and involve guidance in our specific area of a professional field, but it can also be found in the hallways, at social gatherings, and in the spaces that separate our medical moments. The significance of our mentorship encounters is sometimes not appreciated until much later. This casual mentorship creates an inclusive environment that contributes to an atmosphere of advancement and decreases physician burnout [1, 2].

As a junior resident, 33 weeks pregnant on my critical care rotation, waddling between codes, I had no idea that the most profound advice that a cardiologist would share with me would be a non-medical text. I was advised to read a book entitled "Healthy Sleep Habits, Happy Child" by Dr. Marc Weisbluth. My cardiology preceptor was also a mother and she instinctively saw me at the entryway of something much larger than I could even imagine, motherhood in medicine. I remember her scheduling our evening CCU rounds after she did her routine bedtime phone call with her two young children. At the time, I did not appreciate the role modeling that she was doing for me and how impactful it would be in my own life.

Now, we also have access to social media which allows for informal peer mentorship in the form of online group forums and blogs. These provide peer mentorship through shared interests and challenges, offering peer–peer advice and support. And while maintaining confidentiality and ensuring a safe space in these types of environments remain a challenge, there are a myriad of benefits from the social inclusion and support one can receive from these groups.

The significance of finding a mentor early in one's career has been emphasized in qualitative studies of mentorship [3], from increased promotion opportunities [2]

A. Mirza (✉)
Grey Nuns Community Hospital, University of Alberta, Edmonton, Alberta, Canada
e-mail: amirza@ualberta.ca

R. P. Olympia et al. (eds.), *An Emergency Physician's Path*,
https://doi.org/10.1007/978-3-031-47873-4_39

to job satisfaction and decreased burnout [1]. For this reason, physicians in every stage of their career should seek mentorship early and frequently. Formal and informal mentee–mentor relationships should be prioritized during career development. Some studies suggest that the ideal space between a mentor and mentee is 10 years [4]. Others suggest that there is a role for peer mentorship, which occurs among individuals of similar rank and mutual goals, and steps beyond the hierarchal model of mentorship [5]. It is never too late to reach out for mentorship for ourselves and or to also provide guidance to incoming colleagues.

Benefits to the mentee include personal development, guidance in career choice, and research productivity [2]. Having someone, who has already successfully navigated something you are only beginning, as a guide can be invaluable for our own success. We can often learn from the mistakes that previous generations have already made. Younger physicians often need guidance in understanding the toll of taking on too many responsibilities or the disconnect in not getting involved enough in our medical communities at the outset of our careers [3]. Benefits to the mentor may not be as obvious. However, leaving a legacy of goodwill and guidance will often create an intrinsic reward that will be protective against burnout and cynicism in medicine. Seeing medicine from the fresh eyes of incoming physicians can bring joy and meaning to the routine of senior practice.

Qualities of a Good Mentor and Mentee

It can be a real challenge to identify a mentor and establish an effective relationship. Finding someone with whom you vibe and can find mutual reward is not an easy task, but it is well worth the effort.

The key elements of a good ***mentor*** involve these five characteristics according to Patel et al. [6]:

1. Expectation management and direct performance-based feedback
2. Active listening
3. Motivation
4. Showing respect
5. Maintaining contact

Some residents have many mentors and others might have none. This might be because some residents are easier to mentor because of their higher social and emotional IQs. However, the most profound and effective mentorship relationships often involve those physicians who struggle to develop relationships. These are the residents who are in most need of mentorship and are likely to benefit the most. Underrepresented groups, including women and those with health disabilities, also lack mentorship opportunities that address their specific needs and challenges [1, 7]. We are at risk of losing the very diversity that our patients seek for holistic care.

According to Patel et al. [8], the five key communication skills that make a good ***mentee*** include:

1. Taking initiative
2. Being honest
3. Realistic goal setting
4. Showing respect
5. Checking in regularly

Case Studies

I share with you the case of Sera, Salter, and Sordid, three young physicians who are beginning their careers in Emergency Medicine (EM).

Case 1: Sera and her Workplace Interactions

Sera had just graduated from her residency and landed a coveted position at Home Town Hospital where she was a former resident. She was excited and nervous to independently practice emergency medicine. The medicine was challenging and she was not sure which staff she could approach for help without fear of judgment. She was also concerned that allied health professionals did not support her new role as staff. She felt her decisions were challenged often and faced criticism from others regarding her professional relationships at work. She was instructed to "be nicer to the unit clerks and nurses" by her chief of emergency medicine.

Literature shows that young women get over-mentored on leadership styles, communication styles, and how to carry themselves like leaders [1, 9]. They are often given vague feedback to their detriment [9]. Sera reached out to a senior physician colleague in the department for coffee and to discuss some of her challenges and the feedback she received. She felt empowered to do this because this senior colleague had previously reached out to her and created a safe psychological space between them by stating "I'm so glad to have you on the team, it's nice to have another woman in the group." At their informal meeting, Sera and her mentor intentionally discussed the unique obstacles women face in the workforce. Strategies and coping mechanisms were put into place so that Sera could effectively respond to interactions as they arose. One of the strategies Sera found most helpful was assertively calling out inappropriate requests as they arose, "I am not in this patient's circle of care so I cannot help you with this, I recommend you ask Dr X who is the main responsible physician."

Sera learned to mentally reframe her interactions with nurses that questioned her orders, into a teaching opportunity. She now saw it as an opportunity to share her knowledge base, making her less resentful of the questions that were asked. This allowed her to build relationships in a positive manner with her nursing colleagues and she in turn realized that they also had valuable experiences to share regarding patient care. At times when decisions needed to be made quickly, she was supported to defer the interaction with, "I'll be happy to discuss with you afterwards my reasoning, but right now I want this completed in a timely manner for patient safety." And finally, she escalated to a supervisor if her concerns were not respected.

Furthermore, when patient interactions involved personal questions (regarding her youth or personal life), she felt empowered to say "We are here to focus on you and x problem, let's refocus our discussion."

The key elements of successful mentoring foster accountability, help-seeking, and self-awareness over time.

Case 2 Sordid and a Whole New Beginning

Sordid had just graduated from his residency and was starting his first shift at Academic Hospital ER, in a brand new city. He was new to the area and new to the hospital. He assumed he would have a tour of the department and orientation on shift. None of this occurred. He was disoriented on his first shift and had no knowledge of the administrative and practical aspects of providing emergency medicine care in this new site. He felt inefficient and frustrated during his shift in the emergency room. He was not sure who to turn to for advice on difficult medical cases.

Workplace distress is a precursor to a lack of physician retention. If physicians do not feel supported, they will often leave and find a community that better suits their needs. A lack of retention of diverse physician populations can be a source of harm to our diverse patient populations. Furthermore, studies on physicians' suicide rates compared with the general public collectively show an elevated suicide rate ratio [10]. One study demonstrated that physicians who identified a mentor in their career showed less imposter syndrome and burnout, as well as increased self-compassion [1].

Having a system in place for mentor/mentee relationships for new physicians allows a safe place for professional, social, and emotional growth and support. In one community hospital where I worked, all new hires had a 6-month reprieve from solo shifts, so they always had an experienced colleague available as they navigated their role. Furthermore, they were also formally introduced to another physician who could provide a peer mentorship model.

Case 3: Salter and Their Dream Job

Salter was a new medical school graduate who joined the EM residency program at Tertiary Hospital. The Chief Resident of Emergency Medicine had oriented them to the department prior to their first day and had an informal social gathering for all the residents to meet each other. Furthermore, Salter was assigned a senior resident in the department to act as their official mentor. Salter left the orientation and social gathering feeling they had officially joined an exclusive club that was invested in helping them to succeed.

Mentorship both formal and informal should aim to enhance the quality of life and quality of care for both physicians and their patients. Mentorship focuses on the transference of discrete skills from a senior physician to a junior physician. However, this mentorship can be elevated when the mentor also has the attributes of a coach and a sponsor. Coaching has similar elements to counseling, as it involves a targeted and collaborative effort to nurture organic growth, but differs in that it is prospectively rooted in the future and not in the past. Coaches aim to impart awareness of existing strengths [1]. While a mentor speaks directly to you, a sponsor speaks on your behalf, using their influence to champion opportunities for you when you are not present [7, 11]. In this manner, our mentors/coaches/sponsors provide us stepping stones to elevate our careers, help build our confidence, and provide us with opportunities we would not otherwise encounter.

Mentoring fosters important skills that improve wellness and professional development within the individual physician. Under-represented groups, including women and minorities, are at most risk of a lack of mentorship in the medical community. Administrators, program directors, and mentors should be aware of this challenge and encourage mentorship in formal and informal ways. Having diverse mentorship opportunities will ensure the retention of our diverse physicians which will ultimately support our patient population.

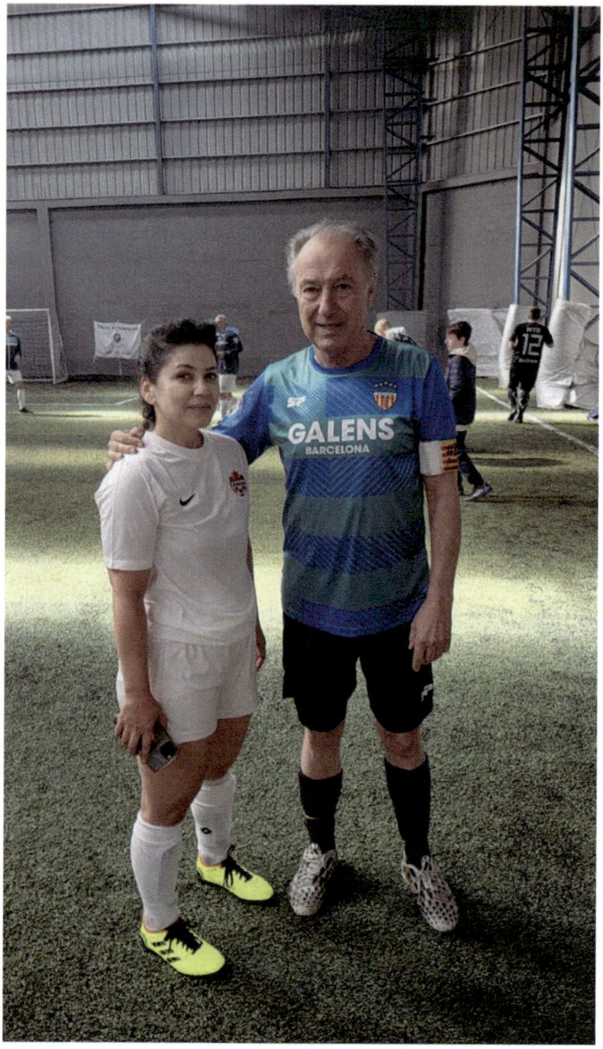

Dr. Aisha Mirza, the first woman to score a goal at the World Medical Football Championships (WMFC), poses with its founder Dr. Ferran Morell while at their game (Canada v Cataluña, WMFC September **2022**) in **Argentina**

References

1. Ott MC. Coaching reduces resident burnout. J Pediatr. 2022;249:117–20.
2. Fainstad T, Mann A, Suresh K, Dieujuste N, Thurmon K, et al. Effect of a novel online group-coaching program to reduce burnout in female resident physicians: a randomized clinical trial. JAMA Netw Open. 2022;5:e2210752.
3. Sambunjak D, Strauss SE, Marusic A. Mentoring in academic medicine: a systematic review. JAMA. 2006;296:1103 15.
4. Lopez, Tai. TED Talk, "Why I read a book a day (and why you should too): the law of the 33%" 2015.
5. Cree-Green M, et al. Peer mentoring for professional and personal growth in academic medicine. J Investig Med. 2020;68(6):1128–34.
6. Patel K, Gupta Y, Patel A. Key communication skills for mentors. J Am College Radiol. 2022;19(7):903–4.
7. Whitson B. Mentorship, sponsorship, and the emerging role of social media. Ann Thorac Surg. 2022;114(2):598–9.
8. Patel K, Gupta Y, Patel A. Key communication skills for mentees. J Am College Radiol. 2022;19(7):901–2.
9. Corell S, Simard C. Research: vague feedback is holding women Back. Harv Bus Rev. 2016;4. April 29, 2016. https://hbr.org/2016/04/Research-Vague-Feedback-Is-Holding-Women-Back.
10. Ventriglio A, et al. Suicide among doctors: a narrative review. Indian J Psychiatry. 2020;62(2):114–20.
11. Mathew A. In a world of mentors, aspire to be a sponsor. J Am Pharm Assoc. 2022;62(4):915–6.

Chapter 40
The academic ladder: demystifying the promotion process

Robert P. Olympia

An important day in my academic career was May 5, 2017, as it represents a lifetime of hard work and perseverance, supported by mentors, colleagues, family, and friends. The road toward promotion to Professor in the Departments of Emergency Medicine and Pediatrics at the Penn State University College of Medicine began the day I decided to become an academic Pediatric Emergency Medicine physician.

Pop-Quiz

1. Do you consider yourself a teacher, and enjoy educating and mentoring your learners?
2. Do you find satisfaction in conducting research, presenting your data at scientific meetings, or publishing your data in peer-reviewed journals?
3. Are you a life-long learner, constantly challenging yourself to be the best clinician you can be?
4. Do you enjoy being in a leadership position, or working within a team construct to serve your community or profession, and improve the lives of your patients?

If you answered yes to any of these questions, you may have a future in academic-based emergency medicine.

R. P. Olympia (✉)
Department of Emergency Medicine & Pediatrics, Penn State Hershey Medical Center, Hershey, PA, USA
e-mail: rolympia@hmc.psu.edu

R. P. Olympia et al. (eds.), *An Emergency Physician's Path*,
https://doi.org/10.1007/978-3-031-47873-4_40

What Is Academic Medicine?

A career in academic medicine involves *demonstrating scholarship, gaining knowledge, and providing education. Demonstrating scholarship* involves imparting knowledge that results from study and research in a particular field and the dissemination of this knowledge, thus becoming an expert in a particular field. *Knowledge* is the sum or range of what is perceived, discovered, and learned over time, therefore practicing "life-long learning." Providing education is the act of imparting knowledge and skill to another person/group or to cause them to learn by example or experience, thus becoming a teacher and mentor.

Climbing the Academic Ladder

The goal of any academic physician is to climb the academic ladder, from Clinical Instructor to Assistant Professor to Associate Professor and ultimately Professor. Although the road may be long and difficult, at times sacrificing other non-academic interests, in the end, the benefits and impact are numerous. While there may be nuances in the promotion and tenure process among academic institutions, criteria for promotion often involve achieving professional excellence in a combination of the following four mission areas, in accordance with your effort allocation:

- *Teaching and Learning*
- *Research and Creative Accomplishments*
- *Patient Care Activities (clinical responsibilities)*
- *Service and the Scholarship of Service to the University, Society, and the Profession*

Promotion is commonly based on performance rather than time-in-rank. Performance is evaluated using the *Dossier*, a standardized format for reporting activities and scholarship. Dossier reviews are conducted independently by faculty committees and administrators of each institution. Performance expectations increase as you advance in academic rank, developing mastery and independence in your field, increasing scholarly accomplishments, growing your regional and national reputation, and demonstrating professional leadership. At each rung of the academic ladder, performance since the last promotion review is evaluated.

What Are the Components of a Promotion Application?

Promotion applications often include the following:

- Narrative statement (personal statement)
- External (outside your institution) evaluations

- Patient/clinical care evaluations (internal, within your institution)
- Pieces of scholarship
- Curriculum vitae
- Dossier

The *narrative statement* is usually a 1–3-page *first-person* statement about your scholarship in the context of your overall goals and philosophy, highlighting professional excellence in the four mission areas.

External evaluations are letters of recommendations from experts in your academic field/specialty, often at an academic rank higher than your current rank, from a variety of external institutions, and without a conflict of interest (i.e., no former students, teachers, mentors, colleagues, or *significant* research collaborators).

Patient/clinical care evaluations are letters of recommendation from colleagues, referring physicians, or subspecialty physicians who can comment on your clinical performance, as well as patient feedback and comments.

Pieces of scholarship are published research articles that support your overall research goals and that are cited/referenced frequently in the medical literature. Based on your academic institution, the minimum number of publications for promotion will vary but often exclude case reports, review articles, and book chapters and frequently require you to be the principal investigator or first author.

The format of your *curriculum vitae* (CV) will depend on your academic institution. The CV is a comprehensive record of your academic career, highlighting in a chronological fashion your involvement with the four mission areas.

The *dossier* is a record of your accomplishments in the four mission areas and is used by internal reviewers to evaluate your performance and scholarship. The information required is more detailed than a CV and must be submitted in a specific format, typically including the following documentation:

1. *Teaching and Learning:* (a) Lectures, seminars, and courses given (both internal and external, documenting attendance numbers), (b) research supervised, (c) mentoring opportunities (students, residents, fellows, and other faculty), (d) teaching evaluations (quantitative information and summary of comments), and (e) peer review of teaching (letters of recommendation from senior faculty members within your department commenting on your teaching style).
2. *Research and Creative Accomplishments:* (a) Publications [peer-reviewed journal articles (note authorship role on each) and non-peer-reviewed publications (book editor, book chapters, and review articles), including "accepted" and "in press"], (b) research projects [completed, current, planned (note role on each project), and internal and external grants], and (c) other creative products (e.g., educational methods or computer software developed, inventions, and clinical guidelines disseminated).
3. *Patient Care Activities:* (a) Statement of clinical assignment including time commitment and effort allocation, (b) detail on quantity and complexity of cases [patients per hour and RVU (relative value unit) productivity], (c) quality of care (patient satisfaction data and QI activities), and (d) letters from peers, colleagues,

and referring physicians commenting on patient care ability and effectiveness (patient/clinical care evaluators).

4. *Service and the Scholarship of Service to the University, Society, and the Profession:* Demonstrating service through committee work and leadership, both internal to your institution (in your department, in the College of Medicine, or in your hospital/health system/university) or external to your institution [within your Profession (journal editorships and reviews, study sections, organizing conferences for professional associations, offices held in professional associations, government advisory groups, etc.) or within your Community (citizen/client groups, outreach activities, volunteerism, etc.)].

Pearls from an Academic Climber

My journey to Professor began the day I decided to become an academic pediatric emergency medicine physician. Here are some pearls to make your journey successful:

Find your passion and seek out your niche: Do you remember why you chose emergency medicine or pursued a career in your subspecialty? Allow this passion to motivate your career in academia. For me, my passion is emergency and disaster preparedness, trauma and sports medicine, urgent care medicine, school-based health, and the impact of media on children. Most of my research accomplishments, education and mentorship, and patient care activities have involved these passions. I still love what I do because of these decisions.

Surround yourself with greatness: Find advisors and mentors who will guide you not only through your career in academia but also with life. I was blessed to have Drs Magdy Attia, Steven Selbst, and Jeffrey Avner train me as a resident and fellow, and even after so many years, also serve as role models and mentors throughout my career. Having an all-star team around you is better than being the only all-star.

Become a hoarder: Save letters and emails that document excellent patient care. File away lecture evaluations, and if there are not formal evaluations for educational opportunities, develop one and collect the data. Seek letters of recommendation from learners, colleagues, or mentees who can comment on your teaching skills, mentorship abilities, or clinical acumen. It is not really hoarding if you keep things organized.

Stalk strategically: As you will need external evaluations from "non-biased "physicians in your specialty, try to meet as many experts in your field. Go to Emergency Medicine conferences (such as the American College of Emergency Physicians, Society for Academic Emergency Medicine, American Academy of Emergency Medicine, National Association of EMS Physicians, etc.), both regionally and nationally. Introduce yourself to experts in your field, ask questions, invite them to your institution, and hand out business cards. Build your professional network and make a friend.

Keep lecturing and writing and become a scholar: Seek out educational opportunities – lectures at your institution will turn into Grand Rounds regionally and then expert panels nationally. Turn lectures into review articles or book chapters, turn clinical questions into research ideas, and turn quality improvement ideas into scholarship. Lectureships and publications will increase your reputation and in turn lead to multicenter research collaborations, opportunities to serve within your specialty, and means to improve the care of children globally. A laptop, pen/paper, and thinking outside the box will be your best friend.

Delegate your work: The amount of time and effort to become promoted can be overwhelming. Utilize medical students, residents, fellows, and other colleagues in the development and implementation of research projects. Collaborate with other departments and institutions for educational and research opportunities. Make friends with the Institutional Review Board, biostatisticians, librarians, and institutional leadership and committee members. Teamwork makes the dream work.

Volunteer your time and efforts: Provide service to your department, institution, profession, and community, but make sure it aligns with your passions. Do you like quality improvement? Medical education? Global health? School-based health? Whatever it may be, just get involved. And seek leadership positions if possible.

Update your CV and dossier regularly: I update my CV and dossier monthly. This may seem pathologic, but it allows me to visually see where my deficiencies lie in the four mission areas and organizes all the data that I have been hoarding over the years.

I believe my career in academic-based emergency medicine has enriched my life, given me purpose and provided professional satisfaction, shaped the future of medicine in the learners that I have educated and mentored, and ultimately impacted the health and well-being of pediatric and adult patients regionally, nationally, and globally. What an honor and blessing.

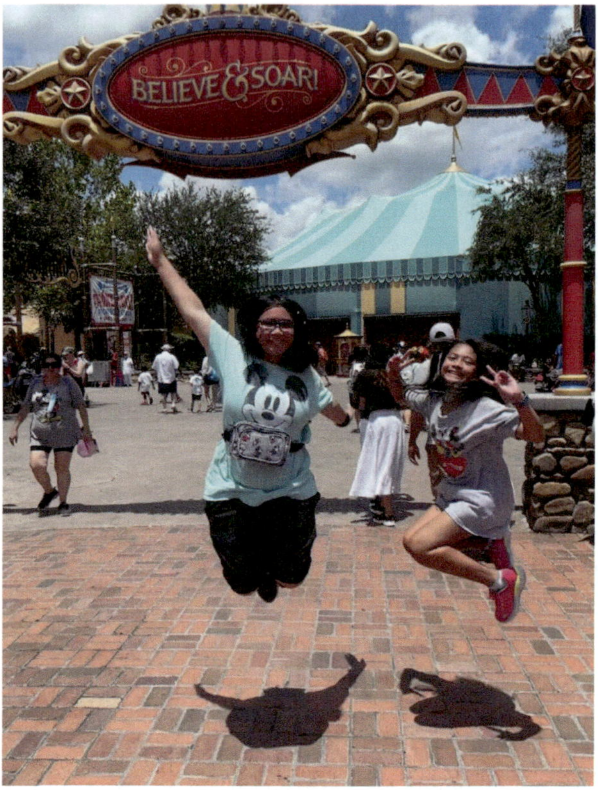

Believe and Soar. My daughters Abigail and Madelyn at the Magic Kingdom, Walt Disney World, Orlando

Chapter 41
Your Curriculum Vitae

Kimberly M. Rathbun

What Is a CV and How Is It Different than a Resume?

Curriculum vitae (CV) is Latin and translates to "course of life." A CV comprehensively details your academic and professional history. As such, the CV of a graduating resident may only be a page or two in length, whereas a senior researcher may have a CV nearly 100 pages long. In contrast, a resume is 1–2 pages in length and highlights skills as opposed to accomplishments. Additionally, a resume is tailored to a specific position.

Why Do I Need a CV?

In addition to job applications, CVs are used for yearly evaluations and as part of promotions packets.

How Do I Build a CV?

Building your CV from scratch can be a daunting task. CV templates and examples can be found online. Many institutions have their own CV templates. The Association of American Medical Colleges (AAMC) has a downloadable template that is a great starting point. Ask for CVs from colleagues and mentors. By looking at other CVs,

K. M. Rathbun (✉)
Department of Emergency Medicine, AU/UGA Medical Partnership, Athens, GA, USA
e-mail: krathbunmd@augusta.edu

R. P. Olympia et al. (eds.), *An Emergency Physician's Path*,
https://doi.org/10.1007/978-3-031-47873-4_41

you can get an idea of the formatting options and you can see how certain activities are worded and into which category they are placed.

In each category, items are listed in reverse chronological order – most recent experiences listed first. Dates are sometimes just listed by year, but, sometimes, a month/year format is required.

Sections of a CV

Contact Information

Start with your name at the top – use your official name. Also include a physical address, phone number, and email address. Be sure that the phone number and email address will work. If you are leaving an institutional job in the near future and will lose access to your associated email account, consider using a personal email address. It is acceptable to use a personal email address, but be sure it is professional!

Education

Here you list all formal education – undergraduate degree(s), postgraduate degree(s), residency training, and fellowship. Include the title of the degree earned, the institution name and location (city, state), and years attended.

Academic Appointments

This section includes only appointments as faculty at a teaching institution. A chief resident year would be included here ONLY if it required an extension of residency. List your current position at the top and list others in reverse chronological order. Include your title, the institution name and location (city, state), and the years you held this position. A change in rank at the same institution would be listed separately from the initial rank. For newly graduating residents or those who are in community practice, this section likely will not apply to your situation and can be omitted.

Professional Experience (or Non-Academic Appointments)

Here you will include any relevant employment experiences that are not listed in the previous section, such as positions at non-teaching hospitals. Any research, volunteer work, and so on done during a gap in your training will be included here. Frequently, an academic physician will have an academic appointment at a medical school and an attending physician designation at one or multiple hospitals. The attending physician designations are listed here. The current position is at the top and list others in reverse chronological order. Include your title, the facility name and location (city, state), and the years you held this position.

Certification and Licensure

This section includes specialty and subspecialty certifications as well as state licensures. If you are not yet board-certified, but board-eligible – this can be included and should be noted. Often, the license number is included with each state license. If you hold a training license, this should be indicated. You may also include any other relevant professional certifications, such as EMT, paramedic, ATLS, ACLS, PALS, and so on.

Professional Development

List in reverse chronological order any training you have done to improve your ability to perform your job. This section includes courses, workshops, bootcamps, and so on which are generally focused on one skill. Many professional conferences offer such options in the days leading up to large national meetings.

Professional Memberships

List any professional societies or groups in which you hold membership. Include national as well as state and local organizations. Indicate the sections in which you are a member. Be sure to indicate any positions held in these organizations.

Committee Assignments

List any committees you have been a part of. This section is often broken down into subcategories. If you have changed institutions, you may want to indicate which activities were at each institution. If you are on hospital, medical school, and departmental committees, you might choose to separate those. Regional and national committees might have their own subsection.

Educational Activities

This section contains any activities that involve learners – faculty, residents (from your or other departments), medical students, graduate students, and undergraduate students. Depending on your situation, subsections might be helpful to designate which activities were delivered to which group. Be sure to indicate if you were a course director, curriculum developer, group facilitator, lecturer, and so on. Any mentoring can also be included in this section. Your list of teaching activities may become so long that you choose to summarize many activities on one line (e.g., "Resident lectures and procedure labs") and note that a full list is available on request.

Honors and Awards

This section includes any scholarships or awards you have received. You may also list programs or courses you were accepted to if they had a competitive selection process. If you receive the same honor more than once, you can list the years with a comma on the same line or list them on separate lines keeping them in reverse chronological order.

Research Activities

You will often see a "Publications" category followed by other similar categories, but using a "Research Activities" category with subheadings is often clearer and easier to use. Items in this category should be numbered and formatted as if they were in a "references" section of a manuscript using a standardized format such as the AMA format. Bold and/or underline your name in each list of authors. The first subcategory should be "Refereed Publications" or "Peer-reviewed Publications." Additional subcategories that might be used are as follows: "Published Abstracts," "Poster Presentations," "Oral Presentations," "Book Chapters," "Non-peer-reviewed Publications," "Patents," and so on.

Community Activities

This section is a place to list any community outreach activities you have participated in. Typically, this category is for activities that are related to your career; however, it is not uncommon to list unrelated activities.

Next Steps

Once you have added all your information to your CV, the next step is to check the formatting. Be sure your margins, spacing, and indentations are consistent from one category to the next. If you choose to bold or underline your category heading and/or subheadings, make sure it is consistent. Your CV is often the first impression a potential employer gets of you – make sure it represents you well.

Once your CV is finished, be sure to proofread it carefully. Look for spelling or grammar errors. Have several colleagues look at it critically to ensure that information is presented in a clear and coherent manner. Ask them if anything listed is unclear.

A final point is that your CV should be a living document. Make a habit of updating it regularly – monthly is a good interval. Add anything you do – giving a lecture, mentoring a student, working on a project, and so on. Use a month/year format for dates in your living document because you might need to know the month at a later time. Information can be removed later, but sitting down and trying to remember everything you did in the past year is challenging and you will likely forget things.

expected/required to do telemedicine…

Do you have other tasks within the hospital … of the emergency department (ED)? What have …

Chapter 42
Creating an Educational Portfolio

Lawrence E. Kass

Introduction

A career in academic Emergency Medicine often involves teaching, whether it be of medical students, residents, fellows, or even other attendings. While a curriculum vitae (CV) documents an individual's accomplishments (education/training, certifications, publications, and the like), it is generally not designed to demonstrate your perspective and skill concerning teaching. An educator's portfolio is a structured document that captures these elements [1, 2]. This chapter will describe why, when, and how an academic emergency physician should create this document.

Why Write an Educator's Portfolio?

There are three main reasons for writing an educator's portfolio [3]. The most common is for promotion [4]. Scholarship in education may be more challenging to define than scholarship in research, but it has become more commonly acknowledged in promotion criteria over the last three decades [5, 6]. Each academic institution may have its own specific template for the dossier they require as part of the application for promotion, but a section on education/teaching is fairly universal. Collecting and saving the data needed for this section (more on this below) as it develops is dramatically easier than trying to assemble it years after the fact when you decide it is time to apply for promotion.

L. E. Kass (✉)
Department of Emergency Medicine, Penn State Hershey Medical Center, Hershey, PA, USA
e-mail: lkass@pennstatehealth.psu.edu

R. P. Olympia et al. (eds.), *An Emergency Physician's Path*,
https://doi.org/10.1007/978-3-031-47873-4_42

The second reason to write an educator's portfolio concerns awards and honors. If you are so fortunate as to be considered for a teaching award, the application generally requires the data that would be in a portfolio. Again, it is much easier to save the data as it accumulates than to try and find it years later.

The final reason is more philosophical. Writing an educator's portfolio, especially the statement of your educational philosophy, is an introspective act that encourages reflection and requires a clear articulation of what you have done in the past, what you are currently doing, and what you plan to do in the future as you continue to grow as an educator. Putting this into words will sharpen your focus as you create new learning opportunities and take on new advisees.

When to Write an Educator's Portfolio?

The simple answer is "continuously." Establish a file (electronic or paper) in which you can track your advisees/mentees, teaching activities, and curriculum development. The details needed for these items are described below and can be seen on the template in the appendix.

Educator's portfolios also include a section describing your educational philosophy. I would advise also doing this when you first start creating your portfolio, though for an entirely different reason. This section, usually just a page in length, will require some reflection and introspection. Writing down an explanation of why you teach and how you think individuals learn best will help you make more considered decisions in your subsequent educational activities.

All of these descriptions of your activities, accomplishments, and thoughts will need to be reviewed and updated at the time of your application for promotion or award. However, if you have been collecting the data, that should be a fairly straightforward process.

How to Write an Educator's Portfolio

There are many templates available online, and your institution may have a specific one they suggest you use, but they all have similar features. I have included an example in the appendix, with a detailed description of the components below.

There are three main components to a typical educator's portfolio: the statement of your educational philosophy, the description of your goals as an educator, and a compilation of your educational contributions.

a. **Educational Philosophy**

   This section should be several paragraphs, typically no more than a page or so in length. In it, you should describe your personal philosophy of education. Optimally, you should incorporate principles of educational theory (such as constructivism, behaviorism, humanism, cognitivism, or social learning [7]), but definitely use examples from your own practice.

b. **Goals**

This section should be a few paragraphs, typically a half page in length. In it, you can describe your aspirations for achievement and plans for your own continued learning and growth. This can be broken down into the short-term (about five years) and long-term, if appropriate. You can either do this in a bulleted list or a free-text essay. It is important to include a statement of how you will measure your success in achieving these goals.

c. **Educational contributions**

This section will comprise the majority of your portfolio. In it, you will not only list what you have done but provide evidence as to your success and/or skill in these areas. Feel free to tailor this section to best highlight your accomplishments, but, typically, the following five areas are included:

a. Teaching/Learning

This can be a simple list, often in table form, of the teaching activities you have performed. Include all teaching activities, including lectures, small group sessions, problem-based learning facilitations, workshops, and clinical precepting. In addition to listing the topic and date of the activity, it is important to include who the audience was (medical students, residents, etc.) and approximately how many were in attendance. In the summary of this section, it is also important to include, when appropriate, a learner assessment (i.e., how did you assess the learners?) and a teaching evaluation (i.e., how did the learners assess you?). This can be done in a table fashion, as in the template provided, or incorporated into the text summary. You may want to include a comment as to what you learned from your evaluation by the learners and how it changed your practice. This is also a good place to incorporate Glassick's criteria to show that your approach to education is a scholarly one. Glassick [6] maintained that educational work, if scholarly, included a demonstration of clear goals, adequate preparation, appropriate methods, significant results, effective presentation, and reflective critique.

b. Curriculum Development

If you have engaged in curriculum development, this is the place to include it. A simple list is sufficient. Indicate where and when the curriculum was delivered, and who the target audience was. Be sure to describe the curriculum evaluation tool used (e.g., GNOME: Goals, Needs, Outcomes, Methods, Evaluation). Similar to the teaching/learning section, a summary, with incorporation of Glassick's criteria if appropriate, can be used to show the impact of these efforts, including mention of the adoption of the curriculum by other institutions or presentations/publications of the work.

c. Mentoring/Advising

Start off by describing your mentoring philosophy if you have not already covered that in your Philosophy section. This should be only a paragraph. Then, in a table format, list your advisees/mentees in chronologic order, including their role (student, resident, junior faculty, etc.), the year(s) of involvement, and any evidence of the success of your mentoring (such as publications, presentations, or career advancement).

If you have any letters of appreciation or support from former mentees/advisees, they can be included in this section.

d. Educational Leadership/Administration

If you have been a program, clerkship, or rotation director (or associate or assistant director), list it here. Then, list educational committees you have sat on and indicate any leadership roles. In the summary, you can include a description of the program's or committee's impact and how you measured it.

If you have any letters of appreciation or support from stakeholders (department leaders, learners, peers, etc.), they can be included in this section.

e. Other Relevant Activities

This section allows you to list and describe any reviewing/moderating activities (if specific to education and not covered elsewhere in your CV), educational grants (including date, amount, and source), educator awards, educational professional development, and educational scholarship (such as relevant publications or presentations) you may have.

Summary

It has been 30 years since Boyer [5] first advocated expanding the definition of "scholarship" to include activities other than research. The educator's portfolio is a valuable document that academic physicians can use to capture the essential elements of scholarship inherent in their educational activities to support applications for promotion and awards and to clarify their educational philosophy, goals, and objectives. This chapter describes why, when, and how to craft this essential document.

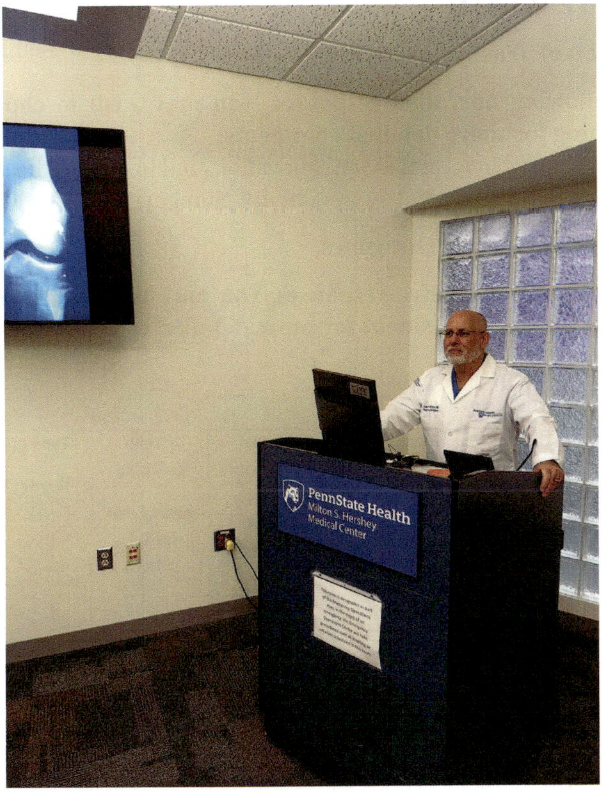

Dr. Lawrence Kass lecturing to emergency medicine residents on orthopedic emergencies

Appendix

EDUCATOR PORTFOLIO TEMPLATE

NAME:

TITLE(S):

PRIMARY EDUCATIONAL ROLE(S):

Date of last update:

STATEMENT OF EDUCATIONAL PHILOSOPHY

GOALS AS AN EDUCATOR

1.
2.
3.
4.
5.

EDUCATIONAL CONTRIBUTIONS

SECTION I: TEACHING

I.1. Description of Teaching Activities

For the following narrative responses, you may wish to choose 1–2 focal areas of teaching for more detailed comments:

Describe the importance, creativity, innovation, and impact of the teaching activities included in Table I.1. (identify by Activity Number).

I.2. Assessment of Learner Outcomes

For the following narrative responses, you may wish to choose 1–2 of the above types of learner assessment for more detailed comments:

Table I.1 Teaching activities

Activity #	**Year(s) and semesters taught**	**Title or topic of activity**	**Teaching strategy and context**	**Where taught** (local, regional, national, international)	**Total teaching hours/year for this activity**	**Type of learner**	**Number learners/year for each activity***
1							
2							
3							
4							
Grand Total							

*If there is a variable number of learners at an activity, provide an average number

Table I.2 Learner assessment

Title or topic of activity (Activity # if applicable)	**Assessment Method**	**Evaluation context** (e.g., # and type of learners, frequency of activity)	**Your role in learner evaluation:** (development implementation analysis/synthesis)	**Evaluation methods and process**	**How did the results of your learner assessments provide evidence of your teaching effectiveness?**

I.3. Evaluation of Teaching

SECTION II: CURRICULUM DEVELOPMENT

Additional narrative details or comments:

Table I.3 Teaching evaluations

Activity number	Who and how many evaluated you? (e.g., 25 learners, 2 peers or educational experts)	Describe the process for evaluating your teaching	List evaluations or note evaluation summaries included in an appendix

Table II.1a Curriculum development activities

CURRICULUM DESCRIPTION(S)					
Activity number	**Curriculum topic and type** (e.g. clerkship module, longitudinal experience, fellowship research component)	**Type and # of learners per yr**	**Is it implemented?** (Yes/No)	**Where is it implemented?** (dept/institution, regional, national, international)	**Your degree of responsibility** (leader or contributor)

Table II.1b GNOME* Analysis of curriculum

GNOME* Elements	Element included? Y/N	Indicators of Quality (example indicators)	Evidence of Quality
Activity number			
Goals/objectives		Goals are appropriate in scope; objectives are specific and measurable/evaluable	
Learner needs assessment		Curriculum design uses learner needs assessment to choose and refine G/O and methods; use learner eval data to refine needs assessment	
Teaching/learning methods		Curriculum design includes variety of methods that address educ goals, and meet needs of diverse learners in specific educational settings	
Learner evaluation and feedback		Curriculum design includes sound learner evaluation methods (valid, reliable, feasible)	
Curriculum/program evaluation		Curriculum is modified periodically using results of learner and program evaluations	
Activity number			
Goals/objectives		See above	
Learner needs assessment		See above	
Teaching/learning methods		See above	
Learner evaluation and feedback		See above	
Curriculum/program evaluation		See above	
For more activities, duplicate 6 lines above			

***GNOME:** G = Goals, N = Needs, O = Objectives, M = Methods, E = Evaluation

SECTION III: MENTORING/ADVISING

III. 1. Description of Mentoring and Advising Activities

Table III.1 Mentoring and advising

Name of mentee or advisee	Dates of mentoring/ advising	Number of years you invested in relationship	Their role/position during the time you were their mentor/advisor	Your role and what you taught them	Their current position	Their significant achievements*

*For example, papers, awards, grants, promotions, and leadership positions. Attach a list if needed

SECTION IV: EDUCATIONAL LEADERSHIP/ADMINISTRATION

IV. 1. Description of Educational Leadership and Administrative Activities

Table IV.1 Description of educational leadership and educational activities

Activity number	Title of program/course(s) directed/co-directed	Scope (Department/Institutional/ Regional/Nat'l/International)	Duration in years
	Name of educational committee(s) and role	**Scope (Department/Institutional/ Regional/Nat'l/International)**	**Duration in years**

SECTION V: OTHER INFORMATION

V. 1. Professional Reviewer/Moderator Activities at the National Level

Activity number	What was reviewed/moderated (Grants, papers, abstracts)	Year/s of review or moderating	Sponsoring organization/institution/agency

V. 2. Educational grants funded
V. 3. Education Awards/Honorable Mentions
V. 4. Publications and Scholarly Products *Related to Education*
V. 5. Workshops and Peer-reviewed/Invited Presentations *on Educational Topics*
V. 6. Professional Development in Education (conferences, certification, degree programs)

Table V.3 Education awards and recognition

Year(s)	Award name	Sponsoring organization (Student group; Department; Institution; Regional/Nat'l/International Org)

Table V.6 Professional development in education

Activity Number	Name and Description (include duration, e.g. 3 hours, 1 day, 1 month)	Dates and Location	Sponsoring organization/institution

References

1. Mayersak RJ, Yarris LM, Tuttle RC, Jones DC, Nelson AM, Bengtzen RR, Kornegay JG, Caretta-Weyer HA. Demonstrating your work: a guide to educators' portfolios for graduate medical educators. J Grad Med Educ. 2021;13(5):635–9. https://doi.org/10.4300/JGME-D-21-00375.1. Epub 2021 Oct 15. PMID: 34721790; PMCID: PMC8527930.
2. Little-Wienert K, Mazziotti M. Twelve tips for creating an academic teaching portfolio. Med Teach. 2018;40(1):26–30. https://doi.org/10.1080/0142159X.2017.1364356. Epub 2017 Aug 17.
3. Kuhn GJ. Faculty development: the educator's portfolio: its preparation, uses, and value in academic medicine. Acad Emerg Med. 2004;11(3):307–11. https://doi.org/10.1111/j.1553-2712.2004.tb02217.x.
4. Gusic ME, Amiel J, Baldwin CD, Chandran L, Fincher RM, Mavis B, O'Sullivan P, Padmore J, Rose S, Simpson D, Strobel H, Timm C, Viggiano T. Using the AAMC toolbox for evaluating educators: you be the judge! MedEdPORTAL. 2013;9:9313. https://doi.org/10.15766/mep_2374-8265.9313.
5. Boyer EL. Scholarship reconsidered: priorities of the professoriate. Princeton: Carnegie Foundation for the Advancement of Teaching; 1990.
6. Glassick CE. Boyer's expanded definitions of scholarship, the standards for assessing scholarship, and the elusiveness of the scholarship of teaching. Acad Med. 2000;75(9):877–80. https://doi.org/10.1097/00001888-200009000-00007.
7. Torre DM, Daley BJ, Sebastian JL, Elnicki DM. Overview of current learning theories for medical educators. Am J Med. 2006;119(10):903–7. https://doi.org/10.1016/j.amjmed.2006.06.037.

Chapter 43
Supervising Medical Student and Residents: Balancing Autonomy and Patient Safety

Brenna M. Farmer

Chapter Content

To ensure the safety of patients and the quality of care provided to all patients in the Emergency Department (ED) when trainees such as medical students and resident physicians are present, there must be an appropriate level of supervision to ensure they learn the practice of Emergency Medicine (EM). However, for trainees to gain confidence and develop trust in themselves and their knowledge and skills, they must also be given autonomy. These two somewhat competing principles can be difficult to balance. The Institute of Medicine and the general public have an interest in resident and trainee supervision to promote patient safety, as do regulatory bodies, like the Centers for Medicare and Medicaid (CMS), when determining reimbursement [1, 2]. This chapter should take some of the mystery out of the balance between autonomy and patient safety and provide ways to supervise while building autonomy for trainees. The term for this balance is *entrustment* and has been the focus of some research in medical education, including for EM training. [3]. In this chapter, the supervision of medical students, the categories of supervision outlined by the Accreditation Council of Graduate Medical Education (ACGME), the factors involved in entrustment, and what entrustable professional activities are in EM will be discussed. Finally, examples of different approaches to entrustment will be included to provide further clarity.

B. M. Farmer (✉)
Weill Cornell Medicine, New York, NY, USA

New York Presbyterian Brooklyn Methodist Hospital, Brooklyn, NY, USA
e-mail: bmf9001@med.cornell.edu

R. P. Olympia et al. (eds.), *An Emergency Physician's Path*,
https://doi.org/10.1007/978-3-031-47873-4_43

Medical Student Supervision

Medical students are classified as "undergraduates" when discussing advanced education, whereas resident physicians fall under "graduate" medical education. In places where medical students and resident physicians both practice, there are likely guidelines and/or policies discussing supervision for "undergraduate medical education" (UME) and "graduate medical education" (GME). GME supervision is outlined by the ACGME, while UME supervision is outlined by the Liaison Committee on Medical Education (LCME) of the Association of American Medical Colleges (AAMC) and the American Medical Association (AMA) [4]. The LCME has a set of 12 standards required for a medical school to be accredited. Standard 9.3 discusses medical student supervision and states that "a medical school ensures that medical students in clinical learning situations involving patient care are appropriately supervised at all times in order to ensure patient and student safety, that the level of responsibility delegated to the student is appropriate to the student's level of training, and that the activities supervised are within the scope of practice of the supervising health professional" [4]. For osteopathic medical schools, Element 5.4 of the Commission on Osteopathic College Accreditation standards states that "a COM must ensure that osteopathic students in clinical learning situations involving patient care are under direct supervision by a licensed health care professional at all times in order to ensure safety. The COM must ensure that all supervised activities are within the scope of practice of the supervising health care professional. Students must have clear guidelines on their role in care and the limits of their scope of authority" [5].

From a patient safety and quality perspective, supervising attendings must be more involved in these cases to ensure no red flags indicating an emergent condition are missed, to ensure quality metrics are met, and to be able to write appropriate orders for whatever is needed as part of the evaluation, treatment, and follow-up for patients seen with medical students. As medical students are new learners, direct supervision allows supervising physicians to provide constructive feedback for history taking, such as wording questions related to sensitive histories for specific clinical scenarios, performing physical examinations in patients unable to comply with the way the examination was taught prior to being in a clinical situation, and introducing quality measures for specific conditions, and so on.

Categories of Supervision

In the education of trainees, there are differing levels of supervision that must be understood (Table 43.1). These levels of resident supervision in EM are clearly defined by the ACGME. They include direct supervision, indirect supervision, and oversight. See Table 43.1 for definitions. For direct supervision, the supervising attending physician is physically present at the bedside in the ED or can be

Table 43.1 Levels of supervision [6]

Direct	Indirect	Oversight
"The supervising physician is physically present with the resident during key portions of the patient interaction." For telemedicine visits, "the supervising physician and or patient is not physically present with the resident and the supervising physician is concurrently monitoring patient care through appropriate telecommunication platform."	"The supervising physician is not providing physician or concurrent visual or audio supervision but is immediately available to the resident for guidance and is available to provide appropriate direct supervision."	"The supervising physician is available to provide review of procedure/encounters with feedback provided after care is delivered."

visualizing the encounter and or procedure through telemedicine [6]. An example of direct supervision is when a trauma-alert patient comes in and the ED attending supervises the entire case and is physically present in the resuscitation bay with the trainees and patient. That way they oversee the history and physical examination in real time and are also present for any procedures that may be necessary as part of the patient's care. For a telemedicine encounter, the attending may be viewing the encounter over a telemedicine platform while the resident is performing a telemedicine visit with the patient. With this direct supervision, the attending can see what the resident sees on physical examination and gets to listen to the history at the same time. If there are any concerns, an in-person visit can be recommended and if necessary, an ambulance can be called. Direct supervision should be used for those procedures that are low frequency but lifesaving, such as placing a transvenous pacemaker, or higher-frequency procedures like endotracheal intubation or procedural sedation where death can occur if complications arise. And all interns must have direct supervision for all patient care until they meet the criteria the residency program has established to allow for other forms of supervision.

The next type of supervision is indirect supervision. During indirect supervision, the supervising attending physician is in the ED but may not be at the bedside at the time a procedure or evaluation is taking place [6]. However, they can come to the bedside immediately if needed. An example of this type of supervision is when the supervising attending is with another patient while the intern or resident is obtaining a history and examining a patient. Another example might be when a senior resident is performing a simple procedure, like suturing a laceration, and the attending is available but providing direct supervision to a junior resident or medical student in the same area of the ED. This example also shows the variable levels of supervision an attending may use depending on the resident involved or the level of postgraduate training of the resident involved. As another example, the attending may be at the bedside for an entire history and physical examination for the first couple of patients that an intern sees. Once trust is built by having the intern demonstrate that he or she can obtain an appropriately detailed history and perform the necessary physical examination elements competently, the attending may switch to indirect supervision where the attending goes to the bedside to confirm the history and physical examination after hearing the presentation and plan from the intern. Most faculty start with direct supervision and then switch to indirect supervision once a resident has proven capable, competent, and trustworthy.

Oversight is less common in the ED. It means that the attending reviews the cases with the trainee and provides feedback but was not physically present at the time of the patient encounter and did not examine or speak with the patient [6]. This type of supervision is not typically seen in the ED while training EM residents and medical students but may happen on off-service rotations or with consulting services coming to the ED. For example, the surgery residents may see and discuss consults with the surgery attending on call, including the plan of care, but the surgery attending does not come to the ED to see and examine every patient requiring a consultation. Oversight may be more commonly used with advanced practice providers seeing lower acuity patients, depending on the culture, reimbursement practices, and expectations of a particular ED and/or EM attending physician.

The above ACGME description of levels of supervision does not always correlate with what CMS or other billing services use to reimburse for medical care provided at teaching institutions. Teaching attendings can bill for direct services they provide, for services that residents and interns provide under the attending's supervision, and for procedures the teaching attending physician directly supervises or when the teaching attending is present for key and critical portions of the procedure [2].

Entrustment

Entrustment is the term used to identify the necessary balance of appropriate supervision while allowing autonomy for the trainee's growth toward independent practice [3]. Supervising physicians must vary their level of entrustment depending on the task and individual patient involved as shown in the examples above [3]. When one EM program reviewed what factors influenced entrustment by attendings, they identified the following factors: the resident, the patient, the environment of the ED at the time, and the faculty involved with entrustment being related to faculty behavior based on the three other factors [3]. For each of the factors involved, subfactors led to the overall impression for what level of entrustment was needed. The level of training, direct observation, performance during previous shifts, information from discussions of resident assessment with faculty, resident self-confidence, and the case presentation and plan were all involved for the resident factor [3]. The supervising attending physician may want more direct observation for an intern than they would for a senior resident since a senior resident would be expected to have more autonomy in their practice as they have more patient care experience than an intern. However, if the attending has never worked with the senior resident, the attending may opt for more direct supervision unless the attending has heard through faculty discussions that the resident is always accurate when presenting and develops plans of care that are always appropriate.

The subfactors for the patient include acuity of the patient's condition, the risk to the patient from necessary procedures, and preconceived view from the supervising faculty [3]. With a critically ill patient, or a patient coming in as an alert of some type (stroke, STEMI, sepsis, trauma, and so on), the level of supervision is likely to be higher. There are likely expectations for the supervising attending to be present for such cases and perform direct observation to ensure specific safe patient care and for quality, regulatory, or other metrics to be met. In addition, if the patient were to require certain life-saving procedures, the supervising attending physician should be present. In this case, the attending may not only supervise but also troubleshoot or even take over the procedure to ensure patient safety, particularly after helping the resident troubleshoot a problem. Certain billing practices may require the attending to be present and document their level of involvement; this may include direct observation of the entire procedure versus key portions, or if they perform themselves, documenting that they were the person performing the procedure. In addition, the "gut" feeling the attending gets from the visitors with the patient may influence how much entrustment occurs. If he or she feels that the rapport with the family could be better, the attending may provide more direct supervision for that case or decide that the resident may not need to be involved in a case if the family is demanding and needs more 1:1 attention from the attending.

The level of activity of the department, what systems factors are required (expectations of faculty to be present at stroke, STEMI, trauma alerts), nursing capability, and what the local departmental expectations are for supervision are the environmental subfactors for entrustment [3]. On a day when the ED is surging due to a high census of boarders and/or a high number of new patients arriving for evaluation, the ED attending may always see patients to ensure that they "don't miss anything" as they know everyone is stretched thin on how much care they can perform. On less busy days, the attending may be doing more bedside teaching with an intern and allow the senior resident more autonomy. In some places, the culture is to always let the residents see the patient first and then hear the presentation and plan before the attending evaluates the patient. In other places, the practice may be that the attending directly observes every case with the interns, and only direct observes the critically ill cases with the senior residents. For the senior resident cases, the attendings see the patients after hearing the plan from the resident and ensure that the patient knows they are working with the resident and supervising the care.

The faculty member's personality and general approach, comfort with his or her own skills and experience, risk aversion, sense of balance between clinical responsibility and educational role, as well as a personal inclination toward micromanagement will determine entrustment. As seen from the descriptions above, all other factors filter to the faculty as "entrustment is a faculty behavior" [3]. Furthermore, residents must have demonstrated specific characteristics to have entrustment from faculty. They must have integrity, reliability, humility, and ability [7]. An attending is not expected to find a resident entrustable if they have been misleading about performing a rectal examination or a pelvic/genitourinary evaluation and so on. The resident needs to show trustworthiness as well as the capability for entrustment to happen.

In addition to the factors associated with entrustment, GME leaders from the Council of Residency Directors in EM have developed 11 EM resident entrustable professional activities (EPAs) that are linked with the EM Milestones as outlined by the ACGME [7]. These 11 core EPAs should be achievable by graduation from residency. The EPAs include transitions of care between healthcare providers, managing low and high acuity patients, managing multiple patients concomitantly, interactions with consulting services, and using recommended processes for patient safety and quality [7]. Each EPA has a list of associated knowledge, skills, attitudes, and behaviors. The list could be individual EM milestones or parts of milestones. They may allow for the supervising attendings to give detailed and more meaningful feedback to the trainees and ensure the supervising attendings know where they should focus autonomy and supervision on shift. For example, if the attending physician is working with a resident needing to improve in interactions with consulting services while already showing he or she is competent in managing multiple patients at the same time, the attending can supervise the resident's conversations, pre-plan the necessary information to present and identify the questions for the consulting service and practice the presentation with the resident prior to the actual conversation with the consultant. This same attending would know that the resident has already proven capable of managing multiple patients, so he or she could allow the resident to see multiple patients prior to hearing the presentations.

Conclusion

Entrustment, the balance of autonomy and supervision, varies depending on the clinical situation and the trainee and faculty involved. This balance is complicated and has many subfactors to ensure patient safety and quality while moving residents to the competency they need prior to independent practice. With the understanding of the different levels of supervision and knowing where residents need further instruction to meet certain EPAs, supervising physicians can focus their coaching and educational efforts, ensuring quality and patient safety, while allowing autonomy in the areas where residents have proven competency.

References

1. Ulmer C, Wolman D, Johns M, editors. Resident duty hours: enhancing sleep, supervision, and safety. Washington, DC: National Academies Press; 2008. Committee on Optimizing Graduate Medical Trainee (Resident) Hours and Work Schedules to Improve Patient Safety for the Institute of Medicine.
2. Centers for Medicare and Medicaid Services. Teaching Physicians, Interns, and Residents Guidelines. May 2022. https://www.cms.gov/outreach-and-education/medicare-learning-network-mln/mlnproducts/downloads/teaching-physicians-fact-sheet-icn006437.pdf. Accessed 2 Oct 2022.

3. Santen S, Wolff M, Saxon K, et al. Factors affecting entrustment in emergency medicine: "how much rope do I give them?". West J Emerg Med. 2019;20(1):58–63.
4. Association of American Medical Colleges and American Medical Association's Liaison Committee on Medical Education. Functions and Structure of a Medical School: Standards for Accreditation of Medical Education Programs Leading to the MD Degree. March 2022. https://lcme.org/publications/#Standards. Accessed 2 Oct 2022.
5. American Osteopathic Association's Commission on Osteopathic College Accreditation's Accreditation of Colleges of Osteopathic Medicine: COM Continuing Accreditation Standards. 2019. https://osteopathic.org/wp-content/uploads/2018/02/com-continuing-accreditation-standards.pdf. Accessed 2 Oct 2022.
6. Accreditation Council for Graduate Medical Education. Emergency Medicine Program Requirements. https://www.acgme.org/globalassets/pfassets/programrequirements/110_emergencymedicine_2022.pdf. Last Accessed 2 Oct 2022.
7. Hart D, Franzen D, Beeson M, et al. Integration of entrustable professional activities with milestones for emergency medicine residents. West J Emerg Med. 2019;20(1):35–42.

Chapter 44
Undergraduate and Graduate Medical Education: Leadership Roles in Medical Student and Residency Education

Eric Chin and Warren Wiechmann

Are you the tortoise or the hare? The practice, or dare I say, the business of medicine, can sometimes challenge the notion of a life-long profession. Pursuing a path in medical education is one way to ensure a fulfilling and long-lasting career. Over nearly two decades as a practicing physician, I have found participating in activities beyond purely clinical practice was essential to maintaining job satisfaction. Furthermore, seeking leadership positions in medical education can help provide a greater sense of purpose and a broader impact on providers and patients.

Why Should I Pursue a Career in Medical Education?

Purpose

Most of us went into medicine to help people. The clinical work we do at the bedside in the Emergency Department (ED) does matter to those we serve. However, the ability to affect many more individuals multiplies with each medical student and physician-in-training you educate and with whom you interact. Your ability to train the next generation of physicians will continue to have an effect after you exit medicine and retire.

E. Chin (✉)
Department of Emergency Medicine, Brooke Army Medical Center,
JBSA-Ft. Sam Houston, TX, USA

W. Wiechmann
UC Irvine Health School of Medicine, Irvine, CA, USA
e-mail: wiechmaw@hs.uci.edu

R. P. Olympia et al. (eds.), *An Emergency Physician's Path*,
https://doi.org/10.1007/978-3-031-47873-4_44

Mentorship

Think back to when you decided to apply to medical school, specialize in emergency medicine (EM), or even complete a fellowship. Was there someone in your life who nudged you forward, or was there someone you aspired to become? Medical students and physicians-in-training are much like pluripotent stem cells looking for guidance on what to become and what to be. Often your experience and expertise can be crucial for identifying characteristics and qualities in a learner that are complementary to a particular career path or position.

Currency

Entering the medical field means committing to lifelong learning. Keeping up with evidence-based practice can be challenging for all but the most efficient physicians, especially when entering private practice and moving away from the academic environment. Working in medical education encourages medical currency to ensure you share the best and most relevant information for a trainee.

Personal Growth

As you progress through your medical career, your priorities can change just as they do in your personal life. Taking on new responsibilities and remaining engaged in the development of others within the medical profession can help you unlock new passions and skills you may not have exercised or realized previously. For example, several positions in medical education leadership helped me identify potential areas of growth which prompted me to pursue a business degree. Surprisingly, many business concepts can be utilized in medical education and have given me valuable tools to be a more effective leader.

Sustainable Career

If you are like me and many other emergency physicians (EPs) I know, a prolonged attention span is not one of our most endearing qualities. Similarly, the passion for and challenge of emergency medicine can diminish over time. Pursuing leadership positions in medical education can extend your career in medicine and provide a counterbalance to the daily grind of working clinically.

Be a Change Agent

Medicine can often feel like trying to change the direction of an enormous iceberg full of dogma and expert opinion. Working with medical students and physicians-in-training challenges how we teach, learn, and practice medicine. When aligned with an institution looking for change or improving health care delivery, being a leader in medical education can be influential and impactful.

What Are Undergraduate Medical Education (UME) and Graduate Medical Education (GME)?

Most simply, UME refers to the years medical students attend medical school in pursuit of a doctorate of medicine. GME encompasses all medical training after graduating from medical school and includes but is not limited to internship, residency, and fellowship programs. Frequently, GME will make a physician-in-training eligible for specialty certification by accrediting organizations such as the American Board of Medical Specialties (ABMS) and its individual specialty boards.

Undergraduate Medical Education

Most emergency medicine physicians identify the Emergency Medicine clerkship director role as the "go-to" (UME) opportunity, but this chapter will introduce some additional opportunities and the more common pathways to attain these roles that may be present at your institution. There are two main categories of opportunities – curricular and student support – that emergency physicians can pursue based on their interests.

Curricular Leadership Opportunities

1. *EM Clerkship*. The opportunity to serve as the assistant, associate, co-director, or sole director of this experience is one of the most common entry pathways for EPs looking to get involved in UME leadership. Appointments to these roles are often primarily driven at the Department of EM (DEM) level with some oversight and approval by the medical school's curricular leadership, which is unique in that the recruitment and filling of most other UME leadership opportunities is managed primarily by the senior UME leadership. In curricula where the EM

clerkship is a "core" or "required" rotation, there may be funding from the medical school to protect faculty time. Similarly, there may be internal support (provided by the DEM) for this role.

2. *EM Clinical Electives*. Outside of the primary EM rotation, some departments offer other electives such as Emergency Medical Services experiences, Point-of-Care Ultrasound, Toxicology, Research, Pediatric EM, Hyperbaric Medicine, and Wilderness Medicine, among others. These appointments are made at the DEM level and there may be medical school funding support or internal support for these roles.
3. *Pre-Clerkship Curriculum Course/Thread Director*. Sometimes referred to as the "pre-clinical" or "basic sciences" curriculum, these are the required courses that occur during the first 12–24 months of medical school. Regardless of whether the curriculum consists of discipline-organized courses (such as Anatomy, Physiology, and Pathology) or systems-based courses or threads (such as Cardiovascular, Gastroenterology, and Renal), leadership opportunities can present themselves as EM physicians get more involved in the teaching of the course. This may start as ad-hoc involvement with individual lectures and progress to providing "clinical correlation" instruction for all topics. These appointments are made at the department level (if the course is discipline-based) or at the senior UME leadership level and may be supported based on the amount of contribution to the course.
4. *Doctoring or Foundations Course Faculty or Directors*. While these courses typically take place during the first half of medical school training, we separate them from the other pre-clerkship courses in that these often utilize a small-group team-based or problem-based learning approach to teaching students the skills to be a practicing physician. These are often longitudinal courses with a high amount of regularly scheduled instruction (several times per week) and therefore receive funding from the medical school. Faculty who excel in these small-group teaching roles could be considered for a course or thread director role. These appointments are made by the senior UME leadership.
5. *Educational Technology (ET) Directors*. ET is a broad term that can be used to encompass any technologies used in support of teaching and learning. Depending on the institution's definition of ET, it could include medical simulation, clinical skills centers, and point-of-care ultrasound. Medical simulation and clinical skills centers are fixtures within most, if not all, UME programs. In addition to staff leadership who keep these centers operational, there are often physician leadership roles in curricular development for these spaces. Experience in medical simulation, especially through a Medical Education or Simulation Fellowship, would be required. Point-of-care ultrasound has become more prominent throughout medical education with almost 100 medical schools offering ultrasound integration in their curriculum, according to the American Institute of Ultrasound in Medicine [1]. EM physicians who have completed an Emergency Ultrasound fellowship may be able to pursue a leadership opportunity here. In all these areas, appointments and funding decisions are made by the senior UME leadership.

6. *Curriculum-Wide Leadership*. Senior UME leadership will often appoint a faculty member who had previously served in one of the above roles to oversee a phase of the curriculum (such as an Assistant or Associate Dean of Pre-clerkship or Clerkship Curriculum) or the entire curriculum (such as an Associate or Senior Associate Dean of Curriculum). These larger administrative roles are often funded to ensure that faculty have time to execute this role.

Student Support Opportunities

Student support is a broad term that can describe divisions or offices of student affairs, student success, student life, and diversity, equity, and inclusion. Each school may adopt its own terminology; however, these types of roles are common to student support:

1. *Advising Roles for Student-Focused Groups*. EM physicians interested in student support roles can first get involved as a faculty advisor for the EM Student Interest Group. This decision is made at the DEM level. Faculty may also consider serving as an advisor for student chapters of larger organizations, such as the Latino Medical Student Association, Student National Medical Association, American Medical Women's Association, Asian Pacific American Medical Student Association, or Medical Student Pride Alliance, in addition to other local non-EM-focused interest groups. The appointment process varies but requires some previous involvement and student engagement within that organization.
2. *Academic Support and Career Advising Roles*. The Liaison Committee on Medical Education (LCME) requires that a medical school "provides effective academic support and career advising to all medical students to assist them in achieving their career goals and the school's medical education program objectives [2]." Faculty may serve as a specialty advisor for students considering applying to an EM residency and expand their advising to a general career advising role. Some schools utilize academic coaching models or academic societies to meet these requirements [3]. As these positions are required for medical school accreditation, appointment and funding decisions are often made by senior UME leadership.
3. *Admissions and Outreach*. Additional opportunities for involvement outside of the curriculum can be found in the Admissions Committee or through Outreach efforts [4]. Interested faculty can get involved first by conducting prospective medical student interviews and later serving as members of the Admissions Committee. This committee membership is often overseen by an Associate Dean of Admissions, who appoints members (in consultation with the senior UME leadership) based on previous involvement. Many schools often offer outreach programs focusing on K-12 and undergraduate students and involvement can

range from advising to directing these programs. These programs are often overseen by the Student Support leadership.

4. *Student-Support Leadership.* Similar to the curriculum, senior UME leadership will often appoint a faculty member who had previously served in one of the above roles to oversee all of these student-focused efforts (such as a Senior Associate or Associate Dean of Student Support/Affairs) with supporting roles of assistant or associate deans who may focus on a specific area (such as an Assistant Dean of Advising and Assistant Dean of Outreach). Depending on the structure of the school, Admissions will have its own faculty leader (such as an Associate Dean of Admissions). These larger administrative roles are often funded to ensure that faculty have time to execute this role.

Senior UME Leadership Opportunities

Within UME, there is often an individual that oversees all of the Undergraduate Medical Education efforts and has the title of Senior Associate Dean or Vice-Dean of Undergraduate Medical Education. Individuals in this role will often have served in another significant curriculum or student support role. In some instances, this role oversees UME and GME and has the title of Senior Associate Dean or Vice-Dean of Medical Education. This senior position often reports directly to the Dean of the medical school. As with other larger leadership roles, this significant administrative role is often funded.

Graduate Medical Education

Similar to UME, there are innumerable leadership positions available in GME from directing a specific component of a graduate training program, such as a curriculum director, to program director of a residency or fellowship, all the way to the Designated Institutional Official and Dean. The only limitation for leadership opportunities in GME is the number granted by an institution or funded by a Department Chair. Frequently each position serves as a stepping stone to a higher level of leadership, with greater responsibility and scope, within an institution or organization. The Accreditation Council for Graduate Medical Education (ACGME) is a non-profit organization that "sets and monitors voluntary professional educational standards essential in preparing physicians to deliver safe, high-quality medical care to all Americans [5]." ACGME is widely recognized as a major accrediting organization for many, but not all, GME programs and identifies specific leadership positions. In this section, we will discuss ACGME and other common leadership roles in GME.

Leadership Opportunities

1. *Curriculum Director.* ACGME EM residency programs are required to provide an average of 5 hours of didactic experiences per week, which can be a daunting task for residency leadership [6]. Serving in this capacity can be an effective way to develop your curriculum-building skills while ensuring EM residents develop a foundation in medical knowledge necessary to pass their written certifying exam and provide high-quality care.
2. *Clerkship Director* (see "*EM Clerkship*" under UME section).
3. *Program/Fellowship Director (PD).* This position provides the overall authority and accountability for a residency or fellowship program. Assuming that all applicable ACGME program requirements are met, the PD has the ability to set the tone and define the character of a training program.
4. *Assistant/Associate Program Director (APD).* This position assists the PD with the oversight and management of a training program and is a great way to develop the knowledge and skills necessary to assume the role of PD in the future. Depending on the program's size, the APD can have variable administrative duties, mentoring, and clinical responsibilities.
5. *Vice Chair.* This role varies from department to department ranging from purely administrative and operational aspects of an ED to specific areas of focus within medical education, such as a Vice Chair of Education or Research.
6. *Department Chair.* As the head of a department, they possess the overall authority over the administrative and educational aspects of an ED. Involvement in GME can vary based on the number, size, and scope of the training programs within the department.
7. *Higher Levels of Leadership.* Depending on the size and complexity of an institution, many other leadership positions may exist. For example, sites with ACGME-accredited programs will have a Designated Institution Official (DIO), who has the authority and oversight over all institutional training programs. Other leadership roles may include various flavors of Deans typically with institutional responsibilities and oversight.

Tips for Success

Start Small and Get Involved

The easiest path to breaking into medical education and then a role in leadership can begin with something as simple as offering to teach, mentor, or lead a piece of the curriculum. Active and successful participation can open up additional roles and responsibilities within a program. Other ways to be more competitive when looking for a leadership position include completing a fellowship or subspecialty training program, such as critical care, emergency medical services, ultrasound, or even a medical education/teaching fellowship. As your leadership roles and responsibilities grow, be sure not to overextend yourself. Think about obtaining protected time and funding to enable you to participate fully in your interests.

Academic Promotion

At more traditional academic institutions, your academic rank (e.g., Assistant, Associate, and Full Professor) can directly impact your compensation and protected time for medical education. To promote through the academic rank structure requires persistent and well-documented accomplishments over time. To climb the promotion ladder most efficiently, consider leveraging an activity that can serve many purposes. For example, developing a curriculum piece and then spending a little more time developing a research question can provide multiple products from a single activity.

Find a Mentor

Even for individuals not new to medical education, seeking a mentor to help provide guidance and input on career decisions can help you achieve your professional goals.

Time Is Valuable

As you establish your career in medical education, being proactive about protecting your time and securing funding for your leadership roles is critical to your success and longevity.

Final Thoughts

Pursuing leadership roles in medication education is a great way to extend and diversify your professional career as an emergency physician. It is never too late to start, and leadership roles can be one way to have a broader impact on society than can be achieved by seeing one patient at a time. Start small and work your way up to increasing levels of responsibility and you will be surprised how different life as an EP can be.

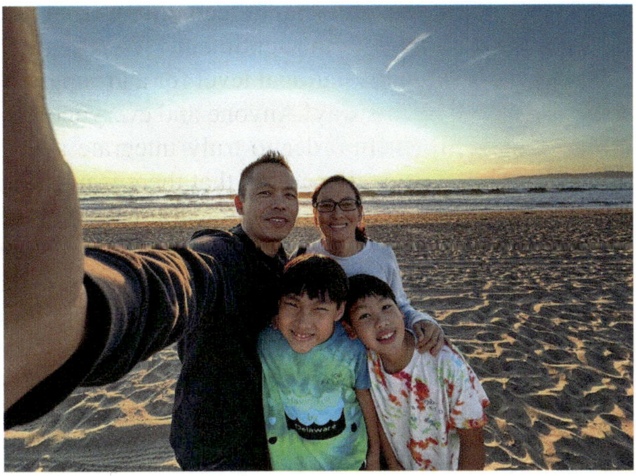

Returning to old stomping grounds from fellowship training in Southern California

Disclaimer The views expressed in this chapter are those of the author(s) and do not reflect the official policy of the Brooke Army Medical Center, Department of the Army, the Defense Health Agency, the Department of Defense, or the U.S. Government.

References

1. Medical Schools. American Institute of Ultrasound in Medicine (AIUM). Ultrasound in Medical Education Portal. http://meded.aium.org/medical-schools. Published 2022. Accessed 31 Aug 2022.
2. Liaison Committee on Medical Education. Functions and Structure of a Medical School. https://lcme.org/publications/#Standards. March 2022. Accessed 31 Aug 2022.
3. Hammoud M, Deiorio N, Moore M, Wolff M. Coaching in medical education. 1st ed. Elsevier; 2022.
4. Visiting student learning opportunities™ (VSLO®). Association of American Medical Schools: Students & Residents. https://students-residents.aamc.org/visiting-student-learning-opportunities/visiting-student-learning-opportunities-vslo. Published 2022. Accessed 31 Aug 2022.
5. Accreditation Council for Graduate Medical Education. About us. https://www.acgme.org/about-us/overview/. Accessed 31 Aug 2022.
6. Accreditation Council for Graduate Medical Education. Emergency Medicine. Program Requirements and FAQs. https://www.acgme.org/globalassets/pfassets/programrequirements/110_emergencymedicine_2022.pdf. Accessed 31 Aug 2022.

Chapter 45
Concepts of Teaching the Adult Learner

Annahieta Kalantari

Most individuals can reflect upon a time in their education when they had an excellent learning experience versus a terrible learning experience. We have all had great teachers and terrible teachers. What made our great educators so great and our poor educators so poor? The answer often depends on us as learners. Where were we in our development? What were our needs at that time and were they met? What emotions were associated with the experience? What was our motivation to learn? Chances are that our great teachers knew where we were in our development, knew our needs and met them in a psychologically safe environment, and knew how to motivate us.

Andragogy Versus Pedagogy

The concept of teaching adults is not novel. The greatest teachers of ancient times, such as Plato and Aristotle, were adult educators [1]. Yet, our classic societal image of teaching and learning is often of elementary-aged children. Pedagogy, the art and science of teaching children, did not develop until seventh-century European monasteries were established to induct young men into priesthood [2]. Pedagogy is fundamentally teacher-centered. In this model, teachers determine what will be learned, how will it be learned, when it will be learned, and if it has been learned [2]. The majority of our current educational systems are based on the model of pedagogy.

A. Kalantari (✉)
Department of Emergency Medicine, Penn State Health Milton S Hershey Medical Center, Hershey, PA, USA
e-mail: akalantari@pennstatehealth.psu.edu

R. P. Olympia et al. (eds.), *An Emergency Physician's Path*,
https://doi.org/10.1007/978-3-031-47873-4_45

Although Plato and Aristotle specialized in teaching adults, the term andragogy, the art and science of teaching adults, was not coined until 1833 by a German educator named Alexander Kapp [2]. The use of the term became more mainstream in 1926 after Eduard C. Lindeman wrote about educating adults. Research on adult education boomed in the 1960s. Malcolm Knowles, an American educator, incorporated the new research, further developed the model of andragogy, and published six basic assumptions of adult learning [1].

1. As a person matures, their self-concept moves from that of a dependent being to a more self-directing being.
2. Experiences are the richest resource for adult learning.
3. An adult's readiness to learn is linked to the developmental tasks of his/her social role.
4. Adults are more problem-centered learners rather than subject-centered learners.
5. Adults are mostly internally motivated to learn rather than externally motivated.
6. Adults need to know the reason for learning something [1].

The model of andragogy is in stark contrast to that of pedagogy. Andragogy puts the learner at the center rather than the teacher. In this model, a teacher is a facilitator who sets a psychologically safe environment for learning where adults participate in selecting what and how is learned in addition to determining if it was learned. This environment respects learners' prior experiences and invites them to contribute what they have learned from those experiences. One of the first steps in being a successful adult medical educator is shifting your lens from the classic pedagogical model to an andragogical model.

Adult Learning Theories

There are five traditional learning theories that are foundational to pedagogy and andragogy: behaviorism, humanism, cognitivism, social cognitivism, and constructivism. The teacher role, student role, purpose of education, and guiding principles vary between each of them. Multiple other educational theories draw from the basic tenets of these five theories. Understanding each of these will assist a medical educator in developing their educational philosophy and how to approach each learner in various settings [3].

Behaviorism identifies learning as an observed, desired behavior. The teacher is central and must create an environment that supports or reinforces a desired behavior. The most classic example of behaviorism is that of Pavlov's dogs. However, behaviorism is very much central to medical education today in the form of entrustable professional acts (EPAs) and competencies [4]. Additionally, reward systems are rooted in behaviorism [1].

Humanism is the exact opposite of behaviorism. Learning is not an observable behavior. Rather, it is the process that allows humans to grow and develop to meet their full potential. The role of the teacher is to facilitate this process so that every individual has learned what they require to become fully functioning and independent. The classic example is that of Maslow's pyramid of human needs [5]. In modern days, humanism is developing the self-directed and life-long learner [6].

Educational theories that discuss how the brain and mind process and retain information fall under cognitivism. Learning occurs when the brain processes information that has been interpreted and assigned meaning. The learning can then be used for future applications. Cognitive development, instructional design, and memory processing are rooted in cognitivism. Cognitive load theory is also a cognitivist learning theory [1, 6].

The prior theories focus on the individual learner: their behavior, development, and processing. Social cognitive theory, however, focuses on the social and contextual influences on learning. Individuals acquire knowledge, rules, skills, strategies, and beliefs through the observation of others and interactions with the social environment [1]. The teacher's role is to model and guide behaviors and provide opportunities to practice new roles and behaviors [7]. Communities of practice fall under the social cognitive theory [6].

Constructivism is a learning theory that integrates the individual and the social environment. Learning is considered the construction of meaning from experiences. Knowledge is formed when learners reflect on an experience and assign meanings to it. That meaning is influenced by the environment and context of the experience in addition to preexisting beliefs and values that were formed through prior experiences [1]. The teacher's role is to assist learners in understanding how they developed certain assumptions and question learners on the validity of their assumptions. Narrative medicine and reflective journaling are examples that utilized constructivism [7].

Knowledge, Skills, and Attitudes

Medical educators must be keenly aware of the three fundamental learning domains: knowledge, skill, and attitude. Knowledge focuses on the facts, information, and data. Skills are psychomotor and behavioral actions. Attitude includes the beliefs, mindset, and feelings of an individual. A well-rounded physician will have the appropriate knowledge, skills, and attitude required of him/her to accomplish their role [8].

Each of these domains is addressed by different learning theories and subsequent teaching strategies. Behaviorism is useful for demonstrating technical or psychomotor skills. Cognitivism is a useful learning theory if a learner has a knowledge deficit. Learners can assume responsibility for their own learning under the humanism theory. Role modeling attitudes and behaviors utilize a social cognitive approach. Reflective exercises in the learning environment are constructivist strategies [7].

Having a basic understanding of the educational theories and aligning them with the desired teaching domain is important for successful adult learning. For example,

Table 45.1 Integration of learning theories with practice

Theory	Defined learning	Assumptions	Example
Behaviorism	Observable, desired behavior	Environment shapes behavior Reinforcement is central to the learning process	Procedural competency through simulation
Humanism	Human development to reach full potential	Self-initiated Learning is evaluated by the learner	Problem-based learning
Cognitivism	Brain processing	Focus on thought processes Knowledge is applicable to other learning situations independent of the topic	Concept maps
Social cognitivism	Occurs through observation	Observation is enough to learn Environment influences learning	Role-modeling
Constructivism	Assigned meaning to experiences	Fosters critical reflection Questions validity of assumptions	Reflective journaling

if a medical educator wishes to teach procedural skills, it does not make sense to ask learners to read and reflect on a chapter of a textbook that discusses that procedural skill. This incorrectly selects a cognitive approach to teach a skill that is behavioral. If the learning domain is attitudinal one, a constructivist reflective exercise would likely yield better learning than an assigned reading. If the goal is to teach how to have a difficult conversation with a patient, role modeling, a social cognitive approach, may be the best strategy. Table 45.1 provides a brief summary of the five traditional learning theories and provides an example of their integration in medical education.

The path to being a successful medical educator begins with a passion for teaching and a basic understanding of adult learning theory. Creating a psychologically safe environment that respects the autonomy, competing responsibilities, and prior experiences of your adult learners will make you one of those unforgettable, great teachers.

References

1. Merriam SB, Bierema LL. Adult learning: linking theory and practice. Wiley; 2013.
2. Ozuah PO. First, there was pedagogy and then came andragogy. Einstein J Biol Med. 2016;21(2):83–7.
3. Tisdell EJ, Taylor EW. Adult education philosophy informs practice. Adult Learn. 2000;11(2):6–10.

4. Ten Cate O. Nuts and bolts of entrustable professional activities. J Grad Med Educ. 2013;5(1):157–8.
5. McLeod S. Maslow's hierarchy of needs. Simply Psychol. 2007;1:1–18.
6. Taylor DC, Hamdy H. Adult learning theories: implications for learning and teaching in medical education: AMEE Guide No. 83. Med Teach. 2013;35(11):e1561–72. https://doi.org/10.3109/0142159X.2013.828153.
7. Torre DM, Daley BJ, Sebastian JL, Elnicki DM. Overview of current learning theories for medical educators. Am J Med. 2006;119(10):903–7. https://doi.org/10.1016/j.amjmed.2006.06.037.
8. Thomas PA, Kern DE, Hughes MT, Chen BY. Curriculum development for medical education: a six-step approach. JHU Press; 2016.

Chapter 46
Giving Feedback and Filling Out Evaluations for Medical Students and Residents

Monisha Bindra and Elizabeth Barrall Werley

Feedback through primary and secondary school education is often in-the-moment for students. When learning to write your letters in elementary school, your first-grade teacher likely corrected you on the curvature and linearity of each letter to correctly compose words in the moment. Similarly, as each of us continued through the elementary years and advanced onward through secondary school and then college, we accepted commentary from our teachers and professors when they returned our essays or exams within a few days of the assignment. Evaluation was often in the form of grades for individual assignments, as well as interval and end-of-year scores. However, what previously worked at earlier levels of education does not necessarily translate to medical education. Taking into consideration the content involved (patient care) as well as differences in generational learning styles for medical students, residents, or even practicing physicians, traditional models of feedback may not always be the most effective approach, and the learner and teacher need to find a balance in the relationship in order to make the feedback effective.

Feedback for medical students and residents can be provided by both clinical and core faculty members (those with combined patient care and academic/educational responsibilities), senior residents, nursing staff and other personnel, and even patients. Most of the direct feedback provided to medical students is through the clerkship director and supervising, often senior, residents. They often gather

M. Bindra
Department of Emergency Medicine, Tower Health-Reading Hospital,
West Reading, PA, USA
e-mail: Monisha.bindra@towerhealth.org

E. B. Werley (✉)
Department of Emergency Medicine, Penn State College of Medicine/Penn State Health Milton S. Hershey Medical Center, Hershey, PA, USA
e-mail: ewerley@pennstatehealth.psu.edu

R. P. Olympia et al. (eds.), *An Emergency Physician's Path*,
https://doi.org/10.1007/978-3-031-47873-4_46

responses on a medical student's performance from shift evaluations and interactions in didactics or other educational activities. Resident learners may similarly receive feedback contemporaneous to clinical activities, but they will also receive feedback and evaluation of their clinical and academic progress based on ACGME, institutional, and program-specific requirements.

Feedback and evaluation are part of the educational process, and it has been ongoing as long as there has been medical education [1, 2]. Efforts to improve or even standardize feedback go back decades or more. In 1983, Ende made a valuable point relevant to this discussion. He acknowledged that, while feedback and evaluation are often used interchangeably with some admitted overlap, the key difference is that feedback provides objective metric or observational data in a more neutral tone, whereas evaluation often is more descriptive and in relation to established norms and expectations and typically involves some element of judgment [3]. As Ende noted, "In clinical medical education, the importance of feedback extends beyond pedagogy. The goal of clinical training is expertise in the care of patients. Without feedback, mistakes go uncorrected, good performance is not reinforced, and clinical competence is achieved empirically or not at all" [3]. Van de Ridder et al. argue that there is no set definition of feedback in the world of medical education. Their team performed an extensive literature search for the definition of feedback within the social sciences and medical education literature, and attempted to define feedback in the clinical environment as, "Specific information about the comparison between a trainee's observed performance and a standard, given with the intent to improve the trainee's performance" [2]. This makes the assumption that key elements are in place, including but not limited to the performance of an observable task (including both mental and physical tasks), a learner and an educator relationship (any combination of a more experienced person working with a learner), a standard to which the learner's performance can be compared, as well as direct observation of the task performance [2]. This clinical feedback is perhaps what is most commonly experienced by learners in medical education.

The intertwined topics of feedback and evaluation have generated much discussion over the years. A quick literature search might generate numerous publications on the efficacy of unique or individual tools, but that is beyond the scope of this chapter. We will instead focus on several different common elements of feedback and evaluation pertaining to your medical training and your future career, including myriad types of feedback, timing of feedback, and what is required of learners throughout their training. As faculty and other supervising staff work to improve the quality of their feedback, it is imperative that a learner gains skills in both receiving and providing feedback, as both help you improve as a physician and prepare you for the practice of medicine in the real world.

Timing and Context of Feedback

When feedback is provided to a student or resident learner, the timing of when that feedback is given can be directly related to the willingness and ability of the resident to receive it and the supervising educator's time and ability to provide it. Real patient care occurs while clinical education takes place, and it can be challenging to complete patient care tasks such as disposition, documentation, pending procedures, and so on, especially at the end of the shift or if a patient decompensates, all while leaving time to give effective feedback. Overlap of outgoing and incoming shifts can be useful to conclude aspects of patient care and create built-in time that can be utilized for feedback. Whether this is part of the culture within a department or not, the challenge is still in making time and the willingness of all participants to give and receive feedback. The "educational alliance" is a framework that may help combat this issue. The educational alliance takes away the unidirectional and traditional supervisor-to-learner feedback model and instead becomes more bidirectionally conversational and interactive, with agreed-upon expectations and goals, action plans to obtain those goals, and opportunities to incorporate feedback in new encounters [1]. This can be done quickly and deliberately in short-term situations, such as at the beginning and end of a paired shift, or on a more longitudinal basis.

Timing of feedback is also critical in terms of how it affects the learner. Some feedback needs to be given immediately if it directly impacts patient care, such as procedural guidance, if a dangerous action or omission is about to occur, or there is a key missing element on a differential diagnosis or management plan; other times feedback is better served after there has been time to reflect on recent performance. After a major resuscitation or difficult case, debriefing may provide ample learning opportunities for discussion. Other times, if a learner is distraught or upset, the conversation may, and probably should, be delayed as the learner may not be in the proper mindset to receive and process any feedback. At this point, the educator may acknowledge that the learner is distressed, and together they agree upon a time in the near future to discuss the events pertaining to an encounter [4]. As time lapses between an educational encounter and the provision of feedback, specific details may not be remembered as clearly, hence a need for timely discussion. Delays are not always intentional on the part of the educator though; learners can also greatly influence the timing of such a discussion. Learners may also strategically seek feedback, targeting educators more likely to give positive feedback or avoid feedback from faculty after perceived negative encounters. Learners may also specifically target feedback from an educator based on that educator's expertise on a topic, ease of access, or even perceived mood [5].

Similar to timing, the location and context need to be considered. If an educator is providing feedback to a group of learners, that educator needs to be mindful of both the learner receiving specific feedback as well as the educational level and expectations of the other learners present. This can be done successfully and may even generate discussion and further feedback amongst the learners [6]. However, if there is any doubt, private conversations may be a more safe environment for critical feedback [6]. In fact, in addition to the group versus individual dynamic, educators should consider other contextual factors when providing feedback, including the level of experience of the learner(s), established level of rapport with the learner(s), and if the feedback is meant to be more formative or evaluative [6].

In terms of educational expectations, the ACGME Program Requirements for Graduate Medical Education in Emergency Medicine recommend providing feedback frequently during a clinical rotation [7]. The ACGME requires that, for rotations lasting longer than 3 months or longitudinal experiences, a learner must be evaluated at a minimum every 3 months and upon completion of that rotation [7]. For an off-service rotation, this may be weekly or bi-weekly or at the minimum at the end of the rotation. For the emergency department or similarly scheduled rotations, this may be divided by shift, weekly, or other established frequency at the discretion of the program. The ACGME recommends increasing the frequency of feedback to resident learners that may have one or more deficiencies that need improvement [7]. This may include direct observation in patient care settings or simulation of procedures or case scenarios to emphasize areas to be improved.

The International Association of Medical Colleges, with the Liaison Committee on Medical Education (LCME) as the accrediting body of allopathic medical schools in the United States and Canada, highlights the LCME Accreditation Standards which mirror those standards put forth by the ACGME. Course directors and clerkship directors are required to develop a system for both formative and summative evaluation of medical students. Similar to the aforementioned ACGME requirements, early evaluation and feedback is strongly encouraged to permit time for remediation of any issues [8, 9]. Medical students are required to be assessed and provided with formative feedback, at a minimum no later than halfway through a course or clerkship. Exceptions are made for shorter courses and clerkships (i.e., less than 4 weeks), where course and clerkship directors may develop alternate means for medical students to be assessed and provided this vital feedback. Although the timing is less clearly defined, the American Association of Colleges of Osteopathic Medicine also addresses the need for the provision of "timely, sensitive, instructive feedback" to other team members, as well as an expectation of a respectful response to feedback from the learner [10].

Types of Feedback and Evaluation

The ACGME Common Program Requirements (Residency) nicely summarizes the difference between formative and summative evaluation. Formative evaluation occurs during the learning process, either in the context of patient care or other educational activities, and benefits both learners and those responsible for their education. Learners should self-reflect on their personal strengths and opportunities for improvement. Supervising faculty and program leaders can also use this as an opportunity to intervene early when issues are raised with a learner [11]. Summative evaluation compares the resident's growth and accomplishments to the set expectations for an event, whether that is a specific rotation or a certain level of training, and is used at key intervals, such as promotion to the next post-graduate year of training or successful completion of the training program. As medical education is a life-long continual learning process, it is not uncommon that there are elements of both formative and summative evaluation during the same feedback session or review document. "Feedback, formative evaluation, and summative evaluation compare intentions with accomplishments, enabling the transformation of a neophyte physician to one with growing expertise" [11].

Programs must also provide objective data regarding resident performance in addition to data from multi-source evaluations (shift evaluations, other faculty evaluations, peers, nurses and other staff, self-evaluations, and patients) to the Clinical Competency Committee (CCC) [7]. The CCC then compiles and reviews all of this data to guide formative evaluation of resident performance along specialty-specific Milestones [11]. The Milestones represent subsets of the ACGME Competencies across five levels and are progressive responsibilities and skills representing multiple aspects of resident performance as one advances throughout training. The goal for graduation for each milestone is to attain a level four, with level five being considered expert-level performance; it is worth noting that level four is a goal and should not be considered a graduation requirement [12]. These data, and the input from the CCC, are then provided to the program director. The program director, or a designee under their direction, then meets with each resident formally at required semi-annual evaluations [7].

Medical students have similar formal feedback. Data from shift evaluations are typically compiled and incorporated into their rotation grade. At the start of their rotation, each medical student typically meets with the clerkship director to understand the goals and expectations of the rotation. As noted earlier, depending on the length of the rotation, there may be a meeting midway through the rotation to both gain and give feedback on how the rotation is going and to help the medical student achieve the best overall educational experience. The clerkship director consolidates the shift evaluations throughout the rotation and should review this with each medical student at the end of the block. There are several forms of evaluations that programs may use, but often they all monitor growth in similar categories. The program may utilize a specialized form like the National Clinical Assessment Tool – Emergency Medicine (NCAT-EM), where each medical student is evaluated on their abilities to complete a focused history and physical exam, generate a prioritized differential diagnosis, formulate a patient care plan, reassess patients and follow up on patient care, recognize a medical emergency and then manage that emergency, and communicate with the patient and the patient care team members. Professional behaviors are also taken into account including compassion, sensitivity and respect toward patients and team members, dependability and accountability, initiative, work ethic, and ability to receive constructive feedback and incorporate it into future interactions [13]. In addition to these evaluations, some clerkship sites may utilize other data points that are incorporated into a student's final evaluation, such as participation in didactics and simulation sessions, presentations, or an exam.

Letters of recommendation for medical students applying to residency are another form of faculty evaluation, although this is a tricky issue, as they are typically confidential. The student and letter writer may meet ahead of time to discuss topics to be included such as future career goals, but the student waives their right to see the final letter, which is then uploaded centrally with the remainder of the student's application. The Council of Residency Directors in Emergency Medicine (CORD) worked to develop a more standardized letter of recommendation, now called a standardized letter of evaluation (SLOE). This way clerkship directors are all speaking the same language when evaluating and providing recommendations about students, and programs are interpreting similar information [14]. Over the years since implementation, the form has been updated including a new electronic version, as well as versions for students who perform subspecialty rotations, rotations at sites without an affiliated residency program, and even off-service rotations [15]. The weight a SLOE carries varies between each residency program, but it is considered to be an honest and informative evaluation that residency programs utilize in the interview selection and ranking process. Within the narrative section, some SLOEs may include specific comments from resident or faculty feedback, patient care metrics, standardized test scores, information on presentations given, and/or participation in educational activities. The SLOE provides a comparison of each medical student with other emergency medicine-bound learners who also complete a rotation in that department, including a projected ranking. While this evaluation of student performance is particularly useful to residency programs during the application and interview season, the drawback is that it provides little to no information to the actual learner because of the associated confidentiality.

Just like the various forms of more formalized feedback listed above, informal feedback can similarly come in myriad ways while on shift or during educational sessions. A high five or verbal kudos are typically appreciated by most, and minor celebrations deserve to be had. However, it helps if some identifying feature of the event is tied to feedback so a learner does not just hear that they did something well, but they also learn what they did well. While a discussion over repositioning with a towel roll or having second- and third-line options available for anticipated difficult intubation may be more obvious, informal feedback may be as subtle as an attending or senior resident giving praise on the successful lead of a team, highlighting closed-loop communication with clear direction during a code, or recommending that the resident make a subtle corrective action to improve first-chance success on a procedure. This similarly holds true for medical students. Feedback can also be more informally incorporated into on-shift teaching with medical students and residents through a discussion and reorganization of a differential diagnosis, a change in management for orders or medications, or when and how to utilize various clinical decision rules to guide medical decision making. As this type of feedback is often incorporated into conversations over patient care, it is less likely to be documented or formally structured. At times, learners may not even recognize it as feedback.

As students become residents, and residents transition into independent practice, traditional feedback opportunities evolve further. There may be regularly scheduled performance reviews where individual metric data and other topics are discussed with a medical director or department chair. Some objective data may be provided for self-comparison to peers, such as department metrics or resource utilization. Some feedback may be more casual, such as input from the inpatient team that admitted your patient, or your colleague to whom you signed out or who took care of your bounce back. Other feedback is likely to be self-directed, as physicians review and follow up on recent cases. While residents may have some initial exposure during training, patient satisfaction scores and comments are typically directed at the attending physician of record. Chart documentation and patient care may also be reviewed as part of a department's peer review process, with subsequent feedback on proposed personal or system-wide improvements to be made, or even at times confirmation of the care you provided. As emergency medicine physicians, we need to embrace that we are in a profession that is ever changing with clinical advances and that the only way that we can continue to improve is to be willing to accept and give feedback. While feedback and evaluation start in elementary school, they evolve over time and by no means stop when we are done with our formalized education.

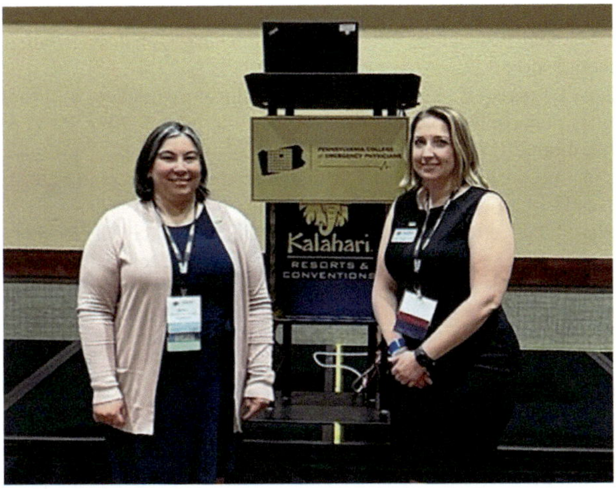

Dr. Bindra and Dr. Werley presenting together at Pennsylvania College of Emergency Physicians (PACEP) Scientific Assembly 2022

References

1. Telio S, Ajjawai R, Regehr G. The "educational alliance" as a framework for reconceptualizing feedback in medical education. Acad Med 2015;90(5):609–614.
2. van de Ridder JM, Stokking KM, McGaghie WC, ten Cate OT. What is feedback in clinical education? Med Educ. 2008;42(2):189–97.
3. Ende J. Feedback in clinical medical education. JAMA. 1983;250(6):777–81.

4. Roze des Ordons A, Cheng A, Gaudet J, Downar J, Lockyer J. Adapting feedback to individual residents: an examination of preceptor challenges and approaches. J Grad Med Educ. 2018;10(2):168–75.
5. Crommelinck M, Anseel F. Understanding and encouraging feedback-seeking behavior: a literature review. Med Educ. 2013;47(3):232–41.
6. Shaddel F, Newell-Jones K, O'Leary D. Providing contextually apt feedback in clinical education. Int J Med Educ. 2018;9:129–31.
7. ACGME Program Requirements for Graduate Medical Education in Emergency Medicine. Accreditation Council for Graduate Medical Education. https://www.acgme.org/globalassets/pfassets/programrequirements/110_emergencymedicine_2022.pdf. Accessed 13 Aug 2022.
8. LCME Accreditation Standards. International Association of Medical Colleges. https://www.iaomc.org/lcme.htm. Accessed 28 Aug 2022.
9. LCME Functions and Structure of a Medical School: Standards for Accreditation of Medical Education Programs Leading to the MD Degree. Association of American Medical Colleges and American Medical Association. October 2021.
10. Osteopathic Core Competencies for Medical Students. American Association of Colleges of Osteopathic Medicine. August 2012. https://www.aacom.org/docs/default-source/core-competencies/corecompetencyreport2012.pdf?sfvrsn=179c6097_4. Accessed 28 Aug 2022.
11. ACGME Common Program Requirements (Residency). Accreditation Council for Graduate Medical Education. https://www.acgme.org/globalassets/pfassets/programrequirements/cprresidency_2022v3.pdf. Accessed 28 Aug 2022.
12. Beeson M, Carter W, Cooney R, et al. Emergency medicine milestones. Accreditation Council for Graduate Medical Education. https://www.acgme.org/globalassets/pdfs/milestones/emergencymedicinemilestones.pdf. Accessed 30 Aug 2022.
13. Jung J, Franzen D, Lawson L, et al. The national clinical assessment tool for medical students in the emergency department (NCAT-EM). West J Emerg Med. 2018;19(1):66–74. https://doi.org/10.5811/westjem.2017.10.34834.
14. Keim SM, Rein JA, Chisholm C, et al. A standardized letter of recommendation for residency application. Acad Emerg Med. 1999;6(11):1141–6.
15. CORD Standardized Letter of Evaluation (SLOE). Council of Residency Directors in Emergency Medicine. https://www.cordem.org/resources/residency-management/sloe/. Accessed 31 Aug 2022.

Part V
Career Options as an Emergency Medicine Physician

Chapter 47
Administration and Leadership

Justin Grill and Steven VanRees

Walking through the door of the Emergency Department (ED) post-residency is the start of a new chapter in your career. Along with your patient care duties and continued honing of your skills as a physician, there is an expectation of taking an active role in leadership. In fact, the AMA Code of Ethics points out an expectation for physicians to go beyond team leadership roles and to take on institutional leadership roles. "What is leadership?" you may ask. "Do I need to be in administration to be a leader?" Although the two are often thought to go together, especially in the world of medicine, you do not need to be in administration to be a leader. However, in order to be an effective administrator, you need to be an equally effective leader.

What does "being a leader" mean? Being a leader does not mean that you are the hero who comes up with all the solutions to the problems that are encountered. Being a leader is more about teamwork and making those around you better. Ronald Reagan once said, "The greatest leader is not necessarily the one who does the greatest thing. He is the one that gets the people to do the greatest thing." If you are able to help facilitate success for those around you, you will distinguish yourself as a leader. A formal title is not required to be a physician leader, but they will often end up in "leadership roles" because others recognize their value, whether serving in system-wide administration, hospital-based administrative roles, departmental leadership, and even team leadership roles. I consider myself fortunate that I have been afforded opportunities throughout my career to serve in multiple leadership positions, most recently as the Medical Director of the Emergency Department.

Throughout our early medical career, we are often primarily focused on individual recognition, accomplishments, and self-promotion. A complete mindset shift is required to be successful as a leader, more specifically as Medical Director. It is

J. Grill (✉) · S. VanRees
Department of Emergency Medicine, Trinity Health Muskegon, Muskegon, MI, USA
e-mail: grillj@trinity-health.org; Steven.vanrees@trinity-health.org

R. P. Olympia et al. (eds.), *An Emergency Physician's Path*,
https://doi.org/10.1007/978-3-031-47873-4_47

important to understand that the role of the Medical Director is to foster collaboration within all departmental areas and to be open and encouraging of ideas from all team members. Seeking this broad input from all areas will enable you to determine the most important and pressing issues that may be affecting the department and assist your decision-making process to create a thriving, well-functioning Emergency Department instead of a dysfunctional, inefficient nightmare that will cause staff and patients to suffer. Leaders cannot possibly know the intricacies of each team member's job functions, so fostering an "open-door" policy will allow getting things right the first time and not having to suffer through regrets and revisions.

Some of the first areas that I focused on in my role as Medical Director were appropriate staffing of the department to meet the needs and demands of the patient population and identifying bottlenecks within the department that slow flow or prevent optimal efficiencies and experience. Both are challenging to accomplish, even more so when a system is already in place. There is an expectation of "buy-in" from all levels of the team in order for the changes to take place and be successful. Add to that the ever-changing environment of healthcare, including a worldwide pandemic and the challenges that even the most experienced directors and leaders never saw coming.

Many people enjoy departmental leadership such as ED directorships for their careers, however, some people have an interest in transitioning to a hospital-based administrative position such as those in Medical Affairs, Medical Education, Quality, or serving as a Chief Medical Officer (CMO). These positions come with their own difficulties and rewards, and we will begin with a brief discussion regarding the transition of a career into hospital-based administration.

During residency, a wise attending told me to join the hospital peer review committee wherever I got my first job. He said that it would rapidly teach me common pitfalls, allow continued learning about other specialties (which always helps in EM), and also give me insight into how the hospital and medical staff operate from the inside. In retrospect, that was also what led me to a career in administrative medicine. While it is understandable that the vast majority of physicians have little interest in administration (it is often why we went to medical school, after all), most would agree that abdicating the mantle of healthcare leadership has not led to better healthcare or an improved work environment. Thus, for the EM physicians who do have an interest in administrative medicine, hospital committee work is often the first place to begin. Prior to choosing which committee, it is reasonable to consider your interests. The organized medical staff is very much different than hospital-based operations. Committees are formed by the Medical Executive Committee (MEC) to serve the needs of the medical staff. Likewise, the hospital will form committees to serve their needs, and often there is overlap. If your passion is quality or safety, it is nearly certain that there are committees with a particular focus on these topics. If education is more your passion, both undergraduate and graduate medical education (UME and GME) are always looking for assistance with the training of future physicians.

Once you begin to gather experience, it will become clear where your administrative passion may lie. A very common next step is elected medical staff office or appointment by a hospital to some sort of administrative position, and this step often differentiates the pathway forward. Moving through the elected medical staff structure allows the unique ability to help shape medical staff process and procedure, support fellow physicians in difficult times in their career, work in dyad relationships with nurses and other hospital-based staff, and, critically, help assure broad quality and safety of patient care. Truthfully, as a profession, one of our greatest duties is self-governance and assurance of high-quality patient care; the organized medical staff is the major mechanism by which we do that.

Outside of work within the organized medical staff are administrative positions hired by the hospital. These can be full- or part-time. Due to the nature of our work in Emergency Medicine, we often have the ability to maintain clinical work while serving in an administrative capacity. Many hospital-based (or medical school-based) positions are addressed in other chapters of the book. This section of the chapter will be focused on the position of Vice President of Medical Affairs (VPMA) and CMO. Indeed, it is not uncommon for these to be combined into one position or found as interchangeable names. In larger systems, you may find them separated. When separate, the VPMA tends to focus their work on quality, safety, recruitment, physician development, and policy/procedure. The CMO often focuses their work on strategic planning with the hospital executive team, finance, clinical service line development, accreditation, and supervision of quality and safety. Perhaps the most difficult part of the CMO's position is serving as a liaison between the hospital executive team, who are often non-clinical, and the medical staff. This position often finds itself with one leg on the clinical side of medicine and one on the administrative side, often being pulled in opposite directions and adjudicating differences between those two groups of people who do not speak the same language.

While the role of a hospital-based VPMA/CMO is amazingly difficult, it is likewise amazingly rewarding. It is not uncommon for that individual to be the only physician on the executive leadership team, possibly one of few on the governing board. It provides the unique ability to shape high-quality and safe healthcare in their community. As noted above, it is not uncommon for CMOs coming from Emergency Medicine to continue some degree of clinical practice (this author included).

It has been published that hospitals run by physicians have 25% better quality outcomes as compared to those run by non-physician administrators [1]. As a profession, we have a duty to take on the mantle of leadership in administration. As physicians, we have a unique and patient-centered perspective on how healthcare should be delivered. As emergency physicians, we are the front door of the healthcare system, which affords us an even more unique perspective. Fortunately, our professional societies have built-in structures to assist in preparing us for this endeavor. ACEP and AAEM have focus areas in leadership. Additionally, organizations such as the American Association for Physician Leadership (AAPL) are devoted to leadership training for physicians. It is our hope that many of you will consider leadership and administrative positions and help drive quality healthcare forward into the future.

Reference

1. Stoller J, Goodall A, Baker A. Why the best hospitals are managed by doctors. Harv Bus Rev. 2016. https://Hbr.org/2016/why-the-best-hospitals-are-managed-by-doctors

Chapter 48
Advocacy

Daniel Freess

If Not Me, Who?

I once counseled a graduating resident who had done some "advocacy" activity during her residency years. In uploading her CV into a preformatted (and somewhat limited) online template for a specific job, she asked me for help deciding in what category to place her activities. I advised her to place them under "Community Service." After all, the whole reason for advocacy activities is to serve your "community." The goal is to enact changes and programs that help your local, professional, hospital, patient, and personal communities. Sometimes you are working on behalf of a specific group, but more often, your efforts seek to improve multiple communities within your medical and professional environment.

Why does our state have such a poor professional liability climate? Why is our reimbursement falling when others are seeing increases? Why does the Department of Anesthesia dictate our ED sedation and intubation decisions? Why do our substance use patients have so few resources on discharge? Why do we have more CME requirements every single year? While we often ask these and other similar questions to ourselves in a depersonalized sense, the answer to all these questions is the same: because we, as a community of emergency physicians, have not sufficiently or effectively advocated for ourselves and our patients to a level at which we are comfortable and satisfied. This does not mean that we have control of every decision or situation, that there is funding for every priority, nor that we are able to immediately create our idealized work environment overnight. With that said, if you are not

D. Freess (✉)
Department of Emergency Medicine, Hartford Hospital, Hartford, CT, USA

Integrated Residency In Emergency Medicine, University of Connecticut, Hartford, USA
e-mail: Daniel.Freess@hhchealth.org

R. P. Olympia et al. (eds.), *An Emergency Physician's Path*,
https://doi.org/10.1007/978-3-031-47873-4_48

helping to advocate for yourself, your patients, and your community, you are partially to blame for your concerns and struggles.

Who Are You Advocating For?

Advocacy comes in many forms and venues. Before initiating or defining an advocacy effort, you must first ask, "Whose interests are being addressed?" Is it for ourselves, for our hospitals, for our patients, for our communities, or some combination of all these entities? On the local level, it is critical to advocate for the needs and goals of the individual emergency department and its patients. Just a couple examples are as follows:

- Setting up community resources for post-discharge care
- Addressing local issues of social Emergency Medicine such as homelessness, substance abuse resources, poverty, education, and mentorship
- Maintaining or defending the autonomy and independence of emergency physicians with the hospital community and infrastructure
- Protecting and ensuring due process rights for physicians and medical staff
- Ensuring fair reimbursement for care provided in the Emergency Department

On the state or regional level, emergency physicians need representatives at the Capitol advocating for them and their patients in both the legislative and regulatory arenas to:

- Ensure fair and equitable insurance standards for patients and physicians
- Testify on bills that affect the health of the community
- Work to improve the professional liability environment to protect and recruit physicians
- Assist with EMS and healthcare regionalization to maximize or optimize resources and coverage

Finally, on the national level, it is critical to set standards for Emergency Medicine practice across the country and the world, as well as advocate for our rights and interests within the greater healthcare landscape. Emergency physicians might:

- Provide testimony and education on issues related to Medicare and Medicaid and how they affect Emergency Medicine
- Help create policies and legislation that work toward universal coverage and access for our patients
- Create national practice standard for emergency care and evaluation
- Work with national Emergency Medicine organizations to maximize knowledge translation and Emergency Medicine practice improvement

What Is In It for Me?

Simply put, advocacy work can be frustrating and often thankless. It requires a lot of work, ongoing dedication, a "glass is half full" attitude, and more than anything else, patience. While some efforts are quick and easy, most are slow and can be equated to moving mountains. Personally, I have been working on the same insurance and professional liability issues on the state level for the past decade and little has changed. This does not make these efforts a failure, simply issues in need of constant attention and ongoing effort. As a result, it can be easy to ask yourself, "what's the point?" or "why do I do this?"

In my personal experience, there is great career fulfillment and a feeling of honor in advocating for others. Even when only small victories are obtained, or no victory is obtained at all, but you successfully educate others on issues in Emergency Medicine, there is a feeling of accomplishment and fulfillment that carries you to the next fight or effort. Also, if not you, then who? Even if you are only fighting to maintain the status quo, your colleagues will appreciate your time, your effort, and the fact that you are sacrificing your time and energy on their account. Similarly, there is self-satisfaction in working toward a goal, particularly one that helps your everyday work life and clinical environment. While there is no research that I can find, anecdotally those whom I have talked to all mention that their advocacy work enhances their clinical career by giving it perspective, meaning, and value knowing what went into supporting and protecting the work environment. Finally, it is thought that working on advocacy issues as well as holding leadership roles within Emergency Medicine leads to decreased burnout and job-related stress.

Your Second Family

Though not unique to advocacy work, once you get involved, you quickly find that you are part of a small and connected community. While we do not usually think about "professional" work for the purpose of making friends, like joining a local sports league or civic organization, when you are working on similar issues and/or work together, there is an inherent camaraderie and respect that comes with combined effort. As a result, when you go to various events and advocacy forums, you are surrounded by like-minded individuals who typically are different and/or separate from your normal clinical colleagues. This provides for a venue and resource where you can gain perspective on mutually experienced issues, share stories of success and failure, and voice honest concerns in a constructive and objective manner without the pressure of being within your own colleague network or work environment.

Integrating Advocacy into Your Career

Adding advocacy into your career can be as simple as a few emails a month to as involved as a few trips each month. Regardless, it helps to start small. Find an area you care about and/or are passionate about. You will not find a niche or joy in advocacy if you do not believe in what you are doing. While it is often recommended to "just say yes" at the beginning of your career or as you try to develop within a field, this does not work well in advocacy when your heart, mind, and energy need to all be aligned along a single idea or mission. Second, it is critical to find mentors. They can keep you motivated, guide you on good starting points, and keep you engaged in the process both actively and passively until you are able to fly and advocate on your own.

Once established and/or active in the areas of leadership and advocacy, it is important to recognize both your worth and your time investment in advocacy efforts. Unfortunately, advocacy efforts and work are often viewed by others and administrators as a "hobby" or "extracurricular activity," in a way separate from your primary career or work. When I first started being involved in advocacy efforts and held some national-level positions, I sought recognition from my organization/group for my efforts and was met with the sentiment, "We already have someone doing that." "That" is advocacy on the national level for a group of more than 1000 physicians. It does not have to be this way! Anyone and everyone should and needs to be involved in advocacy efforts. In order to truly integrate advocacy into your career though, you must fight against this notion that there is no "space/time" to go around or that advocacy is separate from the clinical arena. No one would deem work in emergency ultrasound, resident education, or ED quality programs to be an "extracurricular activity" or something emergency physicians do in their spare time, yet advocacy work often takes a back seat to other niches and activities. Instead, you must account for the time and energy spent on advocacy efforts in order to obtain credit and time allowances commensurate with other academic pursuits and activities.

Getting Started

There is no "right way" to get started in advocacy. It can begin organically when someone asks you to help out with a project or effort, or you can take a more direct approach by researching different activities and reaching out to those involved to offer your time and energy. Some places to seek information include looking up your State Medical Society and their activities, contacting members of your State ACEP Chapter, or searching the ACEP website (acep.org) where there is an entire heading/section on the main page dedicated to "Advocacy," with a sub-section on how to "Get Involved." Now it is up to you!

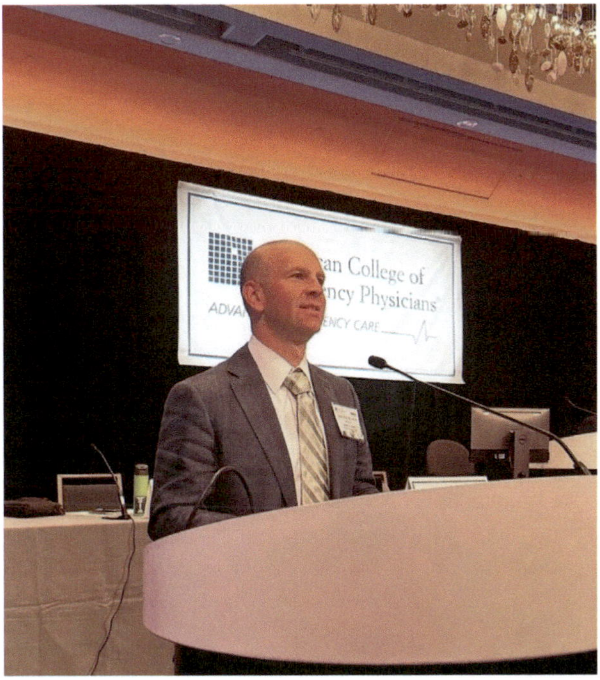

Leading a Reference Committee presentation of resolutions to the ACEP Council. Every resolution written in some way advocates for our fellow physicians, our jobs, and our patients

Chapter 49
Patient Safety and Quality Improvement

Brenna M. Farmer

All leaders in Emergency Medicine (EM) must have some awareness of quality and patient safety (QPS). In part, this awareness is due to the attention QPS has gained since the first Institute of Medicine report focused on QPS, "To Err is Human: Building a Safer Healthcare System," was published in 2000 [1]. QPS principles and training are now a standard part of medical student and resident education. For an academic career in EM, physicians with a role in QPS can be educators, departmental, hospital, or healthcare system leaders, or work in other aspects of the healthcare industry such as pharmaceuticals, device development, technology, and so on.

Education

A career in QPS also provides the ability to educate all healthcare providers along the continuum of medical school, residency, and fellowship education on QPS topics. For undergraduate medication education (medical students), most medical schools have an introduction of QPS terminology and principles as part of classes related to health care quality, social determinants of health, and health disparities. For graduate medical education, QPS basics are emphasized and expected as part of the Clinical Learning Environment Review (CLER) process of accreditation [2]. In addition to the education of QPS concepts, participation in QPS is expected and evaluated during the CLER visit for teaching hospitals as part of maintaining

B. M. Farmer (✉)
New York Presbyterian Brooklyn Methodist Hospital, Brooklyn, NY, USA

Weill Cornell Medicine, New York, NY, USA
e-mail: bmf9001@med.cornell.edu

R. P. Olympia et al. (eds.), *An Emergency Physician's Path*,
https://doi.org/10.1007/978-3-031-47873-4_49

accreditation from the Accreditation Council of Graduate Medical Education (ACGME) [2]. Moreover, a core part of the EM curriculum for every residency program is the EM milestones. They include QPS as part of systems-based practice [3].

Within education, there is a need for QPS leaders to ensure that learners have a basic understanding of QPS as outlined by the EM milestones from the ACGME. The specific EM milestones focused on QPS are sub-competencies of the system-based practice core competency [3]. Residents should participate in case reviews, morbidity and mortality conferences, reviews of grievances and complaints, and root cause analyses (RCAs). Active participation in these different QPS spaces ensures that residents have exposure to all aspects of QPS, allows for a better understanding of the EM milestones related to QPS, and may spark interest in further study to gain greater expertise. These exposures also allow residents to contribute to corrective actions, process improvement, and sustainability of any changes made for QPS. The contributions residents bring to QPS are very valuable, especially as they are providing frontline care and know the processes and workarounds to take care of patients, often better than the supervising attending physicians. Additionally, for the ACGME CLER program, QPS leaders can contribute to the education and discussions for two of the six focus areas (patient safety and health care quality) for their local graduate medical education office, which oversees all resident and fellow education for QPS [2].

To provide an example for how QPS education is a career opportunity, I will highlight some of my work as an assistant residency program director (APD). When I became an APD, the CLER visit and EM milestones were newly implemented as requirements from ACGME by the Residency Review Committee (RRC) for Emergency Medicine. Our local program needed to add curricular pieces to highlight the new QPS emphasis and decide what we would consider as meeting each level for systems-based practice 1 (Patient Safety) and systems-based practice 2 (Quality Improvement) after our gap analysis of all of the current curricular initiatives[2]. I led other QPS leaders from our department to develop basic lectures on terminology, process improvement, the QPS process at our hospital, and root cause analysis. To allow our residents to apply the knowledge we imparted, a mock root cause analysis (RCA) was implemented during one of our usual conference days. An example case from our curriculum is here: https://www.cordem.org/globalassets/files/curricular-toolkit/root.cause/rca.instructors.guide.pdf [4]. This QPS scholarly activity demonstrates expertise for academic advancement. For further resident education and for faculty development of coaching, mentoring, and supervisory skills, outside of usual resident didactic time, a QPS leader should include residents in departmental QPS meetings, RCAs, ad hoc meetings to develop process improvement around newly identified issues, and answer grievances and complaints submitted by patients and their advocates. This educational aspect for residents is best done as part of an administrative rotation.

Departmental Leadership

If education and curriculum development are not your forte, there are QPS opportunities in departmental or divisional leadership. The best way to start is to show interest and let your boss know of that interest. One of the easiest ways to show your interest is to ask to attend QPS meetings for your department. Attendance there will provide exposure and allow you to identify the QPS goals, strategies, and concerns for your department. Seek out mentorship from current QPS leaders in the department, and if you are newly appointed to a QPS leadership role, from other physicians in other departments in the same role or from other institutions with the same departmental role. As a part of the QPS team for your department, you can do quality reviews, formulate responses to grievances and complaints, and work with the operations leadership to address quality metrics reported to different regulatory bodies.

Within a department, QPS can be a sub-focus for leaders in different divisions as well. For example, in toxicology, there may be a need for improved medication safety in the ED and evidence-based guidelines for medication use in certain situations. For emergency medical services, there is always a need to review pre-hospital care and evaluate for any QPS issues. For emergency ultrasound, there must be a quality review program in place to allow for review of each study performed in the department to ensure it meets quality standards. A QPS ultrasound leader can also develop guidelines with other services on acceptable point-of-care ultrasound studies to drive clinical decision-making and decrease time to definitive care. Any EM sub-specialty will have similar QPS needs.

Hospital/Health System Involvement

For a hospital or health system to have a meaningful QPS program, they need manpower. This manpower comes from all disciplines and is often focused on teamwork, as healthcare is provided in teams and is multi-disciplinary. Committee involvement may be as broadly labeled as QPS or executive QPS with subcommittees focused on medication safety, falls, stroke, STEMI, trauma, and the like. Within these committees, there are leadership opportunities for the local hospital or for the more extensive health system with multiple hospital or campus locations. These leadership positions may include chair positions of committees such as medication safety, significant events review, root cause analysis, and so on.

There are also QPS hospital or healthcare system roles such as in the executive suite as a Chief Quality Officer or a Vice President of Quality and Patient Safety. While these roles may have slightly different titles depending on the institution, they perform similar duties. These QPS leaders not only develop the QPS strategy for the hospital: deciding which national patient safety goals (NPSG) from the Joint Commission[5] the organization will focus on for the year, what additional areas of QPS must be included in the local goals based on local needs and RCAs, identified gaps, state requirements, and so on. They ensure that the hospital is meeting requirements from multiple different regulatory agencies, reporting incidents to regulatory and governmental bodies, and can discuss specialty or service-line specific goals based on national organizations, special recognitions, and certifications such as stroke, STEMI, and trauma. In fact, EM physicians are ideal for such roles as a lot of areas and certifications involve care in the ED in some way. Furthermore, EM physicians are regularly interacting with many different services and service lines, given that the ED is one of the main front doors to care for any hospital.

Industry

There are many opportunities outside of clinical care for QPS careers. There are quality and safety officers or roles for pharmaceutical, device, health technology, and other aspects of the broad healthcare industry. Oftentimes, companies like to have physicians in these roles because of the previous bedside clinical knowledge that others in the same field may not have. This clinical experience allows for the companies to understand the impact a QPS concern should or could have and whether a new drug or device should move forward or be changed.

Training

To get started in QPS, all you need is a basic understanding of the terminology and concepts. That initial education is usually provided in the residency curriculum as part of the EM milestones [3]. On-the-job training by participating in different aspects of case reviews for quality and committee work is helpful. This work provides you with an understanding of how QPS works at your divisional, departmental, and hospital or health system level. Mentorship from current QPS leaders is very valuable as you move forward into QPS leadership. In addition, there are options for additional trainings, certifications, and fellowships to help eliminate any knowledge gaps, build a deeper understanding of QPS, and meet with others experiencing similar QPS challenges. Your local institution may have a quality academy or other educational program to build up knowledgeable QPS leaders. You can participate in specialized EM QPS or administrative fellowship programs after residency or in non-specialty specific fellowships offered by national organizations. These fellowships are non-ACGME accredited fellowships and sometimes offer advanced degrees as part of the program. Online certifications such as the IHI's Open School are a very good primer for new QPS leaders or those looking to become QPS leaders [6].

A QPS Career Example

My journey into QPS, as a career focus, started when I was a medical toxicology fellow. My fellowship director invited me, as a guest, to our local hospital's medication safety committee and to a root cause analysis (RCA) meeting concerning a real case related to a medication error. These exposures to QPS principles and discussions of corrective actions piqued my interest. The avoidance of blame and concentration on the prevention of future such events were always highlighted during the discussions I witnessed. I wanted to learn and do more.

After my fellowship and with my newfound medical toxicology background, I joined the medication safety committee at my hospital. There I learned about the hospital's event reporting system (ERS), summative data reviewed by a hospital from the ERS, retrospective chart reviews, and much more. I gained knowledge about how a hospital or healthcare system approaches single cases from the quality and safety reviews performed and one approach used to identify patterns of concern from multiple sources of QPS data. I also learned what outside sources were used to help develop overall QPS strategies, guide policies, and develop guidelines. The knowledge gained during my initial participation on the medication safety committee allowed me to reach out to my local ED leadership and ask how to become involved in broader the ED QPS program of my department.

As I became more engaged in QPS, I identified my own knowledge gaps and decided to pursue additional training. Through a fellowship in patient safety leadership, I learned about goal setting, trends, improvement science, and qualitative research approaches to QPS. I heard national and international QPS leaders teach about their areas of interest and best practices for different aspects of QPS, whether it was medication, equipment, knowledge, or skills related. The focus on multidisciplinary and inter-disciplinary aspects of QPS was emphasized. I participated in group projects to solve QPS problems to show how multiple roles, disciplines, and specialties providing many different viewpoints impact the development of robust solutions and QPS initiatives for process improvement.

After a few years of QPS experience, I became a director of patient safety for my department. My major projects and initiatives focused on improving medication safety by working with pharmacists in the ED, standardizing shift change and sign-out process, and QPS leadership rounding to hear from the frontline team about concerns that had not made it into the ERS or come up with case reviews. When the department was looking for more oversight as more hospitals with EDs were added to our health system, I was promoted to Vice Chair for Quality and Patient Safety.

The goals of such a role were to standardize our QPS strategy across our multiple EDs, to ensure implementation of any process improvement was disseminated across the sites, and to mentor each director of QPS with local initiatives.

Academic Promotion

When considering QPS as an academic niche, you must consider the requirements needed for academic promotion if that is your desire. In most medical school promotions, written scholarly activity must be demonstrated. Some institutions may have very rigorous requirements with the need for grant funding, research, and publishing in peer-reviewed journals on the efforts the grant supported. Most institutions have modified titles to allow for a clinical or educator or other tract for promotion. These modified tracts tend to not have the same rigorous research requirements or require as many peer-reviewed publications. QPS can fit under any such promotion pathway for an academic EM physician. The key is taking QPS work implemented or completed and publishing it in some way. These publications can include rigorous research, or by promoting locally developed QI protocols, guidelines, and outcomes from those guidelines and publishing in peer-reviewed and non-peer reviewed ways including journals, newsletters, free open access medical education (such as the mock RCA curriculum mentioned above), and so on. From a peer-reviewed publication standpoint, I have published an initiative to increase paracentesis to decrease the time to identify spontaneous peritoneal bacteremia in cirrhotic patients [7]. An example of a non-peer-reviewed work is seen with my publications and collaboration for society position statements for medication safety during the COVID-19 pandemic or the role pharmacists play in patient care in the ED [8, 9].

In addition to scholarly activity, more and more promotion committees are including mentorship as a criterion. QPS can allow many such opportunities for mentorship. And any EM physician should be able to look at how they have impacted others through mentorship, coaching, and sponsorship. Again, using myself as an example, I have worked with students, residents, advanced practice providers, and junior colleagues to coach and mentor them in whatever stage they were in their careers. One of my former residents leads QPS initiatives for her residency program, for the Council of Residency Directors in Emergency Medicine, and with the ACGME. Her work is leading the way in QPS education for EM. Other junior colleagues are directors of QPS in their local departments. An advanced practice provider I worked with is participating in a multidisciplinary fellowship for QPS from a regional organization. He is now working with our institution on several QPS initiatives for EM and beyond. These mentees and colleagues will be my legacy. Hopefully, they will impart some of my teaching and my examples in mentorship and coaching to their mentees continuing my future legacy.

Summary

QPS is a great niche for any EM physician. Whether you want to be an educator, a divisional, departmental, or hospital leader, or pivot to industry, QPS opens those options. The necessary training starts in medical school and continues in residency. Through mentorship, coaching, and sometimes fellowship or certification programs, it is easy to gain the knowledge for working in a QPS and becoming a leader.

References

1. Institute of Medicine (US). Committee on quality of health care in America. In: Kohn LT, Corrigan JM, Donaldson MS, editors. To err is human: building a safer health system. Washington, DC: National Academies Press (US); 2000.
2. Accreditation Council for Graduate Medical Education. Clinical learning environment review. https://www.acgme.org/what-we-do/initiatives/clinical-learning-environment-review-cler/cler-site-visit/. Last Accessed 2 Oct 2022.
3. Accreditation Council for Graduate Medical Education. Emergency medicine milestones. https://www.acgme.org/globalassets/pdfs/milestones/emergencymedicinemilestones.pdf. Last Accessed 2 Oct 2022.
4. Fant A, Farmer B, Lock B. Mock root cause analysis instructor's guide and associated materials. https://www.cordem.org/resources/education%2D%2Dcurricula/curricular-toolkit/medicolegal/. Last Accessed 2 Oct 2022.
5. The Joint Commission. National patient safety goals. https://www.jointcommission.org/standards/national-patient-safety-goals/. Last Accessed 2 Oct 2022.
6. Institute for Healthcare Improvement. IHI Open School. https://www.ihi.org/education/ihi-open-school/Pages/default.aspx. Last Accessed 2 Oct 2022.
7. Jesudian A, Barraza L, Steel P, Shen N, Schneider Y, Bodnar D, Farmer B, Dargar S, Del Toro C, Sharma R, Brown RS, Lee JI. Quality improvement initiative increases total paracentesis and early paracentesis rates in hospitalized cirrhotics with ascites. Frontline Gastroenterol. 2020;11(1):22–7.
8. Farmer BM, Hayes B, Rao R, et al. The role of pharmacists in the emergency department. J Med Toxicol. 2018;14(1):114–6. PMID: 29075954.
9. Farmer BM, Cole JB, Olives TD, et al. ACMT position statement: medication administration and safety during the response to COVID-19 pandemic. J Med Toxicol. 2020;16(4):481–3. PMID: 32617893.

Chapter 50
EMS Medical Director

Daniel Johnson and Jeffrey S. Lubin

Background

The inception of emergency medical services (EMS) in the United States was prompted by the development of the U.S. highway system and the subsequent burden of traumatic injury that resulted. Despite the many motorists being injured in accidents, the country lacked a coordinated system to care for these victims. In 1966, the National Academy of Science–National Research Council published a paper entitled *Accidental Death and Disability: The Neglected Disease of Modern Society* which is largely credited for prompting the development of EMS programs in this country [1]. As these systems became more advanced, physician medical oversight became a necessity and thus, was borne the role of the EMS Medical Director ("medical director").

The role of the medical director was initially filled by any physician who was eager and willing to oversee care in the out-of-hospital environment. Prior to Emergency Medicine (EM) being declared a medical specialty in 1979, many medical directors were family physicians, surgeons, or other specialists. As the field of EM has grown, so has the percentage of medical directors trained in the specialty. In 1985, the National Association of EMS Physicians was established and paved the way for the definition of EMS Medicine as its own unique subspecialty. In 2010, EMS Medicine was recognized as a subspecialty by the American Board of

D. Johnson
Department of Emergency Medicine, Penn State College of Medicine, Hershey, PA, USA
e-mail: djohnson18@pennstatehealth.psu.edu

J. S. Lubin (✉)
Departments of Emergency Medicine and Public Health Sciences, Penn State College of Medicine, Hershey, PA, USA
e-mail: jlubin@pennstatehealth.psu.edu

R. P. Olympia et al. (eds.), *An Emergency Physician's Path*,
https://doi.org/10.1007/978-3-031-47873-4_50

Emergency Medicine, and the first diplomates were board-certified in EMS medicine shortly thereafter.

Even before an emergency occurs, many EMS agencies take responsibility for educating the lay public on the signs and symptoms of life-threatening medical conditions such as heart attacks and strokes, how to access the 9-1-1 system, and how to perform basic first aid. When someone calls 9-1-1 during a medical emergency in the United States, this triggers a chain of events resulting in prompt evaluation, treatment, and transportation if necessary. Often, the first contact with emergency services is with a 9-1-1 dispatcher. They are able to provide initial care instructions to bystanders over the phone and dispatch appropriate resources to the scene. Commonly, the first units to arrive are first responders, such as police officers or firefighters, who can provide initial stabilization and first aid. This is followed by the dispatch of an appropriate EMS unit (i.e., ambulance) to provide more advanced care and transport the patient to the hospital. Occasionally, patients may require transportation between hospitals for specialty care and services. Each element of this chain of survival described above demands the oversight of physicians with particular knowledge of care in the unique, pre-hospital environment.

This chapter outlines the various roles and responsibilities of medical directors. It should be noted that there is a distinction between providing online medical control/direct medical oversight and being a medical director. Nearly all EM physicians will be required, as part of their clinical duties, to provide guidance to EMS units transporting patients to their emergency departments. In some states, this comes with formal training and certification. For example, in the Commonwealth of Pennsylvania, EM physicians are required to complete training and become certified as a "Medical Command Physician" by the Department of Health. Though nearly all medical directors would be expected to be medical command physicians, the corollary is not true; medical command physicians are not required to provide medical direction for EMS agencies, and so on.

EMS Agency Medical Director

The most common role to be referred to as a "medical director" would be that of an EMS agency. EMS agencies that provide advanced life support, basic life support, and quick response agencies in certain areas of the United States are required to have medical direction. Many non-EMS agencies that have a role in providing medical care such as police departments and fire departments have medical directors as well. The role of the medical director is variable and is largely determined by the complexity of care that is provided. Agencies that utilize first responders to provide immediate first aid and stabilization require much less oversight than complex, critical care transport teams. Although some components may be added or removed based on the level of care that is overseen, the primary roles of the agency EMS medical director include credentialing EMS personnel, overseeing quality improvement and quality assurance, process improvement, field supervision, and provider wellness [2].

Credentialing of EMS Personnel

EMS providers go through a process of certification, licensing, and credentialing before they are able to care for patients independently. The certification process, which serves to ensure that the EMS providers have mastered the educational content to fulfill their role, is generally performed by accredited educational institutions. After certification, providers go through a process of licensure which grants them the ability to provide care up to their level of training, usually granted by a governmental body. Finally, before the provider is able to "hit the streets," they must be credentialed by the EMS agency medical director. This process, broadly, ensures that the provider has the knowledge and skills to function within their given EMS system. Usually, this process is revisited on an annual basis to ensure that skills are maintained [2].

If a provider no longer demonstrates the knowledge or skills to safely care for patients, they may require de-credentialing by the medical director. This is an unfortunate but necessary role of the medical director to ensure the safety of the community and an area of potential liability for the medical director. De-credentialing must be performed in a way that it does not unduly interfere with the ability of the provider to find employment elsewhere or lose their certification, which is considered an extension of their personal property. Medical directors must work closely with those in the operational sector of their agency and not to confuse their role as a medical authority with that of human resource officers [2].

Quality Improvement, Quality Assurance, and Process Improvement

The cornerstone of providing high-quality care to the community is the process of quality improvement and quality assurance. It is the responsibility of the agency medical director to ensure that the care provided is meeting the standards set by national guidelines and local/regional protocols. Various metrics must be tracked and closely monitored. Often, the medical director will randomly sample patient care reports for review to ensure that care is appropriate. Many will more closely review high-risk patient encounters such as cardiac arrests, endotracheal intubations, cases utilizing new or updated medications or protocols, or refusals of medical attention. The medical director must also analyze their system's metrics compared with national benchmarks for cases such as trauma, cardiac arrest, and stroke care, reporting this data to national databases when appropriate.

Concerns about negligent supervision comprise a significant portion of the legal liability for an EMS agency medical director. However, because only in rare cases do EMS providers technically operate directly under the license of the medical director, there is some protection for the medical director should the EMS providers provide negligent care. However, the medical director is responsible for recognizing trends among EMS providers who may be providing consistent, substandard care. If the process is not in place to recognize and address alarming trends, the responsibility for patient harm can fall on the shoulders of the medical director [2].

Field Supervision

While this is not necessarily a mandatory job responsibility of all medical directors, many will argue that to provide appropriate medical oversight the medical director must understand the environment in which their EMS providers operate. Medical directors can provide direct medical oversight in the form of field response to emergency scenes. In some cases, they operate their own emergency vehicles designated to the medical director. This provides an opportunity to observe their crews in action while also providing immediate feedback and education. Physicians who choose to include this in their practice must be trained in all aspects of scene safety; in some states, certification as a prehospital EMS physician and/or emergency vehicle operator may be required [2].

Provider Wellness

Medical directors are physicians, so it would be expected that they should also be the authority for the providers' physical and mental wellness. EMS is a stressful profession, and the mental health of EMS providers is something that should be monitored closely and be able to be intervened on if necessary. EMS providers, at times, work under hazardous conditions, are exposed to life-threatening substances, and may be required to wear protective equipment that may interfere with their health. The medical director should act as an authority on programs and policies that keep their providers safe [2].

Medical Director for Educational Programs

With the advent of modern EMS systems also comes a robust system to educate, train, and evaluate EMS personnel to ensure they are providing high-quality care to their patients. The process begins with certification, a process in which an accredited EMS education program ensures that the providers have gained the minimal necessary knowledge to fulfill their roles. Many accredited EMS training programs are required to have medical directors as part of their faculty. The medical director has a responsibility to recruit and ensure the quality of faculty that provides instruction to the students. Additionally, they may be responsible for curriculum development and implementation. While generally not the primary role, the medical director may be called upon to teach and provide educational content. Ultimately, the medical director of an education program is the final authority to review student performance and ensure that they have met all knowledge-based requirements for graduation prior to becoming certified as an EMS provider.

Medical Director for Critical Care Transport Programs

A medical director for a critical care transport program is responsible for the ambulance and helicopter transportation of critically ill or injured patients. This includes medically complex patients and sometimes neonates, who may be particularly vulnerable to complications during transport. Similar to other EMS agency medical directors, a critical care transport medical director ensures that all staff involved in transport are properly trained and equipped to deal with any potential emergencies. This may involve being familiar with equipment not typically carried by an EMS ambulance (e.g., ventilators, medication pumps, intra-aortic balloon pumps, neonatal isolettes, etc.) and the development of transport protocols and policies outside the scope of typical EMS ambulances (e.g., rapid sequence intubation, blood administration, titration of vasoactive infusions, etc.). Medical directors of critical care transport agencies may need to interface with multiple specialists, such as intensivists and neonatologists to develop these protocols.

Medical Director for Tactical Teams and Special Operations

Within the realm of EMS is tactical medicine. Law enforcement agencies that perform tactical operations often embed EMS providers within their team who are adept at treating immediate life-threatening traumatic injuries, sometimes while under fire or in extremely hostile conditions. These so-called "tactical medics," just like any other, require medical direction. Care in this arena is unique and requires a medical director who understands the nuances of care under duress. Other care that would generally fall under the category of special operations include emergency care at the sites of special events. In many cases, EMS crews and medical personnel are stationed at locations of special events and mass gatherings to care for the attendees and take some of the burden off of the local EMS and health systems. Planning for these events and the care provided during the event require medical oversight with particular knowledge of mass-gathering and event medicine.

Becoming an EMS Medical Director

There is more than one way to prepare to become an EMS medical director. The most formalized and thorough way to prepare is by pursuing subspecialty certification in EMS through the American Board of Emergency Medicine. There are also less intensive programs, such as the Foundations of Medical Oversight Course offered by the National Association of EMS Physicians. This course covers topics such as understanding the role of the medical director, developing policies and procedures, managing quality improvement initiatives, and working with other members of the EMS team. Different states may have different requirements for training and licensure of EMS medical directors, and may even require certain coursework to be completed; it is important to understand the rules around this in your particular state to ensure compliance with any necessary regulations. You might also consider first working with a local EMS agency to shadow a current medical director and gain experience and mentorship.

Conclusion

The EMS system in the United States has seen dramatic changes in the past 50 years. As the system has grown and developed, the need for physician medical direction of these services has grown with it. From complex critical care transport programs using helicopters to transport critically ill neonates, to tactical EMS programs skilled in caring for patients under duress, to small volunteer EMS programs, being an EMS medical director requires a commitment to understanding the prehospital environment and providing the oversight for EMS providers to best serve their communities.

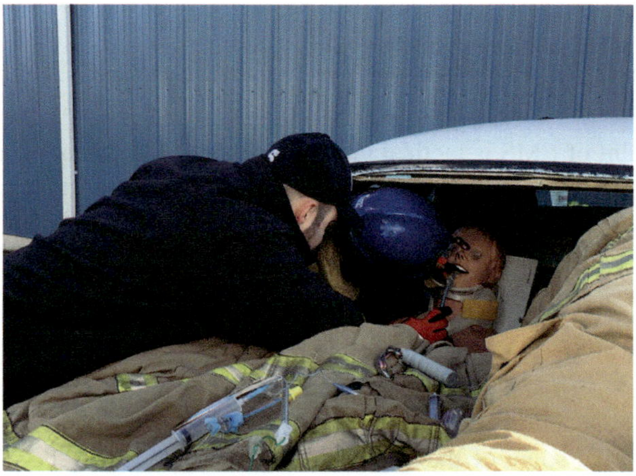

EMS physicians training to perform advanced procedures on a simulated patient trapped in a vehicle

References

1. National Academy of Sciences (US) and National Research Council (US) Committee on Trauma; National Academy of Sciences (US) and National Research Council (US) Committee on Shock. Accidental death and disability: the neglected disease of modern society. Washington, DC: National Academies Press (US); 1966.
2. Cone DC, Brice JH, Delbridge TR, Myers JB. Volume 2, Chapter 8: Medical oversight of EMS systems. In: Emergency medical services: clinical practice and systems oversight. Hoboken: Wiley; 2021.

Chapter 51
Informatics

Farah Z. Dadabhoy, Andrew Marshall, and Adam Landman

F. Z. Dadabhoy · A. Marshall
Brigham and Women's Hospital, Harvard Medical School, Boston, MA, USA
e-mail: farah.dadabhoy@mgh.harvard.edu; amarshall8@bwh.harvard.edu

A. Landman (✉)
Brigham and Women's Hospital, Mass General Brigham; Harvard Medical School, Boston, MA, USA
e-mail: alandman@bwh.harvard.edu

R. P. Olympia et al. (eds.), *An Emergency Physician's Path*,
https://doi.org/10.1007/978-3-031-47873-4_51

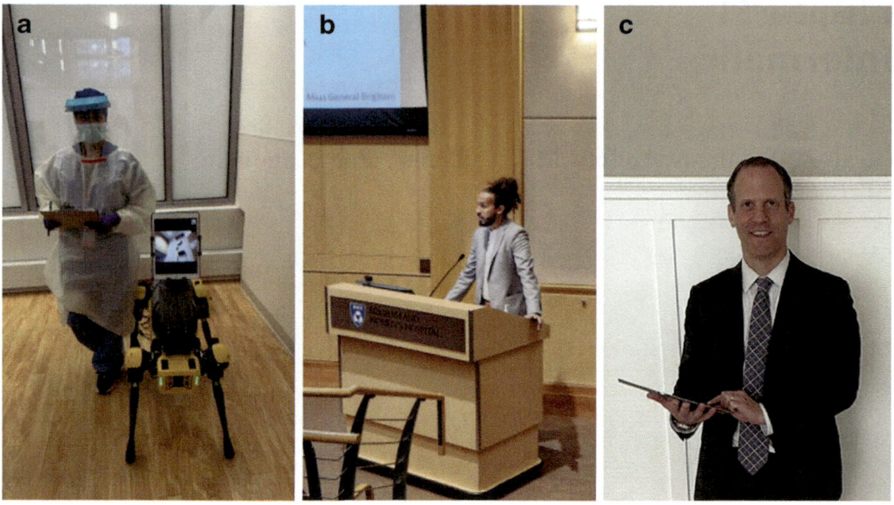

(**a**) Farah Z. Dadabhoy, MD, is an emergency medicine attending and clinical informatics (CI) fellow who worked with a team of clinicians and engineers at the Massachusetts Institute of Technology to develop and deploy telepresence robots in the ED capable of obtaining contactless vital signs to interface with patients. (Photo credit: Greg Howarth). (**b**) Andrew Marshall, MD, MBI, is an Emergency Medicine Physician and Clinical Informaticist at Brigham and Women's Hospital in Boston. Dr. Marshall's research is driven by industry partnerships and focuses on innovation as a means to address health disparities. (Photo credit: H. Mark Zhang, DO, MMSc). (**c**) Adam Landman, MD, MS, MIS, MHS, is an emergency medicine attending and Brigham and Women's Hospital's Vice President and Chief Information Officer and Digital Innovation Officer. Dr. Landman is responsible for maintaining a focus on excellence while developing system-wide strategic IT initiatives, with the goal of evolving the next generation of information systems across the organization. (Photo Credit: Adam Landman)

What Is Informatics?

According to the American Medical Informatics Association, clinical informatics (CI) is "the application of informatics and information technology to deliver healthcare services" [1]. Clinical informatics integrates principles of health information technology, data science, and medicine to improve human health. While this definition may seem broad, it is intentionally so. The widespread availability of consumer-facing health technologies, federally incentivized adoption of electronic health records, and growing numbers of connecting medical devices have made more data available than ever before. Thus, opportunities in informatics are vast, and the demand for physicians with training and experience in informatics (clinical informaticians) is rising.

Relevance to Emergency Medicine

The combination of expertise in clinical medicine and information technology (IT) is increasingly needed in all avenues of healthcare. Informaticians have the ability and expertise to propel healthcare transformation by harnessing data to impact care decisions and improve health systems, with many applications in Emergency Medicine (EM). Emergency medicine informaticians lead a diverse range of endeavors, including electronic health record (EHR) adoption and optimization, workflow automation, and clinical decision support [2]. Increasingly, EM informaticians are leveraging machine learning models and precision medicine to enable high-quality, equitable care [2]. Examples of such applications include health information exchange to reduce ED costs, clinical decision support, patient photos in the EHR to reduce wrong patient orders, and utilization of artificial intelligence (AI) for triage, organizational planning (admission prediction), and controlled substance monitoring [3–9].

A Brief History of Informatics and Emergency Medicine

Clinical Informatics is one of the newest medical subspecialties. Much like Emergency Medicine in the twentieth century, clinical informatics has taken years to develop into its current form. Over a span of roughly 50 years, the field of informatics in medicine has developed alongside the integration of computers and information technology into the everyday practice of medicine (Fig. 51.1). The widespread adoption of EHRs has furthered the development of the subspecialty and brought it to the forefront.

In 1978, the International Medical Informatics Association (IMIA) was formed. IMIA represented international efforts to promote the application of information science in the field of medicine. A little more than a decade later in 1989, the American Association for Medical Systems and Informatics, the American College of Medical Informatics, and the Symposium on Computer Applications and Medical Care merged to form the American Medical Informatics Association (AMIA). In 2005, AMIA began the process of making clinical informatics a medical

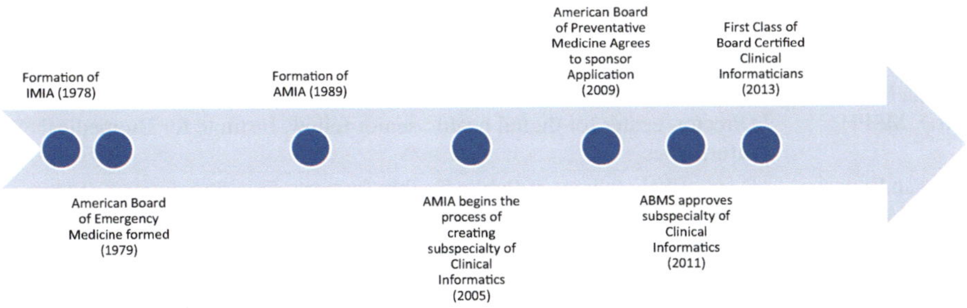

Fig. 51.1 A timeline of Clinical Informatics and Emergency Medicine

subspecialty. In 2009, the American Board of Preventative Medicine agreed to sponsor the subspecialty, and by 2013, the first board-certified clinical informaticians were recognized. Clinical Informatics is now a subspecialty with more than 2000 board-certified clinicians, many of whom practice Emergency Medicine as their primary specialty.

Clinical informatics is a subspecialty that has become integral to the practice of medicine. Emergency Medicine clinicians not only generate and consume large amounts of data during their day-to-day practice [1], but they also rely heavily on electronic systems to help manage patient flow into and out of the hospital. Electronic tools that provide clinical decision support and information exchange between hospitals are essential to practicing safe and effective emergency care.

To foster the growing community of emergency physicians interested in informatics, the American College of Emergency Physicians (ACEP) formed a Section of Emergency Medicine Informatics and the Society of Academic Emergency Medicine (SAEM) has an Informatics and Data Science section. Emergency physicians have held major leadership roles and made substantial contributions to informatics. Table 51.1 highlights a sample of influential Emergency Medicine informaticists.

Table 51.1 Sample of influential emergency medicine informaticists

Name	Role(s) and contribution(s)
Carrie K. Baker, DO, MS, FACEP	Clinical informatics fellowship program director, Kettering health network; AMIA 10x10 faculty; ACEP section of emergency medicine informatics (SEMI) chair-elect
Craig Feied, MD	Chief scientist, WhisperSom corporation; professor of emergency medicine, Georgetown University; former, chief health strategy officer, Microsoft; former, director of informatics, MedStar health
John D. Halamka, MD, MS	President of Mayo Clinic Platform, former CIO of Beth Israel Deaconess Medical Center (1998–2019), International Healthcare Innovation Professor at Harvard Medical School, Advisor to Bush and Obama Administrations
Jonathan Handler, MD	Senior fellow, innovation, OSF healthcare; former VP of digital innovation at Baxter Healthcare Corporation; former CMIO at M*modal
John Lumpkin, MD, MPH	President, blue cross blue shield of North Carolina foundation; former senior vice president, Robert Wood Johnson Foundation; former board member, American College of Emergency Physicians
Kenneth Mandl, MD, MPH	Director of the computational health informatics program at Boston Children's hospital, creator of SMART on FHIR; Donald A.B. Lindberg professor of Pediatrics and professor of biomedical informatics, Harvard Medical School
Raina Merchant, MD, MSPH	Chief transformation officer, Penn medicine; Director, center for digital health; senior fellow, Institute for Biomedical Informatics
Megan Ranney, MD, MPH	Dean of Yale School of Public Health; formerly founding director of the Brown-lifespan center for digital health; formerly appointed member of the HIMSS' mHealth physician taskforce

Table 51.1 (continued)

Name	Role(s) and contribution(s)
Todd Rothenhaus, MD	CEO of Cohealo, former Chief Medical Officer of Athenahealth
Don Rucker, MD, MS, MBA	National Coordinator for Health Information Technology, U.S. Department of Health and Human Services (2017–2021); Adjunct Professor of Emergency Medicine, Ohio State University; Chief Strategy Officer 1upHealth
Jonathan Teich, MD, PhD	Chief medical information officer and director of product management at InterSystems; led development of one of the first electronic ED tracking systems; expert on clinical decision support.

Clinical Informatics: Areas of Focus

Clinical informaticists operate at the intersection of clinical care, information technology, and the health system. Technology is advancing rapidly and offering new and exciting opportunities to improve healthcare delivery. Clinical informatics started with a focus on the electronic health record – helping healthcare delivery organizations adopt these systems. While the core clinical system remains the EHR and work on EHR optimization continues, informaticists are increasingly focusing on data science, virtual care/telehealth, and innovation.

Electronic Health Records

The growth of informatics in Emergency Medicine can be directly linked to increased use of electronic health records. The 2009 Health Information Technology for Economic and Clinical Health (HITECH) Act introduced the Meaningful Use Program aimed at improving quality, safety, efficiency, and health equity using EHRs. EHRs are now such an integral part of the day-to-day practice of Emergency Medicine, that the American College of Graduate Medical Education (ACGME) recognizes documentation, record review, and systems improvement as metrics that contribute to mastery of the specialty. Widespread adoption of EHRs and efforts to improve interoperability have made it possible to share records across institutions, greatly improving the safety and efficacy of emergency care. Furthermore, informatics solutions, such as the state-by-state implementation of prescription drug monitoring programs, have been instrumental in addressing public health crises, such as the opioid epidemic, that affect emergency care.

The practice of Emergency Medicine is rooted heavily in operational efficiency. Metrics used to evaluate the Emergency Department are often gathered from time-stamped data in the EHR. Large quantities of information generated, coupled with advancing technologies for processing those data, have moved Emergency Medicine beyond simply retrospective research and operational analysis of data into the realm of predictive analytics and data science. EHRs are also associated with increased administrative burden and provider burnout. There is an increased focus on making EHRs more usable and supplementing EHRs with tools that make documentation more efficient, such as voice recognition, scribes, and ambient documentation.

Data Science

Data science provides the tools by which physicians and researchers manage, analyze, and assimilate large quantities of clinical data. In the Emergency Department, real-time analysis of data can take the form of clinical decision support (CDS). These suggestions or alerts (e.g., allergy warnings, drug–drug interactions, or more complex, artificial intelligence/machine learning models that predict the likelihood of sepsis) are built into the EHR. It is the role of the clinical informatics specialist in the Emergency Department to ensure that these warnings and alerts are appropriate and non-obtrusive to clinical workflow and create the desired effect on clinical practice.

Advances in data science have begun to move emergency care into the realm of precision medicine. Precision medicine is medical care designed to optimize efficiency or therapeutic benefit for a specific patient or group of patients. Researchers at Stanford use a form of precision medicine, coupled with machine learning, to monitor deviations from the standard of care by comparing similar cases across their large health information exchange [10]. As techniques for analysis of individual pharmacokinetics, genomes, and metabolisms evolve, there are signs that these techniques might soon play a role in helping emergency physicians treat strokes, heart attacks, and other common emergencies.

Virtual Care/Telehealth

Telehealth is an important and evolving part of emergency informatics. In 1924, the magazine *Radio News* foreshadowed the development of telehealth by depicting a "radio doctor" linked to patients by sound and a live picture. By the late 1940s, the first radiographs were being sent via telephone wire for interpretation by a remote physician. Emergency Medicine is a specialty that relies heavily on picture archiving and communication systems (PACS), teleradiology, and software, such as LifeImage, to share images between institutions. In smaller healthcare facilities, telehealth has enabled the use of "virtual consults" to augment specialist coverage. Examples include tele-neurology evaluation of acute stroke, tele-cardiology evaluation of electrocardiograms, or tele-intensive care evaluations for ICU admissions. Some rural facilities plagued with physician shortages have even turned to tele-emergency care, with emergency room physicians positioned in a remote facility hundreds of miles away examining patients via high-definition camera and audio [11]. Furthermore, the COVID-19 pandemic has driven the relaxation of regulations governing telehealth, which rapidly furthered its use in the Emergency Department [12]. The ability to rapidly gather and synthesize clinical information and make critical triage decisions makes emergency physicians the natural choice to work in and develop telemedicine applications for acute care (and beyond).

Innovation: Emergency Technology

As software and hardware technology continues to rapidly accelerate (i.e., robotics, AI, drones, and extended reality), there are new opportunities to apply these tools to help address unmet challenges in healthcare. Clinical informaticists who understand the technology as well as the clinical needs and workflows are essential to matching the technology with unmet needs. Emergency physicians operate on the frontlines of the healthcare system and are often faced with medical cases that can be seen as the result of failures of a complex healthcare system. This unique perspective on problems within a healthcare system, coupled with the operational knowledge of the hospital and flexibility of Emergency Medicine shift work, often allows emergency practitioners to take a lead in innovation.

While technology is an important component of clinical informatics, successful informatics implementations need to strongly consider people and processes (workflows). Dr. Enrico Coiera put it well when he wrote, "medical informatics is thus as much about computers as cardiology is about stethoscopes" [13]. Informaticists not only need to have knowledge of technology but also need strong skills in leadership, negotiation, project management, and change management.

Career Path for Informatics

There is a wide range of job opportunities available for emergency physicians with informatics training and skills, including roles in academic, healthcare delivery operations, industry, and government settings. Informaticists may also pursue hybrid careers where they divide their time in one or more of these settings at a given time (or over the course of their career).

Academic roles in informatics might include basic science or health services research where informatics tools for data management and analysis are heavily leveraged. Alternatively, some researchers may build and evaluate informatics solutions on quality, safety, and experience impacts. For example, researchers developed and evaluated clinical decision support for whether a computed tomography (CT) angiogram of the chest is beneficial for pulmonary embolism evaluation [14]. Researchers are required to find financial support for their work, most commonly in the form of federal grants, foundation and industry awards, or philanthropy.

Healthcare delivery organizations need clinical informaticists to be a bridge between technology teams and clinical operations to advance the use of technology to improve care delivery. Over the past 10 years, informaticists have focused on the implementation of electronic health record systems. With most hospitals and Emergency Departments now having EHR systems, the role of the operational informaticist has shifted to optimizing the EHR and using the data to improve quality and population health [15–17]. Informaticists also support additional clinical technologies, such as virtual care tools, as well as the growing field of data science, using advanced machine learning algorithms for diagnosis, treatment, and follow-up [18]. There are a variety of operational informatics roles available in healthcare delivery organizations at the division/department levels and hospital levels. For example, a Director of Emergency Medicine Informatics role focuses on informatics support to the ED, and a Chief Medical Information Officer role extends the scope and breadth across the hospital/delivery system. Some systems may have specialized operational informatics roles that focus on telehealth, data science, or innovation.

Industry, ranging from startups to Fortune 100 companies, is also increasingly seeking clinicians with informatics training. Technology, diagnostic, and therapeutic companies employ clinical informaticists in a variety of roles from clinical content expert and product development to leadership roles, such as medical director and chief medical officer. Emergency Medicine informaticists are often highly sought after in the industry given their breadth of clinical expertise.

Clinical informaticists also have career options in the **government** at the federal, state, and even local levels. The Office of the Coordinator for Health Information Technology is the primary federal agency responsible for Health Information Technology and employs many informaticists. Opportunities are also available in other Department of Health and Human Services (HHS) operating divisions, such as the FDA, CDC, and NIH. For example, during the COVID-19 pandemic, specialists in public health informaticists were critical in tracking COVID-19 infection and vaccination rates across the country. The Department of Veterans Affairs also provides opportunities for informaticists in operations and research (as well as clinical opportunities for emergency physicians).

The biggest career opportunity challenge clinical informaticists are likely to face is the wide range of available job options. In addition to available positions at the time of the search, personal factors are critical considerations and should include role/responsibilities, geographic preferences, and professional development opportunities. Overall, it continues to be an exciting time in health technology with a strong demand for clinical informaticists to work in a variety of settings.

Training

Physicians interested in clinical informatics can begin to get exposure to the field as early as medical school and residency training. For example, Harvard Medical School and the National Institute of Health offer student rotations, and Mass General Brigham and Vanderbilt University Medical Center offer resident rotations.

While relatively new, board certification in clinical informatics may become an expected credential for those seeking a career with a significant focus on informatics. Board certification for clinical informatics is offered through the American Board of Preventive Medicine. There are currently two pathways available to become board-certified in clinical information: (1) the practice pathway or (2) completion of a 2-year ACGME-accredited fellowship. The practice pathway requires at least 3 years of informatics experience (with at least 0.25 full-time equivalent effort each year) and ends in 2025 [19]. Therefore, most readers of this chapter seeking clinical informatics board certification will require fellowship training.

Most ACGME-accredited clinical informatics fellowship programs consist of a practical or applied component and an educational or didactic component. While all programs cover the same core curriculum, there can be variation in the focus of the programs. For example, some programs focus heavily on EHR development and applications, while other programs focus on data science. All programs offer didactics, and some offer formal certificates or Masters degrees. When considering programs, consider location, quality and delivery of didactic education, faculty depth and breadth, required projects, flexibility, rotations, and mentorship.

Importantly, ACGME-accredited fellowships are open to all physicians from any specialty of medicine. Programs are hosted by different departments, commonly Internal Medicine, Anesthesiology, Emergency Medicine, Family Medicine, Pathology, and Pediatrics. Most use Electronic Residency Application Service (ERAS) applications and participate in the clinical informatics match program.

Completion of the fellowship offers several advantages, including an accelerated pathway to leadership positions, industry opportunities, protected time for projects, and structured mentorship and growth.

Other informatics training options for EM physicians who may not want to pursue formal fellowship training include the 10 × 10 AMIA-ACEP informatics course and informatics graduate degree programs which can be online, hybrid, or in person. AMIA maintains a searchable catalog of academic informatics training programs, including ACGME-accredited programs, certificate programs, and graduate programs.

In summary, informatics is a rich and exciting field, ripe with opportunities for emergency physicians to transform the future of healthcare. To get started, consider joining Emergency Medicine informatics interest groups and obtaining additional training in informatics. The healthcare system is increasingly being supported by technology; we need Emergency Medicine physicians with informatics expertise to lead this transformation, ensuring that the solutions meet the quadruple aim: improving patient experience, health of populations, improving efficiency, and clinician experience.

References

1. American Medical Informatics Association. What is informatics? (https://amia.org/about-amia/why-informatics/informatics-research-and-practice). Accessed January 1, 2024.
2. Obermeyer Z, Powers B, Vogeli C, Mullainathan S. Dissecting racial bias in an algorithm used to manage the health of populations. Science. 2019;366(6464):447–53. (In eng). https://doi.org/10.1126/science.aax2342.
3. Shapiro JS, Kannry J, Lipton M, et al. Approaches to patient health information exchange and their impact on emergency medicine. Ann Emerg Med. 2006;48(4):426–32. https://doi.org/10.1016/j.annemergmed.2006.03.032.
4. Dutta S, McEvoy DS, Stump T, et al. Clinical decision support reduces unnecessary tetanus vaccinations in the emergency department. Ann Emerg Med. 2021;78(3):370–80. (In eng). https://doi.org/10.1016/j.annemergmed.2021.02.021.
5. Salmasian H, Blanchfield BB, Joyce K, et al. Association of display of patient photographs in the electronic health record with wrong-patient order entry errors. JAMA Netw Open. 2020;3(11):e2019652. (In eng). https://doi.org/10.1001/jamanetworkopen.2020.19652.
6. Salmasian H, Landman AB, Morris C. An electronic notification system for improving patient flow in the emergency department. AMIA Jt Summits Transl Sci Proc. 2019;2019:242–7. (In eng)
7. Raita Y, Goto T, Faridi MK, Brown DFM, Camargo CA Jr, Hasegawa K. Emergency department triage prediction of clinical outcomes using machine learning models. Crit Care. 2019;23(1):64. (In eng). https://doi.org/10.1186/s13054-019-2351-7.
8. McAllister MW, Aaronson P, Spillane J, et al. Impact of prescription drug-monitoring program on controlled substance prescribing in the ED. Am J Emerg Med. 2015;33(6):781–5. (In eng). https://doi.org/10.1016/j.ajem.2015.03.036.
9. Goto T, Camargo CA Jr, Faridi MK, Freishtat RJ, Hasegawa K. Machine learning-based prediction of clinical outcomes for children during emergency department triage. JAMA Netw Open. 2019;2(1):e186937. (In eng). https://doi.org/10.1001/jamanetworkopen.2018.6937.
10. Stanford Department of Emergency Medicine. Harnessing data to improve emergency care. (https://precisionem.squarespace.com/informatics). Accessed January 1, 2024.
11. Saslow E. The most remote emergency room: life and death in rural America. Washington Post; November 16, 2019.
12. Hamm JM, Greene C, Sweeney M, et al. Telemedicine in the emergency department in the era of COVID-19: front-line experiences from 2 institutions. J Am College Emerg Phys Open. 2020;1(6):1630–6. https://doi.org/10.1002/emp2.12204.
13. Coiera E. Medical informatics. BMJ. 1995;310(6991):1381–7. (In eng). https://doi.org/10.1136/bmj.310.6991.1381.
14. Raja AS, Ip IK, Prevedello LM, et al. Effect of computerized clinical decision support on the use and yield of CT pulmonary angiography in the emergency department. Radiology. 2012;262(2):468–74. (In eng). https://doi.org/10.1148/radiol.11110951.
15. DesRoches CM, Charles D, Furukawa MF, et al. Adoption of electronic health records grows rapidly, but fewer than half of US hospitals had at least a basic system in 2012. Health Aff. 2013;32(8):1478–85.
16. Adler-Milstein J, Jha AK. HITECH act drove large gains in hospital electronic health record adoption. Health Aff. 2017;36(8):1416–22.
17. Landman AB, Bernstein SL, Hsiao AL, Desai RA. Emergency department information system adoption in the United States. Acad Emerg Med. 2010;17(5):536–44. https://doi.org/10.1111/j.1553-2712.2010.00722.x.
18. Berlyand Y, Raja AS, Dorner SC, et al. How artificial intelligence could transform emergency department operations. Am J Emerg Med. 2018;36(8):1515–7. (In eng). https://doi.org/10.1016/j.ajem.2018.01.017.
19. American Board of Preventative Medicine. Clinical informatics requirements table. (https://www.theabpm.org/become-certified/subspecialties/clinical-informatics/table/). Accessed January 1, 2024.

Chapter 52
Public Health and Community Medicine

John Westhoff

Introduction

Like many of the readers of this book, I went to medical school to become an emergency physician. By the time I graduated, I was also interested in public health. I knew there were residencies in preventive medicine that would lead directly to a career in public health, but I was not ready to abandon what I had come to medical school to do. I resolved to become a "real doctor" first and then pursue preventive medicine once I had solidified my clinical skills.

As an emergency medicine resident, I told our program director about my interest in public health and mentioned someday doing a second residency in preventive medicine. While he was not dismissive, neither was he supportive. Preventive medicine seemed antithetical to emergency medicine. He saw no reason to bridge two disciplines that were not in his mind related in any meaningful way. This was the almost universal opinion expressed by my friends when, several years after completing training in emergency medicine, I began a preventive and occupational medicine residency. It seemed to them I was "changing specialties." I explained that I did not see myself as leaving Emergency Medicine but as acquiring complementary skills. I wanted a better understanding of epidemiology, risk communication, health policy, informatics, research methodology, and so on — skills that would enrich my clinical practice and could serve as an academic niche.

Eventually, skepticism among my colleagues gave way to understanding. Over the years, I have learned that the community of emergency physicians in public health is much larger than I thought. I have served on the Public Health and Injury

J. Westhoff (✉)
Department of Internal Medicine, University of Nevada, Reno School of Medicine, Reno, Nevada, USA
e-mail: jwesthoff@unr.edu

R. P. Olympia et al. (eds.), *An Emergency Physician's Path*,
https://doi.org/10.1007/978-3-031-47873-4_52

Prevention Committee of the American College of Emergency Physicians (ACEP) for many years now. I ran into my old program director a few years ago at an ACEP Scientific Assembly. Older and wiser, he had since joined a prestigious academic Emergency Department, where he admitted: "everyone is doing Public health."

What Is Public Health?

It is beyond the scope of this chapter to describe in detail all of the activities that could properly be considered public health. Suffice it to say that public health encompasses much more than the population-based efforts of physicians to mitigate disease. In 1994, a steering committee of U.S. Public Health Service agencies and other major public health organizations standardized a list of ten Essential Public Health Services (EPHS). A task force revised the framework in 2020. The current model emphasizes equity and divides the 10 services into three major domains: assessment, policy development, and assurance. Assessment consists of surveillance and hazard investigation. Policy development addresses health communication, community partnerships, policy creation, and regulation. Assurance encompasses issues relating to access, workforce development, innovation, and infrastructure. The EPHS model is the basis for the standards of the Public Health Accreditation Board (PHAB), which accredits public health departments [1].

The most well-established career paths for physicians in public health are in government, the military, the academy, or non-profit organizations. These physicians oversee or advise municipal, county, and state health departments, counsel decision-makers on policy and resource allocation, provide clinical preventive services, design and conduct health-related research, analyze population-level illness and injury data, conduct outbreak investigations, and so on.

Given the breadth of public health services, it is not surprising that, in my own practice, I have led or collaborated with teams of technicians, industrial hygienists, chemists, health physicists, environmental scientists, entomologists, veterinarians, nutritionists, ergonomists, organized labor representatives, safety professionals, exercise physiologists, public relations experts, epidemiologists, translators, attorneys, community health nurses, government officials, and microbiologists.

Public health is a functional area much larger than the medical specialty of preventive medicine. Non-preventive medicine physicians, especially those in leadership positions, sometimes find themselves making decisions that directly impact the health of their communities at large. These de facto public health practitioners are prone to reinvent the proverbial wheel as they often do not "know what they don't know." Not infrequently, it is the task of those with training in public health to advise and influence such deciders. Some medical specialties naturally engage in some form of preventive practice in the course of their routine clinical responsibilities, e.g., infectious disease experts engaging in antibiotic stewardship or outbreak investigations. For emergency physicians, formal training is not a necessary antecedent to a career in public health—but if you are sure that you would like to someday pursue a career beyond the ambulance bay, some additional preparation certainly helps.

Additional Training

Preventive medicine as a second residency or fellowship is common and even desirable. While some physicians go directly into a preventive medicine residency after the required clinical internship, many choose to first complete training in a clinical specialty before pursuing education in public health. My personal experience is not unusual—of the four residents in my preventive medicine class, three had prior residency training: family medicine, internal medicine, and emergency medicine, respectively.

Physicians with clinical specialty training tend to approach public health practice through the lens of their primary specialty. An ophthalmologist might prioritize the elimination of river blindness, while an emergency physician may (as I have) feel compelled to draw attention to significant deficiencies in local EMS services. This is a natural consequence of "knowing what right looks like" by virtue of your background. Many times in my career, I was "at the table" as a public health official but able to make substantive contributions because I had the perspective of a practicing emergency physician. In this way, emergency physicians with public health and leadership responsibilities ensure the hard-won lessons of EM are not forgotten when relevant policy decisions are being made.

Preventive medicine residency programs and related fellowships and graduate programs provide experience in biostatistics, bioinformatics, epidemiology, the provision of health services, management of health care organizations, research, clinical preventive services, and so on. Board certification in public health is available through the American Board of Preventive Medicine (ABPM), which is, like the American Board of Emergency Medicine (ABEM), a member board of the American Board of Medical Specialties. The ABPM certifies physicians in three primary specialties: public health and general preventive medicine, aerospace medicine, and occupational medicine. In addition, ABPM oversees four subspecialties of immediate interest to many emergency physicians: addiction medicine, clinical informatics, medical toxicology, and undersea and hyperbaric medicine. Of note, ABEM also offers subspecialty certifications in medical toxicology and undersea and hyperbaric medicine. ABEM-certified physicians with appropriate training can obtain subspecialty certification by ABPM in addiction medicine and clinical informatics.

There are two pathways to board certification by the ABPM, i.e., the "residency pathway" and the "complementary pathway." Grandfathering into the specialty without specialty-specific residency training ceased to be an option after 2022. The residency pathway requires completing an ACGME-accredited (or American Osteopathic Association or Royal College of Physicians and Surgeons of Canada) residency in the specialty area for which certification is being sought. The complementary pathway accommodates physicians who have already completed at least 2 years of a qualified clinical residency; they must then complete at least 1 year of a residency program in the preventive medicine specialty area of interest and practice in that specialty for 2 years.

Both pathways to ABPM certification require a Master of Public Health (MPH) or equivalent degree, including coursework in epidemiology, biostatistics, health services administration, environmental sciences, and social and behavioral sciences. Schools of Public health offer different MPH tracts and areas of emphasis analogous to undergraduate majors, e.g., epidemiology, occupational and environmental medicine, health services, global health, maternal and child health, biostatistics, genetics, tropical medicine, nutritional sciences, and so on. Enrollment in an MPH program is concurrent with residency training in preventive medicine but can be completed independently, during medical school, or as a part of an unrelated fellowship.

Depending on your interest, other opportunities abound. For example, emergency physicians with an MPH and at least 1 year of full-time public health work experience are competitive applicants for the CDC's Epidemic Intelligence Services (EIS), the famous "disease detectives" renowned for participating in global investigative and emergency response efforts. EIS fellows practice applied epidemiology, working in the field on infectious disease mitigation, injury prevention, and environmental and occupational health.

The Synergy between Public Health and Emergency Medicine

When emergency physicians partner with public health officials on topics of mutual interest, their voice is amplified, and the resultant interventions are more likely to be effective. Emergency physicians have moral authority in the eyes of the public and are powerful advocates for issues related to the injuries and illnesses they encounter firsthand.

Such partnerships also improve clinical practice. We take for granted how "epidemiologically located" we are until we are called upon to practice in a setting or population alien to us. Even within the United States, differences in epidemiology can be striking. Fever in the Pacific Northwest does not have the same differential as fever in the Midwest. I once investigated the death of a young adult who presented to a small midwestern ED with fever. The providers who failed to diagnose the disease had trained in other parts of the country. They incorrectly presumed the fever to be from a viral syndrome, so they did not prescribe the appropriate empiric treatment. I told a friend native to the area about the case, i.e., fever with mild pancytopenia in the summer—and to my astonishment, he made the correct diagnosis immediately: "Ehrlichiosis," he said, "they would have made the diagnosis at triage [at the nearby medical center where he trained]." The absence of a tick bite history delayed the diagnosis until after the patient required intubation and ticks were discovered in the groin. Ehrlichiosis—exotic to itinerate providers—was evident to those who understood the local epidemiology and that occult summertime tick exposure was a given.

Biosurveillance is the other side of the epidemiologic coin and another important area of cooperation between emergency medicine and public health. Whereas population-level information informs clinical practice in the form of epidemiology, patient-level information informs public health practice when aggregated via surveillance networks. Near real-time syndromic surveillance has long been seen as a national security priority. Influenza (and more recently, COVID-19) surveillance informs global vaccine development on an annual schedule. Calls to toxicology centers can similarly be considered a form of surveillance in which emergency physician cooperation is essential, e.g., the spike in nicotine-related deaths in children related to electronic delivery systems helped shape new regulations concerning vaping devices.

Emergency medicine can itself be thought of as a public health intervention. In 1966, the National Academy of Sciences reflected the zeitgeist when it published *Accidental Death and Disability: The Neglected Disease of Modern Society* to call attention to the poor state of emergency care at the time [2]. Emergency medicine as a specialty followed, as did the development of EMS systems and programs aimed at addressing knowledge gaps of other physicians, e.g., ATLS, ACLS, and PALS, and improving bystander health literacy and response, e.g., CPR, stroke awareness, and so on. It should come as no surprise then that there continue to be important areas for cooperation between emergency physicians and public health officials—and a great need for physicians who can bridge the gap.

References

1. Center for State T, Local, and Territorial Support. 10 Essential public health services: Centers for Disease Control and Prevention; 2021. Available from: https://www.cdc.gov/publichealthgateway/publichealthservices/essentialhealthservices.html
2. National Academy of S, National Research Council Committee on T, National Academy of S, National Research Council Committee on S. Accidental death and disability: the neglected disease of modern society. Washington (DC): National Academies Press (US), Copyright © National Academy of Sciences; 1966.

Chapter 53
Urgent Care Medicine

Robert P. Olympia

What Is Urgent Care Medicine?

Urgent care medicine (UCM) incorporates clinical services provided at urgent care centers (UCCs) into a growing specialty consisting of administration, education, research and scholarship, and community service. As per the Urgent Care Association, the leading organization for UCM since 2004, urgent care services are defined as (1) a medical examination, diagnosis, and treatment for non-life or -limb-threatening illnesses and injuries that are within the capability of a UCC that accepts unscheduled, walk-in patients seeking medical attention during all posted hours of operation and is supported by on-site evaluation services, including radiology and laboratory services; and (2) any further medical examination, procedure, and treatment to the extent they are within the capabilities of the staff and facilities available at the UCC. Growth of the UCM industry over the past few decades can be attributed to the general population's need to seek convenient, high-quality, low-cost care, in response to overcrowding in emergency departments and limited hours and physician shortages in primary care physician offices.

R. P. Olympia (✉)
Department of Emergency Medicine & Pediatrics, Penn State Hershey Medical Center, Hershey, USA
e-mail: rolympia@hmc.psu.edu

R. P. Olympia et al. (eds.), *An Emergency Physician's Path*,
https://doi.org/10.1007/978-3-031-47873-4_53

What Is the History of Urgent Care Medicine and Urgent Care Centers?

UCCs were developed in the 1970s, seeking to meet the medical needs of the community by providing convenient and affordable care (the "doc-in-a-box" model). The first known use of the term "urgent care" was in 1973. The Urgent Care Association (UCA), established in 2004, consists of 3000 UCCs representing 30,000 urgent care clinical and business professionals. The UCA supports its members through education, advocacy, community awareness, benchmarking, and promoting standards of excellence and provides urgent care certification, accreditations, and commendations. The UCA hosts many educational opportunities, such as clinical and practice management online webinars, a peer-reviewed medical journal (*The Journal of Urgent Care Medicine*), and an annual national convention highlighting educational advancement and research in the field. The American Board of Urgent Care Medicine, which was established in 1997, provides certification to urgent care providers. Several UCM textbooks provide evidence-based management of patients in an urgent care setting and include the Textbook of Urgent Care Medicine (Shufeldt 2014), Urgent Care Emergencies: Avoiding the pitfalls and improving outcomes (Goyal 2012), Urgent Care Medicine Secrets (Olympia 2017), EMRA Urgent Care Guide (Levine 2021), and Essential Procedures for Emergency, Urgent, and Primary Care Settings (Campo 2021).

Some Facts Regarding Urgent Care Medicine and Urgent Care Centers

1. As of June 2019, there are approximately 9279 UCCs in the United States.
2. UCCs have reported a median patient volume of 35 patients per day increasing during late fall and winter, with an estimated total of 112 million patient visits per year in the United States. This represents 23% of all primary care visits and 12.6% of all outpatient physician visits.
3. Notably, 94% of UCCs in the United States report an average wait time of 30 min or less.
4. The majority of consumers presenting to UCCs are millennials (ages 18–34 years) and younger Gen Xers (ages 35–44 years).
5. The presence of UCCs in the community has decreased ED visits by 30%.
6. Notably, 40% of UCCs in the United States are physician-owned, and 37% are hospital-owned.
7. Over the past decade, there has been an increase in the number of pediatric-specific UCCs, employing pediatric EM physicians, such as PM Pediatrics and UCCs associated with children's hospitals in the United States.
8. The majority of UCCs employ family medicine and emergency medicine trained physicians, as well as other licensed healthcare professionals, including physician assistants, nurse practitioners, registered nurses, and radiology tech-

nicians. Notably, 62% of UCCs utilize a hybrid model of physicians and advanced practice clinicians.

9. The majority of UCCS provide the following on-site laboratory testing: complete blood counts, comprehensive metabolic profiles, diabetic testing (hemoglobin A1c), urine pregnancy, urinalysis, rapid strep and throat cultures, and rapid viral testing. Several UCCs offer tuberculosis testing, drug screens, and STD testing.
10. The majority of UCCs provide X-ray imaging, while an increasing number of UCCs offer CT scan, MRI, and ultrasound services.
11. The majority of UCCs utilize radiology and laboratory technologists.
12. Other services provided by most UCCs include pre-placement physicals, urinary drug screening and post-injury testing, annual employment physicals, flu and other vaccine immunizations, and workforce health education on injury/illness prevention.
13. Notably, 8% of UCCs offer telemedicine options, although this service likely has increased due to the COVID-19 pandemic.
14. In February 2019, a 5-year pilot plan was instituted called the Emergency Triage, Treat, and Transport (ET3) program. The program allows partnered EMS providers to transport patients to an alternative site for care, including UCCs, based on their presenting chief complaint in the hope of decreasing overcrowding in EDs. More to come on this program.

As an Emergency Medicine Physician, in Addition to Working Clinically in a UCC, how Can you Contribute to the Field of Urgent Care Medicine?

1. *Providing education in the community regarding when to go to a UCC* versus *an ED:*

   A recently published study concluded that there exists much variability on the websites of the top 30 urgent care organizations regarding acuity-appropriate triage of chief complaints to the UCC or ED [1]. EM physicians working in urgent care are well versed on this distinction and should educate their community on the appropriateness of presentations to UCCs versus EDs based on their presenting symptoms. While most consumers present to the UCC with non-life and -limb-threatening conditions, approximately 2–4% of patients are transferred from UCCs to the ED due to a need for a higher level of care. A single-centered study found that for *adult referrals* from a UCC to an ED, the most common diagnosis for simple referrals (considered unnecessary) and complex referrals (requiring resources not commonly available at UCCs) was nonspecific abdominal pain, laceration, and fracture, and for critical referrals (requiring intensive care, surgery, or invasive procedure) was appendicitis, fracture, and cholecystitis [2]. A single-centered study found that, for *pediatric referrals* from a UCC to an ED, the most common diagnosis for essential referrals was closed extremity fracture, nonsurgical unspecified abdominal pain, and gastroenteritis,

Table 53.1 Mnemonics used to classify chief complaints as either urgent or emergent [1]

"URGENT CARES" (presenting problems that UCCs can evaluate and treat)	"STOP AT AN ER STAT" (presenting problems needing a higher level of care than an UCC)
Urinary/vaginal symptoms Rashes Gastrointestinal complaints Extremity injury Nose bleeds Temperature (fever) Cough and cold symptoms Allergy symptoms Respiratory illness Earaches Skin infections	Shock Trouble swallowing Overdose Pain Altered mental status Tormented thoughts Abnormal walking Numbness Environmental emergency Difficulty breathing Seizures or syncope Trauma Anaphylaxis Tachycardia or tachypnea
Excludes: Any complaints above combined with confusion, poor blood flow to extremities, dehydration, difficulty breathing or swallowing, unbearable pain (especially headache, neck pain, chest pain, and abdominal pain), serious weakness, numbness, lightheadedness, dizziness or changes in vision or speech, uncontrollable bleeding, trauma with significant deformities.	

and for nonessential referrals was gastroenteritis, brain concussion, and upper respiratory infection (Olympia et al. 2019).

Two mnemonics developed by Rothstein et al. to help educate the community are "URGENT CARES" and "STOP AT AN ER STAT" (Table 53.1).

2. *Conducting research and scholarship in the field of urgent care medicine.*

   In general, the field of UCM is in its infancy when it comes to research and scholarship. A recently published bibliometric study found that, between 2000 and 2020, there were 144 published studies pertaining to UCM in 94 peer-reviewed journals, the rate of publication increased over the past decade, the majority of studies were retrospective, 48.6% of studies were considered clinical, and the most common topics were urgent care utilization (specifically effectiveness and disease-based), diagnostic testing (specifically HIV and STD), and antibiotic stewardship (McNickle et al). The authors challenged the urgent care community, including EM physicians working in UCCs, to develop high-quality research, including prospective, multi-institutional/UCC studies, filling in the gaps in both clinical and non-clinical topics.

   Research in the field of UCM can be disseminated through traditional EM peer-reviewed journals and scientific assemblies (see Chap. 78: Scholarship and the dissemination of research), as well as other specialty/subspecialty scholarship forums, and through UCM specific methods, such as *The Journal of Urgent Care Medicine* or the Urgent Care Association's annual national convention.

3. *Spearheading emergency and disaster preparedness in your community:* While UCCs often care for patients with minor illness and injury, patients may present to a UCC with life- or limb-threatening presentations requiring initial stabilization, resuscitation, and transfer. Furthermore, UCCs may be subject to natural disasters and mass-causality incidents affecting their center and the surrounding community. EM physicians working in an urgent care setting can advocate for emergency and disaster preparedness by (a) ensuring certification in basic and advanced life support of all UCC staff members, (b) equipping their UCC with the minimum standards for emergency medications, equipment, and supplies, (c) setting up triage, transfer, and transport agreements with local EDs, (d) establishing organized and structured quality-improvement programs to monitor and improve the care of their patients, (e) participating in disaster planning by coordinating care with their local EMS, police and fire departments, and ED, and (f) providing disaster training to their UCC staff and to their community. Resources highlighting recommendations for preparedness include The American Academy of Pediatrics ("Pediatric care recommendations for freestanding urgent care facilities"), the Journal of Urgent Care Medicine (https://www.jucm.com/developing-an-emergency-preparedness-plan-for-urgent-care/), the Joint Commission (https://www.jointcommission.org/-/media/tjc/documents/standards/r3-reports/final-r3-report-emergency-management.pdf), and the American Academy of Family Physicians (Medical Emergency Preparedness in Office Practice).

What Are your EM Colleagues Saying about Transitioning into a Life of Urgent Care Medicine?

I conducted an informal survey on several EM Facebook pages and asked EM physicians who have made the transition several questions regarding their decision and the positive/negative aspects of UCM. Here is a summary of their responses:

Why did you leave emergency medicine for urgent care medicine?

1. Family – not spending enough time with family and children, limited flexibility
2. Sleep – lost the ability to sleep, many sleepless nights
3. Age/burnout – "realized that EM is a young person's sport and I was no longer young," wanted a less stressful environment to work in

Positive aspects of Urgent Care Medicine compared with EM

1. No nights, sleep in my bed every night
2. Diurnal rhythms
3. Less stressful and easier mentally
4. Much quieter and calmer
5. More work-life balance
6. Patients are generally very nice and appreciative
7. Very infrequent drug-seeking and mental/behavioral health patients
8. Lower liability risk

9. Less worry about RVU's and annual reviews
10. Do not need to argue with hospitalists and specialists
11. Feel a stronger bond with the community
12. Lunch breaks

Negative aspects of Urgent Care Medicine compared with EM

1. Everyone asking/demanding for antibiotics for viral infections, sore throats, and coughs
2. Mind numbingly boring
3. Miss cardioversions and cardiac arrests and intubations
4. Lower acuity
5. Losing all the procedural skills that you spent years to master
6. Not having all resources available to you, limited testing and monitoring
7. Having to decide whether to send someone to the ED
8. Convincing a patient to be transferred by ambulance when they want to go by private vehicle
9. Less pay
10. Felt I was abandoning my ED family
11. Frustrated more by insurance companies
12. Lots of performance pressure not to get a bad review that is easily accessible on the Internet

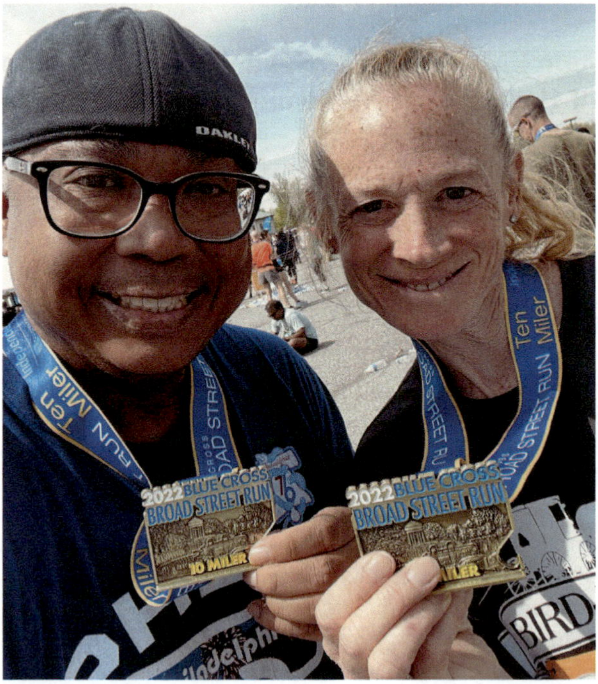

Photo caption: "Crossing another item off the bucket list. Completing the 2022 Broad Street Run in Philadelphia with my wife Jodi."

References

1. Rothstein R, Zhen K, Kim RY, et al. Acuity-appropriate triage of chief complaints found on urgent care center organization websites. Am J Emerg Med. 2021;43:276–80.
2. Siegfried IB, Jacobs J, Olympia RP. Adult referrals to an emergency department from urgent care centers. Am J Emerg Med. 2019;37(10):1949–54.

Suggested Readings

Committee on Pediatric Emergency Medicine. Pediatric care recommendations for freestanding urgent care facilities. Pediatrics. 2014;133(5):950–3.

McNickle LA, Chiang KC, McNulty EM, et al. Publishing trends in the field of urgent care medicine from 2000 to 2020: a bibliometric analysis. Am J Emerg Med. 2021;46:233–7.

Olympia RP, Wilkinson R, Dunnick J, et al. Pediatric referrals to the emergency department from urgent care centers. Pediatr Emerg Care. 2018;34(12):872877.

Toback SL. Medical emergency preparedness in office practice. Am Fam Physician. 2007;75(11):1679–84.

Urgent Care Association. Urgent care industry white paper: the essential role of the urgent care center in population health. Accessed September 9, 2022; 2019. https://www.ucaoa.org/LinkClick.aspx?fileticket=Q4TP7cypW94%3D&portalid=80

Chapter 54
Observational Medicine

Ravindra Gopaul

What Is Observation Medicine?

The traditional approach to hospital care has been medical evaluation in the Emergency Department (ED) followed by admission or discharge within a 3–4-h timeframe. With higher hospital volumes, increasing capacity constraints, and lack of reimbursement for short inpatient stays, hospital systems became more selective of admissions, often accepting patients with an anticipated prolonged length of stay (LOS) and/or meeting specific inpatient criteria. As a result, there was greater pressure on ED physicians to discharge patients who fell in the "grey-zone" of needing an extra 4–24 h of monitoring, testing, or treatment. This practice resulted in an increasing number of missed diagnoses, such as acute myocardial infarction which was missed in 2.5% of patients who presented atypically [1]. A third disposition pathway was needed to provide safe and efficient care for patients requiring a shorter length of stay, which ultimately led to the concept of observation units (OUs) in the 1980–1990s.

Observation Medicine (OM) is a rapidly expanding field as it addresses some major issues facing hospital systems, including overcrowding and ED boarding. In particular, emergency department observation units (EDOUs) serve as a pathway for patients who may need additional testing, treatment, or monitoring without using an inpatient bed. Such patients are moved to a separate space within or near the ED in which they receive protocolized care with plans for disposition within a 24-h timeframe. A perfect example is a patient with chest pain who needs a stress test. Instead of unnecessarily occupying an ED or inpatient bed for this patient who

R. Gopaul (✉)
Department of Emergency Medicine, Penn State Milton S. Hershey Medical Center, Hershey, PA, USA
e-mail: rgopaul@pennstatehealth.psu.edu

R. P. Olympia et al. (eds.), *An Emergency Physician's Path*,
https://doi.org/10.1007/978-3-031-47873-4_54

will likely be discharged within 24 hours, a good alternative is to move the patient to an EDOU under a chest pain protocol where they are managed by a mid-level provider and efficiently discharged after the test.

OUs have been shown to lead to lower costs, shorter lengths of stay, lower rates of inpatient admissions, less diagnostic uncertainty, greater patient satisfaction, better clinical outcomes, and improvements in the use of hospital resources [2]. As such, an increasing number of hospital systems have adopted this approach.

What Does a Career in Observation Medicine Look like?

The most common career option for physicians in Observation Medicine (OM) will be running an observation unit (OU). This can sometimes mean starting a unit from scratch, which is no easy task, but is an excellent crash course in operations. As an OU medical director, you are responsible for protocol development (see below), oversight of OU physicians and/or mid-level providers, and cross-collaboration with other departments as it relates to specific protocols. The role may also entail resident/mid-level education and research in OM.

Other OU medical director responsibilities include keeping track of unit metrics such as daily census, length of stay, admission percentage, protocol utilization, and patient experience. You are generally expected to attend and present at leadership meetings such as Operations and Utilization Management.

In terms of day-to-day operations, the OU medical director works in tandem with an OU nurse manager. You typically receive protected administrative time for OU management responsibilities. If your OU is covered by physicians only, then you may have more clinical shifts in the unit as opposed to the Emergency Department (ED). If your institution has multiple observation units such as an ED and Internal Medicine (IM) OU, you may be expected to oversee both and interface with the hospitalist group. If you are part of a large health system, there may be an opportunity to oversee and manage all units within the system (i.e., Chief of Observation Services). It is not uncommon for physicians who begin careers in OM leadership to transition to ED or hospital leadership positions as there is significant overlap in skill sets.

What Are Observation Protocols and how Are they Designed?

OUs are highly efficient due to protocolized care. As OU medical director, it will be your responsibility to develop and maintain observation protocols that best meet the needs of your department/institution. Each protocol consists of well-defined inclusion/exclusion criteria, a plan of care, and disposition parameters. As of the time of this publication, Penn State Milton S. Hershey Medical Center has 34 adult and 14 pediatric observation protocols. The most frequently used protocols are chest pain, dehydration, and abdominal pain. Some protocols require collaboration with other specialties. A good example is our chest pain protocol, which was developed in collaboration with Cardiology at Penn State. The HEART Score is embedded in this protocol for risk stratification. Patients with a moderate HEART Score (4–6 points) are generally appropriate for stress testing from the observation unit. Patients with a high HEART score ($\geq$ 7 points) require cardiology consultation. Buy-in from consulting services, as they relate to specific protocols, is often necessary to improve efficiency. See below for a list of adult protocols used at Penn State Milton S. Hershey Medical Center.

Penn State Milton S. Hershey Medical Center ED Observation Unit Adult Protocols

- Abdominal pain
- Accidental overdose/alcohol intoxication
- Acute back pain
- Atrial fibrillation
- Allergic reaction
- Ambulatory dysfunction
- Anemia
- Asthma/COPD
- Behavioral health
- Cellulitis
- Chest pain
- Congestive heart failure
- Dehydration
- Dizziness/vertigo
- Deep venous thrombosis
- Electrolyte abnormalities.
- GI bleed
- Headache/migraine
- Hyperemesis
- Hyperglycemia
- Hypoglycemia
- Hypertension
- Influenza
- Joint pain
- Opioid withdrawal
- Pharyngitis
- Pneumonia
- Procedures
- Pulmonary embolism
- Renal colic
- Seizure
- Syncope
- Transient neurologic deficits
- UTI/pyelonephritis

How Do we Select Patients for the Observation Unit?

To be eligible for care in the ED OU, patients must satisfy the following criteria:

- Meet the inclusion criteria of a specific protocol.
- Have a high probability of discharge within 24 hours.
- Must not meet in-patient criteria.

Some units have a call to utilization management embedded in their observation admission process. This is to ensure that patients do not meet in-patient criteria.

What Metrics Do you Track?

Useful metrics include average daily census, length of stay, percent discharge, and protocol utilization. In general, the target census is one patient per bed per day. This number will fluctuate depending on the length of stay, staffing, and unit capacity. The target length of stay is typically less than 24 h to maximize flow and ensure daily turnover of beds. The target percent discharge should be about 80%. If this number is consistently less than 80%, then protocol exclusion criteria may not be strict enough, allowing patients of higher complexity into the unit. If this number is consistently higher than 80%, then the exclusion criteria may be too strict. Some more advanced metrics worth tracking include time from OU admission order to OU arrival, time from OU discharge order to OU departure, and OU return visits. For protocols that involve advanced imaging/diagnostic testing (i.e., stress tests and echocardiograms), it is important to keep track of study delays and turnaround time as this may significantly impact the length of stay.

Why an Observation Fellowship?

With an increasing prevalence of EDOUs across the country, there is a high need for physicians trained in EDOU development, management, and leadership. The broad knowledge base required to be successful in EDOU leadership includes clinical operations, patient flow, quality improvement, patient safety, observation patient selection, observation unit design, and observation billing. To address the need for physician leaders in EDOU management, fellowship programs have been developed which provide broad education in the field.

What OM Fellowships Are out There?

There are currently three fellowship programs in OM (Fig. 54.1). All programs are 1 year and have the option to add an additional year to pursue an advanced degree (i.e., MBA, MPH, or MHA). During the fellowship, you work a specified number of clinical hours as an attending physician while completing an OM curriculum under the mentorship of trained faculty. In addition to a core knowledge base in OM, you will acquire skills in administration, leadership, and research. There is no board certification in OM.

Differences between programs

All three available fellowship programs are very similar:

Program	ACGME Accredited	Duration	Option for Advanced Degree? (+1 year)	Available Positions	Clinical Shifts
Emory	No	1 year	Yes	1	64/mo
John Hopkins	No	1 year	Yes	TBD	800/yr
Thomas Jefferson	No	1 year	Yes	1-2	64/mo

Fig. 54.1 Observation Medicine fellowships currently available (*Source*: https://www.emra.org/books/fellowship-guide-book/16-observation-medicine/) [3]

What Is the Application Process/Timeline?

To apply for a fellowship program, you must be graduating from an Emergency Medicine (EM) residency or be an EM graduate who is board-eligible or board-certified. As all OM fellowship programs are unaccredited, applications are selected on a rolling basis. Each program has details on its website for applying. You will apply to the program directly. Just like the residency application process, you will need an up-to-date CV and personal statement. You will also be asked to complete an interview. Fellowship starts on July 1. Some programs will consider mid-year candidates.

How Can I Be Competitive?

While there are very few fellowship spots (1–2 per program), there is also a very small pool of applicants. Some good ways to stand out are to demonstrate a passion for the field through research/publications, OU rotations, OU committee involvement, and letters of recommendation from observation physician leaders.

Is Fellowship Necessary for a Career in OM?

While the fellowship is available for OM, it is by no means required for a leadership career. Given the limited number of fellowship programs, it should come as no surprise that the vast majority of physician leaders in OM are not fellowship-trained and acquired their skills on the job and through mentorship. Many physicians transition to OM from prior roles in ED operations. Conversely, a career in OM provides an excellent skillset in operations to facilitate a transition to ED or hospital leadership roles.

Why Did I Choose a Career in Observation Medicine?

After completing a combined residency in Emergency and Internal Medicine, a career in OM provided an excellent opportunity to use both of my skill sets and take on a leadership role. The OU population is unique in that it requires a combination of acute care and chronic disease management, which was ideal for my dual training. I have always held an interest in hospital leadership and operations, and the EDOU medical director role provided a crash course in clinical operations, patient flow, quality improvement, and patient safety which is essential to any clinical leadership career.

My other draw to OM was being part of the "solution." OUs have been associated with lower costs, shorter lengths of stay, lower rates of in-patient admissions, less diagnostic uncertainty, greater patient satisfaction, better clinical outcomes, and improvements in the use of hospital resources [1]. OUs provide a third disposition pathway, which frees up ED beds while also conserving inpatient beds. This is essentially a win–win for the ED, the health system, and the patient.

References

1. Lee TH, Cook EF, Rouan GW, Weisberg MC, Goldman L. Ruling out myocardial infarction: prospective multicenter validation of a 12 hour strategy for low risk patents. Clin Res. 1989;37:524A.
2. Ross MA, Aurora T, Graff L, Suri P, O'Malley R, Ojo A, et al. State of the art: emergency department observation units. Crit Pathw Cardiol. 2012;11(3):128–38.
3. EMRA. Emergency Medicine Resident Association fellowship guide: opportunities for emergency physicians. Available at: https://www.emra.org/books/fellowship-guide-book/16-observation-medicine/ (Accessed 19 August 2022).Google Scholar

Chapter 55
Telemedicine

Tae Eung Kim

The telephone has become such a ubiquitous part of modern life that it often does not even register as a significant technological development. Telephony has become so commonplace that it is often derided as an antiquated form of communication with the use of terms like "plain old telephone service" (POTS). However, these technologies overcome time and distance to allow humanity to distribute our intellectual capacities beyond where we can be physically present. Medicine, as a cognitive endeavor, has been a beneficiary and driver of telecommunication technologies for decades since the adoption of the simple landline telephone. Emergency medicine, as a specialty that extends access to care, has used and continues to employ telemedicine for that purpose, or conversely, telemedicine enables emergency physicians to expand access to our care – "the skill set does not change – just the location" [1].

The first time I successfully employed telecommunication as *telemedicine* was almost two decades ago, using a simple POTS line. A local nursing home called our emergency department in the middle of the night to give a report on a patient that they wanted to send to us for evaluation. The nurse explained over the phone that one of their patients with tetraplegia was without complaints but seemed oddly distressed with diaphoresis, tachycardia, and hypertension. Hearing this description prompted me to ask what the patient's urinary output had been and to suggest catheterizing the bladder which revealed a significant retained urine volume and resulted in the resolution of these findings and normalization of their vital signs. After discussion with their physician, the nursing home decided that the patient could safely avoid the discomfort of taking a trip to the hospital in the middle of the night, and this led me to realize I had just remotely diagnosed and treated autonomic dysreflexia.

T. E. Kim (✉)
Corona Regional Medical Center, Corona, CA, USA

R. P. Olympia et al. (eds.), *An Emergency Physician's Path*,
https://doi.org/10.1007/978-3-031-47873-4_55

Emergency Medicine as a specialty has, over the decades of its existence, integrated the use of telecommunications so seamlessly that society as a whole rarely thinks of it as a distinct practice of telemedicine. The development of the 911 emergency telephone number in North America is an everyday example. Base station medical direction for prehospital health care professionals such as paramedics is another. Fans of the television show "Emergency!" from the 70s undoubtedly remember fire-medics Johnny and Roy consulting with Dr. Brackett over their field Biophone and relaying ECG tracings by telemetry, and "radio contact with base" is a part of most emergency physicians' routine work. The use of telemedicine extends to other parts of the quotidian EM practice as well: Many hospitals' stroke programs rely on synchronous (or "real-time") consultation with and evaluation by teleneurologists. Telepsychiatrists are virtually present in many EDs as the need for emergency mental health services has grown. An even more common application of telemedicine in EM is teleradiology, as almost all EDs now have radiologists who remotely interpret studies with asynchronous (i.e., data such as a radiograph are stored and then forwarded or otherwise remotely accessed) telemedicine connections, particularly after hours. There are now also some urban EDs that are trialing "teletriage" visits, often in conjunction with community paramedicine programs, to assess patients remotely and determine if a visit to the hospital can safely be avoided.

So, telehealth is already an integrated part of the daily practice of emergency medicine, but what about telemedicine as a specific career pathway of EM? There is some practice of "teleEM," usually in rural settings, similar to teleICU wherein the EM specialist provides consultation and support in diagnosis and treatment for non-emergency medicine health care professionals (such as midlevel practitioners, or physicians trained in the family or internal medicine) in remote EDs. These types of practices are available to practicing emergency physicians and will undoubtedly increase in demand as rural hospitals continue to contend with the need to staff their facilities.

That style of EM telemedicine is still by far the exception rather than the rule, and the majority of emergency physicians in telehealth practices deliver incidental care through audio–video telemedicine visits for individual patients that can be addressed in a single visit. Even prior to 2020, there were a number of telehealth platforms upon which EPs could practice this type of incidental health care as a "virtual urgent care," a format with which many physicians were already familiar. The pandemic and the resulting need to socially distance and isolate led to a marked proliferation of remote telemedicine services to provide for healthcare visits of all kinds including urgent or even emergent needs.

Emergency physicians and other health care professionals providing incidental care initially worked primarily as employees of telehealth companies, although many now enter into arrangements in which the physicians are independent contractors with their practices on the telemedicine platforms. In exchange, like many "real world" EDs and urgent cares, the contracted telemedicine companies often provide malpractice insurance, as well as the software and other infrastructure for these practices, and so on. Licensure is typically required for the state in which the patient is located, and practices with large, national telehealth companies may necessitate multiple state medical licenses.

Advances in Internet connection speed, data compression, and so on have meant that the equipment necessary for much of the practice of telemedicine has become much more accessible to a broader range of users. Even as recently as 10–15 years ago, telehealth required dedicated computer workstations and T1 Internet lines to maintain stable connections. However, most telemedicine platforms now use cloud-based software that does not require specialized hardware beyond a stable Wi-Fi connection and a computer equipped with a webcam and a microphone which are often included features. Patients accessing telehealth visits can often use the same kind of computer equipment or even more commonly their own mobile devices to access care from virtually anywhere. Most telehealth organizations use an electronic medical record (EMR), which may be proprietary to the platform or one that is more broadly available, to document, write orders, and so on.

Conditions treated by these means are at present usually ones that can be examined and therefore diagnosed by sight. Some limited palpation by the patient or an on-site assistant may be possible. However, concomitant with the increase in telehealth utilization has been the development of remote and at-home monitoring devices and diagnostic equipment. Widely commercially available automated sphygmomanometers and smartwatches can already deliver rudimentary telemetry data about blood pressures and heart rates/rhythms; other Internet-connected devices such as Wi-Fi-linked scales can provide trends in weight for the management of CHF. Near-term developments such as video otoscopy and in-home point-of-care ultrasound promise to improve diagnostic capacity. In the future, prolonged human space flight will require asynchronous telemedicine consultations for the unplanned conditions that will inevitably arise.

Telemedicine, like any other medical practice, requires appropriate remuneration. Compensation varies widely depending on the kind of telehealth organization and contracted services engaged. As mentioned above, most telemedicine practitioners currently work as independent contractors with the telehealth company providing malpractice insurance as well as the necessary software infrastructure in exchange for part of the collected fees. For the most part, just like an in-person urgent care setting, compensation is lower than what an emergency physician would typically receive for a similar amount of time worked in an ED; up to approximately 70% or so of the reimbursement of an ED shift for the lower acuity of a telemedicine workday would typically be considered reasonable to good remuneration. Most EPs consider their clinical telemedicine incomes as supplementary to their primary compensation from the ED, but, as telehealth services expand, more physicians may find the flexibility of the work an attractive option as their main careers.

Since a key advantage of telemedicine is that it enables an EP to apply their abilities outside of the ED setting, most of the skill set required to practice telehealth is already incorporated into our training. Further education in telehealth development, administration, and so on is currently available through courses operated by various institutions. Several non-ACGME boarded telemedicine fellowships are also currently available in the United States, and the fact that they are based out of departments of emergency medicine should be telling with regard to EM's leadership and adoption of the field. Although these programs are by no means required in order to practice telemedicine, one may view them similarly to the development of ultrasound fellowships in EM wherein these tracks provide dedicated time and experience for the development, administration, and leadership in the field. Telemedicine is a way for emergency physicians to practice our ethic of "anyone, anything, anytime," by use of these technologies to extend our skill set outside of the ED.

Reference

1. Hollander JE, Sharma R. The availabilists: emergency care without the emergency department. NEJM Catalyst. 2021;1–13. https://doi.org/catalyst.nejm.org/10.1056/cat.21.0310.

Chapter 56
Cruise Ship Medicine

Erol Kohli and Jeff Baker

Brief History of Cruise Ship Medicine

Medical care aboard passenger ships (carrying 13 or more passengers) including sailboats, yachts, river cruise ships, expedition ships, and ocean cruise liners is designed to provide crew and passengers with timely medical care as comparable as possible with that which is available ashore. The International Labor Organization (ILO) Maritime Labor Convention of 2006 states that ships carrying 100 or more persons for more than 3 days duration carry a qualified medical doctor who is responsible for providing medical care [1]. Ships that do not have a medical doctor on board should have at least one seafarer on board who oversees providing medical care.

In 1951, the World Health Organization (WHO) developed International Sanitary Regulations (ISR) to provide global standards for ship and port sanitation, health surveillance, and response to infectious disease outbreaks to reduce public health risks on ships. The ISR are currently known as the International Health Regulations (IHR) [2].

The American College of Emergency Physicians (ACEP) Section on Cruise Ship and Maritime Medicine has developed Health Care Guidelines for Cruise Ship

E. Kohli (✉)
Attending Physician, Department of Emergency Medicine, BronxCare Health System, Bronx, USA

J. Baker
Associate Professor, Department of Emergency Medicine, University of Louisville, Louisville, USA
e-mail: Jeffery.baker@louisville.edu

R. P. Olympia et al. (eds.), *An Emergency Physician's Path*,
https://doi.org/10.1007/978-3-031-47873-4_56

Medical Facilities and includes the following policy statement (which is followed by the Cruise Line International Association):

> "The American College of Emergency Physicians believes that appropriate emergency care and health care maintenance for passengers and crew members aboard ships sailing in international waters are desirable. The cruise ship industry and its medical departments should retain medical personnel who can:
>
> - Provide quality maritime medical care for passengers and crew members aboard cruise ships.
> - Initiate appropriate stabilization, diagnostic, and therapeutic maneuvers for critically ill or medically unstable patients.
> - Support, comfort, and care for patients on board ship.
> - Assist, in conjunction with the cruise line, in the medical evacuation of patients in a timely fashion when appropriate" [3].

Required Qualifications

Per ACEP guidelines [4], physicians should have at least 3 years of post-graduate experience and be board certified in Emergency Medicine, Family Medicine, or Internal Medicine and have an active license to practice medicine. Furthermore, clinical staff should be certified in advanced life support or an equivalent certification (including ABEM certification), and ships carrying children ≤12 years old should have at least one physician certified in PALS or an equivalent certification. Physicians should be competent in the following skill sets: emergency cardiovascular care, minor surgical/orthopedic care, and procedural sedation.

Common Conditions Encountered on a Ship

Some of the commonly encountered conditions on cruise ships include seasickness, respiratory infections (including COVID), GI illness (including norovirus), and various injuries including sprains, contusions, and open wounds. Although cruise ship passengers come from all demographics, many passengers have one or more chronic medical conditions that might require acute management while on board. The ship's physician may also be tasked with caring for the crew, so elements of occupational health will be frequently encountered.

Cruising during COVID

COVID has drastically affected the practice of cruise ship medicine and infectious outbreaks of COVID among cruise ships are not uncommon. Further complicating the presence of COVID aboard ships is staying up-to-date with the frequently changing policies and procedures for the testing, quarantine protocols, and treatment of COVID among passengers and crew. An additional challenging aspect of cruising during COVID is being aware of and following the national guidelines regarding testing and isolating COVID-positive cases depending on where you are sailing and making sure that guests are aware of these policies and procedures prior to boarding the ship to avoid any confusion/frustration after leaving port.

"A Day in the Life"

8–9 a.m.: Wake up, have breakfast, check in with the medical team, and chief mate aboard the ship. Review the ship's itinerary for the day and become familiar with the locations of local ports (including available medical services) should there be a need for medical evacuation.

9 a.m. to 12 p.m.: The clinic opens for you to see guests and crew who need medical care. The first patient of the day is a crew member who works on the deck and has had a mild cough and sore throat for a few days. You perform a rapid COVID test which is negative and recommend supportive care. The next patient is a guest who fell down the stairs while returning to her cabin during rough seas last night. You examine her, recommend RICE, and place an ace wrap for a suspected ankle sprain. You do not have X-ray available on your vessel, so you plan to reassess the patient the following day. The third patient is a guest who is an elderly male with heartburn. After obtaining a thorough history, performing a physical exam, and obtaining an EKG, you treat for likely GERD with antacids. You then follow up with several crew members you previously evaluated during the previous weeks.

12–1 p.m.: Lunch. Meet with colleagues and staff.

1–4 p.m.: Return to the clinic to see additional guests and crew. In between seeing patients, you work on preparing the medical team for the upcoming man overboard safety drill scheduled for tomorrow morning.

4–5 p.m.: Visit the gym, go for a run around the top deck of the ship, and play a few games of table tennis with fellow crew members.

5–6 p.m.: Shower, zoom/skype with family and friends back home.

6–8 p.m.: Dinner and socialize with guests aboard the ship while sailing past icebergs under the evening sun of the Arctic Circle.

10 p.m.: You are called to the cabin of a guest who has a suspected kidney infection. You place an ultrasound-guided IV, start IV fluids, and administer intravenous antibiotics. You plan to reassess the patient in the morning for possible evacuation. You are hoping to get some sleep, as there are several shore excursions planned the next day.

Benefits of Working as a Cruise Ship Doctor

You get to wake up at a new location every day and get paid while traveling the world. You will have access to complimentary food and entertainment and access to educational activities while aboard the ship. You will have the opportunity to participate in shore excursions at a variety of destinations. Ship physicians enjoy having their own private room where they might also bring their spouse or children at no charge. As an officer aboard the ship, there may be additional benefits and privileges, depending on the cruise line. Although cruise ship medicine can be a full-time career, many emergency physicians work part-time on cruise ships with assignments ranging from a few weeks to a few months.

For emergency physicians interested in a job on a cruise ship, joining ACEP's Cruise Ship Medicine Section is a logical first step. Many job openings are filled primarily by networking. Compensation will vary depending on the cruise ship line, location, and length of the assignment. Larger ships might be salary-based, while smaller expedition ships may only cover expenses and allow a companion to join you on the voyage. You can expect your salary to be generally less than what you would earn working in an emergency department. Malpractice is typically provided by the cruise ship company.

Unique Challenges and Limitations of Working aboard a Cruise Ship

Working on cruise ships is unlike any other work environment. You will experience long voyages, strong oceanic storms with rough seas, and being away from home for extended periods of time; these are just some of the challenges. The stress and pressure of adapting to ever-changing COVID protocols and policies can certainly take a toll. Regular communication with your medical team and the ship's officers is critical to medical operations as you must always be aware of anticipated needs for medical evacuation of patients. This not only includes knowledge of local ports and cities but also being aware of future weather conditions that could affect the ability to safely complete an evacuation. On smaller ships, you will need to be comfortable with limited supplies and facilities, as you may be the only medical provider on board and be on call 24/7. The ship's physician will often find themselves performing the duties of a physician, nurse, and clerk all at the same time.

Equipment on board can be highly variable, although all ships will have basic ACLS equipment and medications, including airway supplies, defibrillators, and IV fluids. Larger ships have dedicated medical clinics with some capable of limited ICU level care and diagnostics such as basic radiographs and bedside ultrasound. Smaller expedition cruise ships will likely have much more limited supplies and focus on the stabilization and evacuation of critically ill patients.

An additional unique aspect to cruise ship medicine is continuity of care and being able to follow up with your patients, especially crew members who may be on assignment with you for weeks to months where you essentially serve as their primary care physician for the duration of the voyage.

Cruise ship medicine is a unique niche in medicine, and Emergency Medicine physicians are well suited to tackle its many challenges. Whether the physician chooses cruise ship medicine as a full-time or part-time endeavor, it can be a rewarding aspect of their career.

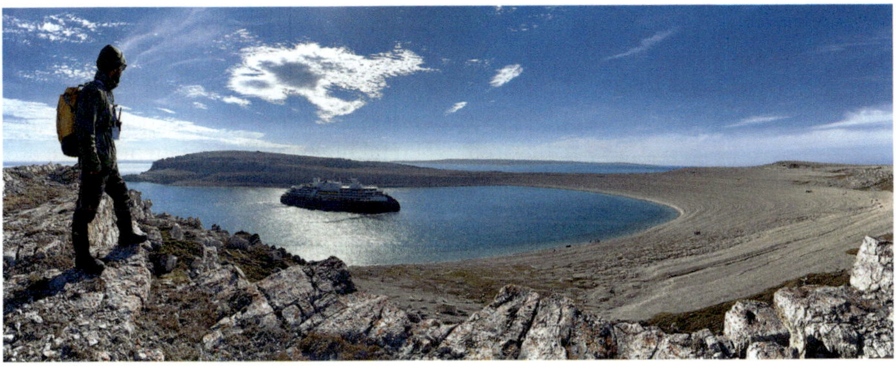

Caption to this photo – "On top of the world." Northwest Passage, Canadian Arctic, 2022.

References

1. World Health Organization. International medical guide for ships: including the ship's medicine chest. 3rd ed. World Health Organization; 2007.
2. Mitruka K, Wheeler RE. Cruise ship travel. Travel Medicine. 2008:351–60.
3. American College of Emergency Physicians. Policy statement: health care guidelines for cruise ship medical facilities. January, 2019.
4. American College of Emergency Physicians. Cruise ship health care guidelines policy resource and education paper. April, 2020.

Chapter 57
Correctional Medicine

Michael Mesisca

How I Found Correctional Healthcare (or How it Found me)

As an Emergency Medicine (EM) resident training at a large, public safety-net hospital in Southern California, I was able to begin moonlighting early in my second year at the county jail affiliated with my hospital. At first, the environment was strangely different and uncomfortable. The first time I walked into the jail, it felt bizarre, like something out of an HBO documentary. I recall the formality of the jail check-in and security process and the meticulous identification validation to get in. I walked through the gates of tall barbed-wire fences, asking myself, "Am I going in the right direction?" and questioning again the decision to enter as large, massive, concrete-secured doors slammed loudly behind me. Yet, once I got to the clinic and began seeing patients, it was a very different and familiar story.

The patients were respectful and appreciative. They were engaged and eager to learn about their often-neglected health issues. I felt safe, having deputies nearby. The nurses and deputies in the clinic were working together, assisting one another to help the inmates. In my second week working there, an older patient was brought to the clinic with chest pain, the staff quickly performed an EKG that showed a STEMI, EMS was called, and he was quickly sent to the ER. Well-run operations delivering timely coordinated care to patients in need ... in jail! Many of the patients I saw had complex medical issues that they had neglected for a long time. Some had abscesses, lacerations, and fractures, which are problems an ER doctor can fix. It was and continues to be very rewarding.

M. Mesisca (✉)
Chairman, Department of Emergency Medicine, Moreno Valley, USA

Medical Director, Disaster Medicine & Clinical Support Services, Chief Medical Officer, Correctional Health, Riverside County, USA
e-mail: m.mesisca@ruhealth.org

R. P. Olympia et al. (eds.), *An Emergency Physician's Path*,
https://doi.org/10.1007/978-3-031-47873-4_57

Several months into my moonlighting time, I was seeing a patient in the clinic when a "man down" was called. I responded to an inmate who attempted to hang himself with a bed sheet. I started CPR, immobilized his c-spine, and guided a medic whom I knew from the ER through an intubation on the floor of a jail cell, and then rode with the patient to the local hospital. While not something that happens too often (fortunately), there is an increasing prevalence of serious injuries and fentanyl overdoses occurring in jails and prisons [1]. Having emergency-trained physicians supporting the jail system's delivery of care can be incredibly valuable [2].

I gained immense experience as a resident. So much so, that years later after becoming the Department Chair of Emergency Medicine for another large county, I would be asked to become the Chief Medical Officer for the county's jails and juvenile halls. In an effort to improve the quality of care for the jails, I brought Emergency Medicine-trained physicians and physician assistants/nurse practitioners into the facilities. The ED team helped take after-hours calls, provided more procedures to the jails to reduce medical transports to the hospital, and integrated the care delivery between the ED, hospital, and the jails. We brought more specialty care to the jails and increased telehealth utilization. Working with the pharmacy, we increased the number of inmates released with their prescriptions in hand to reduce medication non-compliance. We also worked to get the inmates enrolled in insurance programs to reduce gaps in their coverage, and we worked with our health system primary care and behavioral health teams to coordinate clinic appointments for inmates with active health issues being released from custody. Correctional healthcare is complex, challenging, and rewarding.

Inmate Medical Care Continuum

When an individual is arrested for a crime, they are "booked" or registered into a city or county jail or juvenile facility. This can entail a transfer of responsibility from an arresting agency (e.g., local police) to a custody agency (e.g., county sheriff). Before booking, to ensure the safety of the individual, there is a medical clearance process. Many regions have a workflow that details what conditions require an Emergency Room visit (e.g., motor vehicle accident, head injury with loss of consciousness, and blood sugar over 400) and other conditions that can be cleared by the healthcare team at the jail. Once at the jail, new arrests are seen by nurses, physician assistants, and/or physicians who assess the arrestee and determine if they are medically stable to be housed at the facility. The medical team addresses acute medical issues, stabilizes chronic conditions, and performs screening for infectious diseases, alcohol and opiate withdrawal, suicidal ideation, and mental illness. Alcohol- and opiate-addicted inmates are started on withdrawal protocols to address the symptoms and potential decompensation associated with severe withdrawal. Some institutions initiate medical-assisted treatment for opiate dependence. Suicidal patients are placed in safety cells and on suicide watch.

Inmates reside in a county jail pending their trial and, after they are sentenced, they are often transferred to a state or federally operated prison (although now it is increasingly common for federal prisoners to be housed in county jails while they serve their sentence). Hence, individuals in the county system are commonly referred to as *inmates* and those in the state or federal system are *prisoners*. Additionally, the term *detention* is now discouraged and has been replaced by the term *corrections* to emphasize the goal of supporting individuals in serving their sentence and moving toward a more positive future. Once booked into the jail or sentenced to prison, inmates receive access to primary and preventive care and specialty care. Correctional health teams are responsible for providing acute medical care for falls, accidents, trauma, and overdoses onsite as well as providing care for chronic medical and surgical conditions. The advantages of having emergency physicians leading those teams include a reduction in ambulance transports to the local hospital by expanding the care delivery capability on-site [2]. Inmates have a right to receive care that meets or exceeds the community standard. The goal of correctional health teams is to provide quality healthcare. Many individuals in custody have neglected their healthcare. They frequently have untreated mental illnesses in addition to their medical issues. They have acute and chronic conditions that are in need of quality, compassionate physicians willing to treat them with dignity and respect and to encourage them to take ownership over their health and future well-being.

Why Emergency Physicians Should Consider a Job in Correctional Health Care?

The following is a list of reasons that emergency physicians should consider working in correctional medicine:

1. **Professionally rewarding:** Inmates are an underserved population that presents a broad range of medical issues in a unique environment. The ability to help patients who are often very appreciative and have a broad range of medical issues can be very rewarding.
2. **Variety in practice and pace**: While correctional health can be very busy and challenging, the pace of work is lower than most busy Emergency Departments, and it does not have the same stress of a constant influx of critical ambulances or emphasis on documentation the supports billing.
3. **Public health service**: Correctional healthcare is a community public health service. Many correctional sites have robust TB, STD, and other infectious disease screening (e.g., HIV and hepatitis C) and treatment programs. Helping identify and treat these diseases in the jails and providing inmates with education help reduce the transmission of the diseases back into the community.
4. **Leadership opportunities and compensation**: Most correctional sites are in need of physician leaders willing to help improve operations, provide quality

healthcare, and work on integrating care with local healthcare clinics and hospitals. Due to physician shortages in many areas, the compensation often includes hard-to-recruit bonuses and incentives.
5. **Unique challenges**: Inmates with chronic health conditions require unique considerations. For example, those with seizure disorders require a bottom bunk, bottom-tier bed. Additionally, correctional health physicians need to consider the implications of infectious outbreaks (e.g., M.R.S.A., lice, influenza, COVID-19, and mumps) and how to isolate, quarantine, and manage outbreaks [3].
6. **Schedule**: Many correctional sites, given challenges in recruiting, offer schedules to accommodate individual physician preferences. Often emergency physicians find reduced nights or weekends offered at some jails and prisons to be particularly appealing.
7. **Teamwork**: Working in corrections, similar to the Emergency Department, requires a collaborative team. It is tremendously gratifying working with law enforcement, nursing, and administrators to create excellent healthcare operations.

Challenges of Working in Correctional Healthcare

1. **Working in a Correctional Setting**: This environment is not for everyone, but everyone working in Emergency Medicine stands to gain a lot of valuable experience touring their regional jail and/or prison and developing an understanding of their scope of services and workflows. Correctional settings are very different from any other hospital or clinic environment that a doctor can work in. In general, physicians often report that it is much safer than expected and, in many ways, safer than working in the Emergency Room.
2. **Not all correctional settings are providing quality care**. There are some correctional sites that suffer significant shortages in nursing, physicians, and/or correctional deputies. Staffing shortages may not allow adequate support to provide high-quality healthcare. Do your research on the leadership team and reputation of the agency providing healthcare prior to accepting a role working with them.
3. **Legal considerations**: Inmates have a legal right to quality care. Much like working anywhere else, there are sites where the frequency of lawsuits may be higher when working in corrections. Having good legal support and malpractice coverage is important and necessary to working in corrections. Most sites provide this for employed and contracted physicians.
4. **Security Clearance**: Almost all jail and prison systems require extensive background checks. Honesty and disclosure are essential. The process can take weeks to months, and applicants may be surprised by the in-depth questions. Being forthcoming and patient is essential.

How Correctional Healthcare Is Provided and Contracted

There are many things to consider when exploring working in a correctional health, one of which is the organizational structure of the medical system. There are publicly run and operated systems where the physicians are employed by the county, state, or federal governments. Some public systems contract out professional services to a physician group or utilize physicians hired as independent contractors. In other settings, all of the healthcare provision is fully contracted to a private organization (some of which are for-profit entities), and physicians are either employed or hired as independent contractors. Each of the structures listed impacts the way a facility operates, and interested physicians are advised to research the reputation and consult with other physicians who currently and previously work with the hiring/contracting entity to gain information about the quality of care, schedule, compensation, malpractice, and legal support.

Exploring Correctional Medicine:

1. **Find a mentor**: Reach out to a medical director or chief medical officer for the local county jail or state prison system in your region. Ask for a site visit and/or tour if possible (there may be limits on access due to security issues). Find out what compelled them to work in corrections. Ask questions.
2. **Experience**: Familiarize yourself with the current medical clearance process for booking and workflows with your local correctional facilities. Support your Emergency Medicine medical director in streamlining these processes. See what staffing needs exist in corrections in your area and consider working part-time to explore if it is something you enjoy.
3. **Education**: The National Commission on Correctional Healthcare (NCCHC) is a great resource for education and certifications in correctional healthcare. There is a two-step certification for physicians (https://www.ncchc.org/professional-certification/cchp-p/). The NCCHC is also a nationally accrediting agency that performs site visits and quality assessments of jails.

References

1. Kaplowitz E, Truong AQ, Macmadu A, Peterson M, Brinkley-Rubinstein L, Potter N, Green TC, Clarke JG, Rich JD Fentanylrelated overdose during incarceration: a comprehensive review – health & justice. BioMed Central. 2021;9(13):1–11. Retrieved September 8, 2022, from https://healthandjusticejournal.biomedcentral.com/articles/10.1186/s40352-021-00138-6
2. Sanko SG, Terp S, Joseph D, Eiting E, Eckstein M. 78 impact of emergency physician care provided at Los Angeles county jail urgent care clinic on municipal emergency medical services agency. Ann Emerg Med. 2014;64(4):28. https://doi.org/10.1016/j.annemergmed.2014.07.103.
3. Mesisca M, Minahan T, Carl B, Fillman T, Randall MM. Minimizing the impact of COVID-19 in a county jail environment to protect a vulnerable population. J Correct Health Care. 2022;28(2):80–3. https://doi.org/10.1089/jchc.20.12.0110.

Chapter 58
Being a Successful Nocturnist

Olga M. Otter

There is something about the hospital at night. Empty lobby atriums, abandoned workstations in the clinics, and darkened hallways have a hush that you would never experience before 5 p.m. With less staff working, you usually know everyone – if not by name, at least by face. You see them rolling out of their cars in the parking garage with coffee in hand. You share a look, square up your shoulders, and walk into that nighttime groove.

I have always loved being in the hospital when I was not supposed to be there. It feels like being in a secret club, like the cool kids sneaking around learning all the secrets. My father was a surgeon. Sometimes, he would have to take me in when he was covering call, and I would sit in the nursing station and take it all in. Not surprisingly, the ED was my favorite nursing station to be in – the energy, the immediacy, and the way the team played off each other. In college, as a volunteer in the ED on late Sunday nights, I fed on the crazy experiences that were available when the rules were relaxed. At my first job out of residency, I learned that I hated the mid-shift, 3 p.m. to 11 p.m. You walk in, the department is a chaotic mess, and often when you are trying to leave it is still at that same level of chaos. I found it hard to get out on time and to settle my brain once I did get home. So, I launched my nocturnist career quickly right out of residency.

O. M. Otter (✉)
Department of Emergency Medicine, University of North Carolina, Chapel Hill, NC, USA
e-mail: omotter@ad.unc.edu

R. P. Olympia et al. (eds.), *An Emergency Physician's Path*,
https://doi.org/10.1007/978-3-031-47873-4_58

Nocturnist and Family

If you are an orphan and have no plans to have significant others, pets, kids, or friends outside of work, you have my permission to skip this section. Go to the next section. I will not be mad. Good Luck.

For everyone else who is not planning on being a hermit nomad loner who does nothing outside of work, here's some advice on how to manage nightlife and everyone else in your circle.

There are some people in your family that no matter how many times you remind them that you work nights will get upset that you do not answer their calls at 2 p.m. The do not disturb function on your phone was created just for them. Others have suggested calling those loved ones at 2 a.m. "just for a chat" to help drive the point home. For everyone else, they will adapt and adjust well. It does take buy-in from your spouse and kids and reminders as everyone settles into the routine. BUT that is the key – routine. Where else in Emergency Medicine can you have a routine? The normal EM schedule of scattered AM shift, mid-shift, swing shift, night shift, and every combination and permutation in between with complicated calendars is hard to coordinate. In my house, Mom is up at 5 p.m., goes to work at 10:30 p.m., and is available during the day if there is active bleeding or a house fire. With this set schedule, it becomes easier to set up pickups, drop-offs, sitters, and family time.

Health

Health and wellness have always been important, but, after the COVID epidemic and with burnout rates on the rise, it is critical to establish good habits if you are going to be successful as a nocturnist. Everyone has different internal clocks and can sleep more readily at certain points of the day. Find what works for you and stick to it. When I talk with my residents about working a string of shifts, I separate out going into a string and then how to recover afterward (Table 58.1).

Table 58.1 Suggested habits starting, during, and ending a string of shifts

STARTING STRING	DURING STRING	ENDING STRING
Pre-sleep: 4 (or more) hours during your sleepy time	Stick to a set sleeping schedule	Post-sleep: 4 hours and then get out of bed
Prep for your string of shifts: • Grocery run • Clean house • Work on projects you cannot get done at night • Clear the decks	Maintain: • Pack healthy snacks • Keep up on charting • Say yes to activities between waking/work but not every night	Set up tasks to stay up and out of bed: • Personal healthcare appointments • Haircut • Oil change • Schedule the house cleaner

Table 58.1 (continued)

STARTING STRING	DURING STRING	ENDING STRING
Exercise	Exercise	Exercise
Do not: Skip pre-work sleep	Do not: • Pick up your phone in the middle of the afternoon. Hide it from yourself. • Booze it up after your shift. This leads to poor sleep and having to get up to pee	Do not: • Sign important paperwork • Schedule anything that takes deep thought • Go back to bed until it is bedtime

Sleep/Wake

So, there you are, staring at the ceiling, trying your best to summon the sandman and get those sheep organized in a counting line, and it is not working. Or, conversely, you are yawning (did you just yawn? Gotcha!) and struggling to keep your eyes open while Mr. Smith is telling you about his abdominal pain that started in 1975 and brought him to the ER today. How do you manage getting to sleep and staying awake? It is best to have consistent sleep patterns, but most nocturnists do flip back and forth between days and nights with their shift strings. You can have a "better living through chemistry," but this has its pitfalls and should be done consistently and safely.

Shift work disorder is defined as a sleep disorder that commonly affects those who work non-traditional hours, outside the typical 9 a.m. to 5 p.m. workday [1, 2]. As EM physicians, nocturnist or not, this is us. The American Academy of Sleep Medicine has written guidelines for a task force addressing shift work disorder [3]. They recommend, in addition to daytime sleep, a pre-shift nap to help with nighttime wakefulness. Timed light exposure, 20–30 min several times during the shift, with light avoidance in the morning also helps with adjusting the wake/sleep cycle. This can be done with a light box at your desk and sunglasses/blue blockers for the ride home. Not surprisingly, the use of melatonin after your shift is encouraged. Lower over-the-counter doses, 3 mg, versus 10 mg was shown to be as effective (your pineal gland produces about 10–80 μg per night). I do not recommend hypnotics such as benzodiazepines or zolpidem. The sedation carryover risk and concern for dependence outweigh the benefits. For wakefulness, caffeine or modafinil is recommended. I would caution to limit use of caffeine after 3 a.m. so as not to cause problems with sleeping once your shift is over. Modafinil (Provigil) is an alertness aid that can be prescribed by your primary care provider. I find that it can be helpful more when switching to daytime mode. Having a cup of coffee or tablet of Modafinil on the last morning of a shift before sleeping can aid when trying to get up and salvage your "day off."

Create a good environment for sleep. Now is the time to splurge on high thread counts, comfortable mattresses and pillows, and blackout curtains. Keep the room dark and cold. A fan for ambient noise or white noise machine is beneficial. There are many apps that can help you fall asleep with meditations. Box breathing (inhaling for 4 s, holding for 4 s, exhaling for 4 s, and holding for 4 s) or other self-calming techniques will get you into sleepy time mode.

Dark Side of Night

Unfortunately, working nights does have health risks. Studies have shown higher risks of breast, colon, and prostate cancer [4–6]. There have been increased rates of dementia among long-term night workers [7]. Fatigue takes its toll and can lead to earlier burnout. [8] Among those studied, peptic ulcer disease, diabetes, coronary artery disease, and preterm or otherwise compromised pregnancy outcomes were much higher in those working nights [9, 10]. Getting routine physicals, doing self-exams, and working on a healthy lifestyle are keys to longevity.

Eating patterns can be erratic, and the nighttime potluck or frequent late night fast food runs are not in your best interest [11, 12]. Bringing a big meal always seems to mean you will have a busy night and not being able to reheat and eat. Having healthy small snacks that you can graze on while you are charting is more reasonable. For those who follow intermittent fasting, being a nocturnist is very conducive to the timing of your meals.

More immediate is the risk of sleep deprivation and driving. While blasting the radio, having the windows down, and chewing gum may seem to be a good idea at the time, sometimes even all of that is not enough.

If you are finding yourself nodding off behind the wheel, pull over and nap. Better to be home 15 min later than not at all. Yes, it can happen to you. If you find yourself with a long commute, consider getting a nap in a call room or nearby hotel/apartment for ultimate safety.

Contract Negotiations

Knowing what you know now about health risks and difficulties with being a nocturnist, you should feel more equipped to discuss benefits with your employer for taking on the group's night shifts. Most groups will have a night shift differential, which can range anywhere from $100–$400 per shift. Asking to make out your own schedule to provide more flexibility is a reasonable request. This can be tricky when there is more than one nocturnist. Others prefer to have a set schedule of nights that they work each week. Find what works for you and ask for it. If shift differential is not available, you might request a shift buydown, so that you can work less nights for the same money. Other ideas for negotiation include 24-h gym memberships, payment for apps such as Headspace or Time shifter, or meal prep plans. It is OK to be creative – you are providing a valuable service to the group.

Work at Night

As a nocturnist, depending on where you work, you may be the only doctor in the hospital. At the very least, the number of physicians physically present in the hospital is greatly decreased at night. Your group should have guidelines in place for what you might be responsible for in areas outside the Emergency Department. That being said, we have the skills as emergency physicians to care for urgent issues. Do the right thing for the patient in the moment.

Calling a consultant at 2 a.m. can be the hardest part of the job. Although they are on call, the early hour page is never a welcome surprise. Have your pitch about the patient ready and expect to have to repeat it a few times while they wake up. It is best to be brief with a specific question for them soon after the one liner about the patient. You can always give more information once they are invested in the question. For example: Hi – this is Dr. X from the ED. I have Mrs. Jones who is an 80-year-old woman with diabetes, hypertension, and previous MI. She is having chest pain. I would like you to admit. (If only it was that simple every time!) Be strong and know your limitations. I have been asked to do some outrageous things over the years so that the consultant can have a few more hours of sleep. In case you did not know, a badly mangled hand with open fractures should not have a wet to dry dressing applied to follow up in the office the next morning. It is admirable to try to be helpful to the consultants. However, if they have you doing a procedure or other ill-advised recommendation and it goes south, it is only on you for the fall out. I recommend having a recorded line for these conversations if possible. Study up on EMTALA and know your hospital's guidelines for admission and timing of consults.

It is good to have a bag of tricks ready to go. With limited staffing in the hospital, you may be performing tasks and managing conditions that during the day would be covered by someone else. Working at night can be cowboy-esque with MacGyver-like solutions. Being able to think outside the box is the skill set to have. Having someone else to talk through problems, whether that be another EM doctor working at your hospital or at a satellite hospital, has saved the day many times. Did you know a black tea bag applied to an oozing post-dental extraction can stop the bleeding when Surgicel, epi, and Combat Gauze have failed? My work bag contains alligator forceps and a tiny camera I got off amazon to better extract roaches from ears, peppermint essential oils for my mask and extra-long ring forceps in case of a retained tampon removal, and a Urology guidewire for difficult to replace suprapubic catheters. When you find a good tool that is hard to find at night, stash it for later.

Your work family will include the staff in the ED as well as elsewhere in the hospital. Cultivate these relationships. Find out about your CT techs' family and pets. Know your hospitalists' likes and dislikes. Participate in Secret Santa and baby showers. Go out after work for breakfast with the crew. The people that work nights are the most loyal and fun in the hospital. They will save you on more occasions than not. They are the biggest reason to work at night.

References

1. Sack RL, Auckley D, Auger RR, Carskadon MA, Wright KP Jr, Vitiello MV, Zhdanova IV, American Academy of Sleep Medicine. Circadian rhythm sleep disorders: part I, basic principles, shift work and jet lag disorders. An American Academy of sleep medicine review. Sleep. 2007 Nov;30(11):1460–83. https://doi.org/10.1093/sleep/30.11.1460. PMID: 18041480; PMCID: PMC2082105
2. Auger RR, Burgess HJ, Emens JS, Deriy LV, Thomas SM, Sharkey KM. Clinical practice guideline for the treatment of intrinsic circadian rhythm sleep-wake disorders: advanced sleep-wake phase disorder (ASWPD), delayed sleep-wake phase disorder (DSWPD), non-24-hour sleep wake rhythm disorder (N24SWD), and irregular sleep-wake rhythm disorder (ISWRD). An update for 2015. J Clin Sleep Med. 2015;11(10):1199–236.
3. Morgenthaler TI, Lee-Chiong T, Alessi C, Friedman L, Aurora RN, Boehlecke B, Brown T, Chesson AL Jr, Kapur V, Maganti R, Owens J, Pancer J, Swick TJ, Zak R. Standards of practice Committee of the American Academy of sleep medicine. Practice parameters for the clinical evaluation and treatment of circadian rhythm sleep disorders. An American Academy of sleep medicine report. Sleep. 2007;30(11):1445–59. https://doi.org/10.1093/sleep/30.11.1445. Erratum in: Sleep. 2008 Jul 1;31(7):table of contents. PMID: 18041479; PMCID: PMC2082098
4. Liu W, Zhou Z, Dong D, Sun L, Zhang G. Sex differences in the association between night shift work and the risk of cancers: a meta-analysis of 57 articles. Dis Markers. 2018;26(2018):7925219. https://doi.org/10.1155/2018/7925219. PMID: 30598709; PMCID: PMC6287141
5. Hansen J. Night shift work and risk of breast cancer. Curr Environ Health Rep. 2017 Sep;4(3):325–39. https://doi.org/10.1007/s40572-017-0155-y. PMID: 28770538
6. Ward EM, et al. Carcinogenicity of night shift work. Lancet Oncol. 2019;20(8):1058–9.
7. Moreno CRC, Marqueze EC, Sargent C, Wright KP Jr, Ferguson SA, Tucker P. Working time society consensus statements: evidence-based effects of shift work on physical and mental health. Ind Health. 2019;57(2):139–57. https://doi.org/10.2486/indhealth.SW-1. Epub 2019 Jan 31. PMID: 30700667; PMCID: PMC6449637
8. Torquati L, Mielke GI, Brown WJ, Burton NW, Kolbe-Alexander TL. Shift work and poor mental health: a meta-analysis of longitudinal studies. Am J Public Health. 2019;109(11):e13–20. https://doi.org/10.2105/AJPH.2019.305278. Epub 2019 Sep 19. PMID: 31536404; PMCID: PMC6775929
9. Harrington JM. Health effects of shift work and extended hours of work. Occup Environ Med. 2001;58(1):68–72.
10. Knutsson A. Health disorders of shift workers. Occup Med (Lond). 2003 Mar;53(2):103–8. https://doi.org/10.1093/occmed/kqg048. PMID: 12637594
11. Hemmer A, Mareschal J, Dibner C, Pralong JA, Dorribo V, Perrig S, Genton L, Pichard C, Collet TH. The effects of shift work on cardio-metabolic diseases and eating patterns. Nutrients. 2021;13(11):4178. https://doi.org/10.3390/nu13114178. PMID: 34836433; PMCID: PMC8617838
12. McHill AW, Melanson EL, Higgins J, Connick E, Moehlman TM, Stothard ER, Wright KP Jr. Impact of circadian misalignment on energy metabolism during simulated nightshift work. Proc Natl Acad Sci U S A. 2014 Dec 2;111(48):17302–7. https://doi.org/10.1073/pnas.1412021111. Epub 2014 Nov 17. PMID: 25404342; PMCID: PMC4260578

Chapter 59
Digital Scholarship and Social Media in Emergency Medicine

Andrew Little

What Is Digital Scholarship?

Digital scholarship is a new and emerging field of academic inquiry that uses digital technologies to enable further research, teaching, and learning methods. Digital scholarship encompasses various activities, from using social media to disseminate research findings to develop new data collection and analysis methods. Digital scholarship can potentially transform how we do academic work by making it more collaborative, open, and accessible.

Digital scholarship has roots in various disciplines, including library and information science, computer science, education, and the humanities. In recent years, there has been an increasing focus on using digital technologies for academic research, teaching, and learning. This has led to the development of new tools and methods for conducting research, managing data, and collaborating with others. Digital scholarship also encompasses a variety of activities that are not traditionally considered scholarly work, such as developing websites or blogs, creating online courses or massive open online courses (MOOCs), or using social media to engage with the public about research findings. As digital scholarship becomes more prevalent, it is essential to consider its implications for the future of academic work.

Digital scholarship has the potential to transform how we do academic work. By making research more open and accessible, digital scholarship can help break down traditional barriers to both knowledge production and dissemination. It also can make academic work more collaborative by enabling interaction among scholars. Additionally, digital scholarship can help increase the impact of research by making it more visible and easily discoverable online. However, digital scholarship also presents some challenges, such as ensuring the quality and credibility of digital

A. Little (✉)
Advent Health East Orlando, Orlando, USA

R. P. Olympia et al. (eds.), *An Emergency Physician's Path*,
https://doi.org/10.1007/978-3-031-47873-4_59

resources, managing copyright and intellectual property issues, and protecting user privacy. As digital scholarship evolves, it is important to consider its potential and challenges.

There is no precise answer to the question of when digital scholarship started existing, as digital scholarship can be said to have started at different times for different people and disciplines. However, we can narrow it down to a few key historical moments. One crucial moment was the release of the first personal computer in 1981. This event made computing power and storage capacity more accessible to individuals, making it easier for them to engage in digital scholarship [1].

The launch of the World Wide Web in 1991 gave scholars new ways to access and share information, which made digital scholarship more widespread and influential [2]. Fast forward to now, where social media platforms such as Twitter, Instagram, and Facebook have significantly impacted its reach, and you have digital scholarship as we know it today. What remains to be decided is how digital scholarship can play a role in educational promotion at prominent universities and their affiliates.

When we describe digital scholarship, it is impossible not to include free open-access medical education (FOAMed). FOAMed describes the growing movement of freely available online medical education resources. These resources include blogs, podcasts, and social media platforms providing medical content for clinicians and patients. The goals of FOAMed are to (1) increase the accessibility of medical education, (2) provide accurate and up-to-date information, and (3) promote collaboration among healthcare professionals [3]. One of the advantages of FOAMed is that it allows clinicians to stay up-to-date on the latest medical advancements without having to pay for expensive continuing medical education (CME) courses. In addition, FOAMed can be used as a supplement to traditional CME courses.

A podcast is a digital audio or video file made available for download, typically via syndication, and can be played on a computer or portable media player. Podcasting has become a popular way to distribute content, primarily due to the ease of subscribing and listening to podcasts. Podcasts are usually episodic, with new episodes becoming available periodically. They often include features such as interviews, commentary, or other types of supplemental information. Many podcasts are free to listen to, but some require a subscription fee. Podcasting has recently seen a surge in popularity, with more people than ever tuning in to their favorite shows.

There are many medical blogs, but they all have one common goal: providing information and resources to help people better understand and manage their health. Some medical blogs focus on specific conditions or diseases, while others offer general health information. Still, others offer advice and tips, from choosing the right doctor to staying healthy during pregnancy. No matter their focus, all medical blogs are committed to providing accurate, up-to-date information that can help people make informed decisions about their health. A medical blog can be a great resource if you are looking for reliable health information.

Vlogging is a type of blogging that focuses on video content. Vloggers create and share videos on various topics, from personal experiences to current events. Many vloggers use their platform to build an audience and connect with viewers personally. While the term “vlog” was coined in the early 2000s, the practice of vlogging has only become popular in recent years. With the rise of social media and easy-to-use video editing software, anyone can start a vlog [4].

Vlogging can be fun and rewarding to share your thoughts and experiences. If you are thinking about starting a vlog, here are a few things to remember: Find your niche. What topics are you passionate about? What do you want your vlog to be known for? Figure out what makes your vlog unique and use that to attract viewers. Be consistent. Upload new videos regularly so that viewers have a reason to come back. A schedule will also help you stay organized and on track. Engage with your audience. Vlogging is all about building relationships with viewers. Respond to comments, follow other vloggers, and collaborate with others in your niche.

In recent years, digital scholarship has increasingly been recognized as a valuable and essential form of scholarly activity. As a result, the impact factor of digital scholarship has risen significantly. Digital scholarship encompasses a wide range of activities, from traditional academic research published online to more innovative forms of scholarship that use digital technologies in new and creative ways. Although digital scholarship takes many forms, all share a common goal: to use digital technologies to advance knowledge and understanding in a particular field or discipline. The increased recognition of digital scholarship has led to a corresponding increase in the impact factor of digital scholarship. In fact, according to a recent study, the average impact factor of digital scholarship is now nearly twice that of traditional scholarly work [5, 6]. This increase in impact factor is due, in part, to the fact that digital scholarship is often more accessible and easier to disseminate than traditional scholarly work. Additionally, digital scholarship often uses new and emerging technologies, attracting a wider audience and leading to more citations.

The increased impact factor of digital scholarship is having a positive impact on the field. As digital scholarship becomes more widely recognized and respected, more scholars will likely engage in this type of scholarly work. This, in turn, could lead to further increases in the impact factor. Ultimately, the increased impact factor of digital scholarship is likely to benefit both scholars and society.

There are many reasons why someone might want to consider participating in digital scholarship. For one, it can help you reach a larger audience for your work, and it can also help you connect with other scholars and researchers working on similar topics or in related fields. Additionally, digital scholarship can also help you preserve your work in a format that is more accessible and easier to share. Finally, digital scholarship can also help you keep track of your research progress and ideas over time. Ultimately, the decision to pursue digital scholarship should be based on what will best suit your needs and goals as a researcher and educator.

References

1. The Birth of the IBM PC. IBM Archives: The birth of the IBM PC. https://www.ibm.com/ibm/history/exhibits/pc25/pc25_birth.html. Accessed January 1, 2023.
2. Fischels J. A look back at the very first website ever launched, 30 years later. NPR. https://www.npr.org/2021/08/06/1025554426/a-look-back-at-the-very-first-website-ever-launched-30-years-later. Published August 6, 2021. Accessed January 1, 2023.
3. Burkholder TW, Bellows JW, King RA. Free open access medical education (FOAM) in emergency medicine: the global distribution of users in 2016. West J Emerg Med. 2018;19(3):600–5. https://doi.org/10.5811/westjem.2018.3.36825.
4. Hurtubise L, Martin B, Gilliland A, Mahan J. To play or not to play: leveraging video in medical education. J Grad Med Educ. 2013;5(1):13–8. https://doi.org/10.4300/JGME-05-01-32.
5. Husain A, Repanshek Z, Singh M, et al. Consensus guidelines for digital scholarship in academic promotion. West J Emerg Med. 2020;21(4):883–91. Published 2020 Jul 8. https://doi.org/10.5811/westjem.2020.4.46441.
6. Langdorf MI, Lin M. Emergency medicine scholarship in the digital age. West J Emerg Med. 2016;17(5):511–2. https://doi.org/10.5811/westjem.2016.8.32283.

Chapter 60
Locum Tenens

William Saunders

Locum Tenens or "locums," as it is often called, is a viable career path for those interested in travel, learning new environments and workflows, supplementing income, or winding down a career. By definition, a locums job is temporary. However, this should not dissuade you from pursuing locums as either a primary or supplemental career path. Locums work can be very rewarding. It allows an emergency medicine physician to expand their work options while also providing experience across diverse patient populations and workflows. Additionally, locums work can be financially beneficial as the hourly rates are often higher than traditional positions.

One of the greatest benefits of locums work is that it gives the physician maximum flexibility. You choose when you work, where you work, and how much you work. This flexibility can take you across the country or even internationally. Because of the flexibility, many physicians chose to augment their careers with additional locums work. For those looking for a new adventure, supplemental income, or just want to wind down their career, locums is a great option.

Emergency department groups may seek to hire locums staff to help cover shifts due to physician vacations, leaves of absence, physician-related health issues, physician turnover, or to combat physician burnout. The locums physician can provide the needed relief to the group by filling gaps in their clinical schedules and working some of the less desirable shifts. The group will contract with a locums company to hire a physician to fill these needs.

At some point in every emergency medicine physician's career, you will get an email or a phone call from a locums company. A quick Internet search will also yield your point of entry into the locums market. Once you have decided on which

W. Saunders (✉)
University of Toledo Medical Center, Toledo, OH, USA
e-mail: William.saunders2@utoledo.edu

R. P. Olympia et al. (eds.), *An Emergency Physician's Path*,
https://doi.org/10.1007/978-3-031-47873-4_60

company to contract with, you supply your credentials. You can give the locums company your specifications such as location, EMR, volume, trauma designation, and pay per hour. The locums company will then try to find the best fit for you. Once they have found a hiring company that meets your specifications, they will present you to the company to see if they are interested in hiring you as a locums physician. If approved, you will then start on credentialing for your new position.

For those who work locums, it is recommended that you have a "credentials folder" with all the pertinent information. You will likely reference this folder many times throughout your career, and it will be invaluable. It should include your life support certifications, medical school diploma, residency documentation, updated vaccination records, continuing education records, and malpractice claims history and certificates of insurance (COI) for all your clinical work. Every time you are presented to a new company, you will be required to supply these documents. Additionally, to broaden your availability consider obtaining multiple state licenses or participating in the Interstate Medical Licensure Compact (www.imlcc.org). You will also need a DEA and prescribing license for every state you work in. This will broaden your chances of obtaining locums work in multiple states.

As part of the onboarding process with your new locums site, you will need to complete hospital and EMR orientation. Any travel or time committed to this process should be compensated to you through the locums company. Once you are fully onboarded, you are ready to start picking up shifts at the location.

Your locums company will reach out to you each month to obtain your schedule requests. They will then submit your requests to the emergency medicine group with which you are contracted. You have the flexibility to work in blocks or single shifts. Once you have worked your shifts, you will then submit timesheets to the locums company, which will then submit the timesheet to the emergency department group for billing. You are usually paid biweekly or monthly.

The benefits of locums work are many, but the biggest benefit for most is the supplemental income. Typically, locums physicians can earn substantially more than their employed counterparts. Many locums contracts can pay upwards of 2–3× the hourly rate of a standard physician employee. The locums company will charge the hospital ~$20–$30 per hour you work. For instance, if your pay rate is $250 per hour, the locums company is charging the hospital $280 per hour, taking the $30 and giving you the remainder. Many physicians use locums income to pay off their medical school loans or other debts.

Another major benefit is an additional retirement savings option. Most locums tenens contracts will designate you as an independent contractor paid through the 1099 form. This designation opens a world of tax and investing benefits. Independent contractors can open a solo 401k and contribute up to the IRS maximum each year. This solo 401k can be in addition to your 401k with your W-2 employment. Locums income can help the physician achieve financial independence and help pave the way for a more comfortable retirement.

Another great benefit of locums is the exposure to different patient populations and workflows. Each emergency department has a unique workflow based on the needs of its patient population. These different workflows will often teach you a different way of practicing emergency medicine based on available resources. You can take these lessons back to your regular employed position. I have often found these workflows beneficial in helping solve process issues within my own department. With each new contract, you will have the opportunity to learn the needs of a new patient population and expand your emergency medicine skills and knowledge.

Despite the many benefits of locums, there are also some downsides. As an independent contractor, you will be responsible for taxes, benefits, retirement funds, and funding your own continuing medical education. This can present itself as a daunting task. However, with some planning, this is easily accomplished and provides you with complete control over how your money is spent and organized. You will need to file quarterly taxes based on your 1099 income. Additionally, if you do not have benefits through other employment, you will need to obtain your own health insurance. Finally, some people find setting up their own retirement funds overwhelming, but this is a great benefit of being an independent contractor and cannot be overstated.

Locums physicians are often not considered "part of the group" to which they are contracted. Depending on the internal dynamics of the group, this may lead to you feeling like you are not part of the team. Additionally, the employed physicians in the group often know you are being paid at a higher rate for the same work. However, locums physicians tend to be more flexible and understanding of these dynamics. Presenting yourself as an easygoing team player ready to help the group can often put these issues to rest. An enjoyable work environment can be achieved through consistency and flexibility. If the group likes you enough, they may even ask to hire you directly or extend your locums contract.

Locums contracts can be very unpredictable depending on the needs of the group that hired you. Your contract could be for only weeks or may last years. For instance, if a group has a physician out for health reasons, they may look to the locums market to fill their staffing needs until the physician returns to work. This variability can make locums work frustrating as your longevity at a location is unpredictable. Good communication between your locums company and the contracting company can help avoid much of this frustration. Additionally, talking with the group members about their needs can open the door to allowing you to pick up extra shifts or stay on a contract longer.

Finally, you may find that a particular location and group are very attractive to you. If the group wants to hire you, they will need to "buy" out your contract. Each locums company contract will have a clause regarding buyout. This means that the hiring group will have to pay the locums company a finder's fee, sometimes around $20,000. Unfortunately, this might mean you lose on getting a $20,000 sign-on bonus, but if the group and location are appealing enough to you, this benefit may outweigh the loss. Be careful about violating your locums contract. Communicate with your locums group about this option.

Personally, I have worked with many variations of locums. Upon graduating from residency, I worked directly with local groups without a locums company, negotiating my own pay rate and schedule. Later, I started using a locums company for locations with which I did not have a direct connection. Each of these positions has been in addition to my main employment as a W-2 physician. This has allowed me to pay off debts, travel, and bolster retirement funds at a faster pace.

Locums tenens has many benefits and few drawbacks. A flexible lifestyle and higher pay are among the top benefits. Locums work can be a primary or supplemental source of income. Either way, locums can be a great career path for the emergency medicine physician at any stage in their career.

Part VI
Critical Skills in Emergency Medicine

Chapter 61
Leadership, Teamwork, and Communication During a Busy Shift

Michael J. Burla

Leadership in the Department

Leadership comes in many forms. Stereotypically, leadership is viewed as a singular individual, with the responsibility to direct others. Or at least this is how it is often portrayed in movies and television series. However, in the clinical setting, I believe leadership is more of a practice. What I mean by this is leadership is more of how an individual (or many individuals) acts (act), as opposed to what their title is. With leadership actions, an individual can influence others to accomplish a common objective. In medicine, the common objective is often to treat the patient. This concept is simple enough; however in the emergency department, there are many barriers and moving parts that may interfere with patient care. These barriers can come in the form of lack of staffing, lack of bed availability, lack of coordination between physician and nursing tasks, or even lack of training from ancillary staff. Within this environment, there are many stakeholders that are affected by these barriers, such as the physicians, nurses, technicians, secretaries, custodians, and, of course, the patients. For this reason, it is paramount to have someone with the highest level of training guide patient care. As an emergency medicine physician, you have the highest level of training in the emergency department.

Just like an old-school 1990s video game, medicine can be like venturing into an unforgiving abyss, especially when, as emergency medicine physicians, we receive undifferentiated patients and are expected to act on limited information. In life-or-death situations, we have to think quickly, and everyone involved in the patient care needs to trust our decisions, just as we need to be able to trust our staff to fulfill the

M. J. Burla (✉)
Department of Emergency Medicine, Southern Maine Health Care, MaineHealth, Tufts School of Medicine, Biddeford, ME, USA
e-mail: Michael.burla@mainehealth.org

R. P. Olympia et al. (eds.), *An Emergency Physician's Path*,
https://doi.org/10.1007/978-3-031-47873-4_61

appropriate tasks. *These types of chaotic scenarios are usually compounded during a busy shift.* This can be a humbling experience, especially when things don't go the way we planned, such as when the patient comes in walky-talky and then the next thing we know he or she is coding. During these situations it is important to keep a level head and resort back to your training.

From my experience, this means leading by example—demonstrating respect to all individuals you come into contact with on a shift and leaving your ego at the door, making sure before the shift starts that you have an idea of how to approach difficult cases that might present themselves. If a stressful situation presents itself, taking a deep breath and walking through the case in your head before acting goes a long way. This can help you maintain poise and confidence, which will garner trust from your staff. Over time this confidence will be embodied with how you present yourself, how you speak to the patient and their family members, and how you treat fellow staff. At the end of the day, your staff members are going to be looking to you (consciously or not) on how to present themselves.

There are myriad leadership training courses out there. If one is interested in this, a great place to start is exploring our national interest groups. The American College of Emergency Physicians (ACEP) has a program dedicated to leadership development [1], and the American Academy of Emergency Medicine has a leadership academy [2]. These resources are geared more toward leadership skills within interest groups or outside the department; however they still can be valuable when approaching to the concept of fostering communication and teamwork. Developing effective communication and teamwork are the pillars of successful leadership, and having a philosophy or technique to approach this development can be vital.

Teamwork

Our next topic is developing and maintaining teamwork. Teamwork is achieved by everyone taking ownership in the task at hand. In the emergency department, this translates to everyone knowing their role when taking care of the patient. There are many examples in the current literature describing how to approach teamwork training [3–6]. Most departments have policies in place outlining the roles of individuals. Sometimes the technicians are responsible for splitting, sometimes students, etc. For stressful or high acuity patients, it is important to be able to have a plan ahead of time, so everyone knows their roles before the patient even hits the door.

A good example of this is applying the TeamSTEPPS concept in a trauma setting [6]. TeamSTEPPS has four learnable skills: communication, leadership, situation monitoring, and mutual support (as illustrated in Fig. 61.1). Within these principles, a team structure needs to be created to understand individuals' roles (performance), develop mutual trust (attitudes), and have a shared mentality (knowledge). For a trauma, the team leader can identify who will be managing the airway, who will be pushing the medications, and who will be monitoring the patient. Communication during these interactions is key, and there are many communication techniques that

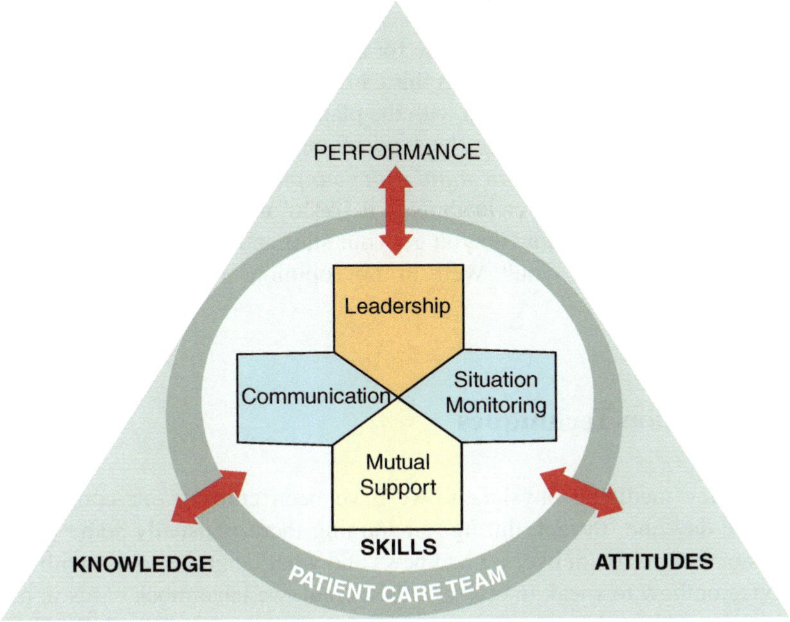

Fig. 61.1 TeamSTEPPS' four learnable skills. https://www.ahrq.gov/teamstepps/instructor/essentials/pocketguide.html#frame

are described in TeamSTEPPS [7]. However, one technique that is easily translatable to other aspects of patient care is closed-loop communication.

Using closed-loop communication can ensure that information conveyed by the sender is understood by the receiver. An example of this is a physician giving a verbal order of "4 mg of morphine" and the nursing staff repeating "4 mg of morphine" back so the physician can verify the order and say "yes, that is correct." Closed-loop communication has been demonstrated to improve speed and efficiency even in difficult situations, such as pediatric traumas [3]. Other aspects of effective teamwork revolve around simple things like being on the same page with patient care.

For me, this means going over the plan with the nurse right at the beginning of an encounter and making sure they are in alignment. Just like setting up patient expectations at the beginning of the encounter, I like to set up nursing expectations as well. For example, a patient with known IV drug abuse might present with back pain. In general, this patient presents often to your emergency department seeking pain medication. This history may predispose the nurse to not take the patient's pain seriously, and be reluctant in general to empathize with the patient. However, when you examine the patient, you realize they have some radicular pain down their left leg and even some objective weakness. At this point you are concerned about an epidural abscess; however if you don't relay this information to the nurse initially, when you order blood work, antibiotics, and even an MRI of the back, the nurse might balk. If you are able to catch the nurse beforehand and explain the plan and the reasoning, he or she will be more likely to buy in and not resent the patient or your plan. Finding the nurse every time for every encounter might be difficult on a busy shift; however for select patients this can save you time in the long run. This is because if the nurse is not on board with the plan, you may face roadblocks later on in the encounter if the nurse comes back questioning orders or medications.

In order for the nurse to get on board with your plan, it starts with trust. As stated earlier in this chapter, effective leadership is based on trust. The same can be said with effective teamwork. How do you get your staff and others you interact with in the department to trust you? Well in my opinion, it starts with successful communication.

Communication Techniques

As emergency medicine physicians, we have been crafting our communication skills since day one. In fact, during our training there is usually some portion of didactics or lectures on delivering bad news and what language to use with patients and advice on how to speak to consultants. In fact, we have mock cases in training and even an oral board exam to test some of these communication skills. However, there aren't always resources out there on how to communicate overall during a busy shift. For these situations, it is important to have a few tricks of the trade to help drive patient care—whether that is improving efficiency with discussing the case with nursing staff or speaking to a difficult consultant. Nevertheless, it is important to review the current techniques out there for certain situations.

For instance, the SPIKES protocol was developed to help deliver bad news [8], such as cancer or the death of a loved one. The SPIKES protocol is a six-step process, which outlines how to approach these difficult situations.

S—set up. This means planning ahead and knowing all the details of the case, making sure you have a private setting to deliver the news to the patient and everyone he or she might want to be present.

P—perception. Ask open-ended questions to assess the patient's current knowledge before explaining anything. This way you can tailor the news to the patient's understanding.

I—invitation of the patient's desire. Figure out how much information the patient would like to know about the diagnosis and prognosis.

K—knowledge. Inform the patient about what knowledge you have on the disease, and use plain language to convey your message, taking caution to avoid medical jargon.

E—empathy. Make sure to express empathy to the patient or loved ones, validating their emotions and any concerns they may have.

S—strategy. Talk to the patient and/or loved ones about the next steps in care or expectations.

I have found that variations of this technique can be applied to communication in situations other than delivering bad news. A good example of this is when speaking to a consultant. It is important to set up the conversation to make sure you have all the information you would need (and nothing more) when speaking to a consultant. Make sure you already have a plan, usually an "A" or "B" strategy that you would like their opinion on. Assess the consultant's perception on your plan, and invite them to ask for more information or insight as needed. Having a strategy when speaking to consultants and being direct will help streamline the process and save time during a busy shift.

For instance, when speaking to a consultant, you have to remember that they generally only think in their silo of specialization. Orthopedics focuses on bones, and cardiology focuses on the heart, and so on and so forth. For most consultants, if all you have is a hammer, everything looks like a nail. Meaning, it is important to keep the discussion straightforward and only keep the pertinent information for the consultant at hand. So if you are calling the orthopedic surgery, try to only talk about the bones. Don't get into the weeds about the patient's complicated past medical history, as it may distract them from the question you have for them. Again, this concept can be applied to other aspects of communication within the department. Being direct with nursing staff and leaving out information that might derail the conversation is just another piece of the puzzle to being efficient on a busy shift. The more puzzle pieces you can put together on shift to streamline patient care, the more effective you will be as an emergency physician.

Overall, it takes time to learn what works best for you and your team during a busy shift. It takes trial and error to know what your staff responds to from a leadership and communication standpoint. Once you have gotten into a rhythm in your department, with your staff, colleagues, and consultants, then you can truly thrive during a busy shift.

References

1. ACEP. Leadership development program. https://www.acep.org/how-we-serve/chapter-services/leadership-development/chapter-leadership-development/.
2. AAEM. Leadership academy. https://www.aaem.org/about-us/leadership/leadership-academy.
3. El-Shafy IA, et al. Closed-loop communication improves task completion in pediatric trauma resuscitation. J Surg Educ. 2018;75(1):58–64.
4. Hamm B, Pozuelo L, Brendel R. General hospital agitation management: leadership theory and health care team best practices using TeamSTEPPS. J Acad Consult Liaison Psychiatry. 2022;63(3):213–24.
5. Alsabri M, et al. Impact of teamwork and communication training interventions on safety culture and patient safety in emergency departments: a systematic review. J Patient Saf. 2022;18(1):e351–61.
6. Capella J, et al. Teamwork training improves the clinical care of trauma patients. J Surg Educ. 2010;67(6):439–43.
7. Agency for Healthcare Research and Quality. TeamSTEPPS. https://www.ahrq.gov/teamstepps/index.html.
8. Baile WF, et al. SPIKES—a six-step protocol for delivering bad news: application to the patient with cancer. Oncologist. 2000;5(4):302–11.

Chapter 62
Multitasking and Rapid Task Switching

Theresa Forty and Jeremy Webb

I remember my first day as a rotating medical student in the emergency department and how it felt as if I was stepping into another world. No longer was I plodding away on highly structured inpatient rounds, seeing patients I had known about, thought about, and presented on for days. Now I found myself in the mix!

Trauma patients rolling through the ambulance bay doors
ECGs shoved in your face with "STEMI" scrolled across the top.
"This guy isn't breathing over here. Can we get some help?!"
Children crying. Patients screaming.
"You have a call from surgery on line 3!"
"Can you set up for a sedation in bay 10?"
"I need that paracentesis done yesterday. We need a dispo!"

It was chaotic.

But it was the sage attending who stood among this cacophony and was somehow able to conquer anything and everything…seemingly all at once. "How do they do it? Can I do it?" I wondered.

Emergency medicine is a specialty with time-sensitive demands requiring rapid inventory and action. It is what drew most of us who practice EM to the field. It is also why this field of medicine remains so challenging yet so fulfilling when we can navigate a busy shift with success. Knowing how to manage multiple inputs of information, organize them, triage our responses, pivot to the next set of to-dos, and do it all in a patient-centered, safe way is what our role is all about.

T. Forty · J. Webb (✉)
Department of Emergency Medicine, LewisGale Medical Center, Salem, VA, USA
e-mail: theresa.forty@hcahealthcare.com; jeremy.webb@hcahealthcare.com

R. P. Olympia et al. (eds.), *An Emergency Physician's Path*,
https://doi.org/10.1007/978-3-031-47873-4_62

Multitasking Vs. Rapid Task Switching. Can You Juggle?

You may have heard at some point "to be good at Emergency Medicine, you need to be good at multitasking." Just look at the example above. Every shift, emergency physicians deal with many unscheduled tasks among frequent interruptions and breaks in flow. The two major ways our minds deal with this deluge are by multitasking and rapid task switching.

Multitasking involves parallel processing and performance of tasks. Rapid task switching, on the other hand, is the ability to move quickly, in series, from one task to the next. Both are complex processes that require access to our working memory (both short- and long-term memory) [1]. They involve split-second attention focusing, inhibition of distracting inputs, maintenance and update of information based on the current environment and previous task outcome, current task integration, and ultimately unification to create new memory that we can then use to tackle the next task at hand [2]. Whew! That's a lot.

Now think about doing that same string of functions for *two* or *more* tasks at the *same* time. One begins to wonder if there is such a thing as multitasking in the first place. Sure, I can chew gum and walk at the same time. I can even pat my head and rub my belly! But can the astute physician really place orders and effectively listen to an update about a patient at the same time? Can I perform synchronized elderly ECG interpretation and pediatric medication order input? Probably not. When presented with two complex, high functioning tasks at the same moment, it is near impossible to do them simultaneously.

Most of the time, when we think we are multitasking, we are more than likely task switching. To the untrained eye, it can seem as though items are being performed simultaneously because the rate of switching can be so rapid. In reality, the mind is juggling its focus from one task to another. But how well can this be done? How efficiently? How accurately? Can I keep all the balls in the air?

The Dangers of Interruptions and Task Breaks

A landmark study found EM physicians may be interrupted up to 31 times every 180 min [3]. That's almost 100 interruptions in a 9-h shift! The cherry on top is that interruptions tend to accumulate with your level of training as workload and managed patient volume increase.

These interruptions may be externally or internally driven and come in many different flavors:

- Messaging/phone calls
- ECG delivery for interpretation
- Nurse questions

- Patient questions
- Resident and/or medical student presentations
- Sudden changes in a patient's acuity level
- New patients presenting to triage/EMS entry
- Electronic health record pop-up screens
- Radio medical command needs
- Procedures that need to be performed
- I could keep going…on and on…forever…

The issue doesn't revolve around the interruption itself, but more so the break in task it produces. Humans have evolved to be monotask oriented. When we have to break one task in order to rapidly switch to another, that can produce errors. We may not return to the initial task we were performing when interrupted. We may also leave out a key step in a procedural task that could lead to error or partial completion. Literature shows that these interruptions directly correlate with physician error. One study among 28 emergency physicians revealed 239 medication orders which contained 208 prescribing errors directly related to rates of interruption and task switching [4]. In our already demanding field, these errors may be serious and potentially life-threatening for the patients we treat. Internal drivers such as emotion, stress, and sleep deprivation only exacerbate the problem.

There is also a time cost to task breaking. It may be just a few seconds or a couple of minutes to stop one task completely, get your head wrapped around the implications of a new task, plan it, and finally start it, but these costs add up. Over a 9–12-h shift, these breaks in action may lead to delays and decreased productivity if not diligent.

Ah, to Be Young Again! Or Not?

There is also the impact of age on the working memory's ability to handle these hurdles. More than once I've heard from my more senior colleagues, "Just wait until you get to be my age. It doesn't get any easier." It has been shown that as we age, we perform worse on working memory-related tasks [2]. So, there may be some truth in my colleague's statement. However, aging isn't all bad. As physicians become more seasoned in their careers, they are presented with similar tasks the mind has sorted through time and time again. The same procedures, the same diagnoses, similar conversations, similar consultations…I have also heard those same colleagues above say "I could do that with my eyes closed." And they probably aren't lying. With experience, certain tasks require less thought to be acted on. Relying on long-term memory for rote performance of tasks may be a sort of "cruise control" where neurons are freed up to process new inputs or even perform a second simple task simultaneously.

Strategies for Success

During my intern year in residency, I remember my senior resident approaching to run my list of active patients with me. At the time, I was beyond overwhelmed. I was multi-failing instead of multitasking. "I don't know if I can ever do this! Maybe I should just run away right now…" Negative thought was sending me into a tailspin. But she was able to stop the downward spiral and stabilize my course. She had clearly translated my body language which was inextricably linked to my internal panic. "Who is your sickest patient? What do you need to do next for them? Look at your stable patients by length of stay. Who can you disposition next? What procedures do you still need to do?"

There it was.

Order.

Now I could calmly and clearly see how to proceed. That was years ago, and I still remember how things could be turned around so quickly. I am not perfect. None of us are. But just like the ABCs in resuscitation, there are safety nets to fall back on when you feel control slipping from your grasp. Here are some strategies you may find useful to deal with the inevitable waves of task breaks and interruptions while avoiding errors and saving your sanity.

1. **Delay when reasonable, but don't forget.**
   - Defer less acute tasks to a later time.
   - However, you must set a reminder (set a stopwatch, ask a nurse, use a sticky note, etc.).
2. **Recognize tasks where an interruption may cause significant harm.**
   - Examples include medication dosing, invasive procedures, immediate care of a severely ill patient, and shift sign-out.
   - Use checklists. Standardized forms to complete "time-out" before procedures and sign-out protocol between shifts (i.e., SBAR) are readily available. These tools help to refocus on important and error-prone tasks at hand [5].
   - If interrupted, complete medication orders before moving on to the competing task if able.
3. **Increase use of long-term memory. Give yourself a cognitive buffer.**
   - Engage in deliberate practice: Regularly participate in simulation/procedural training if available.
   - Mentally prepare for rare procedures: Perform steps in your mind and map out supplies/staff needed for later recall.
   - Simplify multistep tasks into algorithmic concepts (i.e., ACLS) or mnemonics that may be quickly accessed by the brain later.
4. **Delegate.**
   - Cognitively off-load by sharing tasks with other team members. You can't do everything at once. By delegating, you will decrease the number of tasks to

which you would naturally try to switch. This gives you extra time and energy to devote to the most important task at hand. For example, in a busy medical resuscitation or cardiac arrest, you may entrust airway and procedures to a resident or colleague and assign a nurse to run medication timing/dosing while you investigate reversible causes of arrest.

5. **Use closed-loop communication.**
   - Verbal orders on the fly during a break in task may not be the safest method and can be misinterpreted. Closed-loop communication lets everybody hear the plan twice. If a mistake is made by one party, there is a greater chance it will be picked up by another and pointed out.
6. **Circle back at scheduled intervals.**
   - Continually reassess the overall picture. Try this once every hour while on shift. Focus on immediate needs and actionable items. Use these windows to re-triage your to-do list if necessary.
7. **Write it down.**
   - Give your mind one less thing to do, not another task by trying to remember what you were going to do after signing that ECG or what your plan was for that patient you saw 2 h ago.
   - Make a list of each patient you see as you see them. That gives you a running idea about each patient's length of stay.
   - Once I see each patient, I quickly jot down what my plan is for each—labs, EKG, CXR, admit. On the same line, I also write the working diagnoses as I discover them—NSTEMI, acute hypoxic respiratory failure, pneumonia. I already know what I'm going to tell the hospitalist when I call for admission.
8. ***Sprint* to the finish.**
   - You may also want to read about the SPRINT curriculum devised to teach EM residents how to handle multiple competing tasks [6]. The SPRINT workflow follows this succession: *s*tabilize critical patients, *p*erform procedures, *r*ack (see new patients in the chart rack or queue), *i*n or out (reassess and disposition), and *t*ype it up (complete charts). It may help you strategize how to tackle certain actions over others, and it was shown to improve resident confidence in task performance and prioritization.
9. **Take time out.**
   - When all else fails, take a couple of minutes to center yourself. Whether it is deep breathing exercises, stretching, or taking time for a snack, do something that can quiet the mind and soothe the body. You will notice how these brief breaks in action can improve your performance and ability to handle the cognitive load.

References

1. Skaugset LM, Farrell S, Carney M, Wolff M, Santen SA, Perry M, Cico SJ. Can you multi-task? Evidence and limitations of task switching and multitasking in emergency medicine. Ann Emerg Med. 2016;68(2):189–95. https://doi.org/10.1016/j.annemergmed.2015.10.003.
2. Chai WJ, Abd Hamid AI, Abdullah JM. Working memory from the psychological and neurosciences perspectives: a review. Front Psychol. 2018;9:401. https://doi.org/10.3389/fpsyg.2018.00401.
3. Chisholm CD, Collison EK, Nelson DR, Cordell WH. Emergency department workplace interruptions: are emergency physicians "interrupt-driven" and "multitasking"? Acad Emerg Med. 2000;7(11):1239–43. https://doi.org/10.1111/j.1553-2712.2000.tb00469.x.
4. Westbrook JI, Raban MZ, Walter SR, Douglas H. Task errors by emergency physicians are associated with interruptions, multitasking, fatigue and working memory capacity: a prospective, direct observation study. BMJ Qual Saf. 2018;27(8):655–63. https://doi.org/10.1136/bmjqs-2017-007333.
5. Buljac-Samardzic M, Doekhie KD, van Wijngaarden JDH. Interventions to improve team effectiveness within health care: a systematic review of the past decade. Hum Resour Health. 2020;18(1):2. https://doi.org/10.1186/s12960-019-0411-3.
6. Todd BR, Traylor S, Heron L, Turner-Lawrence D. SPRINT through tasks: a novel curriculum for improving resident task management in the emergency department. MedEdPORTAL. 2020;16:10956. https://doi.org/10.15766/mep_2374-8265.10956.

Chapter 63
Successful Patient Handoffs

Rachel Patterson and Holly Stankewicz

Introduction

Transfer of care in the Emergency Department (ED) is one of the riskiest times for both the patient and the physician. It is during this transition between physicians, EMS providers, and nursing staff that all critical information regarding the patient must be communicated to the oncoming treatment team clearly and concisely. Emergency physicians work in an environment prone to various distractions and interruptions, creating inherent barriers to effective communication and increasing the risk of poor patient handoff.

Several potential factors may contribute to poor sign-outs. Some common sources of distraction include the ever-constant noise of alarms, staff, and patients intrinsic to the ED environment. The lack of an organized system for patient handoff also introduces errors via various methods. For example, the relaying of incomplete or incorrect information, disorganized or confusing discussions, failure to provide a clear clinical impression and plan, and inattention or distraction of the recipient of information limit effective listening [1]. Handoffs between specialists and ED personnel have an additional layer of ambiguity stemming from their different perspectives of what is important [2].

Most of us can appreciate that there are shifts where sign-out is difficult for a variety of reasons—whether it is fatigue from working several shifts, a busy department, patients that have been in the department for prolonged periods, social issues affecting dispositions, or uncooperative patients that require our attention. It can be a struggle to follow up on sign-out details when you are seeing your new patients as

R. Patterson (✉) · H. Stankewicz
St. Luke's Bethlehem, Bethlehem, PA, USA
e-mail: Rachel.patterson@sluhn.org; Holly.stankewicz@sluhn.org

R. P. Olympia et al. (eds.), *An Emergency Physician's Path*,
https://doi.org/10.1007/978-3-031-47873-4_63

well, some of which may have their own critical care needs. The following help to identify what makes a good patient handoff and the tools we can utilize to improve communication between physicians.

What Defines an Effective Sign-Out?

We will define sign-out or patient handoff as a transition of patient care and use the terms interchangeably. A transition, as defined in nonmedical realms, occurs when two or more workers exchange mission-specific information, responsibility, and authority for an operation [1, 3]. This transition is when there is a potential source of errors. In medicine, this is true as well and when errors occur, communication errors are deemed to be the root cause in about 70% of cases [1]. Faulty handoffs are specifically implicated in up to 24% of malpractice claims in the ED with communication breakdowns accounting for nearly 80% of medicolegal cases [3]. Due to these issues, in 2006, The Joint Commission recommended patient safety goals to "implement a standardized approach to 'handoff' communications, including an opportunity to ask and respond to questions during the handoff process" [1] with the goal identified by a safe, patient-centered, timely, effective, efficient, and equitable health care [4, 5].

Components of a Strong Sign-Out/Patient Handoff

Perhaps the most important issue with sign-out is ensuring both physicians are paying attention and able to listen to and process what the other physician is saying. The Emergency Department is full of people, alarms, questions, phone calls, etc., but sign-out should be a protected time when the physicians can discuss patient care without distractions.

Previous studies have identified at least four phases of handoffs. These include the pre-turner, arrival, meeting, and post-turnover periods. During these times, the departing physician must gather all pertinent patient information in an organized manner to give to the oncoming physician and then succinctly relay this information for the new physician to take responsibility [1, 3]. When broken down into these stages, one can see how critical all elements of sign-out are to ensure a safe patient transfer.

One of the most common forms of handoffs is a simple narrative of the patient. Here, the physicians have a verbal exchange of pertinent information regarding the patient(s) being handed over. This narrative may be written down on paper, via the Electronic Medical Record (EMR), or simply as a verbal transfer of information.

It is essential that the physician signing out is organized and gives a clear report, including a brief, pertinent history, pending results, code status, disposition plan, and potential issues. Additional information such as primary care physicians or what the admitting service should be is also helpful. If a patient is critically ill, code status is also important to be verified and documented at this time. The physician signing out must ensure that they are signing out every patient they are responsible for at the time of sign-out, regardless of whether or not they were the original physician. Every patient in the Emergency Department must have an attending physician responsible for their care.

Common Problems Identified at End of Shift Handoff

Emergency physicians need to be aware of the multiple potential barriers that exist and may affect the efficiency and accuracy of the sign-out process from the noisy environment, time constraints, frequent interruptions, and communication differences. Overcoming some of these obstacles is possible by creating a space free of most distractions during the handoff process. Given the unpredictability of the Emergency Department, this is not always possible. Still, by creating a quiet space and announcing to others that patient handoff is occurring, we can attempt to limit the environmental distractions and interruptions [6].

Communication styles between different types of medical professionals or specialties are a common barrier in the Emergency Department. This likely stems from differences in training and what is deemed most important at the time of patient handoff. We need to recognize that these barriers exist at the time of patient handoff and that certain physicians may place significance on different components of the medical history, treatment, and plan of care.

Boarding or holding patients has also become an issue in Emergency Departments. Some departments will have patients boarding in the ED for prolonged periods. If the patients have been seen by their admitting service and admission orders have been written, those admitting physicians are technically responsible for their care. However, if there are critical issues with these patients or a potential need for emergency interventions, the oncoming physician should be made aware of these patients. For that reason, the argument can be made that all patients, even those already admitted, should be signed out. Some studies suggest that having an inpatient medical provider responsible for the acute care needs of the boarding patient would help to facilitate the patient's care while not overburdening the emergency physicians and staff [5].

In academic Emergency Departments, the resident physician and the attending physician may sign out at different times. If that is the case, they should agree on their sign-out plans before shift change. Staggered sign-out times may be both an advantage and a detriment since group sign-outs ensure that everyone is in agreement and any ambiguity between physicians is clarified. However, staggered sign-out makes it potentially possible for at least one provider to have continuous care of the patient while in the Emergency Department. Many community settings do not have the staffing resources or residents to aid in the workload. Some institutions will therefore build time into the shift to allow for the completion of work, limiting the need for excessive sign-outs.

Tools to Improve Transition of Care Between Providers

Many tools have been employed to help standardize handoffs, but there has yet to be a consensus on any single system for a structured handoff. For example, we could not find a study that showed clear superiority between bedside rounds, written, and EMR. However, most studies do suggest that regardless of the method employed, the top five rated handoff elements were patient identification, brief history, clinical stability, working diagnosis, and consulting services involved [7]. Utilizing a structured approach to sign-out between members of your team or interdisciplinary teams will create a safer and more efficient method for communication of the most critical patient information.

SBAR stands for *s*ituation, *b*ackground, *a*ssessment, and *r*ecommendations. SBAR is a highly published and cited tool utilized by medical personnel to communicate patient information to various other healthcare team members. It is approved by The Joint Commission and was initially created and implemented by the US Navy. It was first utilized in hospitals by Kaiser in the early 2000s to have more effective and precise communication between physicians and nurses [5, 6]. The SBAR system, however, has since been implemented in many specialties and has been shown to improve the effective communication of critical patient information promptly. SBAR may not be as useful in the Emergency Department because our goal is to relay the most important information succinctly. SBAR may add extra information and does not specifically address important information such as code status, potential issues, etc [8].

I-PASS stands for illness severity (I), patient summary (P), action list (A), situational awareness and contingency plans (S), and synthesis by the receiver (S). I-PASS is another mnemonic that has been validated for use during the physician handoff period and can be easily incorporated into the EMR creating a more easily shared format of sign-out. Therefore, this helps the departing and oncoming treatment teams to have a shared picture of the patient, potentially reducing errors through increased verbal and written communication [9]. I-PASS may be more applicable to the Emergency Department sign-out unless the provider is unclear on what should be in each section as they are somewhat vague.

Another possible tool is a sign-out checklist. In one study, investigators developed a sign-out checklist that included patient diagnoses, patient care tasks to do, patient disposition, admission team, and patient code status [8, 10]. The standardized checklist was shown to improve Emergency Medicine residents' sign-out at the end of their shifts by increasing the frequency of discussion of the critical tasks remaining for patient care and disposition status. Additionally, it improved the subjective assessment of the quality of sign-out [10]. This is a simpler form of organized sign-out and may help streamline the overall sign-out process.

While it may be difficult to mandate the use of a formal sign-out procedure in an Emergency Department, a formal process may ultimately make sign-out safer and easier. Departments could make their own specific procedure, whether that is a checklist or something more formal such as a template sign-out note in the EMR. Some sort of standardization of the process may be beneficial and help providers avoid missing important details for patient care and safety.

A Case

Let's look at a sample case.

The outgoing physician is in a rush to sign out and has a few patients who are still active. During sign-out there are several interruptions. One of the patients that is signed out is a 70-year-old male who came in with chest pain and has labs pending but will likely need admission. No other information was given, no history or code status, and no medication history. Soon after the outgoing physician left, the oncoming physician is called to the room for a patient in distress. The patient is found in the room with agonal respirations and the patient is not on the monitor. The patient then loses pulses and CPR is started. The patient has only one peripheral IV and is noted to have a fistula in his right upper extremity that the oncoming physician assumes is for dialysis. During the code, the nurse shows the physician the original EKG that has what looks like peaked T waves, and she explains that the patient and his family had reported that he missed dialysis this week. The labs that had been drawn earlier revealed critically high potassium. The patient is then given the appropriate medications and a return of spontaneous circulation is achieved. However, due to the prolonged downtime, the patient does not ever return to his baseline neurologic status and requires placement in a long-term care facility. In addition, the family is upset because they and the patient had made it clear to the original physician that the patient did not want CPR or intubation.

This case highlights how communication at sign-out was lost between the outgoing and oncoming care teams. But there are ways to prevent this from happening. Let's take this example and see what happens when the physicians involved implemented one of our aforementioned methods for sign-out. The physicians sit in a designated area of the Emergency Department away from patient rooms and have informed staff that they are doing sign-out. The outgoing physician has prepared for sign-out with a written checklist for each active patient, including a 70-year-old male with a history of end-stage renal disease who missed dialysis this week and came in with chest pain. Labs are pending and the EKG did have some possible peaked T waves, so there is a concern for hyperkalemia, and treatment including albuterol and insulin was given while awaiting official lab results. Because of this, follow-up on potentially critical labs, especially electrolytes, is necessary. The patient has a living will and is DNR/DNI. The family is in the room and aware of the current plan and likely need for admission. The family doctor is Dr. Primary Care and his nephrologist is Dr. Kidney. When the patient decompensates after sign-out, the oncoming physician is more prepared and the patient is treated for hyperkalemia immediately resulting in a better outcome.

Countless examples could be given to help show how effective sign-out will result in safer and better patient care. Patients being treated for psychiatric complaints in the Emergency Department are another example of patients who may benefit from better sign-outs, especially those with other comorbid diseases. As these patients don't have another inpatient physician assigned, they are the responsibility of the emergency physician, and those on chronic medication at home will likely need medications if they are in the ED for prolonged periods. For example, a patient with epilepsy in the Emergency Department for suicidal ideation awaiting placement could start to seize in the department. If the patient was signed out appropriately, the oncoming physician would be more prepared to treat the patient quickly and appropriately.

Conclusion

The process of patient sign-out is a high-risk period. However, if the department can implement a standardized process, including ensuring that the physicians have a private space and a template of critical information necessary for patient care, the process would improve safety and efficiency.

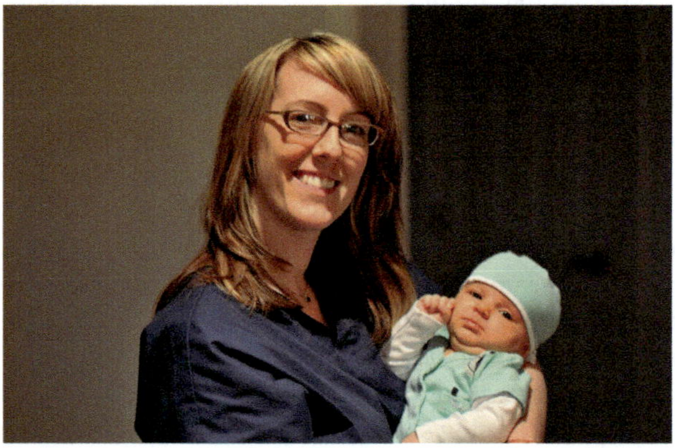

Holly Stankewicz, DO, going back for her first shift after having her first child.

References

1. Committee on the Quality of Health Care in America, Institute of Medicine. To err is human: building a safer health system. Washington, DC: National Academies Press; 2000.
2. Pound A. Effective and safe patient handoffs. Tews M, editor. https://www.saem.org/about-saem/academies-interest-groups-affiliates2/cdem/for-students/online-education/m3-curriculum/communication/effective-and-safe-patient-hand-offs.

3. Cheung DS, Kelly JJ, Beach C. Improving handoffs in the emergency department. Ann Emerg Med. 2010;55(2):171–80.
4. Lardner R. Effective shift handover: a literature review. Offshore Technology Report-OTO 96 003. Health and Safety Executive, 1996.
5. Meisel ZF, Shea JA, Peacock NJ, Dickinson ET, Paciotti B, Bhatia R, Buharin E, Cannuscio CC. Optimizing the patient handoff between emergency medical services and the emergency department. Ann Emerg Med. 2015;65(3):310–317.e1.
6. Shahid S, Thomas S. Situation, Background, Assessment, Recommendation (SBAR) communication tool for handoff in health care—a narrative review. Saf Health. 2018;4:7. https://doi.org/10.1186/s40886-018-0073-1.
7. Alrajhi K, Alsaawi A. Developing an emergency medicine handoff tool: an electronic Delphi approach. Int J Emerg Med. 2019;12:37. https://doi.org/10.1186/s12245-019-0249-4.
8. Bornemann-Shepherd M, Le-Lazar J, Makic MB, DeVine D, McDevitt K, Paul M. Caring for inpatient boarders in the emergency department: improving safety and patient and staff satisfaction. J Emerg Nurs. 2015;41(1):23–9. https://doi.org/10.1016/j.jen.2014.04.012.
9. Blazin LJ, Sitthi-Amorn J, Hoffman JM, Burlison JD. Improving patient handoffs and transitions through adaptation and implementation of I-PASS across multiple handoff settings. Pediatr Qual Saf. 2020;5(4):e323. https://doi.org/10.1097/pq9.0000000000000323.
10. Milano A, Stankewicz H, Stoltzfus J, Salen P. The impact of a standardized checklist on transition of care during emergency department resident physician change of shift. West J Emerg Med. 2019;20(1):29–34. https://doi.org/10.5811/westjem.2018.10.39020.

Chapter 64
Dealing with Difficult Patients and Their Families

Joan Naidorf

Our Instruction Guide for Good Patients

To understand how some patients are judged as difficult, it helps to understand how we decide which patients are good [1]. Most doctors would describe their ideal patients as mature and self-sufficient individuals who are logical and rational in their thinking. They value the good advice and counsel of the physician and make every attempt to comply with the recommended plan.

"Good patients are actually people who reflect what the physician views in him or herself" as desirable characteristics. Many of the traits that physicians judge as most desirable often include shared language and cultural values. Treatment of these patients leads to congenial, effective, and mutually rewarding interactions" [2, p. 10].

When patients or their families do not follow the plan or make the path very hard, they get labelled as difficult. These are some common categories of patients that the ED staff label as difficult:

1. Psychiatric patients—don't follow logical thought patterns and act out
2. Poor compliers—don't take medications or follow up with consultants
3. Dying patients—frequently end of life wishes that have not been discussed or documented
4. Private patients—may want to wait for their own doctors or have their own physician direct care
5. Substance abusers—return frequently with withdrawal, overdoses, and related infections
6. Hostile, abusive patients—demanding people who disrupt the department

J. Naidorf (✉)
Alexandria, VA, USA

R. P. Olympia et al. (eds.), *An Emergency Physician's Path*,
https://doi.org/10.1007/978-3-031-47873-4_64

7. Demanding caregivers/parents—strong opinions held in opposition to the physician's plan
8. Chronic medical patients—often seeking short-term fixes for long-term problems
9. Poor historians—can include non-English speakers, negate diagnostic clues gained from history
10. Patients with inconsistent exams—throw the physician off the right diagnostic trail
11. Non-emergent patients—can divert precious resources from emergent patients
12. Patients with multiple complaints—can cloud the investigation of the most pressing issue
13. Patients dumped by families—inadequate social support and disposition services
14. Covid-19 patients/unvaccinated—can endanger other patients and staff, can cause isolation issues

Fear and Challenges for the Patients

Ill and injured patients have many basic fears underlying their behavior. Basic survival instincts of humans underlie many of these fears. Being part of a tribe or community would increase an individual's chance of survival. Wondering whether they will live or die or sustain permanent injury is understandable. Children and some elderly people will fear strangers and separation from their families.

Good patients must deal with many challenges as they become injured or ill. They are able to maintain emotional balance and can still experience hopefulness and joy during their illness. They can preserve family and social relationships that become strained. "Good" patients can cope with some level of disability and either find ways to get things done or ask for help from family or friends. Uncertainty, painful conditions, and a variety of healthcare personnel can be handled by "good" patients.

Six typical and common behavior patterns are noted in our patients during illness and injury [3].

1. Regression. Regression refers to childlike stages of emotional functioning in response to illness or injury.
2. Denial. Denial can take many forms. It can be an unconscious response to anxiety and help keep worry at bay. One form, suppression, involves pushing the thought of illness out of the mind. Suppression can contribute to better functioning and is considered a relatively healthy psychological defense mechanism. True denial is a deleterious defense mechanism in which the patient contradicts or disbelieves the information or diagnosis received from the physician.
3. Control by Gaining Knowledge. Some individuals have personalities that prompt them to want to control every situation. They believe they can reduce uncertainty and obtain a better outcome by knowing everything there is to know.

4. Anxiety. People may imagine the worst scenarios after a quick internet search of their symptoms and become anxious.
5. Anger. Some chronically ill patients become angry, asking, "Why me?" Healthcare professionals often become easy targets for this displaced anger.
6. Sadness. Sadness is a common reaction to an illness or diagnosis. Extreme sadness can color every aspect of a person's relationship with those around them. Normal sadness allows the anticipation and expectation of pleasurable activities over time. Prolonged sadness with dysphoria may actually be undiagnosed depression, and of course, these patients should be evaluated for major depression and observed for indications of self-harm or suicide.

Medical Literature on Difficult Interactions with Patients

The medical literature on the subject is sparse, but one of the first people to address the issue openly was Dr. James Groves, a psychiatrist on the consultation at Massachusetts General Hospital. In 1978, Groves categorized behavior types that physicians dread in his article, "Taking Care of the Hateful Patient," published as a special article in *The New England Journal of Medicine*.

Dr. Groves wrote, "a few patients kindle aversion, fear, despair and even downright malice in their doctors." In his article, he described his four main classifications of "hateful" patients by their stereotypical personality types and characteristics: dependent clingers, entitled demanders, manipulative help-rejectors, and self-destructive deniers. These are the definitions:

Dependent Clingers—Clingers are excessively needy patients who require endless attention and reassurance. They use flattery and childlike behavior to seduce the physician into giving them constant attention and reassurance.

Entitled Demanders—Entitled demanders resemble clingers in their need for attention, but rather than flattery, they use intimidation, devaluation, threats, and guilt induction to get what they want from the physician.

Manipulative Help-Rejectors—Like clingers and entitled demanders, manipulative help rejectors never seem to get better. They display an endless demand for emotional support from the relationship with the physician.

Self-Destructive Deniers—These people disregard the prescribed treatment regimen or unconsciously engage in self-injurious behaviors such as excessive alcohol, drug, or tobacco use. They take no responsibility for themselves, forcing others to be responsible for them.

For the first time, the emotional responses of the physicians were emphasized and considered during their interactions with their patients. Over the following decades, the role of the physician in mitigating the occasional difficult interactions with patients and their families was recognized. *The Essential Role of Medical Ethics Education in Achieving Professionalism: The Romanell Report* was published in 2015 as part of an analysis of the current state of medical ethics education in the United States, focusing in particular on its essential role in cultivating professionalism among medical learners.

The report proposed a lengthy list of the objectives for medical ethics education. Notable for our discussion regarding "difficult" patients is the statement that "Upon completion of medical school or a residency training program, learners will, with an appropriate level of proficiency…manage challenging patients/family members, including recognition of what the clinician may be contributing to the difficulty" [4].

Common Thought Distortions of Physicians

During our interactions with our patients, we take an extensive history and begin the evaluation of the patient's presenting medical problem. There are some common thought distortions physicians employ.

1. Arbitrary inference—We make assumptions or reach conclusions based on insufficient or incorrect data.
2. All or nothing thinking—We tend to frame solutions in the extremes as if there is only one right answer.
3. Personalization—When we take too much blame or too much credit for what happens when there is no objective reason to do so.
4. Questioning reality—Believing that something that happened should not have happened.
5. Assuming victim mentality—Evading personal responsibility by blaming other people and circumstances for poor outcomes.
6. Mirroring emotions—Mirroring is the behavior in which one person unconsciously imitates the gestures, speech patterns, or attitudes of another person.

Understanding that Thoughts Cause Emotions

Our interactions with challenging patients occur quickly along with many negative emotions. It seems to us that what the patient has said or what the family member has done has caused us to feel frustrated. This is not exactly true. Between the comment or action of the patient and the emotions of the physician, there is a thought. Often the thought goes something like this: He shouldn't have said that or the mom doesn't really know what's best for the baby.

Becoming aware of the actual thoughts that cause our feelings of anger, or frustration, or disappointment can help us put some space between our emotions and any impulsive or dangerous actions. We don't need our patients to change for us to feel better about them. We just need to change the way that we think about them and naturally, we will have better feelings about them (Fig. 64.1).

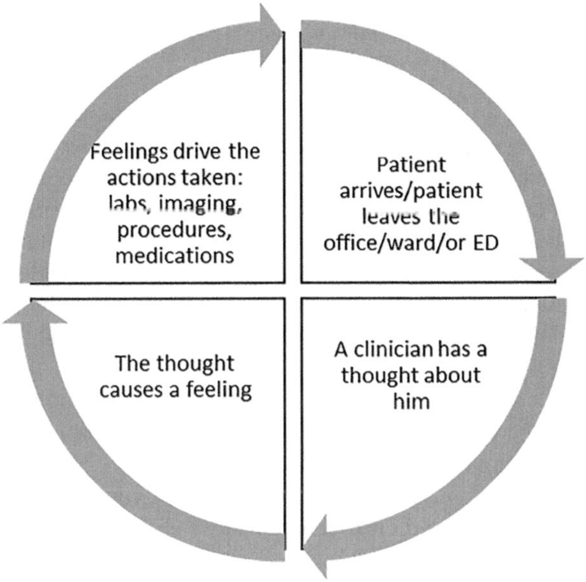

Fig. 64.1 The think-feel-act cycle in the emergency department [2, p. 46]

The arrival of a person as a patient in the ED is a neutral event until a clinician has some thought about the person. Our thoughts cause us to have emotions and those emotions drive our actions or inactions. Our actions in the form of treatments or testing lead to the results we get and whether a person can get discharged or requires admission.

When a patient rejects a plan for admission to treat some diagnosis, your anger may prompt you to have them sign out against medical advice. Many times, signing out against medical advice would not serve either party well. Some common ground or intermediate answer can be found if a physician will admit that their way is not the only way. Of course, one must document in the medical record what the advised course should be.

In a situation of a hostile or aggressive patient, immediate evasive or protective actions need to be taken. One definitive resource is the article "Verbal De-escalation of the Agitated Patient: Consensus Statement of the American Association for Emergency Psychiatry Project BETA De-escalation Workgroup" [5]. The article offers ten domains of de-escalation:

1. Respect personal space.
2. Do not be provocative.
3. Establish verbal contact.
4. Be concise.
5. Identify wants and feelings.
6. Listen closely to what the patient is saying.
7. Agree or agree to disagree.

8. Lay down the law and set clear limits.
9. Offer choices and optimism.
10. Debrief the patient and staff.

How do we change our thoughts about challenging patient interactions?

The negative emotions that physicians have about some of their "difficult" patients should not be ignored just to power through. We just charge through and do difficult things, but giving time to process sadness, grief, disappointment, or guilt will allow the emotions to pass through more quickly. We can intentionally choose thoughts that will lead to feelings of compassion and generosity. We can get to those thoughts by asking questions such as these:

What else is true about this "difficult" person? Are they a mother or someone's son?

Could I be wrong about my approach or solution to this problem?

Where else could a person go to get this problem evaluated? This ED is exactly the setting this person needs.

Can you imagine that the problems of your patients are your own? You can have compassion for their fear and anxiety about some symptom or a diagnosis that they do not yet understand.

Patients who challenge us will never stop coming to the emergency department and we will infrequently get people to change their behavior. The only solution for handling the issue more intelligently is by changing our thoughts about them. They are just people having human emotions in a very chaotic and exciting setting where they are not in control. Nothing has gone wrong here. If we accept them as they are, people with autonomy to disagree and, occasionally, act out, we will feel better about our shifts in the ED.

Our human experience is 50% good and 50% terrible. Some days in the ED feel like the scales are tipped tremendously to the bad side. We have to look hard for the bright spots. The sweet smile one gets from a child who finally feels better near the end of her visit sets up the sweetest contrast, the amazing nurses that we get to work with, the hot coffee that we can enjoy on our break, the amazing welcome you will get from your dog when you walk in the door of your home.

What you think and feel matter as you treat patients in the emergency department. When you feel better emotions, you will get better results. Feeling resentment toward some patients feels terrible and saps the energy out of you. When you come to families with empathy and concern, they will accept bad news from you more graciously. If a patient senses that you care, he will listen to your advice and consider it more closely. It isn't always what you say but it is definitely how you say it.

Quell generosity and kindness will make you feel better and quell feelings of cynicism in a workplace where physicians frequently question themselves. The last piece of dealing with difficult patients has to be our absolute belief in our own abilities and worthiness. You must get to know yourself, to love being in your own company, to want to be with yourself, and to have your own back. You have to be your biggest advocate and support yourself.

You can accept that you are human and humans are imperfect and make mistakes. You are the real deal; you are not an imposter. If you think about the way you want to be and how you want to act, you can love and appreciate yourself. You will not have to look to others for validation. You can accept that some people or patients will not like you. Not everyone will do what we advise. You can feel confident and know that you tried to treat them as you were trained and with the best of your ability. It is your job to think thoughts that get you excited about your job and all your patients, even the ones who don't follow the "good" patient script.

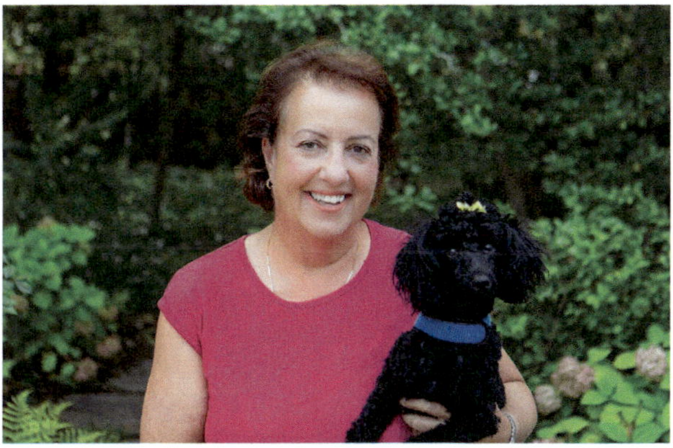

Joan Naidorf and her poodle Dolly photo by Laura Marshall

References

1. Jackson JL, Kroenke K. Difficult patient encounters in the ambulatory clinic: clinical predictors and outcomes. Arch Intern Med. 1999;159:1069–75.
2. Naidorf J. Changing how we think about difficult patients. American Association for Physician Leadership. Washington, DC. 2022.
3. Blumenfield M, Thompson TL. The psychological reaction to physical illness. In: Simons RC, Pardes H, editors. Understanding human behavior in health and illness. 2nd ed. Baltimore: Williams & Wilkins; 1981.
4. Carrese J, Malek J, Watson K, et al. The essential role of medical ethics education in achieving professionalism: the Romanell report. Acad Med. 2015;90(60):744–52.
5. Richmond JS, et al. Verbal de-escalation of the agitated patient: consensus statement of the American Association for Emergency Psychiatry Project BETA De-Escalation Workgroup. West J Emerg Med. 2012;13(1):17–25. https://doi.org/10.5811/westjem.2011.9.68.

Chapter 65
Giving Bad News

Jennifer Maccagnano

The First Time You Give Bad News

Most emergency physicians recall the first time they shared bad news with a patient. As a third year medical student, I was taking care of a patient who presented to the emergency department pregnant with the chief complaint of vaginal bleeding. After reviewing her exam, labs, and ultrasound with the resident and attending physician, we concluded that the most likely diagnosis was a miscarriage. I inquired with the resident if they wanted me to inform the patient of her likely diagnosis. He stated, "sure you can tell her if you feel comfortable." Is anyone ever comfortable giving bad news? Well, I accepted the challenge and reflected on what one of my medical school professors taught me. Prepare your conversation ahead of time, sit down, spend time with the patient (and as a medical student compared to the residents and attendings—I had all the time in the world), and then, listen and provide time for questions.

I walked around our busy ED and reflected on what I would tell this patient and then searched for a stool to sit on and delivered the news. I told the patient that we suspect this is most likely a miscarriage, but further testing was essential. I emphasized the importance of following up in 2 days for a repeat beta-hCG quantitative blood test and ultrasound. I also informed her should the bleeding increase, or should there be severe pain or any other new concerns, to return to the ED immediately. I was surprised how well she took the news. At the end of our conversation, I offered to call someone for her, but she refused any phone calls.

J. Maccagnano (✉)
Division of Emergency Medicine, Department of Clinical Specialties, New York Institute of Technology College of Osteopathic Medicine, Old Westbury, NY, USA
e-mail: jmaccagn@nyit.edu

R. P. Olympia et al. (eds.), *An Emergency Physician's Path*,
https://doi.org/10.1007/978-3-031-47873-4_65

After talking with my patient, I discussed the conversation with my supervising resident, who then checked in on the patient. He told me that I delivered the news well as she had no further questions.

Strategies on How to Give Bad News

When considering how to disrupt the lives of recipients of bad news as they move from their previous world into their new world, there are three common strategies used: forecasting, stalling, and being blunt. Evidence portrays that forecasting appears to be the most effective in delivering life-altering news [1].

Stalling is a strategy where doctors have bad news but avoid sharing it. They skip over the actual news or use analogies or medical jargon which often leads the patient to misinterpret the news. When patients and families suspect a problem and medical professionals stall, people may self-blame for the problem and believe they caused the illness or death [1]. By stalling, patients and families may also speculate (correctly or incorrectly) or deny the severity of their illness, among other reactions. It is impossible for patients to realize the situation when the medical team withholds information, and ultimately this can affect the patient's long term care.

The opposite strategy of being blunt is not the solution either. Bluntness can come as a shock to a patient or family member and can lead to a disorientation or a feeling of being shattered or in disbelief. Bluntness can cause patients and family members to become angry with the physician or ignore the care they need and instead put their efforts on condemning the medical team for their bluntness, which ultimately can have grave consequences for the patient's health [1].

Forecasting serves as an important tool for giving bad news. It indicates to the patient that something bad is coming, and in essence gives them a moment to prepare and anticipate the bad news. There are a few different options to employ forecasting such as non-vocal strategies, vocal preannouncements, prefaces, citing the evidence, and a perspective display sequence [1]. At times, a combination of forecasting strategies may be used depending on the clinical situation and the environment. Some examples include bringing the family into a private room to talk, or telling a patient "It's bad" and then pausing after the preannouncement before giving the diagnosis. Through the perspective display sequence, physicians forecast the bad news and aide patients in grasping the information. With perspective display sequence, the physician initially elicits the patient's view/perspective on the situation; the patient shares their view; and finally, the physician delivers the news [1].

As one is busy navigating the emergency department, it can be helpful to use the ABCDE mnemonic for breaking bad news. The ABCDE mnemonic (see Table 65.1) takes into consideration the strategy of forecasting [2]. Another protocol that can be useful for employing the strategy of forecasting is the BREAKS protocol (see Table 65.2) [2]. There is not one correct way to give bad news, but each memory aide helps physicians prepare to have an empathetic conversation that can be life-altering for their patients.

Table 65.1 ABCDE mnemonic

Advance preparation
What does the patient know/understand already?
Arrange for a support person and appropriate family members
Arrange undisturbed time and place (hand off phones/pagers to colleagues)
Prepare yourself emotionally
Prepare a script
Build a therapeutic environment/relationship
Have a private location without interruptions
Provide adequate seating
Sit close enough to touch, if appropriate
Reassure about pain, suffering, abandonment
Communicate well
Be direct—"I am sorry that I have bad news for you"
Do not use jargon, acronyms
Use words like "cancer," "death" as appropriate
Allow for sitting in silence
Use touch appropriately
Deal with patients and family reactions
Assess patient and family reactions: Physiologic responses, cognitive coping strategies, affective responses
Listen actively
Express empathy
Encourage and validate emotions
Evaluate the news
Address further needs
What are the patient's immediate and near-term plans? Access for suicidality
Make referrals for support as needed
Explore what the news means to the patient

Adapted from Table 65.2 ABCDE mnemonic in Nunn [2]

Table 65.2 BREAKS protocol

B = Background: What led to this moment for the patient?
R = Rapport: Make a connection
E = Explore: Where are they now in their thoughts and feelings?
A = Announce: The bad news
K = Kindling: Draw out the emotional response
S = Summarize: News in a nutshell

Adapted from Table 65.3 BREAKS protocol in Nunn [2]

Interdisciplinary Education

One can employ some techniques that our oncology colleagues use to share life-changing news with their patients. It is estimated that oncologists "give bad news" more than 20,000 times during their career [3], and they have valuable lessons that we can employ in the emergency department.

A skills-based practice called SPIKES (see Table 65.3) is often employed as an additional strategy for giving bad news. SPIKES goes beyond forecasting to set a scene, employ kindness, elicit additional information, and then summarize and strategize [3]. SPIKES is a guideline that helps physicians address individual patient needs in a personalized manner. Although an oncologist's discussion on treatment options or failures will be more detailed than a life-threatening diagnosis given in the emergency department, emergency physicians can use some of the ideas from SPIKES in their discussions with patients.

Table 65.3 SPIKES method

S = Set up the interview
P = Perception: Assess patient's perceptions
I = Invitation for patient's permission to proceed
K = Give Knowledge to the patient
E = Empathy/Emotions: Express empathy to the patient's emotional response
S = Summary/Strategy: Summarize the meeting and strategize on when to meet again for the next steps

Adapted from Table 65.1 SPIKES method in Nunn [2]

The Discussion's Stress on the Medical Team

As caring physicians, it is critical that we recognize the stress we hold when giving bad news. Our personal emotional reactions can affect how the news is delivered along with our fears of being blamed or taking the responsibility for the objective news itself. Part of mitigating our own stress can be to employ mindfulness about one's own emotional reactions and unhelpful attitudes. Being mindful allows one to be aware of one's own feelings in the moment through nonjudgmental observation [3]. Physicians can act on these emotions with calmness, so their psychological reactions do not negatively interfere during critical discussions with their patients.

Special Population: Pediatrics

Although the medical diagnosis and prognosis will be discussed in detail with the parents, it is critical to understand the age of the child and how this affects their interpretation of the problem. For infants, it is important that parents are reminded that they are mostly the ones suffering the psychological effects of the diagnosis—when their dreams of who their child would become are broken. Infants do not know what their parents wished for them prior to their birth. Infants, toddlers, and preschoolers respond well to sensorimotor comfort. These young children need reassurance for their questions "Will it hurt? Will I be alone?" Words are less important than actions that comfort and reassure toddlers they are safe and loved [2]. Two to four-year-olds understand what is happening but not why or what it means. They often blame themselves as the cause of the problem. Giving names to emotions around them is often helpful. Again, early school age children require comfort, relief, and reassurance of safety and companionship [2].

The 8 to 12-year-old population is an age of cognitive generalization about themselves, the world, and the future. They still respond to sensorimotor comfort and relief, but they also worry how their parents will manage if they die and how they can relieve their parents' distress. As children reach puberty, they see life as, if something is wrong, mom and dad can fix it. When bad news is given, they can interpret this as parents' unwillingness or incompetence to fix it. During middle adolescence the shift for comfort moves from family to the friend unit [2]. When treating children and adolescents, we must remember to reach the child/teen at their level in addition to talking with the parents. This may mean simply hugging a young child or explaining the diagnosis to a teenager and anticipating questions from them on how it will affect their education or their activities with friends.

Diverse Cultural Expectations

Many cultures request that serious diagnoses be concealed from patients in order to protect patients from psychological harm. Although diagnostic non-disclosure is motivated by compassion, negative outcomes can occur when bad news is hidden from patients. Survey studies in countries where diagnostic non-disclosure is the norm portray that patients do want to know their diagnosis. In addition, depending on the country, diagnostic non-disclosure can have professional and legal ramifications for the healthcare team [4].

As a global, diverse, international society, diagnostic non-disclosure can be an ethical challenge to physicians when test results portray bad news. Western ethics based on the principles of autonomy, beneficence, and non-maleficence teaches that disclosing serious information to patients is essential [4].

Last year, a patient was sent to the emergency department with the clinical suspicion by their outpatient physician that the patient had cancer. Her daughter informed the triage team that she did not want her mother to be made aware of the potential diagnosis. After examining the patient and ordering her CT scan and blood work, I employed the ARCHES model.

Acknowledging the daughter's request,
Building a **Relationship** with the daughter,
Finding **Common** Ground,
Honoring the patient's information preference,
Providing **Emotional Support**, and
Reaching a **Solution**

to gain rapport with the daughter and address her concerns.[4] As a practicing physician in the United States, ethically and legally, I needed to respect my patient and her personal wishes. Sadly, the patients CT scan returned with signs of peritoneal carcinomatosis. I followed Dr. Beng's model in "Collusion in Palliative Care," and talked directly with the patient [5]. I informed her that I did not have good news. The patient inquired what her daughter and I were talking about. I honestly informed the patient that her daughter "requested I share the results only with her as she is worried about you." I informed the patient, "I want to do what you want as these are your results and you are my patient." The patient said, "It's okay that you just tell her." She then proceeded to ask me a few questions, such as, "When can I go home?" I informed her based on the CT scan that she would need to see some specialists and will need to be admitted for more tests. It was apparent the patient had a strong suspicion of her diagnosis. Afterwards, her daughter thanked me and expressed her understanding that given our ethical standards in the United States, we have a duty to respect our patient's wishes first and foremost.

The ARCHES model allows clinicians to help with conflict resolution between the healthcare system and the family's wishes. It gives appreciation to the family's standpoint, affirms their good intentions, and helps correct misperceptions.

In addition to respecting various cultural ethics and norms, many patients may require interpreter services. This can be very challenging to effectively share bad news in an empathetic manner. When using an interpreter, it is often noted that physicians may want to share less, be more effective in their communication skills, and speak slowly. With patient permission, it may be beneficial to engage their family and friends [2].

Lessons from the Families Who Receive Bad News

The news of a relative's unexpected death is probably the pinnacle of bad news physicians share with families. A survey study given to families of patients who received news that their loved ones died from a trauma highlights some of the qualities valued by family members when they received life-changing news [6]. The survey portrayed evidence that sharing news of a traumatic death requires a caring attitude and a well-informed sympathetic caregiver who is familiar with the patient and is available to answer questions. Families ranked privacy and time as critical components when receiving news of a traumatic death [6]. This survey from TICU and ED patients can be applied to other aspects of medicine when information is given that changes one's life in a negative way.

Parents of newborns with congenital malformations in NICUs in Brazil were interviewed regarding their reception of bad news. Families were satisfied with delicate, careful, honest, and clear communication in which parents were able to have hope for the future. Complaints were noted in the survey on difficult language, haste, nervousness, aggressiveness, and lack of empathy [7]. These studies provide critical information about the communication families desire when receiving life-changing information on their loved ones.

Each patient seeking help has their own values, and each physician has their unique way to address patients' needs. Therefore, although the models such as SPIKES, ABCDE, ARCHES, and BREAKS are helpful guidelines, each time we give bad news, it is critical that a personalized, individual approach is used. As Dr. Nunn clearly states, "good clinicians make islands of quiet and protected time in the midst of medical mayhem to say what must be said without haste and without failing to distinguish between what they know and do not know" [2]. How bad news is given must be done in light of the individual patient and their background which takes into account their emotions, intellect, social skills, and disability, if any. As we grow in knowledge and wisdom as clinicians, it can become easier to share life-changing news, but we must remember that the information will never be easy on the patient who receives bad news. Therefore, we are called to express compassion and integrity in these critical conversations with our patients and families whose lives have been changed forever.

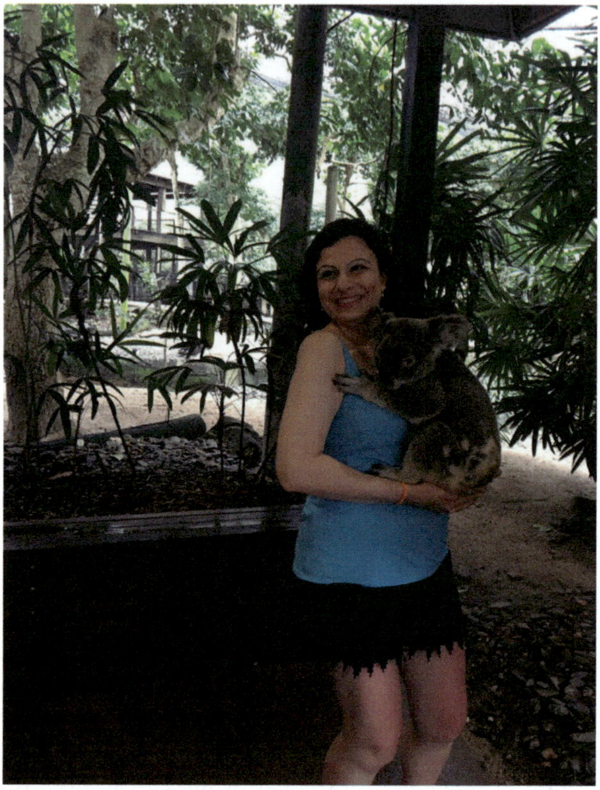

Dr. Maccagnano enjoying some wellness time (cuddling a Koala) on her travels in Australia after attending the SMACC (Social Media and Critical Care) Sydney Conference.

References

1. Maynard DW. Delivering bad news in emergency care medicine. Acute Med Surg. 2016;4(1):3–11.
2. Nunn K. Delivering bad news. J Paediatr Child Health. 2019;55(6):617–20.
3. Baile WF. Giving bad news. Oncologist. 2015;20(8):852–3.
4. Holmes SN, Illing J. Breaking bad news: tackling cultural dilemmas. BMJ Support Palliat Care. 2021;11(2):128–32.
5. Beng KS. Collusion in palliative care. Malays Fam Physician. 2006;1(2–3):62–4.
6. Jurkovich GJ, Pierce B, Pananen L, Rivara FP. Giving bad news: the family perspective. J Trauma. 2000;48(5):865–70; discussion 870–3.
7. Marçola L, Zoboli I, Polastrini RTV, Barbosa SMM. Breaking bad news in a neonatal intensive care: the parent's evaluation. Rev Paul Pediatr. 2020;38:e2019092.

Chapter 66
Ensuring Patient Satisfaction in the Emergency Department

Julia Bonanno, Rachel Patterson, and Holly Stankewicz

Introduction

As in other areas of industry, the medical field has not been immune to the demands of consumer satisfaction. The consumer, or the patient, is looking for high-quality, rapid, and friendly care. The emergency department (ED) is often a patient's first encounter with a hospital system during a time of acute and unexpected illness or injury, making emergency department patient satisfaction scores all the more important for that institution. Patient satisfaction is defined as meeting patient expectations in various elements of care and experience. Emergency physicians are therefore not only expected to deliver medical care, but also to create an environment of comfort with clear and frequent communication despite time constraints, overcrowding, and the loud, often understaffed, environments in which they work [1, 2]. Patient satisfaction is often based on the entire patient experience. This includes everything from the medical treatment to how clean and bright the department appears. Meeting patients' expectations is an important goal for emergency departments as the care rendered as well as the treatment environment often forms a patient's overall impression of an institution and their likelihood of recommending the institution to others. Satisfied patients are also less likely to give poor physician reviews and less likely to enter into malpractice claims [1].

In recent years, there has been a greater focus on patient experience. Many different commercially available survey systems exist. Previous studies have shown that satisfaction is based not only on the perception of the quality of care rendered, but also on other factors. These include the patient's overall perception of an emergency department visit as well as the interpersonal skills of physicians/nurses/

J. Bonanno · R. Patterson · H. Stankewicz (✉)
St. Luke's Bethlehem, Bethlehem, PA, USA
e-mail: Julia.Bonanno@sluhn.org; Rachel.patterson@sluhn.org; Holly.stankewicz@sluhn.org

R. P. Olympia et al. (eds.), *An Emergency Physician's Path*,
https://doi.org/10.1007/978-3-031-47873-4_66

ancillary staff, communication regarding tests/illness, and overall wait time [3]. Hospitals have employed the use of various survey tools to help gauge patient satisfaction and the overall patient experience in the emergency department. Through these surveys, physicians and providers receive data to help guide areas of success and improvement with the overall goal of improved patient and physician satisfaction.

How Do We Define and Measure Patient Satisfaction?

Patient satisfaction can be measured and defined in different ways. There are various scoring methods in place that all assess different outcomes.

It is critical that any survey instrument frame a general satisfaction question by *defining* the chosen satisfaction measure. For example, "in terms of meeting your expectations for treatment and care, rate your satisfaction with your overall care" [1].

Below are listed some of the scores that are utilized in emergency departments throughout the country.

- Hospital Consumer Assessment of Healthcare Providers and Systems (HCAHPS) survey [4]
  - 27 question survey
  - Often utilized by institutions to gauge overall hospital experience
  - Three goals of data gathering:
    - Develop incentive programs
    - Hold hospitals accountable for actions
    - Compare various hospital systems
  - Federal government
  - Limitations
    - Not specific to ED
    - Length of survey
- Press Ganey
  - A voluntary survey, random selection
  - A measure of the quality of service rendered
  - Divided into various quality measures including the overall experience as well as specifics regarding the care environment, nursing staff, radiology services, and physician care
  - Limitations
    - Delayed requests for information, patients may have forgotten the details of the visit
    - Patients may have been seen by multiple providers and it can be unclear as to who they are evaluating

Most hospitals place emphasis on "top box" values, which is the number of fives given, resulting in a score of 4 having the same value as a 1.
Patients may have been seen multiple times in the ED and therefore could be evaluating a completely different visit and provider

- ED CAHPS
  - A voluntary survey, random selection
  - Gathers data about the experience of care
  - Could mean that ED only surveys would be on low acuity patients—generally spend less time on those patients as their chief complaints are generally less time intensive
  - Limitations

    Delayed requests for information, patients may have forgotten the visit details
    Patients may have been seen by multiple providers and it can be unclear as to who they are evaluating
    Patients may have been seen multiple times in the ED and therefore could be evaluating a completely different visit and provider

Barriers in the Emergency Department

One of the most important factors regarding patient satisfaction is communication, especially the quality and timeliness of that communication with the patient. Under normal circumstances, emergency department physicians manage multiple patients of various acuity and often have to prioritize patients requiring a higher level of care, as opposed to patients who have been waiting the longest. The nature of going to an ED for care also tends to be anxiety-provoking for patients, which can influence patient satisfaction. When patients are anxious, they are looking for comfort and reassurance from their physicians. ED physicians do not have the benefit of having an established relationship with their patients, making it harder for them to connect with patients in a time-pressured environment.

In recent years, emergency departments nationwide have suffered from issues of ED overcrowding and understaffing. This is especially true post-COVID-19. As emergency department personnel have become overwhelmed with more patients while also dealing with personal protective equipment availability issues and less staff, it can be a challenge to maintain effective and timely communication as well as provide an overall comfortable environment in the ED.

The passage of the 21st Century Cures Act may have future potential impacts on patient satisfaction as well, specifically communication issues. As patients will have immediate access to charts including notes and laboratory, or imaging results, a new challenge for physicians will be discussing details of the chart with the patient in a timely and concise manner.

How Can We Improve Patient Satisfaction?

Improving patient satisfaction requires a multi-faceted approach that varies depending on the institution and patient demographics. Certain factors such as hospital environment may be difficult to change, while the patient and certain components of provider characteristics cannot be changed at all. However, there are qualities and non-verbal actions that physicians and other ED staff can control, which may have an even more substantial impact on overall patient satisfaction.

The hospital environment includes factors such as parking, cleanliness, overall noise level, and the ability to adjust the lighting in patient rooms. Unfortunately, not all hospitals have private rooms for every single patient, and many patients are seen in hallway beds with little privacy which may be associated with decreased patient satisfaction. While these factors can be adjusted, they are generally not immediately controllable by the ED physician.

Other factors such as patients' age and baseline health level, provider gender, and type of hospital also influence patient satisfaction but cannot be changed [5]. Physicians should be mindful of potentially complex factors such as race and gender concordance between the treating physician and the patient. [6] Simple things such as providing a pediatric patient with a popsicle, blanket or pillow for an uncomfortable patient, or even adjusting room lighting, have all been evaluated for improved patient satisfaction scores showing the promise of higher marks [7].

Therefore, the focus should be on factors that physicians can control shift by shift. We have already identified that one of the main factors contributing to patient satisfaction is that they feel their physician is empathetic towards them. ED providers are accustomed to working in stressful noisy environments while many of the patients cared for are in an unfamiliar environment and nervous that they could be life-threatening, adding the vulnerability of being in a new place without appropriate information only adds to that stress.

The AEIOU approach can help mitigate some of these problems. AEIOU is defined as follows. Addressing patients in their preferred manner and also properly introducing members of the patient care team helps to establish an initial patient-provider relationship. An empathetic statement and simply stating that you understand how nervous they may be and that you are happy to address the questions they have will also help improve your relationship. It is also beneficial to inform patients where bathrooms are, how to reach a nurse for assistance, what the next steps in the plan are, and offer to help them with anything quick at the moment such as getting a blanket or a cup of water. Keeping patients updated with what they are specifically waiting on, and how long that may take, is also more important to patient satisfaction than decreasing wait times in the ED. [8] Empathizing with patients and understanding how afraid they may be can improve their overall satisfaction, however, the steps outlined above are time-consuming. Whether this method is implemented by physicians, nurses, or through the creation of new roles such as an ED patient advocate, following these guidelines is likely to increase overall patient satisfaction [8].

The physician's awareness of how they interact with patients can play a major role in patient satisfaction. For example, introducing yourself as the physician to the patient and allowing them to introduce anyone else in the room with them. Physician body language is also extremely important in helping patients feel comfortable with their doctor. Holding one's arms at their side versus crossing one's arms, simply sitting in a chair or any available surface, and making eye contact with the patient, all contribute to the patient feeling comfortable. The patient will then feel like the physician is listening to them and devoting time to their care in an already stressful situation [4].

The Role Patient Satisfaction Plays on Physician Satisfaction

The role that physicians play on patients' overall experience with their care is also very important. When physicians have greater overall job satisfaction, it improves morale, thereby making physicians more likely to enjoy coming to work each day and an overall improved attitude toward their patients and other staff. This personal physician happiness is then reflected in the attitude physicians have toward their patients. Ultimately, this makes patients more satisfied, more compliant with care plans, and reduces malpractice risk [3].

Conclusion

Patient satisfaction is an important aspect of the ED patient experience. Several factors contribute to this satisfaction, many of which are not within the control of the ED physician. However, there are some steps the ED physician can take to improve patient satisfaction, such as being aware of their own body language, anticipating the patient's needs, and improving communication by updating patients promptly. Communication is essential to improve patient satisfaction. By creating an atmosphere in the emergency department that fosters improved communication and well-being, physicians and patients will both have a greater overall satisfaction.

References

1. Trout A, Magnusson AR, Hedges JR. Patient satisfaction investigations and the emergency department: what does the literature say? Acad Emerg Med. 2000;7(6):695–709.
2. Abass G, Asery A, Al Badr A, AlMaghlouth A, AlOtaiby S, Heena H. Patient satisfaction with the emergency department services at an academic teaching hospital. J Family Med Prim Care. 2021;10(4):1718–25. https://doi.org/10.4103/jfmpc.jfmpc_8_20. Epub 2021 Apr 29.

3. Patient satisfaction—emergency department patient satisfaction surveys. An information Paper. ACEP. June 2011. https://www.acep.org/imports/clinical-and-practice-management/patient-satisfaction/.
4. HCAHPS: Patients' Perspectives of Care Survey. https://www.cms.gov/Medicare/Quality-Initiatives-Patient-Assessment-Instruments/HospitalQualityInits/HospitalHCAHPS. Accessed 22 Sept 2022.
5. Arman D. Are you satisfied with your patient satisfaction scores. EM Resident. 17 Aug 2020. https://www.emra.org/emresident/article/edda-patient-satisfaction/.
6. Takeshita J, Wang S, Loren AW, Mitra N, Shults J, Shin DB, Sawinski DL. Association of racial/ethnic and gender concordance between patients and physicians with patient experience ratings. JAMA Netw Open. 2020;3(11):e2024583. https://doi.org/10.1001/jamanetworkopen.2020.24583.
7. Finn RM, Voelkel J, Bellolio MF, Jeffery MM, Wiswell J. Pediatric ice pop administration to improve patient experience scores. Mayo Clin Proc Innov Qual Outcomes. 2020;4(4):410–5. https://doi.org/10.1016/j.mayocpiqo.2020.04.011.
8. Feuerwerker S, Rankin N, Wohler B, Gemino H, Risler Z. Improving patient satisfaction by using design thinking: patient advocate role in the emergency department. Cureus. 2019;11(1):e3872. https://doi.org/10.7759/cureus.3872. PMID: 30899623; PMCID: PMC6414297.

Chapter 67
Communicating with Consultants

John Westhoff

Background

Patients frequently require services we cannot provide in the Emergency Department (ED) for lack of time, resources, or expertise. Of necessity, we seek the aid of providers of differing backgrounds, training, and temperament. Conversely, we regularly assist clinic providers and pre-hospital personnel who call for assistance. In these ways, we both "consult" and "are consulted," though we do not often frame it this way. When we call for help, we think of our task as getting a reluctant consultant "to do the right thing." When we are asked for help we may, with no sense of irony, complain loudly (after hanging up) of being "dumped on" [1].

Forty years ago, Goldman et al. published "Ten Commandments for Effective Consultations" in the *Archives of Internal Medicine* [2]. The Harvard and Stanford-based authors cited a concerning lack of explicit instruction regarding the consultation process and offered an expert opinion to fill the gap (Table 67.1). In contrast to similar and more recent work in the emergency medicine literature, Goldman and his colleagues wrote from a consultant's perspective.

Subsequent authors have pointed out that changes in the practice of medicine necessitate an updated approach to the "ten commandments" and emergency medicine-focused teaching rubrics have been developed to define taxonomy and standardize the teaching of the consultation process [3]. The "5C's of Consultation" (Table 67.1) has been formally tested in a prospective, randomized, multicenter trial and was found to be both efficient and effective as a method for training medical students [6]. The PIQUED approach (Table 67.1) was developed in Canada via a

J. Westhoff (✉)
Department of Internal Medicine, University of Nevada, Reno School of Medicine, Reno, NV, USA
e-mail: jwesthoff@unr.edu

R. P. Olympia et al. (eds.), *An Emergency Physician's Path*,
https://doi.org/10.1007/978-3-031-47873-4_67

Table 67.1 Commonly referenced models for improving consultant communication

Ten commandments for effective consultations [3]	5C's of consultation [4]	PIQUED [5]
I: Determine the question. The consultant should determine the question that is being asked	**1. Contact.** Introduction of consulting and consultant physicians. Building of relationship	***P*reparation & review.** Initial work up and resuscitation; review investigations
II: Establish urgency. Establish the urgency of the consultation	**2. Communicate.** Give a concise story and ask focused questions	***I*dentification of involved parties.** EM physician, consultant physician, patient and patient-case specifics
III: Look for yourself. Gather primary data	**3. Core question.** Have a specific question or request for the consultant. Decide on a reasonable timeframe for consultation	***Q*uestions.** EM clinical questions; anticipate consultant questions
IV: Be as brief as appropriate	**4. Collaboration.** A result of the discussion between the ED physician and the consultant, including any alteration of management or testing	***U*rgency.** Modify behavior and information based on increasing urgency
V: Be specific. Make specific recommendations	**5. Closing the loop.** Ensure that both parties are on the same page regarding the plan and maintain proper communication about any changes in the patient's status	***E*ducational modifications.** Consider learner needs, hierarchy concerns; remember to teach if you are more senior
VI: Provide contingency plans		***D*ebrief and discuss.** Illicit or provide feedback regarding the case
VII: Thou shalt not covet thy neighbor's patient. Understand your role as consultant in the process		
VIII: Teach with tact. Offer educational information		
IX: Talk is cheap, and effective. Communicate recommendations directly to the requesting physician		
X: Follow-up. Provide appropriate follow-up		

mixed-methods study that analyzed semi-structured interviews and group discussions with residents and attendings from emergency medicine, internal medicine, and general surgery [5].

These instruments are rightly a focus of medical educators. During the first month of my residency, I spent an entire half-day listening to recordings of real (and problematic) telephone conversations with consultants. As we listened, a former department chair led a discussion of what might have been done differently for each call and provided tips, such as always starting with a "hook" or "bottom line up-front" that gets the consultant's attention immediately. This exercise had a major impact and has served me well. Still—miscommunication, mistakes, and lapses in professionalism are inevitable. Sound methodology is necessary but not sufficient in a chaotic, 24-h, high-stakes, time-pressured environment. Over a career in emergency medicine, emotional self-control, situational awareness, and a focus on the long-term cultivation of trust are of greater importance than any specific rubric and, accordingly, are the focus of this chapter.

The High Cost of Disruptive Consultants

We are taught the art of the case presentation early. Communicating accurately and efficiently to supervising residents and attendings is a major emphasis of undergraduate medical education. It is no accident then that when working with consultants, you will inevitably feel at times as if you are back in training..

By definition, the consultant has been sought out because of their relevant expertise. This asymmetry pre-disposes toward a dynamic that can be antithetical to collegiality. If the specialist is abrasive or condescending, it can activate the emotional baggage of formative medical education in the emergency physician—that they are perceived as subordinate, weak, or ignorant. A physician triggered this way is not unlike a combat veteran with PTSD. We are suddenly back on the proverbial battlefield—angry and humiliated. In extreme cases, we can be compromised in our ability to focus for hours. During this time we are more likely to rely on mental shortcuts than more systematic reasoning [4]. Much has been written about managing anger at work, and while it is a skill worth developing, it is beyond the scope of this chapter [7].

The term of art used in the medical literature for a colleague who is so interpersonally dysfunctional as to impact operations negatively is "disruptive physician." Disruptive behavior among physicians has become a high-profile issue in recent years because of growing awareness of the impact this behavior has on patient safety. In the United States, the former Joint Commission on Accreditation of Healthcare Organizations (whose name lost its descriptive utility when it re-branded itself "The Joint Commission" in 2007) now requires hospitals to have an explicit plan for dealing with disruptive providers. An example from my own experience illustrates the problem.

A young woman with abdominal pain presented to the single-coverage ED of our small community hospital. The physician on duty diagnosed ectopic pregnancy and then discharged her with an outpatient follow-up appointment without consulting an obstetrician. The patient deteriorated shortly after discharge, and her family called for an ambulance. She was taken to another facility and had emergency surgery for a ruptured ectopic. As director of the ED to which she initially presented, I investigated the case. My colleague acknowledged he had made a serious mistake, but what was remarkable about his error was the context. He had begun the process of obtaining an obstetrics consult, but when he realized who was on call, he thought "I just can't deal with her today." The consultant was well-known to him. She had berated him many times, aggressively criticizing his presentation and clinical reasoning.

To be clear, the proximate error was his, and previous interactions had likely revealed to the consultant genuine weaknesses in his skillset. But among the root causes of this near-fatal outcome was the toxicity of the consultant. The emergency physician talked himself into what he knew to be a deviation in the standard of care because the emotional implications of talking to a disruptive obstetrician were too great. All of the physicians in our group had had negative interactions with this obstetrician, so I asked to meet with her and her department chair to discuss her professionalism. She was surprised to hear that she had a reputation as being difficult to work with and her chair vouched for her competence. But of course, her skill as a surgeon was not at issue. Disruptive physicians are often gifted clinicians. They hold high standards for themselves and expect others to do the same. They see their demanding nature as a manifestation of fierce patient advocacy rather than an unhealthy degree of perfectionism. Disruptive physicians are often beloved by their patients. It is their coworkers and colleagues that find them insufferable [8].

Problematic peers are not unique to medicine. The Harvard Business Review once devoted an issue to "How to Work with Toxic Colleagues." One article described the work of researchers who had studied the workplace dynamics of competence and likability. They surveyed workers and then observed their behavior. When given a theoretical scenario in which they faced a difficult work-related problem, most people insisted that they would approach an unpleasant expert or over an affable but incompetent peer. In practice, however, workers were more likely to seek the advice of a "lovable fool" than a "competent jerk." While the "fool" might prove useless, there was a chance of getting helpful feedback, and in any event, there was no emotional cost. In contrast, asking a "competent jerk" for help can be a humiliating and potentially day-ruining experience. It is human nature to find another solution [9].

There are two key takeaways concerning toxic consultants. First, recognize the deleterious effects of a negative interaction of this kind on patient care, and be aware of the potential for the emotional fallout to influence your decision-making. If the problem is severe or ongoing, consider addressing it definitively with the consultant when you are off shift or refer to departmental leadership. Second, recognize the very real downside of being abrasive on those ill-timed calls from clinics or nursing homes sending you yet another patient. It is tempting to be curt or condescending when you sense a "dump," but for the sake of future patients, be consummately professional and address important systemic issues later.

Proximity Advantage

Another kind of asymmetry exists in the consulting relationship. The requesting physician is proximate to the patient, while the consultant works on what amounts to professional hearsay. Properly considered, this should engender humility on the part of any consultant. When there is disagreement, the requesting physician is drawing on a rich mental model borne of first-hand experience, while the consulted has access only to an imperfectly communicated verbal caricature.

To understand the pitfalls of this dynamic, it can be helpful to think of a presentation to a consultant as the logical statement "A, therefore, B" (A∴B), where "A" is the description of the patient and "B" is the proposed disposition. This is the essence of the stories we tell one another. For example, "this patient has appendicitis; therefore please remove their appendix," or "this patient has high-risk chest pain, therefore please admit them for telemetry," etc.

When we disagree with another's A∴B formulation, we tend to assume that we have a perfect understanding of "A" (the presentation) and that our disagreement is about "B" (the disposition). Such reasoning can be manifest in statements like: "it doesn't sound like they need to go to the OR tonight." But what if "A," not "B" is wrong? That is, the patient *does* need to go to the OR immediately, but I have imperfectly communicated why. I have erred in "A" rather than "B." Reasonable disagreements about disposition frequently occur, but it is possible that the patient in your consultant's mind is very different from the patient you've examined. When you hear a frustrated consultant say "why didn't you just tell me that at the beginning?"—you have experienced this phenomenon. Similarly, I have learned that when I hear a story from a clinic or ambulance crew that doesn't make sense, it is often the case that the emergent care requested is indeed appropriate, but not for the reasons I (thought I) heard.

Limitations of the Telephone

Miscommunication is sometimes an artifact of the limitations posed by the telephone. During my first deployment to Iraq, our unit chaplain offered a seminar on "How to Avoid a Fight Over the Phone." The class had nothing to do with consulting per se, but it spoke to the serious limitations of the telephone as a communication medium. Without non-verbal cues and with imperfect situational awareness, the signal can get lost in the noise. These conversations happen "in situ" for the consultant, i.e., while they are driving in heavy traffic, when dogs are barking, or babies crying. They interrupt emotionally charged situations—heated financial discussions, romantic moments, or arguments with teenage children. While you are focused on how well you are *crushing* the "5Cs," your consultant, struggling with work-life balance, is processing the fact that their plans for the evening are ruined. It is remarkable that such calls are not *more* prone to acrimony [10]. I once called a neurosurgeon at night about a gunshot wound to the head. He said, "What do you want me to do about it?" I responded, "I was thinking neurosurgery stuff?" He apologized and said that he'd just woken up—and that he'd be right in. Who can blame him? No doubt he had a full schedule the next day.

The Inevitability of Disagreement

Collegial disagreements with consultants are inevitable. They are *inherent* in our role. Consider the gedankenexperiment or "thought experiment" represented by Fig. 67.1. This is a conceptual model, not a representation of real data. The x-axis represents the *spectrum of presentation* for a given disease. To the right are presentations of greater clinical concern. To the left are those that are less so. The larger curve represents the distribution of patients without disease and the smaller curve, those with the disease. The vertical lines represent the threshold of action for a given physician.

In scenario A, the consultant is less likely to consider action appropriate for a given presentation than the emergency physician. Every patient in the stippled domain to the right of the consultant's threshold can be thought of as a referral considered by the consultant to require action (e.g., surgery, admission, etc.). Patients in the hashed domain between the two vertical lines represent cases of concern to the emergency physician that *do not* meet the consultant's action threshold. If the clinical acumen of the emergency physician is thought of as a test for the disease, the emergency physician is "more sensitive and less specific" than the consultant in this case.

In scenario B, the opposite is true. The emergency physician is *less sensitive* than the consultant. One consequence of this arrangement is that the emergency physician will never call the consultant about a patient that does not meet the consultant's threshold for action. The consultant will get fewer calls, and she will never get "inappropriate consults." Of course, this arrangement is also unsafe in that the consultant is never made aware of some patients that meet her threshold for action.

For serious diseases and from the perspective of patient safety, scenario A is better than scenario B, i.e., as a test for disease requiring immediate action, it is better for the emergency medicine physician to be more *sensitive* than a consultant—and so occasional disagreement should be thought of as inevitable and even desirable.

However, in practice, it is prudent to minimize the distance between action thresholds—and physicians in collaborative practice tend toward convergence over time. In the ideal end state, the domain of disagreement has shrunk such that the lines are functionally identical; they overlap. This is perhaps why I cannot recall a serious clinical disagreement with a consultant I knew well. In a state of high trust,

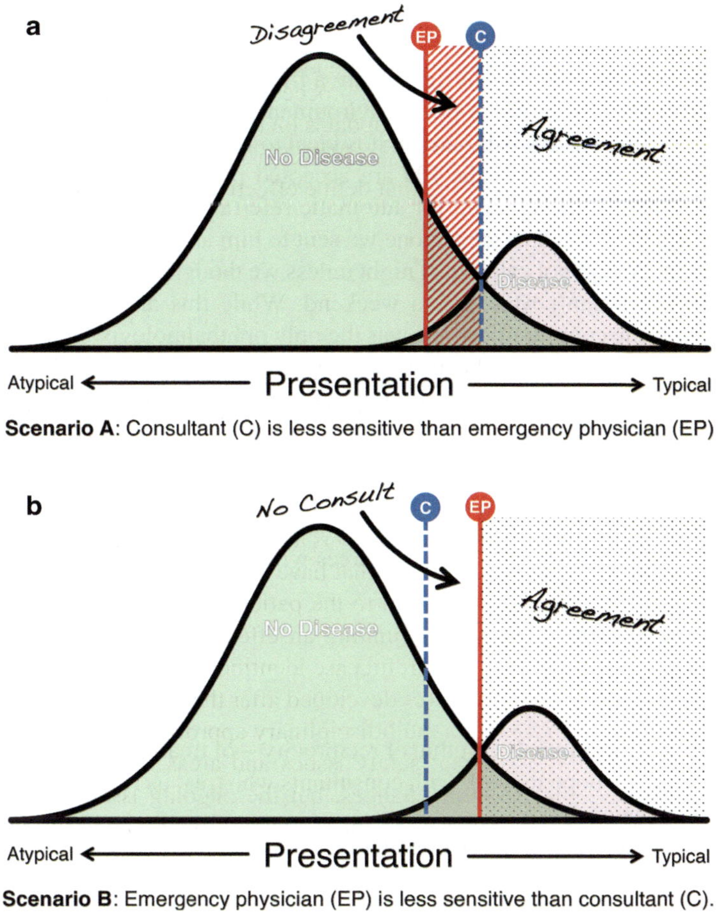

Fig. 67.1 Conceptual model illustrating the spectrum of disease presentation and the thresholds of action for the emergency physician and consultant. Collegial disagreements arise when thresholds differ, highlighting the importance of trust and convergence in collaborative practice. In scenario (**a**), the consultant is less sensitive than the emergency physician, resulting in "inappropriate consults" from the perspective of the consultant. In scenario (**b**), the emergency physician is less sensitive than the consultant, which jeopardizes patient safety but (from the perspective of the consultant) improves the "appropriateness" of the average consultation

the consultant operates under the presumption that "if you're concerned, then I'm concerned," or, in terms of the model, "your threshold is my threshold." The consultant sees the emergency physician as a reliable (but not perfect) test for the disease. This level of Zen is carefully cultivated over time, and sometimes requires deliberate interaction outside of work [9]. Keep the long-term nature of the relationship in mind when you are new or working with a new or unfamiliar consultant. Be careful not to win a battle at the cost of the war.

Protecting Consultants

Consultants, like emergency physicians, are a limited resource and should be dealt with accordingly. In resource-poor environments where consultants are overwhelmed and bear a heavy call burden, it is ideal to build systems where urgent (but not emergent) consults from the ED are accepted presumptively. For example, I once worked out an arrangement for automatic referral with an ophthalmologist in a rural setting. He agreed to see anyone we sent to him at 7 o'clock the next (weekday) morning. We did not call him at night unless we thought a case needed immediate surgery or couldn't wait over a weekend. While this arrangement might be untenable in some communities—he was the only ophthalmologist in town and was de facto on call every day, so the arrangement was a clear "win-win." We spent less time trying to reach him and woke him up less often, which meant we had a much happier colleague when we did need him to come in. We worked out a similar arrangement with the only otolaryngologist in town. Efforts like these will differ in different communities and between specialties, but proactive, good-faith efforts to "protect consultants" go a long way toward building professional trust and increasing the likelihood that these limited resources will be available in the future.

Conclusion

The Golden rule is famously an ethic of reciprocity—of treating others as one wants to be treated. If we hope to work with consultants who treat us respectfully, we must model that behavior.

Early in my career, I remember being quite busy in the ED when I got a call from an internist with a good reputation in an adjacent clinic. I don't remember the details of the story he told me, but I remember thinking he was "weak" and that this was a *classic* 4 o'clock Friday afternoon clinic dump. I (regretfully) told him so, but as EMTALA gave me no choice, I accepted the referral.

As soon as his patient arrived, I recognized my error. The sick patient before me did not match the stable one in my head—the mental caricature I had constructed during our telephone conversation. After I cardioverted the patient, I called the internist back to let him know that his decision to send his patient to the ED was spot on—and, more importantly, to apologize for my lack of professionalism. I had focused on and criticized his "A∴B" story instead of seeing his call for what it was—a cry for help from a colleague proximate to the patient. Only with the patient in my ED, were we finally talking about the same patient. I told him we were here to help, and that I didn't want him not to call during a busy clinic because he remembered me and thought, "I just can't deal with that guy today."

References

1. Apker J, Mallak LA, Gibson SC. Communicating in the "gray zone": perceptions about emergency physician hospitalist handoffs and patient safety. Acad Emerg Med. 2007;14(10):884–94.
2. Goldman L, Lee T, Rudd P. Ten commandments for effective consultations. Arch Intern Med. 1983;143(9):1753–5.
3. Salerno SM, Hurst FP, Halvorson S, Mercado DL. Principles of effective consultation: an update for the 21st-century consultant. Arch Intern Med. 2007;167(3):271–5.
4. Lerner J, Shonk K. How anger poisons decision making. Harvard Business Review. Sept 2010.
5. Chan T, Orlich D, Kulasegaram K, Sherbino J. Understanding communication between emergency and consulting physicians: a qualitative study that describes and defines the essential elements of the emergency department consultation-referral process for the junior learner. CJEM. 2013;15(1):42–51.
6. Kessler CS, Tadisina KK, Saks M, Franzen D, Woods R, Banh KV, et al. The 5Cs of consultation: training medical students to communicate effectively in the emergency department. J Emerg Med. 2015;49(5):713–21.
7. Fosslien L, Duffy M. How to manage your anger at work. Harvard Business Review. April 2022.
8. Feinmann J. "Disruptive" doctors are often found to be perfectionists, agency reports. BMJ. 2011;342:d876.
9. Casciaro T, Lobo M. Competent jerks, lovable fools, and the formation of social neworks. Harvard Business Review. June 2005.
10. Shetty AL, Vaghasiya M, Boddy R, Byth K, Unwin D. Perceived incivility during emergency department phone consultations. Emerg Med Australas. 2016;28(3):256–61.

Chapter 68
Communicating with Surgical Colleagues

Kahyun Yoon-Flannery

"Heads up—I probably have a consult coming up for you soon." These are the most dreaded words to a surgeon on call coming from our colleagues in other parts of the hospital. Thankfully, long gone are the days when as a surgical resident I was on a 24-h call working on admissions and consults from the emergency room. Nevertheless, my record for the greatest number of consults is about 20 in a 24-h call. Having spent years as a medical student and a surgical resident in the same program, thereby knowing every corner and every person staffing the hospital, I was well known and familiar to everyone by the end of my training years. Some days this certainly came in handy. When we found a bat flying about in one of our bedrooms, needing to deal with the rabies shots for my family of five, I did not have to hesitate to call one of my emergency room and infectious disease attendings. But this also meant, that sometimes, if there were even a hint of a surgical situation in the hospital, I was usually the one to field the questions. "This patient just hit the door and has right lower quadrant pain. No labs or CT yet but I'm telling you this is going to be an appendicitis for sure. Just come down and take a look." "I was too afraid to call your senior resident who was on call last night. So there are six consults down here for you this morning." These were typically the questions I had to field on the day to day on the job. I, along with my colleagues and patients, survived intact after the 5 grueling years of general surgery residency, despite many of these requests. In fact, one of my children's godfathers is a dear friend who spent all 5 years of post-graduate training years along with me. He is a phenomenal physician practicing emergency medicine in the sunny state of Florida. But even Claudio, despite my threats of bodily harm, felt no shame in calling me with the "heads ups" during our years of togetherness.

K. Yoon-Flannery (✉)
MD Anderson Cancer Center at Cooper, Cooper Medical School of Rowan University, Camden, NJ, USA
e-mail: yoon-flannery-kay@cooperhealth.edu

R. P. Olympia et al. (eds.), *An Emergency Physician's Path*,
https://doi.org/10.1007/978-3-031-47873-4_68

Here are some helpful hints in guiding us surgeons when facing a potential surgical problem in the emergency department (ED):

1. Keep the data handy. A short presentation on the telephone, rather than a long one fit for a storytelling, is appreciated by those who have been on call for the 15th hour.
2. Communicate to staff what is expected. A tracheostomy fell out of a patient? Calling the respiratory therapist and getting the right tray/supplies is probably going to save the day for all. Sure, the surgeon being there will be helpful, but he/she won't be able to do a thing unless the right equipment/staff are present.
3. Physical exam is still important. We live in the era of CT scans and imaging-guided diagnoses. But we still value the diagnostic skills of our treasured physician colleagues. A peritoneal belly along with a CT result of appendicitis is going to get the attention of your surgeon quicker.
4. Keep the communication succinct and unambiguous.

Pun et al. reported that the communication in EDs is complex, nuanced and fragile [1]. Communication on all levels can come to a palpable result quite quickly and noticeably in a high-pressured setting such as an emergency department. We are all human and mistakes can happen, particularly when one is not in sync with those working around and with them. This is why effective communication with consulting colleagues, particularly those hot-headed folks like surgeons, is crucial in the day-to-day life in emergency medicine. I still remember this one instance where I was called down emergently to the ED when a patient showed up hemorrhaging from a bleeding fistula. When I made my way down to meet the patient, I remember seeing an entire room full of all kinds of people, and a whole lot of blood all over the place. Bloody bandages galore. Then, magically, as soon as I came to the bedside, literally everyone left me to deal. Somehow, I figured out how to throw that figure-of-eight stitch without letting the patient hemorrhage to death, without any help; but any subsequent similar consults, I quickly learned to at least grab one individual prior to the whole room escaping from me again.

I spent 5 long years, some days longer than others, in a general surgical residency, while raising a big family. But I wasn't born a surgeon. Although I trained as a pianist growing up (which supposedly works on our ambidexterity) I had to work hard on perfecting my surgical craft. But while I worked on this, I made it a point to make sure that my communication skills were never in anyone's doubt. Even after so many hours on call, I never refused a consult and always ended the call with a "thank you, I will be right down." I was saved on many occasions, by colleagues in different disciplines, particularly as a junior resident during critical situations. There were times where I could not get that femoral stick, no matter how much I tried. Who saved the day? My senior unit resident. When a critical post-op patient of mine rolled up in the emergency room, my colleagues who were intimately aware of the complex case called me immediately. Some heads-ups are definitely appreciated for sure.

Someone said to me early in my career, “if you find a job that you love, you will never work a day in your life.” Communicating well on a daily basis and making the best out of a situation that most people outside of medicine can hardly fathom can certainly save your sanity. In the end, be honest with yourself and your colleagues and remember that we are all here for the one goal. Save this patient in front of us. Together.

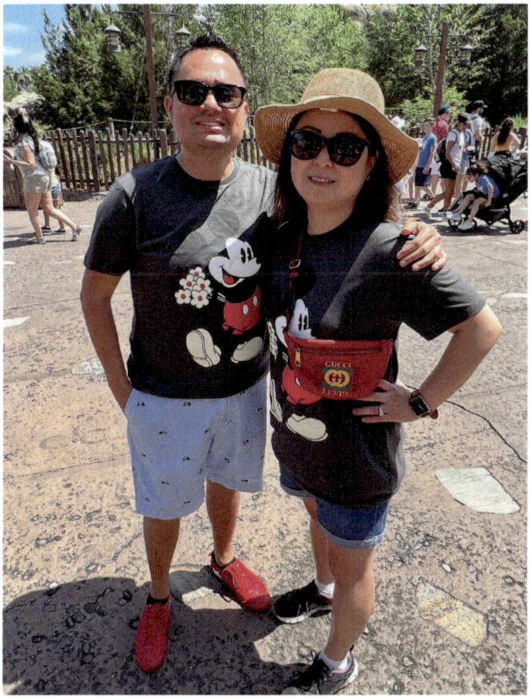

Forever call mates between surgery and emergency medicine, with Claudio Fernandez, DO, Emergency Medicine

Reference

1. Pun JK, Matthiessen CH, Murray KA, Slade D. Factors affecting communication in emergency departments: doctors and nurses’ perceptions of communication in a trilingual ED in Hong Kong. Int J Emerg Med. 2015;8:48.

What are the patient's immediate concerns?
Make referrals for support as needed
Explore what the news means to the patient

Chapter 69
Effective Documentation

Carmen Julia Martínez Martínez and Caroline Molins

Documentation is essential in many aspects of medicine. This is also true for emergency medicine (EM). Therefore, understanding critical aspects of documentation are imperative to all those involved. This chapter will discuss three key points: the purpose of emergency department (ED) documentation, the unique characteristic of ED documentation, and the importance of quality documentation.

How Is the ED Chart Different from Other Charts?

Emergency department visits are complex as they can be seen as outpatient and inpatient visit. In addition, ED visits are usually time sensitive and under high stake environments. Therefore, emergency physicians (EPs) are expected to be thorough, accurate, detailed, and efficient as they capture all the information for high-quality patient care and document this care as well.

The Purpose

Understanding the purpose of documentation is crucial to those who practice medicine. In EM, like other specialties, the purpose can be summarized into three main components: Patient care and communication, Medico-legal, and Billing/reimbursement.

C. J. M. Martínez (✉) · C. Molíns
Department of Emergency Medicine, University of South Alabama, Mobile, AL, USA

Department of Emergency Medicine, AdventHealth, Orlando, FL, USA
e-mail: cmartinez@health.southalabama.edu

R. P. Olympia et al. (eds.), *An Emergency Physician's Path*,
https://doi.org/10.1007/978-3-031-47873-4_69

Patient Care/Communication

Emergency department medical records are foremost a means of communication. It communicates the patient's ED course from when they enter the ED to when they depart. This includes communication between physicians, nurses, technicians, respiratory therapists, social workers, and all of the ED care team. Furthermore, it accurately captures the provided care given at the ED for consultants who will see the patient later. Effectively documenting these communications should be done in an unbiased format. This can be incredibly challenging when difficult situations interfere with the workflow.

The chart should include every action taken to address the patient's chief complaints and abnormal vital signs. In addition, it should include all pertinent details that substantiate the differential diagnosis.

Medico-Legal

All forms of medical documentation are discoverable in medico-legal action. Although there is no standard of care for documentation, the chart must communicate that the care given to the patient adheres to the standard of care for a particular chief complaint/diagnosis.

Billing/Reimbursement

Most medical records are used for billing purposes. Although the exact nature of how billing occurs is in constant flux, particularly in emergency medicine, comprehension of some basic concepts is crucial. This aspect has three main components: History, Physical Exam (PE), and Medical decision-making (MDM). The history component includes a chief complaint, history of present illness (HPI), review of systems (ROS), and past medical/surgical/family/social history (PMFS). Although there is no specific number of components required for billing, it is important to be medically appropriate. The chief complaint is necessary for all ED documentation, regardless of its level of billing. The HPI section should contain: (1) Location, (2) Quality, (3) Duration, (4) Modifying factors, (5) Timing, (6) Severity, (7) Context, and (8) Associated signs and symptoms. The ROS section is divided into the traditional organ systems. Therefore, it is essential to document the pertinent positives and negatives as it relates to the HPI. The PMFS section includes past medical (surgical history, prior hospitalizations, immunizations, medications/vitamins, and allergies), family history (illness and causes of death in family members), and social history (tobacco, alcohol, drugs, sexual, marital status, employment, education). Similar to ROS, PE should be focused and medically relevant.

Although some components are easily understood, others can be elusive, particularly the MDM. The MDM includes identifying diagnosis, assessing the status of the condition, and the management. In addition, three elements define the MDM, the number and complexities of the problems, the amount of data reviewed or analyzed (this includes prior medical records, office records, laboratory tests and imaging ordered during the current ED visit, consultations with other healthcare providers, improvement or worsening of problems) and the risk of complications of patient management decisions.

Quality

ED documentation comes in wide varieties—handwritten, dictated/transcribed, scribed, templated, and electronic medical records. The American College of Emergency Physicians Policy statement on "Patient Medical Records in the Emergency Department" mentions that high-quality ED medical records can promote improved patient care. Therefore, ED medical records are often referenced when discerning quality assessment and improvement initiatives.

Electronic health records (EHRs) gather, create, and store patient information. It both presents benefits and challenges. The centralized nature of the records helps improve patient safety and service quality. In addition, it facilitates communication between all parties involved in a patient's care. However, for some physicians, it can be seen as time-consuming and an impediment to their workflow. Using EHRs tools like templates, dictation, shortcut phrases, and macros will help maximize documentation efficiency. Documentation should be completed as much as possible in real-time. The physician's mind is fresh to remember all the details of the encounter as it is happening. The time that will take a physician to document will double or triple if done at the end of the shift. Furthermore, only some details will be fresh, and the assessments of patients with similar presentations can get mixed, resulting in inaccurate charting. Furthermore, it is important to remember that EHRs keep metadata every time the charts are accessed and if any modifications are made. Suspicious access to gather information or chart amendments can lead to denial of claim by insurance companies and legal ramifications.

Key Tips to Remember

(a) One of the goals of ED charting is to summarize and communicate the patient's ED visit effectively and accurately.
(b) Chart readers (i.e., patients, doctors, lawyers, insurance companies, and administration) will invest hours reading a document that you, the author, wrote in about 30 min.

(c) Addressing vital signs, especially if abnormal, is crucial. Document every reassessment.
(d) ED documentation should be done in an all-inclusive, time-efficient, effective, cost-conservative manner and flow in an easy-reading format.
(e) Complete your documentation in real time. It will take you double or triple the time to complete it at the end of your shift.

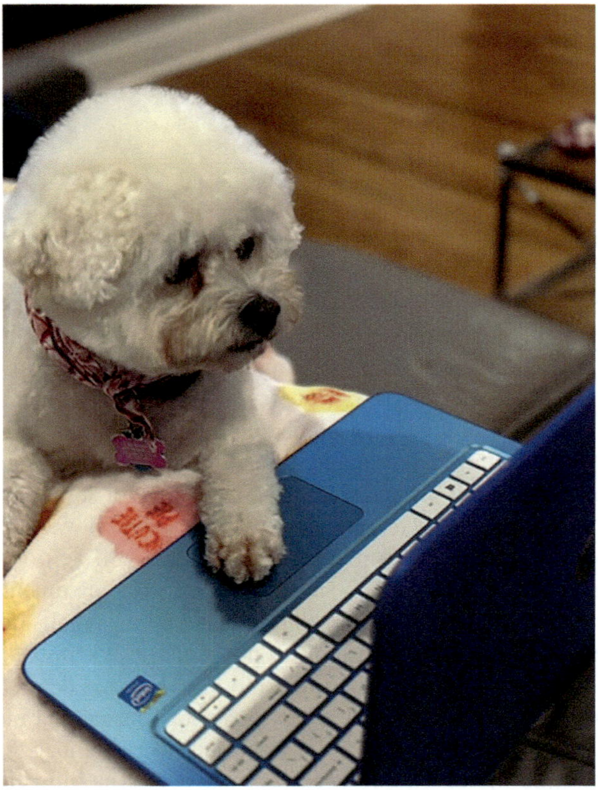

Effective documentation requires organization, reflection, completeness, and a steady paw

Suggested Readings

1. ACEP. Medical decision making and the Marshfield Clinic Scoring Tool FAQ. May 2021. https://www.acep.org/administration/reimbursement/reimbursement-faqs/medical-decision-making-and-the-marshfield-clinic-scoring-tool-faq/.
2. ACEP. Patient medical records in the emergency department. June 2022. https://www.acep.org/patient-care/policy-statements/patient-medical-records-in-the-emergency-department/.

3. ACEP. Medical decision making and the Marshfield Clinic Scoring Tool FAQ. n.d.. https://www.acep.org/administration/reimbursement/reimbursement-faqs/medical-decision-making-and-the-marshfield-clinic-scoring-tool-faq/.
4. Lorenzetti DL, et al. Strategies for improving physician documentation in the emergency department: a systematic review. BMC Emerg Med. 2018;18(1):36. https://doi.org/10.1186/s12873-018-0188-z.
5. Tung S. A guide to charting in the ed. CanadiEM. 15 Apr 2020. https://canadiem.org/a-guide-to-charting-in-the-ed/.
6. Yu KT, Green RA. Critical aspects of emergency department documentation and communication. Emerg Med Clin North Am. 2009;27(4):641–54, ix. https://doi.org/10.1016/j.emc.2009.07.008.

R = Rapport: Make a connection

[illegible]

... patient's overall impression of ...

the institution to others. Satisfied patients are also ...

Chapter 70
Risk Management and Patient Safety

Linda Gangai

What Is Quality in Healthcare?

Quality can mean different things to different people in healthcare. It can encompass risk, infection control, patient safety, and performance improvement. The Institute of Medicine's (IOM) framework includes six aims for quality healthcare. Care should be: Safe, Effective, Patient-centered, Timely, Efficient, and Equitable [1]. These aims provide guidance as you deliver care and serve as a measure when reviewing care. You will deliver some extraordinary, lifesaving care while working in emergency medicine. You will also be involved in cases where the patient did not receive the appropriate care, resulting in a patient safety incident [2]. Patient harm is rarely due to egregious or malevolent behavior on the part of the physician or other team members. Rather, harm is caused by a combination of system factors, human factors, and individual actions together. These events not only harm the patient but also impact clinicians.

Quality improvement and patient safety science helps us to identify, understand, and address the various factors involved in the events to prevent future harm. Some elements of quality improvement include: the Plan Do Study Act (PDSA) cycle (an iterative process), continuous improvement, data, change management, and, in my opinion, the most important element—trust-based relationships [3]. See recommended readings at the end of the chapter for more detailed information on quality improvement and patient safety.

Patient safety science is focused on reducing harm to patients and staff. When either reviewing events or completing a root cause analysis (RCA), the

L. Gangai (✉)
Emergency Medicine, Penn State Health-Milton S. Hershey Medical Center, Hershey, PA, USA
e-mail: Lgangai@pennstatehealth.psu.edu

R. P. Olympia et al. (eds.), *An Emergency Physician's Path*,
https://doi.org/10.1007/978-3-031-47873-4_70

organization's goal is to identify any system issues, fix them and prevent recurrence. Organizations with a robust safety system have active leadership involvement, provide education on human error and the corresponding error prevention tools, and create a culture that supports reporting and interventions to prevent future errors.

You may hear the term High Reliability Organization (HRO) in quality and safety circles. This term comes from the high-risk fields of aviation and nuclear energy. Despite the potential for catastrophic events, they have outstanding safety records and predictable, high performing systems. Healthcare systems are striving to adapt HRO concepts into their organizations, some are further along than others [4]. The HRO principles consist of: (1) preoccupation with failure, (2) reluctance to simplify, (3) sensitivity to operations, (4) commitment to resilience and (5) deference to expertise. Preoccupation with failure is identifying small errors or gaps which can be indicative of bigger problems. Reluctance to simplify is refraining from minimizing or dismissing issues, as in the statement, "we have always done it that way". Sensitivity to operations requires mindfulness of the big picture and knowing a problem in one area can have downstream effects. Commitment to resilience is the capacity to address unexpected events and prevent their spread. Deference to expertise is making sure those with the appropriate expertise are making the decision, even if lower in the organizational hierarchy [5]. See recommended readings at the end of the chapter for more detailed information on HRO concepts.

The Emergency Department (ED) is a chaotic, unpredictable and exciting environment to practice medicine. This chaos creates a "natural laboratory for error" [6]. No discussion about patient safety is complete without mentioning human error, a favorite science of mine. As humans, our actions can go awry. A key component of error is that they are unintentional. Errors can be classified as latent and active. Latent errors are those concealed in a system (design, equipment, policies). Active errors are errors which cause harm either in the design of the action or performance of it [7]. Active errors can be further classified into lapses, slips, and mistakes. For example, if you forget to order a test, that is a lapse. If you pick the wrong side for a hip X-ray, that is a slip. If you order a CXR on a patient with cellulitis of the leg, that is a mistake. If you are interested in learning more about human error and healthcare, there is an excellent resource listed under recommended readings at the end of the chapter.

How Do We Apply the Science, Tools, and Concepts into Practice? Let's Walk Through a Serious Safety Event

Here is the scenario (reality-based): A male patient, 50–75 years old, with history of HTN, CAD, left BKA (secondary to trauma), and cholecystectomy presents to the ED with complaints of abdominal pain. During a brief exam in triage, their HR and BP are noted to be slightly elevated. The patient shares his abdomen was checked for something but does not know what it was. The astute clinician is concerned this could be an Abdominal Aortic Aneurysm (AAA). They order a CXR, labs, and a computerized tomography angiography (CTA) scan of the abdomen. After 2 hours, while waiting for the lab results, the patient experiences a significant increase in abdominal pain. He is taken to the scanner, arrests, and expires despite all efforts. It was a ruptured AAA.

What Happens Next?

The first step is to check in with the clinicians involved. Be familiar with what resources are available in your organization. This is a stressful event not only for the family but also the care team. Most organizations offer a staff debriefing opportunity in some form or another [8, 9].

Second, notify your risk, patient safety, or quality department of the event. Commonly, the details of the event are entered into a patient safety software system, usually tied to the electronic health record. Learn the specific process at your health system. Upon receiving the report, the safety team will classify the event based upon state requirements and the health system's Patient Safety Organization (PSO) criteria. PSOs, required under the Patient Safety Act of 2005, serve to improve care and reduce adverse events [10].

What constitutes a serious safety event (SSE)? An SSE needs to have a gap or deviation in care resulting in patient harm. Consider these situations. First, a patient receives the wrong medication but has no harm; there was an error but no harm. This is not an SSE. Second, a patient gets the wrong medication, has an allergic reaction with a severe rash, leading to scars. This is an SSE. There was a deviation (RN did not scan the medication's barcode) and there was patient harm. Think about our case, what do you think the primary gap was? The answer: a delay in imaging.

After the key information is reported, the medical record is reviewed and clinician feedback is obtained. The safety or risk team will evaluate the severity and permanence of harm. The SSE is classified based upon severity (moderate or severe) and permanence (temporary or permanent). Generally, there is either a numerical or alphabetical severity scale. For our discussion, we will use the numerical scale from 1–5 with 1 being death and 5 being temporary with moderate harm. Our case is classified as an SSE 1.

Root Cause Analysis

After an event is classified and determined to be an SSE, the next step is a comprehensive review of the care. The Joint Commission (and some states) mandates review of SSEs within a specific timeframe as well as specific action items to prevent recurrence. An RCA is the standard for reviewing SSEs. It follows a structured approach and was originally used to analyze industrial events. The goal of an RCA is not to place blame but to identify the active errors (where the system and individual intersect) and latent errors (buried system weakness) that contributed to the event and then make appropriate modifications to prevent recurrence [11]. We look for the "why" this happened, implement system changes to prevent them, and share the lessons learned across the organization.

Who conducts the RCA and what does it entail? This varies by health system but common elements include: trained facilitators, staff interviews, subject matter experts, mapping the sequence of events, identifying staff deviations or systems issues which influenced the staff, and, lastly, producing action items to improve the processes. The RCA team understands this is a stressful experience for the clinicians and attempts to make it as comfortable as possible. Generally, legal counsel is not allowed in the interviews, as this review falls under quality improvement and patient safety.

What about the individual's culpability in the event? Many health systems have adopted the "Just Culture" principle as defined by J. Reason [12, p. 141]. This model represents the middle ground of a blameless (no one's fault) to blaming (it is all your fault) models. It is focused on creating a culture of trust so events are reported and reviewed. It also provides a decision tree to identify culpability, if present. The culpability decision tree puts the clinician's actions through a series of questions or tests [12, p.151]. The RCA team uses the decision tree when reviewing the case and reports on the findings.

Let's put our case through the decision tree. First, was there evidence of malicious intent, substance abuse, or violation of policy? If the answer is "no", then we land on the substitution test. Would someone else, having the same training, in a similar situation, have done the same thing? In this case I believe this is a "yes", which instructs us to coach/console the individual and identify and fix system issues [12, p. 151].

Implementation of Action Items

After the information is collected, the RCA team will identify the root causes and subsequent action items to address them. Getting back to our case, there were several root causes with associated action items. We will discuss one specific action item that I was responsible for: the creation of a guideline to expedite care of patients with a suspected AAA. The guideline is a system-based solution to prevent recurrence. It was a collaborative effort between the divisions of emergency medicine, vascular surgery, and trauma surgery.

Time is critical for patients with a suspected AAA. The overall mortality rate associated with a ruptured AAA is 80–90%. Prompt recognition is key to delivering the appropriate treatment of either open or endovascular repair [13]. Emergency medicine and surgery each play a vital role in this patient's care. Not every patient who presents with a AAA is actively rupturing but the potential of rupture exists.

Our goal is to get images as soon as possible and have a process to quickly get a surgeon to the bedside.

In order to write this guideline, we reviewed available published protocols and then met to create one for our organization. The "we" included EM quality, Chief Vascular and Chief Trauma surgeons. The AAA guideline was drafted and included an algorithm for quick reference to reduce cognitive load in a critical situation. The algorithm is comprised of two arms based on the patient's systolic BP (SBP):

If the SBP >100 mmHg, labs are waived and they are prioritized to the CT scanner.
If the SBP is ≤100 mmHg, the EM physician activates the newly-formed AAA Alert.

The AAA alert sends a page to a key group of staff and includes: vascular surgeons (attendings & residents), radiologist, radiology techs, OR Charge RN, respiratory, ED key staff, and trauma surgeons (attendings & residents). The surgeons decide the next steps whether it is taking the patient directly to the operating room or getting images. What this does from a systems perspective is to deliver quality care with the incorporation of the "Timely" aim from the IOMs 6 aims.

Once the guideline was created and approved by the organization, we moved onto the implementation phase. Implementing system changes can, at times, feel like you are a snail stuck in cement. Guideline approval was very prompt; however, creating the paging group required substantially more time and effort. There is more to pagers and the telecommunications infrastructure at hospitals than meets the eye. I learned more about pagers than I wanted to know. There are different types including: short range, long range, and my favorite, the ghost pager. Once the pagers were programmed, we conducted two test pages and were ready to go live.

The protocol was ready and went live in under a year, an impressive feat in some organizations. Our first AAA Alert was called 10 days after the go live. The appropriate staff responded, the patient went to the OR, had a repair and was discharged home. Two months later, the second AAA Alert was paged, which was technically an over call but based upon the patient's history and presenting symptoms, was reasonable. The third AAA Alert followed about 3 months after the go live. This one did not work entirely as expected but did not cause any patient harm. It did allow us to identify and correct errors, both human and technical. This is why it is so important to have redundancy in processes and practice the HRO principles we discussed earlier.

We reviewed the three AAA alerts to understand (1) what went well, (2) what went wrong and how was it caught, and (3) what system factors influenced the various individuals. As discussed earlier in this chapter, quality improvement is an iterative process; we are always looking to improve. The following were our findings from our third alert that did not go as intended as well as the type of error involved.

1. Context: The first two alerts went off on weekdays, during daylight hours. The third alert occurred on the weekend, during the nighttime hours.
2. Humans: The operator incorrectly paged the AAA alert as a Trauma alert. This is an example of active error, a *mistake*. Thankfully, Trauma alerts bring significant resources to the ED including surgeons. The operator's coworker noted the

error and corrected the page within 1 min. This is a good example of the HRO principle: *sensitivity to operations*.

3. Pagers: The programming of the pagers (yes, the clunky bricks of a bygone era) is an example of active error. The ED and Trauma team (already in house) assemble and wait for the patient to arrive. As they are caring for the patient, the team notices the vascular surgeon has not arrived (not in house). This is an example of HRO behavior, specifically the *principle of sensitivity to operations*. They decide to call the vascular surgeon to make sure they are on their way. The vascular surgeon (very close by) arrives quickly and joins the team. The patient agrees to surgery and is taken to the OR. It turns out when the long-range pagers were programmed, a step was missed. This is an example of active error-a *slip and mistake*. Since they were in house when tested, the error was not observable. This is an example of *latent error*. Once identified, the pagers were corrected immediately. After, all pagers were tested multiple times on the weekends and in the evening hours and functioned appropriately, I applied multiple principles of HRO including *pre-occupation with failure, sensitivity to operations, reluctance to simplify*, and *practicing resilience*.

To summarize, we put the process in place, identified gaps, closed the gaps and now we monitor for success, unintended consequences, and any gaps yet to be found.

10 Parting Pearls

1. Data is important but relationships are crucial; make friends and improve the care together. Work on a project with a service you interact with on a regular basis.
2. Look to improve, not to defend.
3. Fear and caution, in the correct amount, will keep you and your patients safe.
4. SLOW DOWN and PAUSE, the 30 seconds you take can save your patient from serious harm.
5. Be receptive to feedback when your cases are reviewed, because they will be reviewed.
6. Respect and listen to the concerns brought forward from other team members, no matter their credentials.
7. Call out unsafe behavior or practice when you see it and escalate appropriately.
8. Strive for well-designed systems. Well-designed systems make it easy to do the right thing and hard to do the wrong thing.
9. Evaluate your organization's commitment to safety and quality.
10. Read the chapter in this book on "Multitasking and Rapid Task Switching".

References

1. Six domains of health care quality. Content last reviewed Nov 2018. Rockville: Agency for Healthcare Research and Quality. https://www.ahrq.gov/talkingquality/measures/six-domains.html.
2. Croskerry P, Campbell SG. A cognitive autopsy approach towards explaining diagnostic failure. Cureus. 2021;13(8):e17041. https://doi.org/10.7759/cureus.17041. Erratum in: Cureus. 2021 Sep 13;13(9):c48.
3. Plan-do-study-act (PDSA) directions and examples. Content last reviewed Sept 2020. Rockville: Agency for Healthcare Research and Quality. https://www.ahrq.gov/health-literacy/improve/precautions/tool2b.html.
4. Sutcliffe KM, Paine L, Pronovost PJ. Re-examining high reliability: actively organising for safety. BMJ Qual Saf. 2017;26:248–51.
5. Rotteau L, et al. Striving for high reliability in healthcare: a qualitative study of the implementation of a hospital safety programme. BMJ Qual Saf. 2022;31(12):867–77.
6. Amaniyan S, Faldaas BO, Logan PA, Vaismoradi M. Learning from patient safety incidents in the emergency department: a systematic review. J Emerg Med. 2020;58(2):234–44. https://doi.org/10.1016/j.jemermed.2019.11.015.
7. Sameera V, Bindra A, Rath G. Human errors and their prevention in healthcare. J Anaesthesiol Clin Pharmacol. 2021;37(3):328–35.
8. Cantu L, Thomas L. Baseline well-being, perceptions of critical incidents, and openness to debriefing in community hospital emergency department clinical staff before COVID-19, a cross-sectional study. BMC Emerg Med. 2020;20(1):82. https://doi.org/10.1186/s12873-020-00372-5.
9. Rose S, Cheng A. Charge nurse facilitated clinical debriefing in the emergency department. CJEM. 2018;20(5):781–5. https://doi.org/10.1017/cem.2018.369.
10. Frequently asked questions. Content last reviewed July 2021. Rockville: Agency for Healthcare Research and Quality. https://pso.ahrq.gov/faq.
11. AHRQ root cause. https://psnet.ahrq.gov/primer/root-cause-analysis#.
12. Clapper C, Merlino J, Stockmeier C. Zero harm: how to achieve patient and workforce safety in healthcare. New York: McGraw-Hill Education; 2019.
13. Hoornweg LL, Storm-Versloot MN, Ubbink DT, Koelemay MJW, Legemate DA, Balm R. Meta analysis on mortality of ruptured abdominal aortic aneurysms. Eur J Vasc Endovasc Surg. 2008;35(5):558–70. https://doi.org/10.1016/j.ejvs.2007.11.019.

Recommended Readings

Human Factors

14. National Center for Human Factors in Healthcare. https://www.medstarhealth.org/innovation-and-research/national-center-for-human-factors-in-healthcare.

Quality Improvement

15. Institute for Healthcare Improvement. https://www.ihi.org/resources/Pages/HowtoImprove/ScienceofImprovementTestingChanges.aspx.

Patient Safety

16. Institute for Healthcare Improvement. https://www.ihi.org/Topics/PatientSafety/Pages/default.aspx.
17. Agency for Healthcare Research and Quality. https://psnet.ahrq.gov/.
18. Edwards MT. An organizational learning framework for patient safety. Am J Med Qual. 2017;32(2):148–55. https://doi.org/10.1177/1062860616632295.

High Reliability

19. Agency for Healthcare Research and Quality. https://psnet.ahrq.gov/primer/high-reliability.

Chapter 71
Peer Review/Presenting Morbidity and Mortality Conference

Nkeiruka N. Onyenekwu

Years ago, as a senior resident, I supervised a very zealous intern who discharged a patient after what appeared to be an uneventful admission. The patient returned some time later with a complication. I wish we had received those fearful words, "Remember that patient…" Instead we were blindsided by a case review during a Morbidity and Mortality conference. My intern, upon listening to the opening remarks, 'conveniently' received a page and did not return for the entire hour, leaving me to explain what might have gone wrong. Hot seat is an underestimation, try a sauna or Sahara seat. By the end of the hour, I felt like my colleagues had placed hot iron on my behind while I had to bend over, pretending not to be burned. Although there were many factors that resulted in the patient returning to the hospital, it felt like all eyes were on my team.

Present-day morbidity and mortality (M&M) conference has moved from the traditional surgeon-specific case review experience to various specialties working on quality improvement (QI) initiatives. Typically, cases were selected from those who volunteered an 'interesting' diagnosis and/or posed potential hospital liability. Now, M&Ms. are prevalent among Emergency Medicine (EM) residency programs and are an indispensable piece of quality improvement initiatives. Studies emphasize the significance of not only presenting a portrayal of weird cases, or cases in which death could be attributable solely to co-morbidities [1]. A selective presentation introduces bias, prevents objective analysis of methods and mitigates research and interview of participants. This often discourages engaged learners and/or faculty from reporting errors or unsafe conditions in fear of retribution. It also did not provide a case pool of "near misses" and health care disparities which hold value in education and QI implementation. Near misses, defined as events that have potential

N. N. Onyenekwu (✉)
Department of Diagnostic Medicine, Second Opinion Consultants, New Orleans, LA, USA

R. P. Olympia et al. (eds.), *An Emergency Physician's Path*,
https://doi.org/10.1007/978-3-031-47873-4_71

harm but are detected prior to reaching the patient, have particular value for discussion in these conferences from a patient safety and systems perspective [1]. Given the new focus on patient safety and QI, there is a shift from analysis of incidents that may or may not be preventable to those that have system-wide implications of failure, even in the face of no actual harm to the patient [1]. Continuing medical education (CME), obviously the longest stage of medical education, has traditionally been out-of-town medical conferences with an instructor at the front of the room. The teacher-driven nature of CME gives little attention to the concept of professional development [2]. One of the purposes of M&M is to promote professionalism and ethical integrity.

The following three themes emerged as the key components of running an effective morbidity and mortality conference: the importance of (1) careful case identification/selection, (2) case presentation/structure and (3) derivatives developed after the conference in the form of QI implementation. To help standardize care, Emergency Departments (EDs) should hold regular case-based error reduction conferences (CBERCs) with a system focus. "Programs should ensure that their CBERCs reflect sound educational goals and move away from the perceptions of "shame and blame" associated with the traditional M&M conference" [3]. How this translates will depend on the presenter. "Knowledge translation is defined as exchange, synthesis, and ethically sound application of knowledge—within a complex system of interactions among researchers and users—to accelerate the capture of the benefits of research…through improved health, more effective services and products, and strengthened health care system" [2]. Knowledge translation can draw on people from many disciplines to join evidence and practice of medicine. All physicians should be trained in the science of patient safety and QI. Compliance with this requirement relies on the M&M conference to expose physicians to quality-related issues such as the Pathman-Preceed Model.

Case Selection

The first stage of preparing for M&M is case selection. Most hospitals have some form of incident identification. Cases should be deliberately chosen for their benefit in securing the goals of process and performance improvement. Four weeks prior to M&M allows sufficient time for preparation [4]. Productive discussion is more likely to occur if selection of cases stem from system failures. To not divert attention from system failures, case analysis should be separate from peer review. "Feedback from involved providers should be sought early and in detail as the health record may not accurately reflect the care episode and to avoid recall bias" [3].

Case Presentation

Each M&M begins with a plain outline of patient safety and education. In order to facilitate discussion, it is the duty of the presenter to succinctly convey the pertinent details of events. Programs should institute a standardized, structured, and systems-based approach to case presentation as this allows presenters to concentrate on the most important details while ignoring irrelevant issues. Using a standardized methodology, error analysis should be performed by a group review. This evaluation includes the cause of medical error as it applies to judgment, knowledge, communication, documentation, process, workflow, and technique. Completing the tables related to the Pathman-Preceed (Table 71.1) and Association of Litigation and Risk Management (ALARM) (Table 71.2) Models also aid in developing a discussion. SBAR which stands for (Situation, Background, Assessment, Recommendations) is a framework for presenting cases at M&M conferences. "This framework, adapted from other high-risk industries, is designed to facilitate clear and consistent communication, leading to higher quality presentations with improved educational value" [3]. Originally in the Emergency Medicine and Trauma departments of an Ottawa hospital, the Ottawa M&M Model (OM3) standardized and gave structure to these departments [1, 5].

Table 71.1 Pathman-preceed model for knowledge translation

Method types/stages	Awareness	Agreement	Adoption	Adherence
Predisposing				
Enabling				
Enforcing				

Table 71.2 ALARM model

Factor types	Influencing contributory factors	Examples
Institutional context	Economic and regulatory context; national health service executive; clinical negligence scheme for trusts	Inconsistent policies, funding problems
Organizational and management factors	Financial resources and constraints; organizational structure; policy standards and goals; safety culture and priorities	Lacking senior management procedure for risk reduction
Work environment factors	Staffing levels and skills mix; workload and shift patterns; design, availability, and maintenance of equipment; administrative and managerial support	High workload, inadequate staffing, or limited access to essential equipment
Team factors	Verbal communication; written communication; supervision and seeking help; team structure (consistency, leadership, etc.)	Poor communication between staff
Individual (staff) factors	Knowledge and skills; competence; physical and mental health	Lack of knowledge or experience of specific staff

Studies show development of fact presentations through visual aids, e.g., a PowerPoint presentation, with little disturbances from the M&M audience. M&M presentations should preserve anonymity to reduce fear of reporting. Presenters can either issue a summary to the group of system failures or ask the audience to brainstorm areas of improvement. The former allows for greater evaluation of the presenter's understanding of the case. However, the latter allows for input across the healthcare professions, disciplines, and other specialties, which has been shown to identify more issues needing improvement. Therefore, the latter would be the structure of choice with respect to advancing QI and patient safety [1].

QI Implementation

Once systemic failures are identified, it is important to address the deficiency immediately. A group of organizers (preferably multi-disciplinary and inclusive of physicians) should meet post-CBERC. This meeting is to unite on error types, strategy and discussion of the deficiencies identified by root cause analysis. The specific recommendations should have a detailed plan which includes time frame, responsible person(s) to lead, inclusion of existing QI team and a list of less urgent QI issues that cannot immediately be addressed [1]. Some studies show sharing previous QI successes to attendees 5 to 10 min proceeding every M&M is impactful [1]. If this is not feasible, consider periodic updates on the progress of QI improvements or summary of meeting minutes of post CBERC group. In conjunction with the QI team, determine measurable factors that define effectiveness of implementation.

Conclusions

The M&M conference is a form of incident analysis that has been present in medicine since 1904. However, M&M often is absent of standardized structure to adequately train residents in performance improvement and establish a benefit in continued medical education. Given the new focus on patient safety and QI, M&Ms. may show benefit in continuing medical education and in programs without residency programs. The focus on patient safety is a shift from analysis of incidents that may or may not be preventable to those that have system-wide implications of failure, even in the face of no actual harm to the patient. The following three themes emerged as the key components of running an effective morbidity and mortality conference: the importance of (1) careful case identification/selection, (2) case presentation/structure and (3) derivatives developed after the conference in the form of QI implementation. In addition, a multidisciplinary approach and inclusion of hospital QI staff can expedite patient safety issues and areas for improvement. The result is QI initiatives and policy changes, but the ongoing issue focuses on the inability to measure the effectiveness of these changes to the M&M format.

References

1. Churchill KP, Murphy J, Smith N. Quality improvement focused morbidity and mortality rounds: an integrative review. Cureus. 2020;12(12):e12146.
2. Davis D, Evans M, et al. The case for knowledge translation: shortening the journey from evidence to effect. BMJ. 2003;327(7405):33–5.
3. Chathampally Y, Cooper B, et al. Evolving from morbidity and mortality to a case-based error reduction conference: evidence-based best practices from the Council of Emergency Medicine Residency Directors. West J Emerg Med. 2020;21(6):231–41.
4. Tapper EB, Leffler DA. The morbidity and mortality conference in gastroenterology and hepatology: an important cornerstone of patient safety and optimal care. Gastroenterology. 2016;150:19–23.
5. The Ottawa M&M model: a guide to enhancing morbidity & mortality rounds. https://emottawablog.com/wp-content/uploads/2018/03/OM3-Guide_2018-1.pdf.

Further Reading

ACGME program requirements for graduate medical education in emergency medicine. https://www.acgme.org/globalassets/pfassets/programrequirements/110_emergencymedicine_2022.pdf.

Gregor A, Taylor D. Morbidity and mortality conference: its purpose reclaimed and grounded in theory. Teach Learn Med. 2016;28:439–47.

Szostek JH, Wieland ML, Loertscher LL, et al. A systems approach to morbidity and mortality conference. Am J Med. 2010;123:663–8.

Chapter 72
Dealing with Malpractice Lawsuits

Harrison Wermuth and Kassem Makki

Introduction

As we begin our journey to become physicians, we learn our field is composed of information from the medical and social sciences, demographics, and a smattering of legal bodies of knowledge, specifically case studies on litigation. As undergraduate students, unless the field of study for a degree was in pre-law you gained little to no exposure to the topic of medical malpractice. During my time as a medical student, the discussion of medical malpractice was usually coupled with ethics courses. However, longitudinal learning on this topic remains scarce throughout all medical school curriculums. As resident physicians, we learn through the experiences of our mentors and attending physicians grasping information from cases seen throughout our shifts. As attending physicians, if named in a malpractice claim, advice is taken from our legal counsel. The aspects of the medical-legal jargon and the policies of our malpractice insurance remain a complex topic to comprehend due to the lack of exposure in learning about risk management in preventing medical malpractice litigation.

Of the many causes of medical malpractice throughout all specialties, misdiagnosis remains at the top of the list [1]. Emergency medicine physicians carry a 7.5% annual risk of litigation and a 1.5% risk of secure indemnity payment. In terms of indemnity, it is defined as the total amount paid to the plaintiff, while a closed claim

H. Wermuth (✉)
Department of Emergency Medicine, Saint Barnabas Hospital, Bronx, NY, USA
e-mail: hwermuth@sbhny.org

K. Makki
Department of Emergency Medicine-Brooklyn, New York Presbyterian Brooklyn Methodist Hospital, New York, NY, USA
e-mail: makkikas@msu.edu

R. P. Olympia et al. (eds.), *An Emergency Physician's Path*, https://doi.org/10.1007/978-3-031-47873-4_72

refers to claims that have completed all legal processing and appeals [2]. Critical areas of high-risk litigation include missed acute myocardial infarction, neglected fractures/foreign bodies, abdominal pain/appendicitis, wounds, intracranial bleeding, aortic aneurysm, and pediatric meningitis [2]. These risks have brought about the practice of defensive medicine, which includes performing diagnostic testing that may not offer any additional diagnostic advantages or be in the patient's best interest; however, for the physician, this is motivated on the fear of malpractice risk.

As we move through this chapter, we will discuss the causes of malpractice and the most likely missed diagnosis in the emergency department leading to litigation. Additionally, the preventable causes such as complex patient interactions and shift change will be addressed. Lastly, we will describe malpractice insurance policies and the steps to take when involved in medical malpractice litigation.

Specific Medical Condition & Approaches

Based on Claims History in Emergency Medicine, the medical diagnoses with the highest number of claims paid are Chest Pain, Abdominal Pain, Critical Neurological Problems, Psychiatric Patients, Bone Fractures, Hand Injuries, and Aortic aneurysms. This section is not exhaustive but highlights aspects of these conditions that may be overlooked and lead to increased litigation.

1. Chest Pain and Acute Coronary Syndrome:

   One of the highest paid-to-close ratios of indemnity pay in medical malpractice litigation is Acute Coronary Syndrome, specifically Acute Myocardial Infarction (AMI), due to its mortality [1]. Many emergency medicine providers over-rely on determining disposition on the initial laboratory studies and EKGs done in the ED, despite literature showing in the beginning timeline at AMI that the results may not be diagnostic, thus, leading to misdiagnoses [1]. Clinician should make a it a practice, if the cardiac pain is suspicious, to perform serial EKG studies and Troponins. Some of the other high-risk areas of chest pain deal with patients with atypical symptoms of all age patients, diabetic patients, and any patient, regardless of age, with a history of coronary artery disease [1]. Moreover, a physician needs to always consider aortic dissection in their evaluation of chest pain due to its high mortality and be observant of oxygen saturation and respiratory rate in the diagnosing pulmonary embolism.

   Physicians need to be cognizant of detailed documentation with all complaints of chest pain. The physician should ensure they are documenting the pertinent features of the cause of the pertinent chest pain, any associated symptoms, and the family history of cardiovascular risk factors. Physicians should also ensure comprehensive notes of their medical decision making process; this includes any tools utilized such as Heart Score and the conversation with the patient and their family. Physicians should also ensure the patient has proper follow-up outpatient instructions and follow up with pertinent specialists and providers to obtain further advanced diagnostics as necessary.

2. Bone Fractures & Hand Injuries:

   Although it carries a lower average indemnity, bone fractures or dislocations can be another frequent cause of litigation. Wounds accompanying the fractures can also become infected if left untreated which can lead to further harm to the patient and add an increased risk of being named in a medical malpractice case [1]. Aside from interpreting the radiologist's findings, it is the responsibility of the emergency medicine physician first to decide whether an X-ray or another radiographic study is necessary. When ordering the study, the physician must also provide all information to the radiologist to help guide them to the specific area of pathology. This can include a brief history and the area to be focused on during the examination. If a fracture is found, it is also essential to provide the patient with the appropriate follow-up to establish their continuity of care. If suspicion remains high after a negative study, the physician must also use their clinical gestalt to determine whether they would like a second read, further study, or consultation to a specialist on an inpatient or outpatient basis.

3. Psychiatric Patients:

   An emergency medicine physician's goal when evaluating a psychiatric patient is to determine the patient's cognition and behavior are from an organic or non-organic etiology. To accomplish this task, a physician will utilize the history gathering and physical examination to assess the patient's memory, attention, fund of knowledge, and level of consciousness [1]. Patients with an altered level of consciousness typically have a component that originates from a metabolic, toxic, or non-psychiatric cause [1]. Furthermore, no emergency medicine physician can medically clear a patient in the ED and should only document what they can do and determine if the patient is medically non-emergent.

4. Critical Neurological Problems:

   Strokes/TIA (Transient Ischemic Attack) and subarachnoid hemorrhages are two of the most cited medical diagnosis for neurological malpractice claims due to their high financial burden. However, most prevailing litigation cases resulted from omitted history, exams, hospitalizations, or involvement of neurologists in medical care [1]. The physician needs to complete and have a detailed neurological examination which includes cranial nerves, strength testing, reflexes when appropriate, and any changes during the emergency room course. Furthermore, patients need to be cognizant of the severe pathology versus ordinary headaches that frequently appear in the Emergency Department. Patients with subarachnoid hemorrhage and diseases of cerebral venous thrombosis do not always exhibit neurological deficits or the classical description of sudden onset.

5. Aortic Aneurysm:

   Another high mortality condition that results in indemnity payouts against Emergency Room physicians is aneurism of the abdominal aorta (AAA) often misdiagnosed due to diagnosis complexity [1]. Unfortunately, patient presentations do not always follow the classic description or expression, and it is more novel to find the classic triad of abdominal pain with concurrent back pain, hypotension, and pulsating abdominal mass. The imaging modalities that are the most reliable are Computer Topography (CT) followed by ultrasound which is highly sensitive and specific with an experienced operator and patients of ideal body weight [1]. A physician should always consider the differential AAA in patients with abdominal pain, flank pain, or lower back pain when the patient has a cardiovascular risk factor and age of 50 or greater. Physicians also need to remember that if CT imaging or the US of the Abdomen reveals an incidental finding of a AAA, it is imperative to document the condition in the medical record properly, and the discharge instructions have follow-up information for the AAA.

Difficult Patient Interactions

Some of the highest medical liability risk patient populations are the elderly, non-English speakers, and acutely intoxicated patients. When dealing with geriatric patients, especially patients who have a poor history, we need to reduce the litigation risk that an acute deterioration is most likely not due to underlying Alzheimer's or Dementia and often from an infection or polypharmacy. Regarding non-English speaking patients, the physician must try to use a qualified language interpreter since a language barrier is no excuse in medical malpractice litigation for inaccurate histories or a misdiagnosis. Some of the available resources currently available for physicians are AT&T Foreign Language Hotline and Voyce Translation Services. Furthermore, the physician needs to have an understanding that cultural variations may be an influence which could limit or impact their history. In emergent situations, it may be appropriate to utilize family if available. However, the physician must be aware of socially sensitive conditions such as history that relates to OBGYN. Finally, regarding acutely intoxicated patients, it is imperative to do a thorough physical examination to evaluate for signs of trauma and frequently reevaluate the patient to determine if further diagnostic studies are warranted if the patient is not "sobering" up as expected [3].

Communication

Having an open line of communication is crucial for the patient experience and is one of the most cited ways to reduce medical malpractice litigation. Based on claims analyses, physicians with lower patient satisfaction scores tended to be involved in more medical malpractice litigation. Physicians should try to take time to thoroughly explain their findings to the patient in simple and easily understood language, treatment options, and teaching of the disease state. In most states, in the event of poor outcomes, it is appropriate to emphasize with the patient, express disappointment, and follow steps to build rapport and have an open line of communication [4].

Shift Changes

One of the highest risk times in a physician's shift is during the transfer of care to another colleague. Any physician assuming the care of another physician is equally liable for the patient's care. The outgoing physician should do their best to ensure the oncoming colleague has all essential information in oral and written form, especially in patients with a high risk of clinical decompensation. The oncoming physician should strive to do their brief independent exam when receiving care, review all ordered imaging and laboratory studies, and use their clinical gestalt to change plans when necessary to ensure the patient is comfortable with the clinical course [1, 3, 5].

Discharge and Follow-up

It is paramount in reducing medical malpractice litigation that before discharge, a physician ensures and documents the patient has stable vital signs and addresses all complaints in the triage report and any new complaints that may have arisen during their ED Course. One of the leading areas of medical malpractice litigation is poorly advised and incomplete discharge instructions given by the physician provider. The treating physician should ensure in the discharge instructions that it includes the complete diagnosis, expected clinical course, potential reasons to return to the emergency room, associated complications to be watchful of, education on the proper dosing of all prescribed medications, and potential impact of any remaining test or imaging studies. If a patient leaves before receiving the final laboratory results or radiology imaging review, the physician should make it a practice to follow up on the results and contact the patient with any significant findings. Moreover, physicians should strive to ensure that patients receive prompt follow-up care with a primary care physician or specialist, depending on the ER visit. The patient must confirm that they understand the discharge and follow-up maintenance details, and the physician must document the discharge discussion; this will significantly reduce medical malpractice liability risk.

Leaving Against Medical Advice (AMA)

One of the misconceptions of physicians is that when a patient leaves against medical advice, this absolves the physician from culpability; however, in some medical malpractice litigation, it only connotes contributory negligence. Therefore, when a patient requests to leave AMA, it is imperative to ensure the patient has been fully informed of the risks and alternatives of their condition and has the capacity to fully understand their decision. Furthermore, the provider should document the AMA discussion, which details why the patient is leaving, follow-up instructions, an open invitation to return to the hospital, all attempts the physician made to offer treatment although less than optimal and incomplete, i.e., the patient was going to be admitted for IV Vancomycin Antibiotic therapy, however the physician prescribed PO Clindamycin, Linezolid, or other antibiotics to the pharmacy despite the patient choosing to leave AMA. If a physician follows the above steps, it will substantially reduce their contributory negligence liability [2].

Understanding Your Medical Malpractice Insurance Policy

Today, there are primarily two types of medical malpractice insurance policies in the United States: occurrence basis and claims made basis. The most comprehensive approach is occurrence-based insurance since it covers any claim occurring in the policy period regardless of when it was reported to the insurance carrier. On the other hand, claims made coverage only covers occurred losses that are reported during the active policy period unless the physician has a rider on the policy of nose or tail coverage. Nose coverage has an insurance carrier cover claims that occurred before the policy period, while tail coverage provides coverage for events that happened while the physician was practicing, even if the lawsuit was filed after the policy ended. Furthermore, especially if a claim is filed against the emergency medicine physician, they should understand the maximum liability that will be covered and if there is any specific language in the insurance policy that allows the insurance carrier to settle the claim without the physician's consent [3].

First Steps After Being Served Medical Malpractice Litigation

If at any time you are served a summons in Medical Malpractice Litigation, your first step is to contact your insurance carrier and/or your hospital's risk management divisions. At no time should you access the EMR to review the case or consider making any changes or addendums to the Medical Records. Most medical malpractice insurance carriers have recommendations or contracted defense medical malpractice attorney's they work with or recommend. You should feel comfortable with the attorney representing you and feel they will be a fierce advocate to represent your best interests. Furthermore, you should be open and honest with your attorney and be your best advocate by educating your attorney on the medical question at hand. By following these steps, you are ensuring the best chances of success in medical malpractice litigation [3].

Conclusion

Like most areas of medicine, an unfortunate aspect of practicing emergency medicine is the risk of medical malpractice litigation. Practicing prudent medicine with detailed and accurate documentation will minimize the overall risk of medical malpractice litigation. In the event of malpractice litigation, it is of critical importance to have detailed patient notes to support the course of treatment you provided. A physician's' chances of prevailing in a medical malpractice litigation lawsuit substantially decrease when the event documentation leaves ambiguity. A malpractice case is an anomaly due to the high daily patient volume. However, an emergency medicine physician will likely be sued at some point during their career. The void of detailed documentation is presumed in the American judicial system if it was not documented it was not done. Your best defense against medical malpractice litigation is to gain an accurate, thorough patient history with solid documentation. It is essential to practice emergency medicine consistently, building a strong rapport with every patient, which will provide an open and empathetic line of communication to ensure you gain the necessary facts to make best rapid practice decisions to facilitate the best outcome for each patient.

References

1. Bianchin C, Prevaldi C, Corradin M, Saia M. Medical malpractice claim risk in emergency departments. Emerg Care J. 2018;14(1) https://doi.org/10.4081/ecj.2018.6366.
2. Ferguson B, Geralds J, Petrey J, Huecker M. Malpractice in emergency medicine—a review of risk and mitigation practices for the emergency medicine provider. J Emerg Med. 2018;55(5):659–65. https://doi.org/10.1016/j.jemermed.2018.06.035.
3. Anderson RE. Medical malpractice a physician's sourcebook. Totowa, NJ: Humana Press; 2005.
4. Carlson JN, et al. Emergency physician practice changes after being named in a malpractice claim. Ann Emerg Med. 2020;75(2):221–35. https://doi.org/10.1016/j.annemergmed.2019.07.007.
5. Gurley KL, et al. Comparison of emergency medicine malpractice cases involving residents to nonresident cases. Acad Emerg Med. 2018;25(9):980–6. https://doi.org/10.1111/acem.13430.

Chapter 73
Working with Advanced Practice Providers

Lydia Younger

Advanced practice providers are a key part of the healthcare team. Advanced practice providers can help improve access to care, especially in light of rising patient volumes. They can offer unique perspectives that help to create a multidimensional healthcare team. The goal of this chapter is to explore the advanced practice provider role and discuss strategies for creating a collaborative provider team.

Advanced practice provider is a term that refers to both physician assistants and nurse practitioners. They function very similarly in the emergency department setting, but their training paths do differ. Physician assistants obtain a master's degree prior to taking their certification exams. Their training model mimics the medical school model, consisting of both a didactic portion and clinical rotations in core areas such as pediatrics, internal medicine, emergency medicine, family practice, and psychiatry [1]. Some applicants to programs apply directly after finishing their bachelor's degrees, while for others this is a second career. There are typically at least 500 medical hours required before applying to physician assistant schools, which could involve shadowing, working as a patient care assistant, certified nursing assistant, or as a paramedic, among other things. While there has been a more recent growth of post-master's degree training programs called fellowships (typically 12–18 months of training in a specialized area) as well certificates of advanced qualification (which requires a certain amount of work experience as well as passing a standardized test), physician assistants have the flexibility of generalist training and are not restricted to practicing in only one area of medicine [2]. You may find yourself working alongside a physician assistant who has a background in another area of medicine such as surgery or family medicine.

L. Younger (✉)
Penn State Hershey Medical Center, Hershey, PA, USA
e-mail: lyounger@pennstatehealth.psu.edu

R. P. Olympia et al. (eds.), *An Emergency Physician's Path*,
https://doi.org/10.1007/978-3-031-47873-4_73

In contrast, nurse practitioners have a different training path. Nurse practitioners will typically work for a period of time as a nurse prior to selecting their nurse practitioner track. These years of work experience gives them a skill set and knowledge base that the average doctor or physician assistant may not possess and it also allows them to select their track with certainty that this is the area of medicine to which they would like to commit. There are currently 13 available tracks for nurse practitioners, ranging from psychiatry to women's health [3, 4]. Similar to physician assistants, the nurse practitioner training model also requires an advanced degree, either a master's degree or a doctorate degree and includes both didactic work and clinical rotations [3]. Typically, emergency departments will hire nurse practitioners who have trained in the family medicine track, acute care track, or the adult-gerontology acute care track [4]. There is also the possibility of obtaining the additional certification of emergency nurse practitioner, which is a test typically taken after several years of work experience with a certain amount of procedural experience in the emergency department [5]. Nurse practitioners can also participate in advanced practice provider fellowships, which would occur after they have finished their nurse practitioner training and have passed their certifying exams.

Regardless of whether you are working with nurse practitioners, physician assistants or a mix of the two, it is important to understand the logistics of working with advanced practice providers at your specific institution as well as in the particular state in which you practice. State laws regulate the amount of autonomy that physician assistants and nurse practitioners have and whether they require counter signatures on charts. This can vary from state to state, and each institution will typically have policies regarding countersignatures. To utilize advanced practice providers well in the emergency department, each advanced practice provider should practice to the extent of their license, as determined by the state licensing boards as well as the medical bylaws of each institution. Each institution will have different guidelines regarding procedures and prescribing practices and each state will have their own particular regulations regarding Schedule II medications, such as narcotics [6–8]. It is also important to emphasize that despite the different training models for physician assistants and nurse practitioners, they typically function very similarly in the emergency medicine setting. Depending on the level of supervision that your state and hospital require, utilizing advanced practice providers in the emergency department can expand the volume of patients that a department is able to manage and can enhance throughput.

In general, there are a few common approaches towards the advanced practice provider role in the emergency department. Some departments choose to use advanced practice providers to evaluate and quickly disposition lower acuity patients in a "fast track" model. This can decant some of the volume from the department, since advanced practice providers can typically manage these patients independently. Some institutions employ their advanced practice providers in the triage model to help initiate diagnostic workups. There is some discussion on whether this truly expedites flow through the department or if it simply reduces the time from door to provider [9]. The benefits of this provider in triage model include supporting triage nurses and allowing sick patients to be identified quickly, but it may not significantly improve flow through the department, depending on the root cause of the poor flow [9]. In addition, there are departments that deploy advanced practice providers to function similarly to their physician colleagues in that they are seeing a variety of acuities and working throughout the department. There are also some innovative ways to use advanced practice providers including advance provider response units, which is an EMS team that includes an advanced practice provider [10]. Analysis of the efficacy of an advanced practice provider response unit in Los Angeles at the 18 month mark showed a decrease in emergency department utilization rates and had a 50.5% treat and release rate, in which patients were evaluated, treated, and discharged on scene [10]. Using APPs in the field with EMS is an exciting opportunity and so far seems to have positive effects on connecting patients with diagnosis and treatment in a more efficient manner and mitigating some of the high rates of over-utilization of the emergency department.

Each practice site is different, but there are some general differences in the advanced practice provider role in an academic center versus a community setting. In an academic center, there are typically many learners, ranging from students to fellows. This creates the additional challenge of ensuring a rewarding educational experience for multiple groups. In an academic center, residency training and education is highly important. As an attending, there is an opportunity to directly impact the next generation of emergency medicine physicians. There should be an emphasis on exposing residents to a wide variety of clinical scenarios and procedures so that they meet training requirements and feel confident as they venture out to practice on their own. An emergency department should also seek to balance the educational needs of both the residency program and the advanced practice provider group. An academic center has the educational resources to facilitate both goals in order to create a strong medical work force. APPs are core staff members and can provide year to year consistency, even as residents move onto fellowships or jobs elsewhere upon completion of their training. Additionally, experienced advanced practice providers can be key members in the educational team for both students and residents. Investing in their education allows your advanced practice provider colleagues to build their skill sets and be able to support the medical team in both higher and lower acuity situations. Developing the whole provider team allows a department to function smoothly.

In a community setting, there are typically fewer learners and therefore there are more opportunities for both the physician and the advanced practice provider to be involved in procedures as well as higher acuity patients. In a community setting, both the attendings and the advanced practice providers will draw on the skills and experiences they developed at prior institutions in order to make a positive impact in what is typically a more resource-limited setting. The functionality of an advanced practice provider in an academic center versus a community setting is similar; however, they will likely have more opportunity to care for higher acuity patients. As a result, it is critical to emphasize team building and to invest in your advanced practice provider team since they will be your primary counterparts in a community setting. If you are entering the community setting as a newer attending, there will likely be opportunities to learn from an experienced advanced practice provider who has medical, procedural, and institutional knowledge. Learning from someone who is familiar with the logistics of a particular practice site is invaluable, particularly as you are building your own clinical foundation.

Regardless of the practice setting, the most important component of any high functioning team is open, frequent, and clear communication. This holds true for the attending-APP relationship. It is helpful to be familiar with the background of the advanced practice providers that you work with—what was their work experience before they became an APP? How many years have they worked as an APP and in what practice settings? If they are coming from another institution, what was the attending-advanced practice provider relationship like there? If they are a nurse practitioner, how long were they a nurse before going back to school and in what practice settings? What are their educational and career goals?

It is important to keep in mind that each APP will bring a different skill set and knowledge base to the table, with various clinical strengths, just as every physician does. One of the key benefits of a strong advanced practice provider team includes expanding team-based care through collaboration—this benefit is enhanced when the team is educated regarding the advanced practice provider role and understands how they function as a part of the healthcare team [11]. Additionally, there is the benefit of continuity within the healthcare team—having consistent strong working relationships can be extremely helpful, particularly in a field that can have high turnover and burn out [12]. There is also significant financial cost associated with high turnover of advanced practice provider teams [13]. In general, employees will stay where they are cultivated—emphasizing advanced practice provider educational opportunities and treating them with respect and humility will create reliable, experienced colleagues who can consistently support the department.

It can be expected that as an advanced practice provider gains more experience both in a particular field and also working in a specific department, they will need less supervision and support from their attending. This can increase the amount of time the attending is able to devote to their own patients or to other learners like students or residents. It is important to remember though that in the first few years of practice for an advanced practice provider, they may require more supervision and may lean on their attendings for support and education. As discussed before, take advantage of this opportunity to invest in department education and to develop a strong advanced practice provider who will be able to contribute to the emergency department team. Particularly with newer advanced practice providers, a mentorship program can be invaluable and this can be a great way of getting involved with your colleagues and department. Providing medical education and career guidance can be personally rewarding and creates a strong team-based culture in your department. Every medical provider has had support and guidance throughout their medical journey—becoming a mentor to a new APP can be an excellent way to pay it forward and positively impact the next generation of medical providers.

Over the years the concept of team-based care has had a positive impact both on patients as well as on the medical team. The new healthcare environment should be one where we view all our coworkers as colleagues, regardless of their role and education level. It is important to be open to learning from a wide variety of experiences and skill sets. Approaching patient care with this attitude allows us all to grow as providers and creates more depth within the healthcare team. Creating positive working relationships with your advanced practice colleagues can enhance everyone's learning, create a rewarding workplace environment, and is a key part of a successful emergency department.

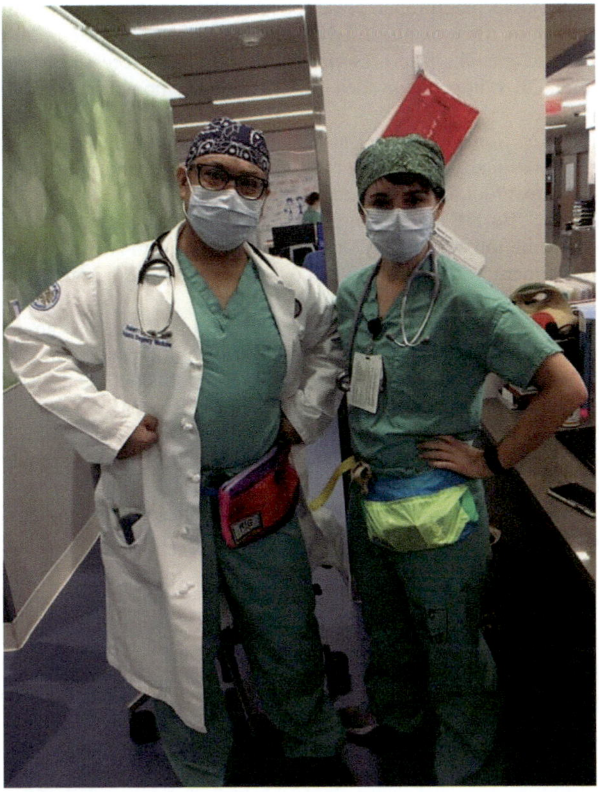

Advanced Practice Provider and Emergency Physician united to battle illness and injury on the frontlines of the COVID-19 pandemic. Lydia Younger and Robert Olympia.

References

1. What is a PA? AAPA. Published July 2022. https://www.aapa.org/what-is-a-pa/#accordion__panel%2D%2D3%2D%2Dwhat-education-does-a-pa-have. Accessed 23 Aug 2022.
2. Specialty certificates. NCCPA. Published 20 July 2022. https://www.nccpa.net/specialty-certificates/#1601111962551-1d87d8d4-6bcc. Accessed August 25, 2022.
3. The path to becoming a nurse practitioner (NP). American Association of Nurse Practitioners. Published 10 Nov 2020. https://www.aanp.org/news-feed/explore-the-variety-of-career-paths-for-nurse-practitioners. Accessed 23 Aug 2022.

4. How to become a nurse practitioner. Nursing License Map. Published Oct 2021. https://nursinglicensemap.com/advanced-practice-nursing/nurse-practitioner/. Accessed 25 Aug 2022.
5. Are you considering a career as an emergency nurse practitioner? American Association of Nurse Practitioners. Published 26 Sept 2019. https://www.aanp.org/news-feed/are-you-considering-a-career-as-an-emergency-nurse-pracitioner. Accessed 23 Aug 2022.
6. PA Prescribing Authority by state - AAPA. AAPA. https://www.aapa.org/wp-content/uploads/2016/12/PA_Prescribing_Chart.pdf. Accessed 23 Aug 2022.
7. State law chart: nurse practitioner prescriptive authority. American Medical Association. Published 2017. https://www.ama-assn.org/sites/ama-assn.org/files/corp/media-browser/specialty%20group/arc/ama-chart-np-prescriptive-authority.pdf. Accessed 23 Aug 2022.
8. Drug scheduling. DEA. https://www.dea.gov/drug-information/drug-scheduling. Accessed 23 Aug 2022.
9. Franklin BJ, Li KY, Somand DM, et al. Emergency department provider in triage: assessing site-specific rationale, operational feasibility, and financial impact. JACEP Open. 2021;2:e12450. https://doi.org/10.1002/emp2.12450.
10. Sanko S, Kashani S, Ito T, Guggenheim A, Fei S, Eckstein M. Advanced practice providers in the field: implementation of the Los Angeles Fire Department Advanced Provider Response Unit. Prehosp Emerg Care. 2020;24(5):693–703. https://doi.org/10.1080/10903127.2019.1666199.
11. Brooks PB, Fulton ME. Driving high-functioning clinical teams: an advanced practice registered nurse and physician assistant optimization initiative. J Am Assoc Nurse Pract. 2020;32(6):476–87. https://doi.org/10.1097/JXX.0000000000000415.
12. Harkins T, Thomas J, Fontenot B, Day J, Faraone M, Borden A, Lomax M, Dranginis D, Krasnosky R, Giardino AP. Utilization and workforce integration of physician assistants. J Nursing Interprofessional Leadership Qual Saf. 2022;4(1). https://digitalcommons.library.tmc.edu/uthoustonjqualsafe/vol4/iss1/6.
13. Ziegler A. Development of an advanced practice provider onboarding structure. Doctor of Nursing Practice (DNP) Projects. 2018;119. https://repository.usfca.edu/dnp/119.

Chapter 74
Dealing with Biases in Emergency Medicine

Joshua Ginsburg

The emergency department has been described as "a natural laboratory for the study of error" [1]. The most common is cognitive error, which is error in eliciting and synthesizing information, formulating a diagnosis, and taking the correct action [2].

Among the many reasons why emergency medicine physicians are so susceptible to cognitive error is that we have high decision density and diagnostic uncertainty, have an unrelenting cognitive load, and are constantly dealing with interruptions and distractions. In an unconscious attempt to deal with these pressures, we often rely on cognitive shortcuts, or heuristics, to provide efficient medical care. While heuristics are necessary and often helpful, the performance of heuristics is altered by our existing biases, and overreliance on heuristics can lead to new biases. In this chapter, we will discuss two types of bias that affect our care: cognitive bias, which affects how we gather, interpret, and act on clinical data; and implicit bias, which refers to our unconscious attitudes and stereotypes about the individuals we treat.

Cognitive Bias

In order to understand how our biases lead to cognitive errors, it is important to understand the Dual Process Theory, which is an imperfect but widely accepted model of cognition. The Dual Process Theory proposes that human thought can be divided into Type 1 and Type 2 thinking. Type 1 thinking is fast, intuitive, and low-effort, while Type 2 thinking is slow, analytical, and high-effort. For many emergency physicians, it is our nature to prefer to use Type 1 thinking, which relies on

J. Ginsburg (✉)
Department of Emergency Medicine, UT Southwestern Medical Center, Dallas, TX, USA
e-mail: Joshua.Ginsburg@UTSouthwestern.edu

R. P. Olympia et al. (eds.), *An Emergency Physician's Path*,
https://doi.org/10.1007/978-3-031-47873-4_74

heuristics and thereby allows us to act quickly when presented with a case rather than analyze the pre-test probability for each potential diagnosis, the performance characteristics of each test we can order, and the post-test probabilities prior to acting. As an example, we may develop a heuristic during flu season that says "fever plus body aches during flu season is probably flu." Such heuristics are crucial for efficient medical practice, useful in many emergency scenarios, and often lead to accurate diagnosis and treatment. But consider how the performance of these heuristics for diagnosis and treatment is altered by cognitive biases. Anchoring bias—in which one prematurely settles on a diagnosis based on the initial presentation, then fails to seek out or adjust to new information—is one of the more well-known cognitive biases. It is easy to see how if one anchors on the diagnosis of flu without considering other diagnoses, the flu heuristic may lead them to miss a more dangerous cause of fever. Table 74.1 lists other common cognitive biases.

Type 2 thinking simply requires that we stop and think things through. It is impractical to suggest that we move completely to Type 2 thinking—we simply cannot practice emergency medicine that way. Rather, we need to learn about the various types of cognitive biases and recognize when we are in situations that increase our risk for cognitive biases that may cause our Type 1 thinking to fail us. In those cases, we should slow down and utilize more Type 2 thinking.

As important as knowing the cognitive biases is recognizing when you are in a high-risk situation for falling victim to them. If you can learn to recognize when you are in such situations, you can remind yourself to incorporate more Type 2 thinking. Ask yourself the following questions regularly during your shift to help identify high-risk scenarios:

1. Is this a high-risk patient triaged to a low-acuity area?
2. Was this patient handed off to me?
3. Was the diagnosis suggested by someone else (e.g., a nurse, medical student, or other physician)?
4. Did I just accept the first potential diagnosis that I found?
5. Did I fail to consider other organ systems?
6. Have I been making the same diagnosis frequently recently?
7. Is this a patient I do not like for some reason?

Now armed with the knowledge of the cognitive biases and an awareness of the high-risk situations for bias, the question becomes, "How can we train ourselves to be less susceptible to bias and make fewer cognitive errors?" Fortunately, several debiasing strategies have been proposed. Admittedly, there is not yet consistent research proving that a single strategy is consistently effective. However, this field of study is in its infancy. It is unlikely that one strategy will work for all, and it is likely best to implement multiple approaches.

1. Learn about cognitive errors. We have already done this.
2. Routinely ask, "What else could this be?"
3. Attempt to refute your diagnosis.

Table 74.1 Common cognitive biases

Bias	Summary	Example
Anchoring bias	Fixation on initial impressions	A patient with a history of alcohol abuse presents with altered mental status. You anchor on the diagnosis of intoxication and miss the evidence of head trauma
Gambler's fallacy	Assumption that past events affect the probability of future events	You have diagnosed two patients today with PEs. When a third patient presents with chest pain, you assume it is unlikely that this patient also has a PE
Base rate neglect	Failure to consider the prevalence of a specific disease	You order a d-dimer on almost all chest pain patients, failing to consider the true prevalence of PE
Triage cueing	Geography is destiny	Your triage nurse assigns all dental pain an ESI level 5. Influenced by this, you miss a case of Ludwig's angina
Blind spot bias	"I am less susceptible to bias than others"	You do not consider cognitive biases as the potential cause of your errors and therefore do not investigate them or try to make changes
Search satisfying	Once something is found, no more information is sought	A patient presents with ankle pain after stepping in a ditch. The ankle x-ray shows a fracture, which you treat. You fail to examine the entire leg, which would have suggested a proximal fibula fracture as well
Zebra retreat	Failure to pursue a diagnosis because it is rare	You are concerned that a febrile patient has bacterial meningitis, but you back away from the diagnosis because you do not want to be seen as an over-tester
Blind obedience	Excessive importance given to expert opinion or test result	You are told over the phone by a specialist to discharge a patient to follow up in their clinic the next day, which you do against your better judgment, leading to a bad outcome
Fundamental attribution error	Blaming patients for their illnesses	You discharge a patient in severe alcohol withdrawal because you think it is "their fault"
Yin Yang bias	Perception that everything that can be done has been done	A patient with chronic abdominal pain has had labs, CT, and endoscopy within the past year. When they present with concerning pain they insist is different, you do not pursue it further and miss acute appendicitis
Availability bias	What most easily comes to mind is most likely	You recently diagnosed an aortic dissection in a patient with isolated back pain. You work up the next few back pain patients for aortic dissection
Feedback sanction	Diagnostic error carries no consequences	Your facility does not have a process for forwarding discharge notes on your admitted patients. You fail to see the diagnostic errors you made
Diagnosis momentum	A previous diagnosis is assumed to be definite	You receive a sign-out on a tachycardic patient you are told is dehydrated. When the heart rate does not improve with IV fluids, you do not investigate further due to the previous diagnostic label

4. Cognitively unload. This can be done by using checklists, looking things up that do not need to be committed to memory, using decision rules (and knowing where to find them online), and delegating tasks as needed.
5. Impose cognitive forcing functions. One way of doing this is by always writing down your differential diagnosis (to enforce the adage that you cannot diagnose what you do not consider). Another is to self-impose cognitive stop points, such as before putting in your orders and before clicking discharge. During these stop points, reconsider the presentation and review the results of the visit to make sure you are not missing anything. Additionally, you can create standing rules for yourself to serve as cognitive forcing functions. For example, a common standing rule we all use is to always check blood glucose level in patients with stroke-like symptoms. A less common standing rule that may be useful is always checking the aorta if you are performing POCUS for a kidney stone to ensure you do not miss a AAA.
6. Improve feedback and accountability. As an example, see if your hospital system can forward you the discharge notes on patients you admitted so that you can avoid feedback sanction and the blind spot bias.
7. Address systemic factors. Although beyond the scope of this chapter, addressing staffing, hours, fatigue, and burnout can help providers avoid cognitive biases and errors.
8. Perform a cognitive autopsy. As soon as possible after a case you would like to review, consider the cognitive biases that may have been contributory.

Implicit Bias

Implicit biases are unconscious, involuntary attitudes towards people or groups of people. As opposed to explicit biases, implicit biases cannot be measured by self-report. Similar to cognitive biases, we often develop implicit biases because they have proven useful in the past, but they very often negatively affect our patient care and relationship with our patients. Two of the more common implicit biases in medicine and examples of their effects on patient care are listed below. Additional biases may pertain to weight, age, religion, and disability, among others.

1. Gender Bias: Medical professionals are more likely to consider women with chronic pain as hysterical or sensitive [3]. In what is likely a related finding, women experience delays in the detection and treatment of acute coronary syndromes relative to men [4, 5]. Additionally, in one study, the mortality rate among women after acute myocardial infarction was higher than it was in men if they were treated by male physicians, but there was no difference if they were treated by female physicians [6].
2. Racial Bias: There is evidence to show that non-White patients are less likely to receive prompt emergency department care, appropriate triage level (which can then lead to cognitive biases such as triage cueing and anchoring), timely and thorough workup for suspected coronary artery disease, and pain control [7–9].

Such racial bias in pain management applies not just to adults. In one study, Black and Hispanic children were less likely than White non-Hispanic children to receive opioid analgesia for limb fractures or appendicitis [10]. Implicit pro-White, anti-Black bias has been associated with Black patients feeling less respect and collaboration with their physician [11].

If these biases are unconscious and involuntary, how can we mitigate them?

1. Awareness and self-reflection: In order to address our biases, we must be aware of them. The Implicit Association Test (IAT) is available for free online and can help you identify the implicit biases that you may have. It is important not to approach your results defensively, as the purpose of the test is not to label you as, for example, racist or sexist based on a single result. Rather, consider that the test reveals subconscious associations that may someday affect the care you provide. Be willing to reflect on these results and discuss them with colleagues.
2. Pay attention to your language: As an example, in one study, providers who reported using the stigmatizing term "sickler" for patients with sickle cell anemia were less likely to provide adequate analgesia [12]. This applies to the medical record as well, as a study showed that Black patients were more likely than White patients to have negative descriptors documented in the electronic health record, as were patients with Medicare or Medicaid compared to those with private or employer-provided insurance [13]. These descriptors can influence the care provided at subsequent visits.
3. Follow guidelines: When used appropriately, clinical guidelines, hospital protocols, and individual care plans may minimize the ability of implicit bias to creep into medical care. For example, hospital protocols regarding workup of patients presenting with chest pain may decrease the time to obtain an EKG. As another example, individual care plans for patients with sickle cell anemia may increase the appropriate use of analgesia when they present with acute pain crises.

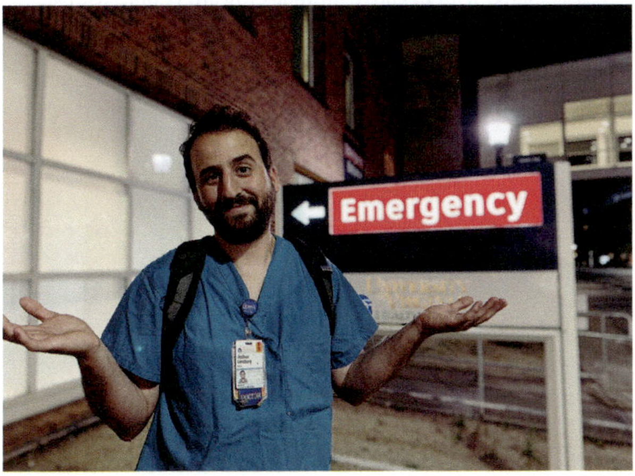

Last shift of residency!

References

1. Croskerry P, Sinclair D. Emergency medicine: a practice prone to error? CJEM. 2001;3(04):271–6. https://doi.org/10.1017/s1481803500005765.
2. Graber ML, Franklin N, Gordon R. Diagnostic error in internal medicine. Arch Intern Med. 2005;165(13):1493. https://doi.org/10.1001/archinte.165.13.1493.
3. Samulowitz A, Gremyr I, Eriksson E, Hensing G. "Brave men" and "emotional women": a theory-guided literature review on gender bias in health care and gendered norms towards patients with chronic pain. Pain Res Manage. 2018;2018:1–14. https://doi.org/10.1155/2018/6358624.
4. Humphries KH, Lee MK, Izadnegahdar M, et al. Sex differences in diagnoses, treatment, and outcomes for emergency department patients with chest pain and elevated cardiac troponin. Acad Emerg Med. 2018;25(4):413–24. https://doi.org/10.1111/acem.13371.
5. Mackey C, Diercks DB. Gender bias in the management of patients still exists. Acad Emerg Med. 2018;25(4):467–9. https://doi.org/10.1111/acem.13394.
6. Greenwood BN, Carnahan S, Huang L. Patient–physician gender concordance and increased mortality among female heart attack patients. Proc Natl Acad Sci. 2018;115(34):8569–74. https://doi.org/10.1073/pnas.1800097115.
7. Schrader CD, Lewis LM. Racial disparity in emergency department triage. J Emerg Med. 2013;44(2):511–8. https://doi.org/10.1016/j.jemermed.2012.05.010.
8. DeVon HA, Burke LA, Nelson H, Zerwic JJ, Riley B. Disparities in patients presenting to the emergency department with potential acute coronary syndrome: it matters if you are black or white. Heart Lung. 2014;43(4):270–7. https://doi.org/10.1016/j.hrtlng.2014.04.019.
9. Lee P, Le Saux M, Siegel R, et al. Racial and ethnic disparities in the management of acute pain in US emergency departments: meta-analysis and systematic review. Am J Emerg Med. 2019;37(9):1770–7. https://doi.org/10.1016/j.ajem.2019.06.014.
10. Guedj R, Marini M, Kossowsky J, Berde CB, Kimia AA, Fleegler EW. Racial and ethnic disparities in pain management of children with limb fractures or suspected appendicitis: a retrospective cross-sectional study. Front Pediatr. 2021;9:652854. https://doi.org/10.3389/fped.2021.652854.
11. Cooper LA, Roter DL, Carson KA, et al. The associations of clinicians' implicit attitudes about race with medical visit communication and patient ratings of interpersonal care. Am J Public Health. 2012;102(5):979–87. https://doi.org/10.2105/ajph.2011.300558.
12. Glassberg J, Tanabe P, Richardson L, Debaun M. Among emergency physicians, use of the term "sickler" is associated with negative attitudes toward people with sickle cell disease. Am J Hematol. 2013;88(6):532–3. https://doi.org/10.1002/ajh.23441.
13. Sun M, et al. Negative patient descriptors: documenting racial bias in the electronic health record. Health Aff (Millwood). 2022;41(2):203–11.

Chapter 75
An Introduction to EMTALA

Jason Jones

Perhaps no law exerts greater influence on the practice of emergency physicians than the Emergency Medical Treatment and Labor Act (EMTALA). Enacted in 1986, the law requires Emergency Departments to evaluate and stabilize all individuals arriving for care, regardless of their insurance status or ability to pay [1]. EMTALA is not a federal malpractice law, and it does not require ill intent, poor quality care, or patient harm to occur to trigger a violation. Rather, EMTALA demands fair and uniform adherence to its federal regulations, which supersede all state and local rules. A single violation can cost tens of thousands of dollars and jeopardize the hospital's participation in Medicare and Medicaid. Thus, understanding the specifics of EMTALA is a critical skill for every emergency physician.

What Is EMTALA?

Until the mid-1980s, common law required physicians to accept a new patient only if both parties agreed. As a result, it was not uncommon for Emergency Departments to turn away patients for lack of insurance or to direct them to other hospitals. In response, EMTALA was enacted as a federal "anti-dumping statute" to combat this discriminatory practice. The law has generated fierce debate since its passage, enduring legal challenges, three major revisions, and frequent clarifications about its interpretation. Though EMTALA forces hospitals to take on a higher burden of uncompensated care, it does not provide funds to provide that care—often called an "unfunded mandate." Nevertheless, EMTALA's central goal—*emergency care*

J. Jones (✉)
Department of Emergency Medicine, University of Florida, Gainesville, FL, USA
e-mail: jasonjones@ufl.edu

R. P. Olympia et al. (eds.), *An Emergency Physician's Path*,
https://doi.org/10.1007/978-3-031-47873-4_75

without discrimination—has been lauded as consistent with the core identify of the specialty of Emergency Medicine.

In a Nutshell, What Does EMTALA Require?

EMTALA applies to any hospital that receives payment from Medicare and has a **dedicated Emergency Department** (ED). If an individual **comes to that ED** and **requests examination and treatment**, the hospital must provide an appropriate medical screening examination. Using any available necessary ancillary services (such as consultants), the ED physician must determine whether an **emergency medical condition** is present. If an emergency condition is not present, EMTALA's requirements end. If an emergency condition is present, the hospital is required to **stabilize** the patient. Patients who have not been stabilized should not be transferred to another facility unless:

1. The patient requests transfer in writing even after being informed of the risks, or
2. The transferring physician signs a certification that the medical benefits of transfer exceed the risks to patient and/or fetus, or
3. The patient refuses to consent to treatment, despite the physician taking "all reasonable steps" to secure informed consent.

Of note, EMTALA and its guidelines have specifically defined many of these concepts (Table 75.1):

Table 75.1 Common definitions regarding EMTALA and its guidelines

Term	Definition
"Dedicated Emergency Department"	"Licensed by the state" as an ED or "held out to the public" as providing treatment for emergencies
	Or
	On 1/3 or more of visits in the past year "actually provided treatment for emergency medical conditions on an urgent basis." This includes many urgent care centers, labor and delivery units, and psychiatric facilities
"Comes to the ED"	Not only patients inside the above-described EDs, but also patients within 250 yards of the hospital's "campus" [2]
"Request for exam and treatment"	Comes from the patient, an individual on their behalf, or is understood to exist if a layperson could identify them as possibly having an emergency
"Emergency medical condition"	A condition with acute symptoms severe enough (including pain) that, without immediate medical attention, the patient (or fetus) may suffer harm to their health or impairment of a bodily function, organ, or part
"Stabilization"	To provide medical treatment such that "no material deterioration of the condition is likely, within reasonable medical probability, to result from or occur during the transfer of the individual from a facility"

What Does EMTALA Require from Emergency Physicians?

Performing a **Medical Screening Examination (MSE)** for all arriving patients is EMTALA's first major requirement [3]. It must be performed by a physician or by qualified medical personnel identified by the hospital's medical staff bylaws. According to CMS (Centers for Medicare and Medicaid Services), the MSE is an "ongoing process" rather than an isolated episode. It may be as simple as a history and physical examination, or as complex as obtaining labs and imaging, calling consultants, and performing procedures like a lumbar puncture. However, similar presentations should receive a similar and consistent MSE process. If the emergency physician is unsure whether an emergency medical condition is present, the evaluation should continue until the question is resolved. This includes transfer to a higher level of care if necessary and appropriate. Of note, CMS has clarified that the **triage** process, which sorts patients into order of evaluation, does not qualify as an MSE as it does not explicitly determine whether an emergency condition is present.

One frequent mistake is the belief that minors must wait for parent or guardian arrival before an MSE can be performed. EMTALA is unambiguous: even if a parent is not present to consent, a medical screening exam should be performed as soon as possible upon ED arrival. Delaying the MSE for parental arrival and consent has resulted in several EMTALA violations.

The second major obligation under EMTALA is a duty to provide "**necessary stabilizing treatment**" to unstable patients. Emergency physicians should use all available and necessary resources to stabilize such patients, including testing and specialist consultation. Available on-call consultants are required to respond to consultation requests *at a time frame set by the emergency physician.* Transfer to another facility should not occur unless the patient requests transfer in writing despite understanding the risks or the physician or their delegate signs a certification that the benefits of immediate transfer outweigh the risks.

Transfers to other medical facilities must be "**appropriate**" by EMTALA statute. Appropriate transfers require that the sending facility provides medical care that minimizes risk of harm to patient (or fetus) due to transfer. They require that the sending facility provides copies of all medical records, including observations, signs and symptoms, preliminary diagnosis, treatment provided, test results, and consent forms. The receiving facility must have "available space and qualified personnel" and agree to transfer and treatment. EMTALA also requires that interfacility transports use "qualified personnel," appropriate equipment, and "medically appropriate life support measures."

The EMTALA duty to a patient with an emergency medical condition ends when:

- The patient is admitted to the hospital
- The patient undergoes appropriate transfer to another medical facility
- The patient refuses hospital admission or interfacility transfer, and a documented Against Medical Advice (AMA) process with informed consent occurs
- The patient's emergency medical condition is stabilized, and no further decline is expected, allowing discharge from the ED

What Does EMTALA Require from Hospitals and Consultants?

Hospitals face a variety of requirements related to EMTALA which are beyond the scope of this chapter. However, several are worth mentioning. First, hospitals must place signs which "specify the rights of individuals with emergency conditions and women in labor" related to EMTALA. These must be placed in the ED and other conspicuous locations likely to be frequented by patients with emergencies. Hospitals may collect insurance information from the patient prior to the MSE, so long as it does not delay or interfere with the MSE. Hospitals must also maintain an accurate list of on-call specialists for use by ED staff (though not *maintained* by the ED staff). This on-call list can be adapted to hospital circumstances, including the use of multi-hospital "community call" for some specialties. Hospitals with specialized capabilities or facilities not available at the sending facility must accept transfers so long as they have available capability and capacity to care for the patient.

On-call consultants are required by EMTALA to respond to ED consults at a timeframe set by the emergency physician unless specified in hospital bylaws. CMS specifies that on-call consultants may not avoid the ED to "refer cases to their offices for examination and treatment" when consulted for an emergency condition. However, some exceptions may exist if specified in advance by hospital bylaws. One frequently cited exception is transfer to an ophthalmology clinic when the ED lacks adequate equipment. As EMTALA only governs the transfer of unstable patients, routine care (such as stable fractures) can be referred for follow-up in subspecialty clinics.

The hospital bears the final responsibility to ensure that its on-call physicians respond to consults in a "reasonable" timeframe. EMTALA requires hospitals to publish policies and procedures to be followed when a specialist is unavailable, or when the on-call physician cannot respond due to unforeseen circumstances. When faced with an unreachable consultant, many authors suggest reaching out to departmental or hospital leadership, such as the Department Chair or Medical Chief of Staff, prior to attempting an interfacility transfer. When transfers occur because an on-call physician failed to appear, an EMTALA violation has occurred, and the sending facility is required by law to provide that physician's name and address to the receiving facility.

What Are the Consequences of an EMTALA Violation?

Two agencies oversee enforcement of EMTALA violations: CMS and OIG (Office of the Inspector General). When an EMTALA violation is sustained, hospitals are given 90 days to correct deficiencies or risk termination from Medicare provider agreements. Individual fines to hospitals and physicians have a ceiling of $50,000 per incident and are not covered by malpractice insurance. Thankfully, sustained

EMTALA violations are generally suffered by the hospital rather than individual physicians. One study found that 96% of EMTALA violations between 2002 and 2015 were borne by the facility, with only one emergency physician fined as an individual [4].

Conclusions

Emergency physicians can avoid EMTALA violations with a uniform medical screening process and an unwavering dedication to patient stabilization. When emergency physicians need additional resources for stabilization, EMTALA is a federal mechanism that compels other hospitals and specialists to help.

References

1. 42 CFR § 1395dd.
2. 42 CFR § 413.65(b).
3. Centers for Medicare & Medicaid Services. State operations manual appendix V—interpretive guidelines—responsibilities of medicare participating hospitals in emergency cases. Baltimore; 2019. https://www.cms.gov/Regulations-and-Guidance/Guidance/Manuals/downloads/som107ap_v_emerg.pdf.
4. Terp S, Wang B, Raffetto B, et al. Individual physician penalties resulting from violation of emergency medical treatment and labor act: a review of Office of the Inspector General Patient Dumping Settlements, 2002–2015. Acad Emerg Med. 2017;24(4):442–6. https://doi.org/10.1111/acem.13159.

Chapter 76
Medical Ethics for the EM Physician

Sajid Khan and Maryam Arshad

Emergency Medicine physicians face a myriad of ethical decisions in everyday practice. Patients arrive with acute illnesses and require immediate care. There is often little time to gather information before decisions must be made. This may mean an inability to speak to the patient or their family members prior to intervention. Patients place their trust in the physicians who work there with the belief that those physicians will care for them based on a set of values, principles, and beliefs to guide their decision-making. Emergency Medicine physicians are uniquely positioned to serve as healthcare providers for many patients who have no other access to care. Knowledge of ethics and practicing ethical behavior is at the center of every good Emergency Medicine physician.

Major Ethical Principles

The physician–patient relationship is based on four major ethical principles:

1. Beneficence

    Beneficence refers to actions that promote the well-being of others. This means taking actions that serve the best interests of patients and their families. For instance, this may mean administering antibiotics to a patient with a bacterial infection or anti-platelet agents to a patient with a stroke. Beneficence does not always mean doing what the patient wants you to do. In situations where a

S. Khan (✉)
University of Missouri–Kansas City, Kansas City, MO, USA

M. Arshad
Emory University, Atlanta, GA, USA

R. P. Olympia et al. (eds.), *An Emergency Physician's Path*,
https://doi.org/10.1007/978-3-031-47873-4_76

person is suicidal or homicidal, the physician may need to act against the patient's wishes in order to protect them. For instance, for a suicidal patient who has inflicted life-threatening injuries on himself and is refusing stabilization and treatment, the physician should act to preserve the patient. Likewise, if a homicidal wants to sign out against medical advice, they may need to be held against their will to receive treatment. These scenarios also constitute beneficence. Part of beneficence is a patient's right to confidentiality. If a homicidal patient plans to harm another person, the physician has an ethical obligation to warn that person [1].

2. Non-maleficence

   Better known by the colloquial phrase, "do no harm," non-maleficence describes a physician's responsibility to make decisions that will not lead to injury or impairment of the patient. For instance, if a patient has a viral respiratory illness and requests certain treatments which have not proven to be effective, the physician has an ethical responsibility to not administer that medication. If a patient with terminal lung cancer has made the decision to not be intubated, then allowing them to remain comfortable and foregoing intubation, even in the event of respiratory failure, may be appropriate.

3. Autonomy

   Autonomy signifies the right of adult patients with decision-making capacity to make informed decisions about their own medical care. This principle underlies the requirement to seek informed consent from a patient before any workup or treatment occurs. Patients have a right to accept or refuse recommended healthcare, and physicians have a duty to respect their choices.

   Decision-making capacity differs from competence, which is a legal term and generally determined by a court. Adult patients should be presumed to have decision-making capacity unless they are cognitively disabled or have significantly altered mental status. The question of a patient's capacity typically arises only when they refuse recommended tests and interventions. Capacity means that the patient is aware of the options available, can articulate the risks and benefits of the options, and why they made the decision they did. For instance, a patient may refuse life-saving blood transfusions on the basis of a religious objection and still possess capacity.

   If the patient lacks decision-making capacity, emergency physicians should turn to an appropriate surrogate decision maker. In the absence of a surrogate, physicians themselves should make decisions for the patient.

   It is important to note that patients may possess decision-making capacity even while intoxicated from drugs or alcohol, having speech or language impediments, or suffering from mild degrees of cognitive deficits. Decision-making capacity can be fluid, depending on the patient's condition. Patients may initially lack capacity but after some type of intervention, such as oxygen, antidotes, or pain medication, capacity may be regained. A person may have the capacity to make relatively simple decisions but the same person may lack capacity to process complex information and make complicated decisions.

4. Justice
   Justice represents being fair and impartial to patients regardless of their gender, race, age, or ability to pay [2].

Informed Consent

Emergency physicians should, to whatever extent time allows, inform the patient prior to initiating diagnostic and therapeutic modalities. There are situations in which informed consent may be bypassed—for instance, in a hypotensive patient who needs a central line, immediate intervention may be necessary to prevent serious harm to the patient. Delaying treatment to obtain consent would be inappropriate. Additionally, an intoxicated patient who cannot make decisions and lacks capacity cannot provide informed consent. Generally speaking, these are rare exceptions and patients should participate in decisions regarding their healthcare.

Some patients, after being evaluated in the pre-hospital setting by EMS providers, wish to refuse further treatment. If it can be determined that the person has decision-making capacity, then they have the right to refuse further care. This can often be difficult to determine over the radio or telephone when paramedics call for assistance in reaching a resolution. If capacity cannot be determined, it may be best to err on the side of caution and further evaluate the situation in person.

End-of-Life Care

Significant ethical issues may arise in the care of terminally ill patients. Emergency physicians should, for example, be willing to respect a terminally ill patient's wish to forgo life-prolonging treatment, as expressed in a living will or by an appropriate surrogate decision maker. Emergency physicians should also honor patient preferences in Do Not Resuscitate (DNR) orders. While family members or surrogates may disagree over treatment choices, it is most important to respect the wishes of the person who is living or dying in the process, and sometimes you need to aggressively advocate for your patient. Not instituting treatments that will prolong someone's life in order to uphold their wishes is practicing non-maleficence [3].

Social Media

Emergency physicians have a duty to protect patient confidentiality. Avoid using social media to post patient information. Confidential data, including the patient's identifying factors, images, and test results can be transmitted over secure electronic servers for the purposes of patient treatment, with the patient's consent.

Mandatory Reporting

Physicians are mandatory reporters, which means that they are legally mandated to report suspected abuse or neglect of the elderly and of children. You do not need to be correct in your presumption and there is no repercussion for wrongful accusation. On the other hand, spousal abuse is not a mandatory reportable offense and if the affected party wishes to remain confidential, you must respect that right. When dealing with such situations, it may be difficult to find a balance between what your ethical principles are and what the legal system dictates. In other words, following the law may not mean making an ethical decision [4, 5].

Minors

In general, treatment of children requires parental consent. Parents have the right to make decisions about the healthcare services that their minor children do, or do not, receive. If a child has a sprained ankle and the parents do not want a prescription-strength pain medication, they can refuse the prescription. On the other hand, if a child suffers blunt abdominal trauma and is hypotensive, parents may not be able to refuse blood transfusion as it may be a life-saving measure. In the case of a potential medical emergency, a physician may treat a patient even without parental consent. There are additional exceptions that vary from state to state, but in general children may be considered "emancipated minors" and be treated without parental consent for sexual health services and pregnancy-related complaints. Additionally, forced alcohol or drug testing on minors is a grey area of ethics and shared decision-making is typically the best course of action [6].

Treating Personal Contacts

Many physicians will face the ethical scenario of a friend, family member, or coworker who requests medical advice. In general, physicians should try to avoid treating such parties for a variety of reasons. Such close contacts may hesitate to share confidential information, physicians may be tempted to treat outside his or her scope of practice to appease, or shortcuts may be taken to expedite care. The AMA Code of Medical Ethics states, "physicians generally should not treat themselves or members of their immediate families…while physicians should not serve as primary or regular care providers for immediate family members, there are situations in which routine care is acceptable for short-term, minor problems" [7]. When it comes to controlled substances, the rules are a little clearer: federal law regulates controlled substances and a written record should be kept in such cases.

The AMA Code of Medical Ethics is a good place to start to develop one's own set of moral philosophies. The very nature of Emergency Medicine means that providers will face a myriad of situations. Many of these will require one to make decisions based on their personal beliefs. Having a groundwork of principles to help guide oneself through such ethical situations is indispensable.

References

1. Derse A. Ethics and the law in emergency medicine. Emerg Med Clin North Am. 2006;24(3):547–55.
2. Iserson KV. Ethical principles-emergency medicine. Emerg Med Clin North Am. 2006;24:513–45.
3. Code of ethics for emergency physicians. Ann Emerg Med. 2004;43:686–94.
4. Iserson KV. Principles of medical ethics. In: Marco C, Schears R, editors. Ethical dilemmas in emergency medicine. New York: Cambridge University Press; 2015. p. 1–17.
5. ACEP code of ethics for emergency physicians. A compendium of ACEP policy statements on ethical issues revised 2002, 2003, 2004, 2005, 2006, 2007, 2008, 2009, 2011, 2012, 2013, 2014. Clin Pract Manage. 2015:1–12.
6. Garrison H, Dinerman N. Ethical challenges in emergency medical services: a special contribution of the ethics committee, national association of emergency medical services physicians. Prehosp Disaster Med. 1993;8(2):179–82.
7. Geiderman JM, et al. Emergency physician care of family members, friends, colleagues and self. Am J Emerg Med. 2019;37(5):942–6.

Part VII
Research and Scholarship in Emergency Medicine

Chapter 77
Getting Involved in Emergency Medicine Research

Robert P. Olympia

You have likely seen it, and I'll even bet you have given it. It's the look of disgust, disinterest, or despair in response to the word "research." As a member of the Medical Student Research committee at the Penn State College of Medicine and Director of Residency Research for the Penn State Health Emergency Medicine residency program, I have seen this "look" often when discussing research as a requirement for medical school or EM residency graduation. And I distinctly remember giving the "look" when asked during an EM faculty position interview: "Describe your research interests and the research niche you hope to establish?" The thoughts of research can be anxiety-provoking and overwhelming, but I hope this chapter encourages you to pursue a career in Emergency Medicine research.

So Why Would Anyone Decide to Do Research in EM?

It is unlikely that you entered medical school or residency wanting to pursue a career in research. Research was definitely not on my radar. But over my career, research went from being a required task to something I truly enjoyed, giving me professional satisfaction and success. Here are some reasons why I became involved in research for your consideration:

1. *Conducting research sharpens your ability to critically evaluate medical literature.* Having personal experience in the performing literature searches, develop-

R. P. Olympia (✉)
Department of Emergency Medicine, Penn State Milton S. Hershey Medical Center, Hershey, PA, USA
e-mail: rolympia@hmc.psu.edu

R. P. Olympia et al. (eds.), *An Emergency Physician's Path*,
https://doi.org/10.1007/978-3-031-47873-4_77

ing research design, completing an IRB application, collecting and analyzing data, and disseminating your results should help you during your career in critically reading the medical literature and practicing evidence-based medicine.

2. *Research is required to climb the academic ladder.* Promotion during your academic career often requires you to achieve excellence in several categories, including the category of Research and Creative Accomplishments (see Chap. 40). Part of this process is conducting research, presenting your research at scientific assemblies, and publishing your research in peer-reviewed journals.
3. *Involvement in research and scholarship is often incentivized.* Most academic EM departments support academic faculty involved in research, providing financial compensation for conducting research, for presenting your research at scientific assemblies (reimbursement of abstract applications, conference registration, travel and hotel expenses, dining, etc.), for publication costs (if necessary), and for end-of-the-year incentive bonuses (based on numbers of scientific assembly presentations and/or publications). Academic EM departments may offer protected time in order to pursue educational research opportunities, to serve on leadership positions in research within the department or your institution, and/or to conduct research.
4. *Going to scientific assemblies to present your research can be fun and good for your overall wellness.* Not only do you have an opportunity to present your research amongst your EM peers, but by going to a scientific assembly you can learn about the current state of EM and network with colleagues in the field, often in desirable locations. Think of it as education, research, and wellness, the best of all worlds. In my career, I may have chosen to present my research at scientific assemblies in warm cities by the ocean, or convention centers near great restaurants and nightlife.
5. *Research can lead to networking and collaboration within your institution and with other academic institutions.* Depending on your research question and design, you may have the opportunity to work with other medical and surgical departments and other healthcare disciplines within your institution or beyond its walls. This research collaboration often leads to stronger clinical relationships, better communication, and improved care of patients.
6. *Research involves mentorship.* One of the reasons I continue to conduct research is that I am able to work with medical students and residents who share a similar passion. I feel like a proud father when one of my mentees presents their research at a scientific assembly or publishes their research in a journal. I have had wonderful research mentors early in my career, and I strive to be a mentor to future academic physicians. It's the research circle of life.
7. *For medical students and residents, involvement in research gives you a glimpse into EM, allows you to interact with EM physicians and other medical and surgical departments, and strengthens your applications for residency, fellowship, and attending physician positions.*
8. *Research can change the world.* We sometimes forget the impact that our research may have on our own patients, for patients both regionally and nationally and internationally, and for mankind in general. Ultimately research is not

about our curriculum vitae or promotion packets, not about incentive plans or conferences in exotic regions of the world, not about networking or mentorship, not about seeing our names on publications or posters or PubMed—it is about being impactful. Isn't this why we entered the field of medicine in the first place?

How to Be Successful in Research, and More Importantly, How to Have Fun While Doing the Work

Research has not always been easy. With each research study I am involved in, I learn something about the process that makes the next project a bit easier. Here are ten pearls I have learned along the way:

1. *Find and pursue your passions*: Research can be boring and feel like a worthless task unless you find out where you passion in EM lies. I assure you that you will be successful in your research career if you pursue research topics that you enjoy and that motivate you to make an impact. My research career started in emergency and disaster preparedness as a direct result of the passion I felt after 9/11 as a PEM fellow in NYC, and continued throughout my career based on the passion I felt for sports medicine/concussions, pediatric trauma, urgent care medicine, prehospital care medicine, and the effect of media on children. Although your passions may change throughout your career, allow your research to follow these passions.
2. *Keep your eyes and ears open:* Some of my best research ideas came from working clinically or from performing literature searches, when gaps in the medical literature were identified. My research on the effect of radiology discrepancies in the ED and the evaluation of after-hour call centers were direct results of questions I could not answer following literature searches from two medical students working clinically on my team. Clinical and research questions surround you daily, it takes curiosity and a bit of time to find them.
3. *Avengers assemble:* I love superhero movies. I love when superheroes, with different superpowers and strengths/weaknesses, assemble into one powerful group. I utilize this concept whenever I start a research project. I collect specialists associated with my research question (both from my institution and from other institutions), as well research specialists—librarians to help with literature searches, biostatisticians to help with research design and analysis, and IT (information technologists) to help with subject identification and data collection. Don't forget to include medical students and residents/fellows, who may be motivated for many different reasons and may have the time to conduct the research. Assemble and delegate, and be prepared to conquer the world.
4. *Be original and seek what is "hot":* The medical profession craves research that is innovative or studies a "hot" topic. You will likely have an abstract or manuscript accepted if your research topic is original or fresh. I was involved in urgent care medicine research when research in the field was lacking and in its

infancy, conducted research on energy drinks, electronic cigarettes, and CDB oil during the peak of their use in the public, and participated in multi-centered, groundbreaking research on the use of salivary microRNA to diagnose pediatric concussions. Develop and seek research opportunities that are innovative and fresh, that will create a buzz in the scientific community, and that create a lasting impression and impact.

5. *Be transformative:* Research ideas can come from scholarly work that you have already prepared and disseminated. Scholarship, such as lectures, panel discussions, review articles, and case reports, often requires a thorough literature search. The very nature of this investigative process identifies potential gaps in medical literature and promotes research. A review article on blunt abdominal trauma in children for *ACEP's Critical Decisions in Emergency Medicine* led to a retrospective study applying PECARN prediction rules for clinically important intra-abdominal injuries in children at our institution, and a lecture I prepared on emergency and disaster preparedness in schools for the National Association of School Nurses conference led to questionnaire-based research on the preparedness of colleges and universities, summer camps, babysitters, child care centers, school buses, and school-based athletics. Scholarship is a beautiful cycle of learning, exploration, education, and dissemination—being involved in this cycle naturally lends itself to research.
6. *Recycle ideas:* After you find a research idea and question that fits into your clinical interests, you conduct a thorough literature search and find out that a similar study has been published previously. Have no fear. Unless the published study is generalizable (multi-centered with a multitude of patients/subject enrolled reflecting all potential demographics), it is likely that you can replicate the study. Although there were two single-center published studies examining predictors for intra-thoracic injuries in children who sustained blunt chest trauma, we replicated the study at our institution (rural/suburban setting, level 1 trauma center) with results that were dissimilar to those published, and well received in the scientific community. As a pediatrician, I have previously adopted research studies that have enrolled only adult patients and modified the study to focus on pediatric patients. I wouldn't call it cheating, it's more like refining.
7. *Time constraints, have no fear:* Work-life balance is so important to those in healthcare, including those who work in EM. Research can be so time consuming, with timelines that overlap with clinical responsibilities and life events, and deadlines that approach at the speed of light. You may not have time to obtain grants, or conduct randomized, double-blind, and placebo controlled studies with $n = a$ billion, but there are research opportunities that may fit into your lifestyle. Consider retrospective studies that utilize patients from your ED or from national/regional databases, consider collaborating with other institutions/EDs, consider systematic reviews, meta-analysis, or bibliometric study designs, consider case reports and case series, and consider questionnaire-based studies that involve accessing Listservs, society membership lists, or email blasts. Research should not compromise your work-life balance.
8. *Find a mentor and be a mentor:* Find research mentors who will guide you, not only through your career in research and academia, but also with life. I was

blessed to have Drs. Magdy Attia, Steven Selbst, and Jeffrey Avner as research and career mentors. After over 20 years, I still look to them for advice regarding research and scholarship. And as your career progresses, seek opportunities to be a mentor to medical students, residents, and junior faculty. It puts a smile on my face when I see former mentees publishing or presenting their research, or obtaining leadership positions that encourage research. "The mediocre mentor tells, the good mentor explains, the superior mentor demonstrates, and the greatest mentors inspire"—Lucia Ballas Traynor. So be inspired, and inspire the future of research in EM.

9. *Take advantage of opportunities to learn about the research process:* For many, research does not come naturally. It takes time and effort, overcoming obstacles and learning from mistakes, in order to become successful. Most academic institutions will have research and biostatistics lectures built into the professional development of their faculty, so take advantage of these educational opportunities. Join the Institutional Review Board (IRB) at your institution, as becoming familiar with the IRB application process and having the opportunity to review IRB applications will be invaluable for your career as a researcher. Volunteer to review abstract applications for scientific assemblies and/or submitted manuscripts for peer-reviewed journals in EM. This experience will highlight what research is being conducted in your field, will help you develop skills in research design and data collection/analysis, and will provide you templates as you develop your own writing styles for abstracts and manuscripts. Lastly, involve yourself in your department's journal clubs, as being able to critically evaluate the medical literature will strengthen your ability to conduct well designed and meaningful research.
10. *Go to scientific assemblies:* Whenever I attend a scientific assembly, I often leave inspired, with a notebook filled with research ideas and contact information of potential research collaborators. Listening to oral research presentations or viewing poster presentations may lead to research ideas (Remember pearl # 2—"Keep your eyes and ears open"). Networking with other researchers that have similar clinical and research interests may lead to multi-centered studies (Remember pearl # 3—"Avengers Assemble"). Being immersed with the innovation of research from all over the world inspires me to become a better clinician and more productive academic EM researcher.

The Anatomy and Physiology of Clinical Research: The Initial Steps

So you have decided to participate in EM research, what are the next steps? Research involves choosing the most feasible, efficient, cost effective, and ethically sound study design that will answer the question most accurately with the least bias. Simplistically, it's defining the anatomy and physiology of clinical research as delineated in the tables below. The anatomy of research (Table 77.1) asks the

Table 77.1 The anatomy of research: steps and questions

	Steps	Questions
Research question	– Starts as a general concern that must be narrowed down to a concrete, researchable question. – Involves conducting a thorough search of published literature in the area of study. – Utilizes the "FINER" technique	– What question does your study address?
		– What is known about the topic at hand?
		– Why is the research question important?
		– Is the research:
		FEASIBLE (adequate number of subjects, adequate technical expertise, affordable with regard to time and money, focused in scope)
		INTERESTING (are people going to care about my results)
		NOVEL (has the study been conducted before)
		ETHICAL (is there a physical/ psychological risk, or invasion of privacy)
		RELEVANT (does the outcome advance scientific knowledge, influence clinical management and health policy, or guide future research)
Research design	Meet with a biostatistician or utilize your own expertise	– How is the study structured?
		– What is your epidemiologic approach (observational vs. experimental design)?
		– What funding do you have, if any, to support your project?
		– What is your time frame?
		– What is your primary outcome?
		– What are your secondary outcomes?
Subjects	Meet with a biostatistician or utilize your own expertise	– Who are the subjects and how will they be selected?
		– What are your inclusion and exclusion criteria?
Measurements	Meet with a biostatistician or utilize your own expertise	– What measurements will be made?
		– What measurement scales will you utilize—Continuous vs. categorical data?
Statistics	Meet with a biostatistician or utilize your own expertise	How large is the study and how will the data be analyzed?
		What is your hypothesis?
		What is your sample size based on power calculations?

Table 77.2 The physiology of research: steps and questions

	Steps	Questions
Draw valid inferences based on your study sample	The goal of clinical research is to draw inferences from the study results about the nature of truth in the universe:	What are the main conclusions from your study?
	1. Design a study plan with subjects and measurements chosen to enhance the process of appropriately answering the research question (DESIGN)	
	2. Carry out the study in a fashion that enhances the likelihood of getting the right answer (IMPLEMENT)	
Make generalizable conclusions to apply to people outside the study	Compare your results with other published studies or your hypothesis	– Do your results agree or disagree with previously published literature?
		– Are your results generalizable to the population outside of your sample, and if not, why not (limitations to the study)?
Minimize errors	Identify potential errors and attempt to minimize them:	– What errors are associated with your study?
	Random (based on chance) or systematic (based on bias)	– What limitations were there to your work?

question "What is the research made of?" and the physiology of research (Table 77.2) asks the question "How does it work?" Before you embark on a research study, ask yourself the following questions:

I hope this chapter has inspired you to become a passionate, productive, and impactful researcher. I would like to end this chapter with quotes from my favorite television show, *Shark Tank*. As I see it, entrepreneurship is much like research:

> "Everyone has ideas. The hard part is doing the homework to know if the idea could work in an industry, and then doing the preparation to be able to execute on the idea." – Mark Cuban

> "Every problem can be solved as long as they use common sense and apply the right research and techniques" – Daymond John

> "A goal without a timeline is just a dream." – Robert Herjavec

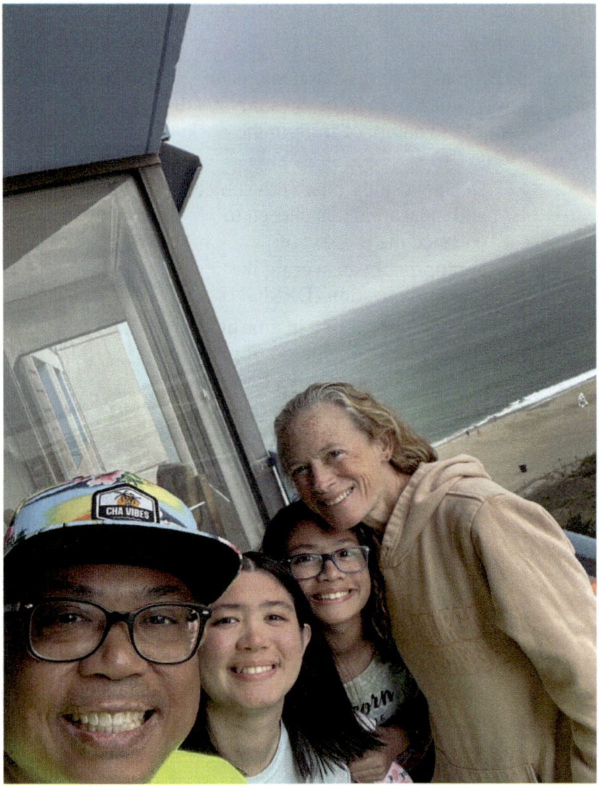

The pot of gold at the end of the rainbow: The Olympia family at Ocean City, Maryland. Feeling blessed.

Chapter 78
Scholarship and the Dissemination of Research

Robert P. Olympia

Initial Steps in Research Dissemination

You have decided to be involved in Emergency Medicine research, and with the assistance of a research mentor, successfully collected and analyzed data to answer your research question. You have organized piles of data spreadsheets and have met with your biostatistician, so what do you do next? Demonstrating scholarship involves imparting knowledge that results from study and research in a particular field and the dissemination of this knowledge. It's time to create the impact that you hoped for with the research you have conducted, but before you do that, here are some questions you want to think about before you decide how to disseminate your results:

1. *Who is your audience?* Who will benefit the most from the research you have conducted? Is it general EM physicians, or other medical and/or surgical subspecialists? Is it nursing, advanced practice providers, or other health care professionals? Is it policy makers, funders, or specific organizations/society leadership? Is it the general public? Defining your audience is an important first step to determine the most effective method of research distribution.
2. *What do you want your audience to learn from your research?* It is likely that once your research project is completed, you will feel overwhelmed with the amount of data you have collected. Step back and think about your hypothesis, your primary and secondary outcomes, and the data that you have collected that supports or rejects your hypothesis. Now select 2–3 main points/conclusions you want your audience to focus on. This simplifies your results and conclusions,

R. P. Olympia (✉)
Department of Emergency Medicine, Penn State Milton S. Hershey Medical Center, Hershey, PA, USA
e-mail: rolympia@hmc.psu.edu

R. P. Olympia et al. (eds.), *An Emergency Physician's Path*,
https://doi.org/10.1007/978-3-031-47873-4_78

and creates a larger impact on your audience—they are more likely to remember and disseminate the results of your study.

3. *Are there any aspects of your research that will make it difficult to disseminate?* Every study faces aspects that may make dissemination difficult. Recognizing these obstacles and addressing their effect on your conclusion is an important step before you disseminate your results. These include:
   (a) Study design limitations
   (b) Obtaining negative or equivocal results
   (c) Results that contradict previously published data
   (d) Type of bias, including information bias, selection bias, and confounding
4. *Is your conclusion interesting or unique?* Hopefully this question was entertained before you decided to pursue your research project, but now that you have collected the data, is your audience going to care about your results? Dissemination of research can be widespread if your results are innovative, interesting, or impactful.

Methods of Research Dissemination

Now that you have answered the questions above, it is time to consider methods of research dissemination. The most common methods include:

1. Publication of your research in a peer-reviewed journal
2. Presentation of your research at a national and/or regional scientific assembly
3. Non-traditional forms of research dissemination

Publication of Your Research in a Peer-Reviewed Journal

Whenever I mentor a medical student or a resident with their research, I reassure them that there will always be a peer-reviewed journal out there that will accept their research, but I challenge them to find a journal that will target their chosen audience, that will create the most "buzz" and reach the most people, and that will create an impact within a reasonable amount of time. Aspects to consider when choosing an appropriate journal include audience, impact factor, traditional subscription journals vs. open access journals, indexing, and timeliness for peer review and publication.

Audience

Most peer-reviewed journals target a particular audience/specialty or are sponsored by a specific society/membership (such as ACEP/*Annals of Emergency Medicine* and SAEM/*Academic Emergency Medicine*). Consider your audience when choosing a peer-reviewed journal to submit to.

Impact Factor

Most journals are designated an impact factor each year. A journal's impact factor for a particular year is calculated by the total number of times articles in the journal were cited during the previous 2 years divided by the total number of citable articles in the journal during those 2 years. In most fields, an impact factor of 10 or greater is considered an excellent score while 3 is considered good, but it is important to remember that these impact factors vary across disciplines. Examples of EM journal impact factors reported in 2021 (Table 78.1):

Table 78.1 2021 impact factors for a select number of emergency medicine journals

Journal	Impact factor (2021)
Annals of Emergency Medicine	6.76
Resuscitation	6.25
Academic Emergency Medicine	5.22
American Journal of Emergency Medicine	4.09
Western Journal of Emergency Medicine	3.98
Prehospital and Disaster Medicine	2.86
Prehospital Emergency Care	2.68
European Journal of Emergency Medicine	2.17
AEM Education and Training	1.62
Journal of Emergency Medicine	1.47
Pediatric Emergency Care	1.25

Traditional Subscription Journals Vs. Open Access Journals

Description of Traditional Subscription Journals

1. Individuals or institutions (university or company libraries) pay subscription charges to have access to the journal's content, so therefore, due to financial constraints, access to your article may be limited or non-existent.
2. Authors can publish their article for free.
3. The journal owns the copyright to the publication, so the author cannot freely distribute their own article or legally publish it on their own web page. Some exceptions include distribution of a PDF version after an embargo period or distribution of a different version of the article, such as a pre-publication version.
4. Subscription journals are more familiar to the medical community.
5. Rejection rates are higher compared with open access journals.

Description of Open Access Journals:

1. Articles are freely and permanently available online, so anyone, anywhere, can read it and distribute it.
2. Journals are less familiar to the medical community and, in general, have lower impact factors.
3. Often the author receives 3–10 times more readers than traditional subscription journals.
4. Articles are free to the reader, and therefore the journals often have a higher citation rate.
5. Authors pay an article processing charge (APC) to publish their article. APC range from $1000 to $10,000, and average $2800–$3000.
6. Authors retain the copyright and it is made available under a Creative Commons license. Readers may use the article in any way they would like to, as long as they attribute the authors of that article.
7. Rejection rates are lower compared with traditional subscription journals.
8. Several open access journals may be considered "predatory" or fraudulent, as they do not provide the same quality assurance and services delivered by reputable journals.

Hybrid journals are fundamentally subscription journals that offer authors the option of making their articles open access. In this model, the author can publish using the traditional model where it's free for the author but not free for the reader, or the author can publish using an open access model where the author pays and it's free for the reader.

Indexing

In order for research to be impactful and discoverable, researchers must consider indexing of journals. Online discovery is the primary way to find articles, and this depends on content dissemination in various indexing and abstracting platforms.

Table 78.2 Types of indexing

Index type	Examples	Features
General search engines	Google	Easily accessible to medical professionals and the general public
	Bing	Any journal can be added to general search engines
Scholarly search engines	Google Scholar	Ensures the websites they index are from academic sources
	Microsoft Academic	
General and discipline-specific scholarly indexing databases	Ulrichsweb	Covers all or multiple disciplines and/or discipline-specific databases
	Directory of Open Access Journals (DOAJ)	
	Scopus (Elsevier)	
	Web of Science (Institute for Scientific Information)	
	Academic Search (EBSCO)	
	PubMed (National Center for Biotechnology Information)	
	IJIFACTOR	
	EMBASE	

There are several indexing options that journals can pursue, from general search engines to discipline-specific databases. Journals go through an extensive process to be included, or indexed, in reputable bibliographic databases. This process evaluates a journal's quality of content published, publishing timeliness, and journal workflow and processes. Once a journal is indexed by a database, it is immediately available to all users of that database. Researchers should consider indexing when deciding on which journal to submit to, as each index type varies in their reach and impact, and offers different levels of detail, from article titles, abstracts, and references to full article files. The types of indexing include (Table 78.2):

Timeliness for Peer-Review and Publication

We live in world where we want things now, and we want them fast. This does not apply to the peer-review and publication process, where there is variability in these processes. Most journals have an initial screening process to determine appropriateness of submitted manuscripts, and decisions are usually made expeditiously (my personal record is rejection 2 h after submission). After the initial screening process, manuscripts are distributed to potential reviewers, and reviewers are often given 2 weeks to 2 months (sometimes longer) to review the manuscript, make a list of revisions/recommendations, and assign a decision. If accepted, your research may be available on the journal's website (published ahead-of print) and/or indexed on scholarly databases within a few weeks to a few months, although it may take several months to years for your research to be in a journal's print form. Consider the timeline you and your research team (especially medical students and residents, who may have requirements for graduation) have adopted when deciding on a journal for submission.

While Chap. 80 describes specifics on turning your research into written form, here are a few pearls, based on years of rejection, and a few acceptances:

1. Read and follow the *Instructions for Authors* provided by each journal carefully. One of the first things that reviewers do, even before they read your manuscript, is assure that the *Instructions for Authors* are abided by. You may have an innovative and impactful study, but if you are not careful enough to follow the *Instructions for Authors*, then reviewers may question the validity of your results, and decide on rejection.
2. I often write the "Results" section first. Choose the 2–3 major points you want the audience to focus on, decide how to present these 2–3 major points (text, table, figure), and then decide which of the other data points you have collected add to your main conclusion. Not every data point you collect needs to be in the manuscript. Simplicity is key.
3. If you have the time, I would recommend submitting your manuscript to a journal with a wide circulation and high impact factor, even if you think rejection is inevitable. Although the acceptance rate is lower than other journals with lower impact factors, rejections are usually accompanied by suggestions from editors/reviewers that, if used to revise your manuscript, result in a better product. Publication decisions are usually decided by a selected few, and you never know what their opinion would be unless you submit your manuscript. You did the work, now shoot for the stars.
4. When choosing a journal to submit to, look through a few years of published studies in that journal to determine if your manuscript would be a good fit, in style and research topic. Another option is utilizing "Journal Finder" tools provided by several medical publishing companies. You simply input your manuscript title, keywords, and the abstract, and they will attempt to match your manuscript with a specific journal (e.g., Elsevier Journal Finder, Wiley Journal Finder, Springer Journal Suggester, etc.).
5. Before I submit a manuscript, I typically give it a few weeks to "rest". I usually have colleagues, medical students/residents, biostatisticians, English majors, and unbiased reviewers, who are unaware of the study, read and review the manuscript for content and grammar. Incorporate their suggestions, perform a final review, and hit the "submit" button.

Presentation of Your Research at a National and/or Regional Scientific Assembly

Another form of research dissemination is presentation at a national and/or regional scientific assembly. Choosing a scientific assembly to submit your abstract to resembles the initial process involved with choosing a journal (determining the audience, defining 2–3 main points/conclusions, identifying limitations and biases, deciding if the conclusion is interesting or unique). In the field of Emergency Medicine, highly regarded scientific assemblies include American College of Emergency Physicians (ACEP), Society for Academic Emergency Medicine (SAEM), American Academy of Emergency Medicine (AAEM), and National Association of EMS Physicians (NAEMSP), and the regional conferences associated with these assemblies. Also, specialty and subspecialty assemblies should be considered based on your research topic. While Chap. 79 describes specifics on turning your research into an abstract and into a presentation for a scientific assembly, here are a few pearls:

1. Although several scientific assemblies have virtual options for poster presentations, the era of having rows and rows of posters pinned onto bulletin boards in a huge convention hall still exist. The key is attracting the horde of audience members to your comparatively small poster to educate and disseminate. There are two types of poster presenters: the "quiet type" who stands to the side of the poster, available to answer questions, or the "salesman", who will walk up to anyone who will listen and start telling you about their research. There is no right or wrong way of poster presenting, but find what you are comfortable with and go with it.
2. When developing a poster, I use the 5 foot rule. If you are standing 5 feet away from the poster, you should be able to easily read the text, tables, and figures on the poster. If you can't read it, then there is potentially too much information on the poster. Also, bullet points often work better than full paragraphs, and usually no more than 2–3 tables/figures per poster.
3. For both oral and poster presentations, make note of comments, suggestions, and questions from audience members. Incorporate these into your manuscript, as often journal reviewers and those who think similarly may be the ones judging the fate of your manuscript submission.
4. As most audience members will only have a few minutes to read your poster or listen to your oral presentation, make copies of your abstract to hand out with your name and contact information on them. Consider handing out business cards. This allows them to read about your research in a less stressful environment, to contact you if they have any questions, and to potentially create networks and relationships for future research, mentoring, jobs, etc.
5. Feel free to submit an abstract to multiple scientific assemblies, both nationally and regionally, and to various specialty and subspecialty conferences. Only a handful of scientific assemblies will discourage or disallow multiple presentations. The goal is to disseminate your research to as many people as possible, and very few medical professionals are able to attend every scientific assembly.
6. Bring a zip drive to the scientific assembly with your poster or oral presentation on it, or email copies of these to yourself. Often assemblies will require you to send a copy of your Power Point presentation or poster (if virtual) to them prior to the conference. Anticipate the worst case scenario. Also, know where the closest print shop is to the assembly … I may have had to print a poster at midnight

in Seattle after realizing that my institution's print shop had shipped the wrong poster.

7. Bribery can be your friend. I have been known to hand out Hershey chocolates to attract the audience to my poster.

Non-traditional Forms of Research Dissemination

In addition to publications and presentations, there are various forms of non-traditional methods of research dissemination, summarized below (Table 78.3). Before you utilize these methods of dissemination, check with your publisher (if

Table 78.3 Non-traditional methods of research dissemination

<table>
<tr><th>Dissemination method</th><th>Examples</th><th>Comments</th></tr>
<tr><td>Workshops and seminars</td><td>ACEP or SAEM or AAEM assemblies, Webinars, TED talks, science festivals, science slams, road shows</td><td>Success of dissemination is associated with knowing the motivation of the learners, building upon the audience's previous experiences, matching the learning approach with the audience background and diversity, and actively involving the learners</td></tr>
<tr><td>News media</td><td>Newspapers, television, radio, online newsletters and magazine</td><td>News stories that are likely to gain attention are associated with the seriousness of the problem, human interest in the form of a personal story, local angle for a national or state headline, timeliness, conflict or controversy</td></tr>
<tr><td rowspan="4">Social media</td><td rowspan="4">Twitter, LinkedIn, Facebook, Personal blogs</td><td>Associated with more downloads and eventual citations</td></tr>
<tr><td>Following people and organizations with similar interest increases dissemination</td></tr>
<tr><td>Use appropriate hashtags to reach relevant audiences</td></tr>
<tr><td>Altmetrics—describes the number of times a scholarly item is mentioned in social media</td></tr>
<tr><td>Issue or policy briefs</td><td>Infographics, research summary document, science comics</td><td>A summary of research information usually enhanced with data visualization (charts, tables, pictures)</td></tr>
<tr><td>E-mail lists and distribution</td><td></td><td>Compile a mailing list that includes funders, your community, other researchers, medical organizations and societies, journalists, politicians, policymakers, and practitioners</td></tr>
<tr><td rowspan="3">Audiovisual clips</td><td rowspan="3">YouTube, Vimeo, Vine clips</td><td>Often picked up by general search engines</td></tr>
<tr><td>Keep clips brief (less than 4 min)</td></tr>
<tr><td>Add clips to your Twitter and Facebook accounts</td></tr>
<tr><td rowspan="2">Post to Wikipedia</td><td rowspan="2"></td><td>Well indexed and optimized for search engines</td></tr>
<tr><td>Widely used and accessible</td></tr>
</table>

Adapted from Brownson RC, Eyler AA, Harris JK, et al. Getting the word out: new approaches for disseminating public health science. *J Public Health Manag Pract*. 2018 Mar;24(2): 102–111.

your research is published in a traditional subscription journal), since copyright policies may limit the method or format in which your research is disseminated.

Hopefully this chapter has inspired you to be a scholar, disseminating your research through traditional and non-traditional methods, in order to be impactful.

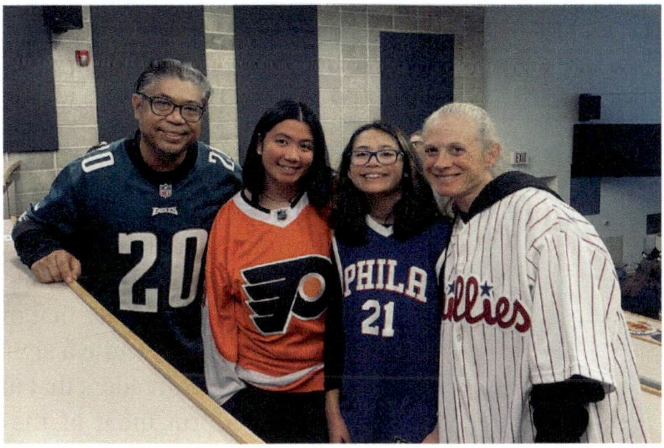

A family of Philly Phanatics: Abigail (Flyers), Madelyn (Sixers), Mommy (Phillies) and Daddy (Eagles)

"extended mandate." Nevertheless, ...

Major Ethical Principles

the provider–patient relationship ...

1. Beneficence

Beneficence refers to action that promotes ...

Chapter 79
Preparing Oral and Poster Presentations

Kimberly M. Rathbun

You've been working on a project, you have data, and now you'd like to share it with the world. Often, the first step is presenting it at a local, regional, or national meeting. This is a great way to get feedback on your project before you submit it as a manuscript. Traditional poster sessions involve dozens of posters hung on bulletin boards in a large room. The creator of the poster stands next to their work. Attendees go around the room looking at posters and speaking with the authors of posters they find interesting. The authors give a brief summary of the project using the poster as a reference and then the attendee asks questions. Now, there are various formats that are used to present your work at meetings: traditional paper posters, ePosters, oral abstracts, lightning talks, etc. Depending on the meeting, you might request a certain format when submitting your abstract or you might be assigned a format once your abstract is accepted. The most important thing to do when creating a research presentation is to follow the specifications given to you by the meeting. The requirements can often be found in your abstract acceptance email. No matter which format you are using, they all contain the same information in limited space. Due to the space limitations, some presenters may wish to develop a handout with their contact information and additional study information to give to those who are interested.

Title

The title conveys main topic(s) and importance of your project. It should be descriptive and can sometimes indicate the type of study (e.g., randomized trial). The title should be interesting enough to attract people, but not complicated. While

K. M. Rathbun (✉)
Department of Emergency Medicine, AU/UGA Medical Partnership, Athens, GA, USA
e-mail: krathbunmd@augusta.edu

R. P. Olympia et al. (eds.), *An Emergency Physician's Path*,
https://doi.org/10.1007/978-3-031-47873-4_79

the title should generally fit within two lines of text on a physical poster or within a given character limit in other formats, an oversimplified title may not attract interest.

Authors

Typically, all authors that will be on the final manuscript should be on the poster. There may be instances in which you are presenting only a part of the entire project and in that case only those authors that contributed to that part should be included. Titles and degrees are generally not listed, but affiliations should be included.

Abstract

There may/may not be an abstract section. This should generally be very similar to the abstract that was submitted and accepted for presentation. Often, there has been more data collected and analyzed since the abstract was submitted and some results/conclusions might change. You should include the most current information in your presentation.

Background and Hypothesis

This section conveys the significance of your work. It also puts your project into the context of work that has already been done. Limit literature review to most relevant previous work. The literature should be succinctly summarized as there is limited space. The last sentence should be the purpose of your study and/or your hypothesis.

Methods

Due to the limited space of this format compared to a manuscript, the methods section often needs to be simplified. You can sometimes even present a flowchart that you verbally explain in greater detail. The methods should still give a thorough and accurate representation of how your study was carried out.

Results

This section is a great place to include graphics: tables, charts, images, etc. You will be presenting this information verbally regardless of format, so the words can be limited. If possible, present all results graphically and use the figure legends to convey the main findings of your study.

Discussion/Conclusion

This is often a combined section in presentations as opposed to separate sections in a manuscript. This section should explain how your study results fit into the context of previous research. You may wish to include a summary sentence. This is also where you can mention future work/next steps, especially if you are presenting an incomplete research study.

Acknowledgments

Usually this is a short section thanking those who assisted with your project, but did not meet the criteria for authorship. An example would be thanking a simulation center and the staff if you used their space and/or equipment. Any financial support you received should be noted here as well.

References

If you have space, you should include references, but this section is often not included.

Now that you know what information needs to be included in the presentation, it's time to work on the formatting. Again, the most important thing to do when preparing a presentation is to follow the instructions set forth by the meeting. Many meetings are very strict with poster sizes and oral abstract time limits while others give more flexibility to authors.

Traditional Posters

If you are presenting a traditional poster, a specified size will be given. Less often, there may be detailed format guidelines. Before creating a poster from scratch, check to see if your institution has a poster template that you should use. Using an existing template can save a lot of time choosing colors and working on formatting. If your institution doesn't have a template, there are plenty of options that you can download from the internet. The easiest way to make a poster is in PowerPoint. The first thing to do is change the size. Click on the 'design' tab at the top and then go all the way to the right, click 'slide size', and select 'custom slide size'. Enter the desired poster width and height—be sure that you have entered them in the correct boxes as some conferences use landscape orientation and others use portrait orientation. Once you have set the size, you can add the content. If not using a template, turning on the grid can help you keep things neatly aligned. When finished, save the file as a PDF.

If your institution does not have a designated format, you will have a lot of flexibility in the design of your poster. You want the poster to be visually appealing and easy to read—keep this in mind when choosing colors and fonts. A solid color background is best as patterns can be distracting. The font should be large enough that it can be read from 5 ft away. Typically, font sizes between 24 point and 36 point are used for the body of the poster with larger sizes used for the author names and an even larger size used for the title. Fonts should be easy to read, so stick with basic fonts such as Arial, Times New Roman, Georgia, or Calibri. Do not use more than two fonts on a poster—instead use bold, underline, or italics to designate headings, etc. Bulleted lists, rather than paragraphs, make sections such as introduction, methods, and discussion/conclusion easier to read and more visually appealing. Use charts, tables, and graphics as much as possible, particularly in the results section, to add color and visual interest. Graphics should be appropriately captioned so the observer can understand them, but during a poster session you will be there to verbally explain them.

Printing a physical poster is another consideration. Many institutions have large format printers and are able to do this for $20–50 . Typical paper posters are generally carried in a poster tube during travel. Some institutions may offer a fabric "paper" that can be folded and later ironed for ease of transport. Another option would be to have the poster printed at the conference location by an office or shipping store, but this can be more expensive.

Poster Examples and Templates

https://phdposters.com/gallery

http://www.craftofscientificposters.com/

Oral presentations almost always involve a slide show. You will be given a time limit (usually 2–7 min) and often a slide limit. The general slide content is often dictated by the meeting organizers; such as title (one slide), background (one slide), methods (one slide), results (two slides), etc. As with a poster, keep your color scheme simple and use easily read fonts so attendees are not distracted from the information being presented. Because this is a slide show, the same general rules apply. Do not crowd each slide with information; hit the important points. Bulleted lists rather than paragraphs are preferred. Results should be presented in graphic form whenever possible and verbally explained by the presenter.

No matter which format is used to present your work, it should be visually appealing and convey the most important parts of the study. More importantly you should understand and be able to explain your work in detail. Poster sessions attendee will ask many questions and oral presentations often leave time for a question and answer session. Be sure you understand the purpose of your study and how it fits into the larger context of your field as a whole.

Suggested Readings

1. Barker E, Phillips V. Creating conference posters: structure, form and content. J Perioper Pract. 2021;31(7–8):296–9.
2. Gundogan B, Koshy K, Kurar L, Whitehurst K. How to make an academic poster. Ann Med Surg (Lond). 2016;11:69–71.
3. Naegle KM. Ten simple rules for effective presentation slides. PLoS Comput Biol. 2021;17(12):e1009554.

Chapter 80
Scientific Manuscript Writing: Original Research, Case Reports, Review Articles

Kimberly M. Rathbun

Scientific manuscripts are used to communicate your research findings with others. They add to the ever-growing body of scientific knowledge, which can then be built upon by subsequent projects. Writing a manuscript can seem like a daunting task. There are probably as many ways to tackle the task as there are authors—a quick internet search will give you multiple strategies of attack. It is imperative that your manuscript be cohesive and tell a single story. Starting with an outline, flow chart, storyboard, blueprint, etc. can be very helpful. Reading lots of papers in your field can help you become familiar with their format and content.

You should start thinking about writing the paper before you submit your IRB or start your experiments. You should have done a literature review while developing your project, so you are able to write the introduction. Writing the introduction can help clarify your hypothesis. Prior to submitting the IRB, the methods should be completely laid out and any survey tools you might want to use should be made. Once the methods are written out for the manuscript, you can have mentors critically appraise your experimental plan and determine if any modifications should be made before the study is begun. Anticipate the results you'll probably get and sketch out the results and discussion sections—you might think of things you can address in your study that you hadn't thought of before. Think critically about limitations and see if any can be avoided/minimized. Have someone read over your prewritten manuscript to look for any methodological problems, etc.

Once you have finished your research project, the next step is choosing a journal. You are probably familiar with the major journals in your field, but your project might be a better fit for a different journal. There is an online tool called the Journal/Author Name Estimator that uses your title, abstract, or keywords to match your

K. M. Rathbun (✉)
Department of Emergency Medicine, AU/UGA Medical Partnership, Athens, GA, USA
e-mail: krathbunmd@augusta.edu

R. P. Olympia et al. (eds.), *An Emergency Physician's Path*,
https://doi.org/10.1007/978-3-031-47873-4_80

work to the most appropriate journals based on what the journals have published previously. Each journal will have its own specific guidelines for authors to follow. Be sure you follow these carefully.

Three types of manuscripts are detailed below.

Original Research

The most common type of manuscript presents original research. This can be observational or experimental research. The IMRAD format has been used since the 1980s. This stands for **I**ntroduction, **M**ethods, **R**esults, **A**nd **D**iscussion. Some manuscripts might benefit from subheadings within these categories and many journals will require a Conclusion section at the end of the manuscript. Other important parts of the manuscript are: title, authors, affiliations, abstract, keywords, references, and acknowledgments.

Introduction

The introduction explains the relevance of your project and puts it into the context of what is already known. It has three main sections: the importance of your project (why should someone care?), what is already known in the field (this is a focused literature review), and how your research will fill some gaps in knowledge. The final sentence of the Introduction is often your hypothesis. The literature review you perform should be extensive so you don't miss important articles, but you should only include those that fit into the context of explaining the purpose/relevance of your study. When performing the literature review, be sure you are able to read the entire article and not just the abstract. Since the literature review is often done early in the research process, another review should be done just prior to submission of your manuscript to ensure that you include the most recent articles on the topic. This section should be written so that an educated person can understand it—it should not be at the level of an expert in the field.

Methods

The Methods section of a manuscript gives detailed explanation of how the study was carried out such that anyone reading the paper should be able to replicate the study exactly. This section is sometimes subdivided. Things to include in the methods section are: the study design, the setting, the study population (with inclusion and exclusion criteria), data collection methods, interventions, the study endpoints/

outcomes measured, and how the data was analyzed. Any established methods can be mentioned and appropriately referenced without having to describe them in detail. Reagents or materials should be identified by name, vendor, and vendor location. For studies involving research involving human or animal subjects, the authors should give information about authorization from institutional regulatory committees. Additionally, if human subjects research his involved, there should be a statement regarding informed consent. This section should be written in past tense and at the level of an expert in the field.

Results

The Results section is where you present what you found. The data is presented factually without interpretation or commentary. This section may be divided into subsections depending on the study. Data should be presented in the same order that the collection methods were mentioned in the methods section. Negative as well as positive findings are reported. Tables, graphs, and images are prominent features in the results section. They should be easy to understand and captioned appropriately. The text should summarize information found in the figures rather than simply repeating it. For example, you might use a table of patient demographics. In that case, you would not list out the demographics in the text; you would refer to the table/figure. Be sure to limit the data you present to information that is relevant to your hypothesis. This section is written in past tense.

Discussion

In this section, you will interpret your results and explain what your findings mean. Typically, the Discussion section begins with a summary of the key results answering the research question posed at the end of the Introduction. The section includes all the main findings of the study and puts these results into the context of previous studies. Your results will agree or disagree with previous findings and you should discuss why this might have occurred. Any limitations and how the limitations may have biased the study should be discussed. Potential areas for further research can be noted.

The Discussion should follow a logical thought process and avoid excessive wordiness. It is important to refrain from over-reaching, or making conclusions that are not supported by your data. Other common mistakes include: mentioning methods or results that are not present in the prior sections, repeating detailed data that is presented in the Results section, and including information that is not relevant to your topic.

Conclusion

The Conclusion is typically a 2–3 sentence paragraph summarizing what you learned from your study. You can think of it as the take-home message for your readers. If the journal does not use a Conclusion section, this paragraph should be the last paragraph of the Discussion section.

Title

The title of your study should be descriptive and attract the interest of the reader. It should not be overly long and complex. Some journals may give a character limit—staying under 100 characters including spaces is a good rule of thumb.

Authors & Affiliations

Authorship and order of authors is best determined at the beginning of a project. Manuscript authorship is a form of academic currency—you may have heard the phrase "publish or perish". As such, heated debates can occur. The International Committee of Medical Journal Editors uses four criteria to establish if someone should be listed as an author. Many journals require that the contributions of each author be listed out during the submission process. The order of the authors is also important. Traditionally, the first author is the person who did the majority of the "work," the last author is the one who came up with the idea and directed the project, and all the authors in the middle also met the guidelines for authorship. At some institutions, only first-author papers "count" for promotion, so in that case the senior author would be listed first and then the next authors listed in the order of their contribution.

An accurate affiliation for each author should be listed; these are published with the manuscript. The affiliation listed should be the location where the work was conducted, which may not be the author's current location. Authors can have multiple affiliations.

Abstract

The abstract is a condensed version of the manuscript. The character limit for the abstract is almost always specified by the journal. Depending on the journal, you may or may not use the IMRAD headings to break the abstract into sections. The abstract should explain the importance of your study, give a very limited idea of how your research fits in to the bigger picture, give a general overview of the methods, highlight the most important results, and end with a brief discussion explaining how your study contributes to your field. It will usually end with a concluding sentence.

Keywords

Journals will often want you to provide 3–5 key words after the abstract. These are the words or phrases that you would type into a search bar when looking for a manuscript similar to the one you are presenting

References

All articles referenced in your manuscript should be listed here. The format can vary by journal so pay close attention to the journal's guidelines for authors. Also, the order of the references can vary—usually it is in the order that the reference appears in the text, but can be alphabetical order. Make sure that the formatting of your references is correct and that all necessary references are listed.

Acknowledgments

This is the section to list any contributors to the work who did not meet authorship criteria. If your work was performed in a simulation center you would acknowledge the support of the center and its staff. If someone helped edit the manuscript or provided technical writing assistance, they would be acknowledged. This section is also the place to note funding that supported the work.

Case Report

A case or case series report is used to communicate an unusual presentation of a known disease, description of a new disease, newly identified effects of new medications, etc. They typically contain five sections: abstract, introduction, case description, discussion, and conclusion. All of these sections except the case description are similar to those described above. The discussion section should connect the case described to the existing literature. The case description is generally presented in chronological order starting with the current condition for which the patient sought treatment. Only relevant demographic information should be included. A detailed history of the current condition and relevant past medical, surgical, and social histories as well as current medications and allergies should be included. A physical exam should be limited to pertinent findings as well as results of all relevant laboratory testing and imaging. The management and clinical course should be described, including any relevant repeat diagnostic testing. A final diagnosis should be given. Images can help facilitate the reader's understanding of the case.

When publishing a case report, it is critical to have patient consent. Many journals have their own forms to be filled out by the patient giving their consent. This can be problematic because when you see the patient, you may not know which journal you plan to submit to. Additionally, if your case report is not accepted at the first journal you try, you might submit to a second journal. It is reasonable to create a generic consent form that includes language found in most consent forms for the patient to sign.

Review Article

Review articles detail the current knowledge regarding a particular topic; so, they can be helpful when creating guidelines or updating personal knowledge. They do not present new data, but summarize existing data. They can also point out areas that need further investigation. Review articles can be broken down into two types—narrative and systematic. The systematic review category can be further broken down into qualitative and quantitative reviews. Meta-analyses are quantitative reviews. Writing any form of review article requires substantial knowledge of the existing literature and the ability to critically appraise these studies. Review articles generally conform to the IMRAD format detailed previously. Additionally, the Preferred Reporting Items for Systematic reviews and Meta-Analyses (PRISMA) statement is a detailed 27-item checklist that is used to guide reporting of systematic reviews.

Be aware that many journals do not publish review articles and some will only publish review articles that are invited—meaning the editors asked a particular individual or group to write a review article on a certain topic.

Suggested Readings

1. Alsaywid BS, Abdulhaq NM. Guideline on writing a case report. Urol Ann. 2019;11(2):126–31.
2. Cohen H. How to write a patient case report. Am J Health Syst Pharm. 2006;63(19):1888–92.
3. Cooper ID. How to write an original research paper (and get it published). J Med Lib Assoc. 2015;103:67–8.
4. Gemayel R. How to write a scientific paper. FEBS J. 2016;283(21):3882–5.
5. Gülpınar Ö, Güçlü AG. How to write a review article? Turk J Urol. 2013;39(Suppl 1):44–8.
6. Huth EJ. Structured abstracts for papers reporting clinical trials. Ann Intern Med. 1987;106:626–7.

7. International Committee of Medical Journal Editors. Recommendations for the Conduct, Reporting, Editing and Publication of Scholarly Work in Medical Journals. http://www.ICMJE.org. Accessed 23 Aug 2022.
8. Liumbruno GM, Velati C, Pasqualetti P, Franchini M. How to write a scientific manuscript for publication. Blood Transfus. 2013;11:217–26.
9. McCarthy LH, Reilly KE. How to write a case report. Fam Med. 2000;32(3):190–5.
10. Page MJ, Moher D, Bossuyt PM, Boutron I, Hoffmann TC, Mulrow CD, Shamseer L, Tetzlaff JM, Akl EA, Brennan SE, Chou R, Glanville J, Grimshaw JM, Hróbjartsson A, Lalu MM, Li T, Loder EW, Mayo-Wilson E, McDonald S, McGuinness LA, Stewart LA, Thomas J, Tricco AC, Welch VA, Whiting P, McKenzie JE. PRISMA 2020 explanation and elaboration: updated guidance and exemplars for reporting systematic reviews. BMJ. 2021;372:n160.
11. The Biosemantics Group. Journal/author name estimator. https://jane.biosemantics.org/. Accessed 24 Aug 2022.
12. Weinstein R. How to write a manuscript for peer review. J Clin Apher. 2020;35(4):358–66.

Chapter 81
Conducting Quality Improvement Research

Christopher J. Wilson, Mark F. Olaf, Eric M. Melnychuk, Judy B. Shahan, and Chadd K. Kraus

Why Is It Important for an Emergency Physician to Participate in QI?

In 2000, the publication, "To Err is Human," [1] estimated that nearly 100,000 patient deaths annually are attributable to medical errors. In 2004, the National Committee for Quality Assurance published "The State of Healthcare for Quality Assurance," that suggested that nearly nine billion dollars were wasted annually in the United States (US) due to inefficiencies in healthcare delivery [2]. Subsequently, quality, safety, and value have become tripartite goals in US healthcare.

Several definitions provide a foundation for understanding quality research. The US Agency for Healthcare Research and Quality (AHRQ), an agency of US Department of Health and Human Services (HHS), defines quality healthcare as "Doing the right thing, at the right time, in the right way, for the right person—and having the best possible results" [3]. Quality assurance is a system for evaluating the delivery of services or quality of products. Quality control is the verification and maintenance of a desired level of quality. The process of continuous quality improvement (CQI) is a combination of quality control and assurance [4].

C. J. Wilson · M. F. Olaf · J. B. Shahan
Department of Emergency Medicine, Geisinger Medical Center, Danville, Pennsylvania, USA
e-mail: cjwilson@geisinger.edu; mfolaf@geisinger.edu; jbshahan@geisinger.edu

E. M. Melnychuk
Department of Critical Care, Geisinger Medical Center, Danville, Pennsylvania, USA
e-mail: emelnychuk@geisinger.edu

C. K. Kraus (✉)
Department of Emergency and Hospital Medicine, Lehigh Valley Health Network (LVHN), Allentown, Pennsylvania, USA
e-mail: chadd.kraus@lvhn.org

R. P. Olympia et al. (eds.), *An Emergency Physician's Path*,
https://doi.org/10.1007/978-3-031-47873-4_81

Emergency Medicine is uniquely positioned to evaluate and analyze quality in healthcare, and emergency physicians are engaged in quality improvement (QI) throughout their career. Beginning with residency training requirements and continuing with practice requirements for maintenance of board certification, emergency physicians participate in QI across the spectrum of their careers and in all practice settings.

What Are Common Strategies for QI Activities and Research?

Langley and colleagues have outlined the steps in the process of QI [5]. First, it is necessary to develop a focused aim and measurable goals for the projects. Next, a time frame and deadline for work completion should be established. Finally, a model or intervention for improvement should be forwarded. To accomplish this process, there are a variety of quality instruments and tools that emergency physicians should be familiar with, including root cause analysis (RCA), plan-do-study-act (PDSA), LEAN, Six Sigma, and value stream mapping.

Root Cause Analysis is frequently employed to investigate a sentinel event. This sentinel event may be a patient death, major complication resulting in morbidity to the patient, or a "near miss" event that could have resulted in morbidity or mortality. RCAs intend to discern the system-level etiology that led to the sentinel event. Frequently sentinel events have multiple contributing factors and confounding variables leading to a specific outcome.

Plan-do-study-act (PDSA) is frequently used in health care as a way to pilot ideas, concepts, or innovations in healthcare delivery in small test "cycles" prior to implementing larger changes. "Plan" involves the introduction of an idea for improvement. The idea is then implemented on a small scale ("do"), and then measured and evaluated for how it is impacting the problem and how it might improve in subsequent cycles ("study"). Finally, the test cycle is repeated and a decision on whether to expand it on a larger scale is made ("act"). The PDSA process can be repeated until an innovation is either adopted on a large scale or abandoned.

LEAN is an instrument for quality, safety, and efficiency that was introduced by the Toyota Corporation in the 1950s as a tool to reduce inefficiency and waste. Initially called the Toyota Production System (TPS), the goal was to reduce or eliminate any activity that does not provide value, with value defined as "positive customer experience or profit margin." The eight wastes of LEAN production are: overproduction/underproduction, overprocessing, inventory, motion, waiting, transport, defects, and unutilized talent. LEAN has been integrated into healthcare models of clinical and operational quality improvement, safety, and value, most notably in patient satisfaction efforts, efficiency, and clinical outcomes. The "5S" model of LEAN is frequently employed in healthcare:

- Sort (Seiri): Sort the work area and keep only what is necessary;
- Set (Seiton): Optimize workflow, clearly identify and label;

- Shine (Seiso): Keep work areas clean;
- Standardize (Seiketsu): Workflows, processes, storage, and labeling; and.
- Sustain (Shitsuke): Equipment and knowledge.

Six Sigma, introduced at the Motorola Corporation in the 1980s, is a quality improvement instrument aimed at reducing variation to approximate perfection [6]. Statistically, "sigma" is the number of standard deviations from perfection, and "six sigma" translates to a nearly error free state. Six Sigma uses a 5-step process: (1) define; (2) measure; (3) analyze; (4) improve; and (5) control. After defining a goal and collecting data, the Six Sigma process measures and analyzes variation from a desired endpoint. Then solutions are aimed at improving that variation. Finally, controls are intended to ensure consistency and efficiency to limit future errors.

Value Stream Mapping (VSM) enhances LEAN and Six Sigma by providing graphical representation of processes and workflows to help identify excess work movements and inefficiencies, lost time, and process variations as targets for process improvement. Staff are included in this process and are asked to identify areas of inefficiency and suggest ideas for improvement. These ideas and suggestions are incorporated into test cycles of potential interventions.

How Do You Convert QI Activities into Research?

Although QI targets processes and research aims for knowledge expansion and translation, these two areas frequently overlap and are complementary. QI work can become research when it creates knowledge and informs the science of how processes improve quality, safety, and clinical outcomes. Often, QI projects include a hypothesis, approximate the scientific method in their execution, directly involve patient care and outcomes, and might result in publication in peer-reviewed scientific journals. For this reason, QI projects that might be viewed as research should be considered for review by institutional review boards (IRB) to protect human subjects as required by ethical principles and mandated by federal law and regulations. Many projects will ultimately not qualify as human subjects' research and will receive IRB exemption. Whether it meets the criteria for human subjects' research, QI research should be aimed at benefitting patients by improving quality, safety, and value, and should be shared broadly.

When planning a QI project or quality research project, it is critical to define a precise and answerable question or solvable problem. In defining the problem, it is necessary to evaluate the existing knowledge and available solutions on a topic. Not all QI research needs to be novel; however, it should build on existing knowledge or provide an innovative approach not previously considered. These exploratory steps should also consider how patient-centered outcomes might be positively impacted. With a question defined, one or more of the tools and instruments outlined above can be applied to the process.

The Standards for Quality Improvement Reporting Excellence (SQUIRE) were first published in 2008 and provide a framework for reporting quality improvement research [7]. This framework and checklist were updated in 2015 with the SQUIRE 2 guidelines [8, 9]. The SQUIRE guidelines provide a foundation for the publication of QI research and can also help as a guide to the QI process.

How Specifically Can QI Research Be Integrated into the Practice of Emergency Medicine?

In 2002 Graff and colleagues provided consensus recommendations for QI activities in Emergency Medicine [10]. These recommendations expanded on prior aims from the Institute of Medicine for improving the safety, effectiveness, patient centeredness, timeliness, efficacy, and equity of healthcare [11]. In Kelly and colleagues [12], outlined key components of an educational curriculum for EM physicians to understand about quality. This framework provides a template for the integration of QI into educational activities, no matter the stage of an emergency physician's career.

References

1. Kohn L, Corrigan J, Donaldson M, et al. To err is human: building a safer health system. Institute of Medicine (US) Committee on Quality of Health Care in America. Washington, DC: National Academies Press (US); 2000.
2. National Committee for Quality Assurance. The State of Health Care Quality. 2004. https://www.ncqa.org.
3. US Agency for Healthcare Research and Quality (AHRQ), An agency of Health and Human Services Department. https://www.ahrq.gov.
4. Varkey P, et al. Basics of quality improvement in health care. Mayo Clin Proc. 2007;82(6):735–9.
5. Langley GJ, Nolan KM, Nolan TW, Norman CL, Provost LP. The improvement guide. San Francisco: Jossey-Bass; 1996.
6. Chassin MR. Is health care ready for six sigma quality? Milbank Q. 1998;76:565–91.
7. Ogrinc G, Mooney SE, Estrada C, et al. The SQUIRE (Standards for Quality Improvement Reporting Excellence) guidelines for quality improvement reporting: explanation and elaboration. Qual Saf Health Care. 2008;17(Suppl 1):i13–32.
8. Goodman D, Ogrinc G, Davies L, et al. Explanation and elaboration of the SQUIRE (Standards for Quality Improvement Reporting Excellence) Guidelines, V.2.0: examples of SQUIRE elements in the healthcare improvement literature. BMJ Qual Saf. 2016;25:e7.
9. Standards for Quality Improvement Reporting Excellence (SQUIRE) Guidelines. Available online at: http://www.squirestatement.org. [Last accessed 12 December 2023].
10. Graff L, Stevens C, Spaite D, Foody J. Measuring and improving quality in emergency medicine. Acad Emerg Med. 2002;9(11):1091–107.
11. Institute of Medicine. Crossing the quality chasm: a new health system for the 21st century. Washington, DC: National Academy Press; 2001.
12. Kelly JJ, Thallner E, Broida RI, et al. Emergency medicine quality improvement and patient safety curriculum. Acad Emerg Med. 2010;17:e110–29.

Chapter 82
Conducting Educational Research

Arlene S. Chung and Annahieta Kalantari

Introduction

Although an extensive body of literature exists on both the history of medical education and education research generally, the much younger field of medical education research has received relatively little attention. The concept of scientific inquiry as applied to the education of physicians was not considered a serious area of study until the late 1950s [1]. This occurred in parallel with the broader societal emphasis on scientific research and scientific progress in the United States. While early medical education research was conducted in the tradition of experimental psychology and cognitive science by non-physician behavioral scientists, medical educators increasingly took on the roles of principal investigator and infused the field with new research methodologies and theoretical perspectives [2]. Accreditation policy changes for medical schools, the explosion of medical knowledge for the diagnosis and treatment of disease, and greater accountability to the public all led to the need for a rigorous, methodological, and outcomes-driven approach to the development and implementation of curricula for medical students and residents [2].

Today, medical education research is defined as research that "aims to advance the knowledge, skills, and professionalism of medical students [and residents] by understanding and evaluating educational ecosystems. These ecosystems include policies related to admissions and curriculum, people who serve as teachers and

A. S. Chung (✉)
Department of Emergency Medicine, University of Vermont Health Network, Burlington, VT, USA
e-mail: Arlene.Chung@uvmhealth.org

A. Kalantari
Department of Emergency Medicine, Penn State Health, Milton S. Hershey Medical Center, Hershey, PA, USA
e-mail: akalantari@pennstatehealth.psu.edu

R. P. Olympia et al. (eds.), *An Emergency Physician's Path*,
https://doi.org/10.1007/978-3-031-47873-4_82

mentors, instructional technology and other resources, the attitudes that pervade a given institution or educational experience, and even the [learners] themselves" [3]. Medical education research is a broad discipline and includes investigation into areas such as assessment and evaluation, curriculum design, educational methods, faculty development, and the clinical learning environment.

Medical education research is unique from other fields of scientific inquiry in many important ways. The study population of learners is often limited and can be considered inherently vulnerable. Principles of fairness come into play when considering intervention and control arms for randomized controlled studies of educational programs. Many important educational and clinical outcomes cannot be fully described with quantitative data and methods alone. These considerations and more have resulted in the development of a rich, complex, and ever-evolving area of study.

Here we discuss best practices for conducting medical education research, using Glassick's Criteria as a framework. Building on Edward Boyer's landmark 1990 publication, *Scholarship Reconsidered*, that expanded the definition of education scholarship, Glassick and colleagues proposed a set of six standards by which scholarship may be assessed: clear goals, adequate preparation, appropriate methods, significant results, effective presentation, and reflective critique [4]. In this chapter, we use these same six standards as a guide for education research.

Clear Goals

Developing Research Questions

Similar to any other type of scientific inquiry, all medical education research starts with a good question. Setting a clear goal requires the identification of important questions in the field and defining objectives that are realistic and achievable. Most medical educators are already heavily involved in different aspects of curriculum design, implementation, assessment, and program evaluation. This day-to-day work with learners and faculty easily lends itself to questions of efficacy and innovation—i.e., is this working and how can we do this better? The acronym FINER (feasible, interesting, novel, ethical, relevant) can help education researchers to narrow their area of focus. A literature search may help to identify similar questions that have already been used to drive prior research in order to avoid redundancy.

At minimum, a good research question clearly defines the subjects and the outcomes of interest in one concise statement without overstating the goals of the study. As an example, say that you have an interest in team dynamics during the resuscitation of critically ill patients. A clear research question might ask, "Does participation in simulated resuscitations with interdisciplinary team members improve the leadership skills of senior Emergency Medicine residents more than simulated resuscitations with peers alone?"

Adequate Preparation

Once a clear goal has been identified, adequate preparation is required to ensure the success of the study. The researcher should reflect on their own knowledge and skills and consider whether additional investigators with expertise in a particular area should be invited to join the study team. Other team members may include research assistants, statisticians, and grant managers. Additional resources may include access to learners and faculty, classroom space, simulation labs, and medical equipment. Institutions and departments will vary widely in the availability of staff, funding, and other resources to support education research. Several certificate courses and degree programs also exist for medical educators who desire greater foundational knowledge and skill with education research and scholarship.

Appropriate Methods

Institutional Review Board Considerations

All human subjects' research requires advance review and approval by the Institutional Review Board (IRB) prior to the commencement of any study. The purpose of the IRB is to assure that appropriate steps are taken to protect the rights and welfare of humans participating as subjects in biomedical research [5]. The IRB has several types of review processes in place depending on the nature of the proposed human research study. The majority of medical education research studies will fall under the category of "exempt" or "expedited" review.

A study is considered to be "exempt" if it is determined to be of minimal risk to its subjects and also falls into one of eight federally defined categories of human subjects' research [6]. These categories include research that involves normal educational practices, educational tests or surveys, or benign behavioral interventions with the collection of verbal or written responses or audiovisual recordings. Medical education research studies that fall under the category of exemption must still be submitted to the IRB prior to beginning the research but do not require ongoing monitoring or approval.

If a study is determined to be of minimal risk but does not fall into one of the eight categories that define exemption, the study may be a candidate for expedited review. Expedited review similarly allows approval of a study without convening the full IRB but will require ongoing monitoring and compliance with IRB policies and procedures [7].

Study Population

Learners and their teachers serve as the study population for almost all medical education research. We use the term "learner" broadly to mean any individual participating as the subject in an educational curriculum, intervention, or experience. Learners may be medical students, residents, or faculty members. Similarly, "teachers" may also be students, residents, or faculty depending on the nature of the study.

Recruitment of medical students and residents for the purposes of medical education research is challenging for several reasons. Due to the hierarchical nature of medical training, an ongoing relationship and inherent power differential often exists between the subjects and investigators. A student may be reluctant to refuse to participate in a study being conducted by his professor who is ultimately responsible for his final grade in the course. This power differential may also influence the results of the research itself. For example, residents may not truthfully disclose verbal or written feedback about a specific educational intervention to their program director who is also the lead investigator.

There is a limited supply of students and residents enrolled in a given class or training program. Infinite recruitment toward a minimum sample size in order to demonstrate adequate power is simply not feasible in most cases. Multi-institutional studies can help to boost the number of available learners but are frequently confounded by cultural differences in the respective educational ecosystems. Students and residents also speak to one another and may influence the results of subsequent interventions.

Study Design

The traditional gold standard methodology of a double-blind randomized controlled trial is difficult to implement and may not actually yield practical findings in the clinical learning environment. In many cases it is impossible to blind learners and teachers to the intervention. Additionally, it may not be fair or ethical to withhold certain educational experiences from some learners and not others, especially in a high-stakes field such as medicine. The process of learning to become a physician is nuanced, complex, and influenced by a whole host of individual and system factors that do not easily reduce themselves to numerical values. For example, on an assessment of professional values, it is difficult to distill the difference between a "4 out of 5" for one resident compared to a "5 out of 5" for another and we have to ask ourselves if that difference is even meaningful at a clinical level.

In order to address these methodological challenges, educators can use different techniques for conducting medical education research studies. A pre/post design, in which learners serve as their own controls, is intuitive, easy to implement, and readily accepted by most students and residents. This is commonly seen in studies assessing medical knowledge or specific procedural skills in which learners complete a pre-test prior to the educational intervention followed by a post-test to determine the impact of the session. Tests may be written multiple choice questions, oral board cases, simulated procedures, or some other form of assessment. This design can be strengthened by conducting a post-test later in order to demonstrate retention. The primary downside to this design is that learners become sensitized to the relevant content during pre-testing and will tend to score higher than they might otherwise on the post-test, particularly if the two tests are similar.

Cross-over designs help to mitigate some of the limitations inherent in pre/post design studies. In a cross-over design, learners are divided into two groups. One group participates in the educational intervention while the second group does not. An assessment is performed to determine the difference in learning between the two groups. The two groups then switch places so that the second group also has the opportunity to participate. The first arm of a cross-over design mimics a randomized controlled trial and statistical analyses are only performed after the first iteration of the educational intervention. The purpose of the second iteration is to ensure that all learners have the chance to participate and is not relevant for research purposes. The primary downside to a cross-over design is that it effectively cuts the number of study participants in half, further exacerbating the problem of small sample sizes common to medical education research.

Survey designs are another commonly used method in medical education research. With the easy and widespread availability of online forms, the temptation to whip up a quick survey to answer a research question can be irresistible. Surveys that measure quantitative data in the form of Likert scales and other numerical inputs are appealing to many novice education researchers because they allow for traditional and also familiar statistical analyses. When used correctly and developed according to sound research principles, survey studies are a powerful tool for assessing the landscape of broad swathes of learners, teachers, and programs. They can identify important trends that are generalizable to large populations, which is often difficult to achieve with other types of research designs. High-quality survey studies require a rigorous approach to question development, involving multiple iterations and pilot testing. In addition, a clear description of the study population eligible to participate (the "denominator") and an adequate number of respondents (the "numerator") is critical to the accurate interpretation of the survey findings. Many peer-reviewed journals will not accept a response rate of less than 70% for publication.

While quantitative measures are commonly used in each of the study designs described previously, it is worth considering that exploration of the educational ecosystem of medical school and residency training often lends itself well to qualitative analysis as well. Qualitative research is the systematic inquiry into social phenomena in natural settings [8]. Study designs using qualitative methods often employ focus groups, structured or semi-structured interviews, and observations of learners and faculty in the clinical learning environment. The data in this case are words rather than numbers, which can be coded line-by-line, cross checked by two or more investigators, and then organized by themes for analysis.

Lastly, literature reviews provide a method for researchers to examine the published evidence. This is useful when conducting a needs assessment for a new curriculum or research question. Several types of literature reviews exist, each with their own level of rigor. Narrative reviews, also known as traditional literature reviews, are useful for a superficial overview of a topic or as background information to develop a new research question. However, the methodology is not structured and is limited by the authors' biases. Narrative reviews also represent the lowest level of evidence. In contrast, systematic reviews are conducted according to strict methodological guidelines in order to minimize bias and are designed to test a specific hypothesis [9]. They represent one of the highest tiers of evidence, second only to meta-analyses. Scoping reviews have emerged as an accepted methodological approach in circumstances where systematic reviews are unable to meet the objectives of the research question. Similar to systematic reviews, scoping reviews follow rigorous guidelines that allow for replication of results but answer much broader questions [10]. For example, a systematic review is designed to answer a defined question such as, "Does this educational intervention improve knowledge in resident physicians more than attending physicians?" A scoping review might answer a related question such as, "What is the nature of the evidence supporting the utility of this educational intervention?"

Significant Results

Data collected using any of the previously described study designs may be either quantitative or qualitative in nature. For example, survey studies may employ free text response boxes and focus groups can be used as an assessment tool in a crossover design.

When reporting the results of quantitative data analysis, it is important to recognize that statistical significance may not reflect clinical or educational significance [11]. This is important to consider when designing a study and specifically when deciding which assessment measures to use. For example, Likert scale responses are simple to collect and analyze but ideally, we should also ensure that there is a meaningful difference between a four and a five. Additionally, while a significant p value (typically <0.05 in medical education research) can tell readers that an effect exists, reporting the effect size (e.g., odds ratio) will inform them of the magnitude of impact. In general, due to the challenges of medical education research as described in previous sections, it can be difficult to demonstrate either statistical significance or meaningful effect size that is generalizable to different populations of learners.

One way in which medical education researchers can show meaningful results is by using the Kirkpatrick Model of Educational Outcomes [12]. The Kirkpatrick Model describes four levels of evaluation: reaction, learning, behavior, and results. Level 1 describes the degree to which learners engaged and were satisfied with their participation in the activity. This is usually assessed using a simple post-session survey with questions such as, "On a scale of 1–5, how likely are you to recommend this to a colleague?" Level 2 describes the degree to which learners achieved the intended knowledge, skills, or attitudes and is typically assessed using pre/post testing. Level 3 describes the degree to which the activity changed the learners' behavior. This might be assessed using simulation or direct observation in the clinical setting. Level 4 describes changes in patient outcomes due to learner participation in the activity and is the highest standard of outcomes for medical education research. The overwhelming majority of published medical education research demonstrates Level 1 or Level 2 outcomes.

Effective Presentation

Dissemination of knowledge is a required component of adequate scholarship. Multiple forums now exist for the presentation and publication of medical education research. Dedicated journals such as *Academic Medicine*, *the Journal of Graduate Medical Education*, *Medical Teacher*, *Medical Education*, and others, all serve as potential avenues for education researchers to share their findings. Online platforms such as *MedED Portal* allow educators to publish peer-reviewed curricula in their entirety, including handouts, slides, and other resource materials required for successful implementation.

In 1990, Edward Boyer shook the academic community with his reimagination of scholarship. Prior to publishing *Scholarship Reconsidered*, the honorable work of educators frequently went unrecognized due to the relative importance placed on original research. He proposed that the term "scholarship" be given a broader meaning to include four separate but overlapping areas of academic work: the scholarship of discovery, the scholarship of integration, the scholarship of application, and the scholarship of teaching [13]. The expanded definition was well-received by the academic community. The explosion of published high-quality medical education research as seen today reflects this critical cultural shift. Dissemination of scholarly work related to the teaching and training of physicians is an important responsibility of all medical educators.

Reflective Critique

Ideally, the findings from one education research study should serve as the targeted needs assessment for the next. Following the successful publication of a research study, educators should reflect on lesson learners and consider the implications for their next cohort of learners and teachers.

Conclusion

In summary, medical education research is a relatively young field as compared to both the history of medical education and education research. Educators face many different challenges unique to the study of learners, such as limitations inherent in sample size, study design, and clinically important measurable outcomes. Medical education research is a complex and evolving area of study that is increasingly being approached with the methodological rigor characteristic of other fields of research. Advancing the quality of published evidence available to guide educators in the process of teaching and training the next generation of physicians is critically important to the future health of the public.

References

1. Kuper A, Albert M, Hodges BD. The origins of the field of medical education research. Acad Med. 2010;85:1347–53.
2. Norman G. Fifty years of medical education research: waves of migration. Med Educ. 2011;45:785–91.
3. Atluru A, Wadhwani A, Maurer K, Kochar A, London D, Kane E, Spear K. Research in medical education: a primer for medical students. American Association of Medical Colleges. April 2015. https://www.aamc.org/media/24771/download#:~:text=Medical%20education%20research%20aims%20to,as%20teachers%20and%20mentors%2C%20instructional.
4. Glassick CE. Boyer's expanded definitions of scholarship, the standards for assessing scholarship, and the elusiveness of the scholarship of teaching. Acad Med. 2000;75(9):877–80.
5. Office for Human Research Protections. 2018 requirements (2018 common rule). U.S. Department of Health and Human Services. 30 Aug 2022. https://www.hhs.gov/ohrp/regulations-and-policy/regulations/45-cfr-46/revised-common-rule-regulatory-text/index.html.
6. Office for Human Research Protections. Exemptions (2018 requirements). U.S. Department of Health and Human Services. 30 Aug 2022. https://www.hhs.gov/ohrp/regulations-and-policy/regulations/45-cfr-46/common-rule-subpart-a-46104/index.html.
7. Office for Human Research Protections. Expedited review: categories of research that may be reviewed through an expedited review procedures. U.S. Department of Health and Human Services. 30 Aug 2022. https://www.hhs.gov/ohrp/regulations-and-policy/guidance/categories-of-research-expedited-review-procedure-1998/index.html.
8. Teherani A, Martimianakis T, et al. Choosing a qualitative research approach. JGME. 2015;7(4):669–70.
9. Preferred reporting items for systematic reviews and meta-analyses. 31 Aug 2022. https://prisma-statement.org/.
10. PRISMA for scoping reviews. 31 Aug 2022. https://prisma-statement.org/Extensions/ScopingReviews.
11. Sullivan GM, Feinn R. Using effect size—or why the p value is not enough. JGME. 2012;4(3):279–82.
12. Kirkpatrick DL, Kirkpatrick JD. Evaluating training programs. 3rd ed. San Francisco: Berrett-Koehler Publishers; 2006.
13. Boyer EL. Scholarship reconsidered: priorities of the professorate. San Francisco: Carnegie Foundation for the Advancement of Teaching; 1990.

Chapter 83
Conducting Operations Research

Mark F. Olaf, Christopher J. Wilson, Eric M. Melnychuk, Judy B. Shahan, and Chadd K. Kraus

Why Do Operations Research?

The Institute for Healthcare Improvement (IHI) Triple Aim of reducing costs, improving patient experience, and improving population health is the goal for every setting where patient care is provided [1]. How to ensure that the IHI aims are being achieved in the operational processes of an Emergency Department (ED) is the focus of this chapter. Federal laws and regulations for Medicare, broader healthcare regulations, the presence of commercial health insurers, and the evolution of integrated healthcare models that provide insurance coverage and clinical care in one system have brought quality and value to the forefront of healthcare delivery, often through financial incentives and penalties. The more recent iterations of this evolution include the measurement of value-based care, including bundles of care [2]. Largely these forces have been externally driven with healthcare organizations largely responding to incentives. Internal attention to quality and value is the preferred mechanism to meet the Institute of Medicine's quality aims of safety, effectiveness, patient-centeredness, timeliness, efficiency, and fairness [3].

M. F. Olaf · C. J. Wilson · J. B. Shahan
Department of Emergency Medicine, Geisinger Medical Center, Danville, Pennsylvania, USA
e-mail: mfolaf@geisinger.edu; cjwilson@geisinger.edu; jbshahan@geisinger.edu

E. M. Melnychuk
Department of Critical Care Medicine, Geisinger Medical Center, Danville, Pennsylvania, USA
e-mail: emelnychuk@geisinger.edu

C. K. Kraus (✉)
Department of Emergency and Hospital Medicine, Lehigh Valley Health Network (LVHN), Allentown, Pennsylvania, USA
e-mail: chadd.kraus@lvhn.org

R. P. Olympia et al. (eds.), *An Emergency Physician's Path*,
https://doi.org/10.1007/978-3-031-47873-4_83

Measuring Operations

Measuring the operational efficiency in an Emergency Department (ED) is inherently tied to measuring the quality of care provided. Broadly, these measures can be categorized as elements of structure, process, or outcome [4]. Measurable outcomes include the efficiency and timing of processes, as well as the experiences of the stakeholders providing and receiving the care, including patients, families, and ED staff. In EDs, there are a variety of operational research opportunities. Some examples include diagnostic accuracy, resource utilization, pharmacotherapy, procedures/procedural competency, patient flow and care (throughput, triage, communication, experience), departmental staffing, education, information technology (computerized order entry, error prevention, and documentation/coding), patient referral/discharge documentation, and appropriate referral for psychiatric/substance use disorders.

Some measures are physician or administrator centered and seek to improve the quality of the physician or administrator experience or perspective. Other measures seek to inform compliance with local, state, and federal regulations and guidelines. Elements of structure include the physical and organizational structure of the ED and the hospital and are often the focus of certain regulatory bodies. Process measures refer to repeatable ED practices which may be analyzed for efficiency, are often amenable to change and continuous measurement. Outcome measures focus on the effects upon the ED and patient after a patient leaves.

Measures of quality can also be categorized in dimensions such as clinical, service, or cost related. Clinical data measure the safe, effective, timely, and equitable treatment of patients. Service data are patient centered and seek to measure satisfaction. Cost related data seek to determine the degree of benefit in proportion to a given cost.

Selecting Measures

The depth and volume of data available to measure care in the ED can be a challenge for focused operational change. To mitigate this challenge, various organizations make recommendations on important measures of quality, often linked to payment. The Center for Medicare and Medicaid Services (CMS), for example, has historically selected core measures for acute myocardial infarction (MI), stroke, pneumonia, atrial fibrillation, and congestive heart failure. An example of a measurement of compliance is the time to reperfusion in patients undergoing percutaneous intervention for acute MI. Although these measures often have input from peer-reviewed literature and medical societies, there is sometimes misalignment of measures and outcomes.

The measurement of process data in the ED should be guided by evidence of impact and importance in the existing scientific literature. Data should be easily abstracted, indicate an opportunity for improvement, be influenced by limited barriers to change, and be applicable to the ED patient population.

Obtaining Data

A paradox often exists between the quality of data and the availability of it. Frequently, inexpensive, easily available data do not contain the detail that is required for a thorough or complete analysis, and the data that do contain such detail are scarce. Acquiring data can be a significant barrier, particularly when organizational leadership does not emphasize or value quality measurement. Information technology (IT) resources, including the acquisition, aggregation, and analysis of data can limit QI efficacy. When appropriate resources are dedicated to the measurement of quality through an organizational business strategy, the IT barrier can be reduced and replaced by provider compliance responding to quality initiatives. A particular example of this paradox is data abstraction from a medical chart. Electronic health records (EHR) are largely oriented towards billing. Although billing parameters are well defined, physicians document in various ways to meet these standards. Abstracting data from narratives in the ED EHR is labor and time intensive, and variability in data entry can impact data quality.

Emergency Medicine Operational Improvement Challenges

Quality improvement (QI) initiatives in the ED face several unique challenges compared to other clinical departments. The variety and types of patients seen in the ED creates a heterogeny in data. Further, effective treatment of a condition, and outcome data related to such, is contingent upon an accurate diagnosis in the ED, a challenge in a population of patients with undifferentiated illnesses and injuries. The selection of quality measures must be informed by these challenges. Quality measures must be clearly defined, and the effects of such measurement must be anticipated.

Sharing current performance data, demonstrating opportunities for improvement, and highlighting the goals or standards to be achieved are critical to getting physician buy-in, and meeting the expected goals. Physician behavior is difficult to change when educational materials are not coupled with practice-enforcing strategies [5]. Another important element of behavior change is the selection of a "physician champion" to lead the project. Experts, sometimes both in the ED and outside of it, are required to oversee the project and guide measurement and strategy. Lastly, involvement of all of those involved in the process change, including physicians, nurses, ancillary staff, and administrators, is necessary for success.

The choice of what must be changed in a QI project is critical to its success. A problem area or opportunity gap must first be identified. This often happens through a collaborative process but may also be influenced by a regulatory body or administrative mandate. Then, possible solutions (change concepts) are considered by the group making the change. Once a change concept is selected, examples of the concept are solicited and reviewed. Finally, a specific intervention is selected that represents the concept change.

Barriers to Change

The barriers to quality improvement in ED operations are broad and may include: a lack of goals or targets, a lack of adequate support (leadership, clinical, or technical), limited scope, poor target choice, inadequate data collection or analysis, and even the proportion of under- or un-insured patients in an Emergency Department population [2, 4].

Success Stories

Despite the challenges in Emergency Department operational research, there have been successes. For example, standing orders for obtaining electrocardiograms (ECGs) in patients with chest pain has resulted in a reduction of time to EKG acquisition, which was correlated with improved outcomes in patients with acute MI. QI processes have led to a reduction in the time to antibiotic administration for pneumonia, for which delays are associated with increased mortality [4]. Process improvements that include the use of an ED observation unit are associated with lowered rates of missed MI and missed appendicitis [4]. Emergency Department efficiency has been addressed with enhanced staffing models, increased space, improved radiology processes, and other interventions which were associated with improved waiting room times and increased patient satisfaction. Procedural success in quality improvement has been shown with increased first pass success in Emergency Department endotracheal intubation when rapid sequence intubation methods were introduced. The long-term success of quality improvement in EM relies on the future physician leaders, and EM provides robust opportunity for QI training. Therefore, it is critical for graduate medical education training to incorporate QI skills development [6].

Ongoing Needs and Opportunities

Building on successes, there are several priority areas for future operations research in the ED, including attention to equity in healthcare delivery, particularly among the elderly, women, patients without health insurance, and racial and ethnic minorities. Evidence suggests poorer health outcomes among patients facing certain social determinants of health including, but not limited to, food insecurity, lack of reliable transportation, neighborhood blight. Public data demonstrate increased vulnerability to poor health outcomes among those individuals who face financial challenges, and among those who reside in particular zip codes or neighborhoods. These challenges reflect barriers to accessing healthcare resources, sometimes leading populations to disproportionately access emergency services as the only means of obtaining care. Communication with the health care system, or the lack of means to effectively communicate, can lead to further challenges in accessing quality health care. Quality improvement efforts focused on delivering equitable care to these vulnerable populations is one way by which Emergency Medicine can lead the charge to right this injustice. The needs of each community are unique, even if certain themes are constant throughout a region, state, or our nation. Therefore, quality improvement projects aimed at systematic improvements, prevention, patient centered communication and education, and psychosocial support demonstrate promise in reducing healthcare inequities [4]. Attention to process monitoring is a recommended quality initiative that can be impactful. Process monitoring tends to be sensitive, demonstrates early indicators of success or failure leading to opportunities for interventions, and allows projects to address systematic features of accessing care. Areas for measurement in these vulnerable populations should reflect existing measures, such as satisfaction and patient outcomes, to allow for comparison to national and other existing measures [4].

References

1. Berwick DM, Nolan TW, Whittington J. The triple aim: care, health, and cost. Health Aff (Millwood). 2008;27(3):759–69. https://doi.org/10.1377/hlthaff.27.3.759.
2. Kelly JJ, Thallner E, Broida RI, Cheung D, Meisl H, Hamedani AG, et al. Emergency medicine quality improvement and patient safety curriculum. Acad Emerg Med. 2010;17:e110–29.
3. Institute of Medicine. Crossing the quality chasm: a new health system for the 21st century. Washington, DC: National Academy Press; 2001.
4. Graff L, Stevens C, Spaite D, Foody J. Measuring and improving quality in emergency medicine. Acad Emerg Med. 2002;9(11):1091–107.
5. Davis DA, Thomson MA, Oxman AD, Haynes RB. Changing physician performance: a systematic review of the effect of continuing medical education strategies. JAMA. 1995;274:700–5.
6. Mondoux S, Chan TM, Ankel F, Sklar DP. Teaching quality improvement in emergency medicine training programs: a review of best practices. AEM Educ Train. 2017;1(4):301–9.

Chapter 84
Grantsmanship

Eric M. Melnychuk, Judy B. Shahan, Mark F. Olaf, Christopher J. Wilson, and Chadd K. Kraus

You cannot disguise a weak idea with great grantsmanship. But bad grantsmanship can disguise a good idea [1]
—Dr. Valerie Durrant, NIH Center for Scientific Review

Introduction

As a specialty, Emergency Medicine (EM) has traditionally had low levels of federal grant funding [2]. A variety of factors contribute to this paucity of funding, including the historical development of the EM as a community-based, clinically focused specialty, EM's relatively recent arrival as a full academic department in many medical schools, and the broad scope of clinical topics in EM that is unique compared to the narrow focus of many federal funding agencies, particularly individual institutes within the National Institutes of Health (NIH). In 2012, the NIH introduced the Office of Emergency Care Research, that facilitates efforts across the 21 institutes and 6 centers of the NIH to promote emergency care research [2]. Despite these and other initiatives to increase federal funding, EM ranks last among

E. M. Melnychuk
Department of Critical Care Medicine, Geisinger Medical Center, Danville, Pennsylvania, USA
e-mail: emelnychuk@geisinger.edu

J. B. Shahan · M. F. Olaf · C. J. Wilson
Department of Emergency Medicine, Geisinger Medical Center, Danville, Pennsylvania, USA
e-mail: jbshahan@geisinger.edu; mfolaf@geisinger.edu; cjwilson@geisinger.edu

C. K. Kraus (✉)
Department of Emergency and Hospital Medicine, Lehigh Valley Health Network (LVHN), Allentown, Pennsylvania, USA
e-mail: chadd.kraus@lvhn.org

R. P. Olympia et al. (eds.), *An Emergency Physician's Path*,
https://doi.org/10.1007/978-3-031-47873-4_84

major specialties in terms of the percentage of NIH-funded principal investigators and NIH-funded specialties [2]. This history and context make it increasingly important that Emergency Medicine researchers become successful in receiving grant funding that can build and expand Emergency Medicine-specific research goals and objectives.

What Is Grantsmanship?

"Grantsmanship" is the art and practice of obtaining peer-reviewed grant funding to perform research activities. Grant writing is unlike other forms of writing familiar to physicians. A grant application includes a review of the current available evidence on a topic, the identification of gaps in current knowledge, and a clear and focused description of how rigorous scientific methods will be applied to fill those gaps. This competitive process takes a detailed, scientific approach, and the grant writer and collaborators need to create a vision and focus for the research that is to be funded, while communicating clearly and concisely.

Grants and Career Development

Successfully obtaining internal and external grant funding is essential to the career development of an Emergency Medicine researcher. Developing expertise and a research focus in a specific topic area is often a requisite to promotion, tenure, and future grant funding. This track record consists of related publications and may include local or internal funding of smaller projects leading up to larger academic or scholarly pursuits. Frequently, professional societies and specialty organizations sponsor workshops, panels, and courses, and offer peer support to develop grant writing skills.

Writing the Grant

Identify Funding Opportunities

It is critical to find a funding opportunity that aligns with your research interests. Most funding agencies can be contacted to confirm whether your research would be eligible for specific grants. These inquiries are not a guarantee of funding but can help to focus your efforts to opportunities that align with your research interests and expertise. In some cases, these inquires might also inform you of additional funding opportunities that are available. When possible, seek feedback from other colleagues who have received funding from similar sources.

It is important to consider a range of funding sources for research, including those within the local health system such as an endowed hospital fund for research, and pilot funding available within medical schools and universities. Most universities and academic medical centers have funding programs support investigations on pilot projects that have the potential to be expanded into larger bodies of work. An investigator may also seek out state, regional or private foundations for funding opportunities to support investigative work accomplished with grant funding. It is often necessary to combine several small sources of grant funding to accomplish the work of a research project.

In addition to traditional NIH funding, there are other sources of federal agency funding including:

- Agency for Healthcare Research and Quality (AHRQ).
- Centers for Disease Control and Prevention (CDC).
- Veterans Administration (VA).
- Department of Defense (DoD).
- Patient-Centered Outcomes Research Institute.
- Health Resources and Service Administration.
- Substance Abuse and Mental Health Services Administration [2]..

Private foundation grants related to Emergency Medicine are also available from:

- Emergency Medicine Foundation (EMF).
- Society for Academic Emergency Medicine Foundation (SAEMF).
- American Heart Association.
- Robert Wood Johnson Foundation.

Seek Peer Feedback

Finding peers who have been successful (and unsuccessful) in securing grant funding is helpful to avoid pitfalls and to gain insights into the most effective and efficient approach to submitting a grant application. When available, critiques of past grants from funding agencies can provide insights into pitfalls and pearls of strong grant submissions.

After reviewing past submissions, create a concise one-page summary of your idea(s) to share with colleagues, and the funding agency, for feedback on whether your ideas are interesting and feasible. Having a group of individuals who have experience with grants and can mentor you through the process can be invaluable—they can help with editing for content and strategy. Grantsmanship is a team sport!

Details Matter!

Details matter in a grant submission. Meeting the requirements for length of submission, components of the grant, spacing and layout are essential to having the submission even considered. Failure to follow instructions could cast doubt on the validity of your research ideas. Finally, it is critical to create a timeline and assign tasks to yourself and others on your team to meet your submission deadline.

Set up a Meeting with Your Office of Extramural Funding (Grants Office)

Early in the process, contact your grants administration office to assist you in determining who will be submitting the grant for you. They will need your completed application before the deadline to peform necessary administrative and regulatory tasks and to prepare the grant for submission by your institution. They will also give you another set of often rigid deadlines to follow, so be sure to include them in your preparation timeline.

Completing and Submitting the Grant Application

Develop a Clear Justification for the Project

Communicate the significance of your project within the context of the current science and the controversies surrounding it. Your research needs to have significance to the granting agency, and you need to communicate to them why they should care about, and why they should ultimately fund, your specific project. Specific aims and objective are key parts of a grant submission. Aims are the broad goals for the research while objectives are specific and measurable ways to accomplish those aims. Also important is outlining any potential pitfalls or anticipated challenges and your rationale behind the mitigation and fixes of these pitfalls or challenges. This is fundamental to showing your insight into the project, and displaying this to the reviewers such that it will improve their confidence in your thoughtful approach.

Create an Accurate Budget

You will be expected to propose a budget that will likely include the following four categories: direct costs that encompass personnel and labor costs; indirect costs that are institutional facility and administrative overhead charges; equipment and materials that include physical items needed for the project; and travel and other expenses for training, fees, etc... Confirm that your budget aligns with the project narrative and that all expenses can be accounted for and supported by the budget justification required for each line item. Ensure that each budget item is necessary to achieve the aims of the project along with how the estimated costs in the budget were calculated.

Make it Easy for the Reviewers

Many review committees incorporate a broad and interdisciplinary panel of reviewers with different backgrounds, so some reviewers will not be content experts in the science proposed in your application. Outline and repeat key messages in your application. Since your expertise is within the field of study that you are writing about, tell the reviewers what is special about your application; clearly tell them what is original and innovative. If not readily apparent in the grant instructions or on the additional information available from the funding agency, inquire about the review criteria and tailor your application to these criteria. You can use the review criteria to critically evaluate your grant or have another set of individuals review your grant using the criteria. Make sure you have addressed every item in the review criteria.

Sell Yourself

You and your experience are part of the application. It is your job to convince the reviewers that you know how to execute the project and have the skills and experience to do so. Find other experts in the field and collaborate with a senior investigator. Be sure to incorporate your excitement for the project as readers and reviewers will key into your passion for the project and desired outcomes.

Proofread

Errors in grammar and syntax and use of informal language and colloquialisms can lead to poor reviews as your colleagues may see these errors as a sign of lack of attention to detail. A specific reviewer may not be experienced in what your application is detailing, so your application needs to be written in a way that a non-expert would understand (clear, concise, easy to read and understand). However, avoid spending too much time explaining principles that are common in the biomedical sciences. Be cautious about getting bogged down in details and adding too much additional information into the appendices. A disorganized application may equate to representing yourself as a disorganized researcher to the reviewers. Additionally, the abstract and summary pages need to be comprehensive enough to stand on their own as some reviewers will allow these pages to guide their final impression of your proposal.

After Submission

Take some Time for Yourself

The process of writing and preparing the grant application is rigorous and time consuming. Once submitted, it is time to congratulate yourself and attempt to re-align yourself. Your work is now off to the reviewers to evaluate and critique.

Don't Give Up!

It is common to not be funded on the first try and it often takes one (or more) resubmissions before a successful review, especially for competitive grants and for funding agencies that receive a large number of submissions. If you are not successful the first time, take some time for yourself, carefully read the critiques and feedback provided by the reviewers, revise and resubmit. If there are questions about the review, contact the funding agency for clarification.

Paying it Forward Helps you

Serve on a grant review panel to gain insight on how to write a good application. As you become more experienced, be willing to share your writing to help others learn from you.

Ethical Considerations

Last, but not least, are ethical considerations. Recognizing and optimizing diversity, equity, and inclusion in medical research at every level, from researcher to clinical trial participant, is essential [3]. A grant application should include how vulnerable populations will be included and how individuals will be protected in research that involves human subjects.

References

1. Durant V. Insider's guide to NIH peer review for applicants. February 25, 2016. Accessed July 25, 2022. https://www.youtube.com/watch?v=DuNYjugBMXM.
2. Neumar RW, Blomkalns AL, Cairns CB, et al. Emergency medicine research: 2030 strategic goals. Acad Emerg Med. 2022;29(2):241–51.
3. Boulware LE, Corbie G, Aguilar-Gaxiola S, et al. Combating structural inequities—diversity, equity, and inclusion in clinical and translational research. N Engl J Med. 2022;386(3):201–3.

Further Reading

ACEP Resident Research and Scholarly Activity—A Primer. https://www.acep.org/globalassets/sites/acep/media/sections-documents/research/acepresearchprimer.pdf

How to write an NIH Grant Application. https://grants.nih.gov/grants/how-to-apply-application-guide/format-and-write/write-your-application.htm

Monte AA, Libby AM. Introduction to the specific aims page of a Grant proposal. Acad Emerg Med. 2018;25(9):1042–7.

NIH Grant Writing Tips. http://grants.nih.gov/grants/grant_tips.htm

NIH Insider's Guide to Peer Review for Applicants. https://public.csr.nih.gov/ForApplicants/InitialReviewResultsAndAppeals/InsidersGuide

NIH Office of Emergency Care Research. https://www.ninds.nih.gov/current-research/trans-agency-activities/office-emergency-care-research

Society for Academic Emergency Medicine Research Resources. https://www.saem.org/research

University of Pittsburgh Grantsmanship Links and Tutorials. https://www.oorhs.pitt.edu/application-assistance/grantsmanship-links-and-tutorials

Part VIII
Being a Teacher in Emergency Medicine

known disease, description of a new ...

be considered for review by institutional ...
subjects as required by ethical principles and ...

Chapter 85
Effective Bedside Teaching for Medical Students, Residents, and Other Learners

Christopher E. San Miguel

Find a Teaching Framework that Works for You

If you are feeling really lost and need a good starting point, I suggest finding a bedside teaching model that fits your personality and your workflow. One of the more commonly cited frameworks is called the "One Minute Preceptor." [1]. Although it was designed to be used in a family medicine clinic, this framework translates very well to emergency medicine. This framework provides the instructor with five specific tasks to complete after the learner has given their patient presentation. This allows the instructor to gain an assessment of the learner's knowledge and clinical reasoning and to provide the learner with timely feedback.

1. Get a commitment: Especially with more junior learners, the first step is encouraging them to commit to a diagnosis or a treatment plan. Leaners are more likely to remember information if they are tested on it and then forced to provide an answer, even if their initial answer is incorrect [2]. It also provides you with a specific learning point to discuss. This can be accomplished by a simple statement like, "You've provided a great differential diagnosis for this patient with a cough. If you had to commit to a final diagnosis right now, what would it be?"
2. Probe for supporting evidence: In this step, the preceptor can assess the learner's clinical reasoning by asking the learner to provide supporting evidence for their decision. Did they incorrectly diagnosis pneumonia because they don't know the diagnostic criteria for pneumonia, or did they fail to ask about fever, or did they fail to identify crackles on their lung exam? This can be accomplished by simply asking, "What about this patient's presentation supports your diagnosis of pneu-

C. E. San Miguel (✉)
Ohio State University Wexner Medical Center, Columbus, OH, USA
e-mail: Christopher.sanmiguel@osumc.edu

R. P. Olympia et al. (eds.), *An Emergency Physician's Path*,
https://doi.org/10.1007/978-3-031-47873-4_85

monia?" Alternatively, you can also ask "Is there anything about this patient's presentation that doesn't support your diagnosis of pneumonia?"

3. Reinforce what was done well: Positive feedback is just as important as corrective feedback. Learners need to know what they have done well. "You did a great job of noting the patient's abnormal vital signs and incorporating that into your decision making."
4. Give guidance about errors/omissions: This is your opportunity to discuss areas of continued growth for the learner. For junior learners focus on history taking, physical exam skills, and presentation skills. "This patient's chief complaint was shortness of breath. Be sure to incorporate the patient's respiratory exam into your presentation, since even a normal exam is likely going to impact our decision making." More senior learners often benefit from feedback related to their medical decision making. "I agree that right now that patient is likely stable enough to go home. However, she lives alone and has no transportation to the pharmacy, so I am concerned with how she is going to obtain her antibiotics. If we can't be sure she'll have access to those medications, we may need to admit her."
5. Teach a general principle: This is your opportunity to really share your clinical acumen and experience with the learners. At this point, you've already provided the learner with some specific feedback, so this general principle can be anything you think is important or interesting related to this case. "The trickiest thing about diagnosing pneumonia is that we're taught, and we often act like a chest x-ray is the definitive test for diagnosis. In reality, a chest x-ray only catches about 70% of pneumonias. So if your clinical suspicion is high, it can be appropriate to treat even if there are no focal findings on the chest x-ray."

Elicit or Set Goals at the Beginning of the Shift

Working with your learners to set goals for the shift is a great way to frame your time together. Because of the shift-work nature of emergency medicine, you may only work with an individual learner one or a few times during their time in your department. Consequently, it can be hard to know your learners' strengths and weaknesses. By asking for one or two learning goals at the beginning of the shift, you gain an area to focus on during the shift. Furthermore, adult learners tend to be more engaged when they are given some degree of control over their educational experiences. Ideally, you will be able to take a few minutes in the middle of your shift and provide your learner with targeted feedback related to their shift goal including some concrete next steps to take. For example, "I wanted to take a minute to check in with you about your goal to be more efficient. I have noticed that you get up and down from your workstation quite a bit and often only accomplish one task at a time. I find it more efficient to make sure there are three things I am going to do every time I stand up. Try to consciously complete three tasks each time you get up and see if that makes you more efficient." Also, make sure you end the shift by discussing the shift goals with the learner. Again, it's always helpful to provide your perspective on their progress and any concrete steps they can take to continue to improve.

Change from the Traditional Format

One of the biggest challenges in clinical teaching is providing education while maintaining clinical efficiency. One of the main reasons for this is that the traditional clinical staffing model is inefficient. The learner goes and sees the patient, the learner presents the patient to the supervising physician, the supervising physician goes and sees the patient, the supervising physician touches base with the learner to let them know of any changes to the plan, the patient undergoes their work up and interventions, the learner checks on the patient, and finally the learner talks to the supervising physician again to review the results of the work up and determine a disposition for the patient. While this perhaps provides the most independence for learners, it is a lot of steps carried out in sequence rather than in parallel. Fortunately, it is not the only way to care for patients with learners.

Consider examining the patient before the learner sees them. This allows you to place orders and get those completed while the learner completes their assessment. It also gives you the opportunity to provide immediate feedback when the learner presents the patient and provides an incorrect history or physical exam finding. This works especially well with junior learners who may not be allowed to enter orders in the electronic medical record and rely on you to do so.

For more senior learners and very critically ill patients, consider seeing the patient together. While they are eliciting a history, you can start your note and enter orders on the computer in the room or on a computer on wheels. When you leave the room, you can skip the presentation of the history and physical exam, and just go straight into a discussion of the differential diagnosis and the plan with the learner.

When in Doubt Think out Loud

One of the concerns I hear most often from new educators is that they don't know how to interact with a learner when they themselves are unsure of the next best step in patient management. While I certainly understand the desire to avoid embarrassment and "miseducating" learners, these can be great learning opportunities. We are all going to come across puzzling cases and be faced with new (or old information) that we are unfamiliar with. The lesson here is not so much what the clinician doesn't know, but rather how does an experienced clinician handle that scenario. The easiest way to continue engaging your learner is to simply think out loud. This turns your internal thoughts into external behaviors that you are modeling for the learner. "Ok this patient who is here for leg pain just became hypoxic. We have corrected that with oxygen and the vitals are stable, so we have a minute to think. The most obvious answer would be that a DVT just turned into a PE. But she's not tachycardic and her work of breathing didn't increase. And her leg pain appears to be an abscess from intravenous drug use. Maybe she just overdosed on an opioid? Let's check her pupils and see if they are pinpoint." In just a few seconds you have demonstrated to your learner a) to focus on interventions when the patient is unstable, b) to review the differential diagnosis when there is a change in clinical status, and c) it's ok to revisit the physical exam and history to help revise your differential diagnosis. Thinking out loud can also become a collaborative exercise with your learner as you both talk through the case together.

Debrief after Critical Cases

There may be times during critical cases when you are unable to talk directly to your learner, especially if they are less experienced and unable to independently complete patient care tasks. It is ok if this happens, and you haven't lost all educational value of that experience. After the case concludes, it is best to take a few minutes and debrief with your learner. "I'm sorry I couldn't check in with you in real time. There was certainly a lot of things going on at once, but do you have any questions about the case?" If the learner doesn't have any of their own questions, I usually try and provide a brief synopsis of the case and my thought processes throughout. This is also a good opportunity to check in with your learner from a more humanistic perspective. Especially with junior learners, this might be the first code they have witnessed, the first death they have experienced as a healthcare provider, and/or they may have found the case otherwise triggering of a traumatic memory. Allowing learners to express and examine their emotions in these cases is a crucial first step for maintaining their personal well-being. On that note, make sure you make whoever is in charge of your learner's rotation aware of any particular traumatic events that may involve your learner. They will be able to provide further resources for the learner that can help them process the experience.

Just-in-Time Role-Playing

The practice of emergency medicine is full of difficult conversations. These can range from delivering bad news, to discharging patients against medical advice, to declining to refill opioid prescriptions. While learners have often been taught some basic framework to approach each of these scenarios, a quick refresher course right before going into the room can be quite helpful. Especially if you have never seen this learner have this conversation with a patient, it can be very helpful to role-play the conversation with the learner. This allows the learner to practice their phrasing and also gives you the opportunity to talk about potential patient responses and how best to address them before you are in the patient's room. If you are not pleased with the learner's performance after a couple of rounds of roleplaying, you should lead the conversation with the patient with the learner in the room and debrief afterward.

Find a Set of Resources to Help You

Thanks to the FOAMED (Free Open Access Medical Education) trend there are numerous resources online to help you educate learners. For some of your more frequent topics of discussion, it can be far more efficient for you to find a good resource and share that with your learners rather than doing all the educating on your own. This works particularly well for procedures. You can pull up your favorite lumbar puncture video on YouTube, have your learner watch it, and then you can discuss it together with the learner reviewing the procedure step by step. Then you can go perform the lumbar puncture together. This also works well when you come across a topic you may not know much about. You can have your learner take 10 min and read all they can about Addison's crisis. Then you can review the findings and see if the new information fits well with the case in front of you.

References

1. Neher JO, Gordon KC, Meyer B, Stevens N. A five-step "microskills" model of clinical teaching. J Am Board Fam Pract. 1992;5:419–24.
2. Metcalfe L. Learning from errors. Annu Rev Psychol. 2017;68:465–89.

Chapter 86
Beyond PowerPoint Presentations: Utilizing Nontraditional Methods of Education

John R. Barrett, Nick Schoenmann, and Dan McCollum

Introduction

There are multiple ways to educate without relying on slide software such as PowerPoint. While it has its uses, an overreliance on slides can lead to a loss of interaction with the learner and distract from the key message being conveyed. Despite its popularity, there is only a small amount of research about the efficacy of slide software in education. Studies have shown lower test scores in a class taught with PowerPoint compared with a traditional lecture format [1, 2]. Another showed that even slides with multimedia elements could lead to lower test scores [3]. Beyond test scores, there is an absence of quality research that demonstrates improved knowledge retention with the use of PowerPoint [4].

Fortunately, there are alternatives to using traditional slides to educate that incorporate more active learning methodology. In addition to being more enjoyable to learners, active learning has demonstrated improved scholastic success, critical thinking, and retention [5–7]. Brown and colleagues in their 2014 book *Make It Stick* recommend frequent, low-stakes testing and other activities that require active and purposeful retrieval of information [8]. The authors discuss that active retrieval of information from memory has been shown to be a powerful educational tool, which more effectively promotes long-term retention of information in comparison to passive rereading of a textbook or notes. In this chapter, we will give a brief introduction to three compelling alternatives to passive learning modalities such as

J. R. Barrett (✉) · N. Schoenmann · D. McCollum
Department of Emergency Medicine, Medical College of Georgia at Augusta University, Augusta, GA, USA
e-mail: jobarrett@augusta.edu; nschoenmann@augusta.edu; dmccollum@augusta.edu

R. P. Olympia et al. (eds.), *An Emergency Physician's Path*,
https://doi.org/10.1007/978-3-031-47873-4_86

PowerPoint. Teaching can be made more interactive by utilizing questions to engage learners, especially when incorporating game elements to capture learner attention. Alternatively, a flipped classroom strategy can maximize time to discuss the material. Lastly, simulations can be utilized to reinforce the practical application of knowledge in a clinical situation.

Low-Stakes Quizzing and Gamification

The general goal of educators is to convey information effectively and promote future retrieval. The classic idea of rote repetition and repeated exposure to a topic has not panned out in education literature as an effective learning modality. Brown and colleagues note that low-stakes testing improved class attendance and decreased higher-stakes testing anxiety, along with improved knowledge retention [8]. *Make It Stick* also discusses the concept of interleaving in education, which they define as covering varying topics rather than focusing on a core block or theme. This mixing of topics, especially when combined with spaced repetition of learning objectives over time, has been shown to be a more effective learning method than single-minded focus on one educational topic at a time [8]. *Make It Stick* discusses that this runs contrary to both lecturer and learner preferences. Switching topics frequently during a lecture block requires more effort from the learner. Thus, it is not surprising that when questioned about preference, learners and instructors disliked the interleaving method in favor of more grouped topic schedules. Yet, *Make It Stick* effectively demonstrates that long-term knowledge acquisition is superior with interleaving strategies, and the authors of this chapter have incorporated interleaving in their emergency medicine residency curriculum. Rather than an entire morning, or month, of didactics on related topics such as cardiology or trauma, each lecture topic varies and is unrelated to the one before or after it.

Combining the educational tools of interleaving and routine quizzing, gamification is an important modality to use in medical education lectures. In 2003, Nick Pelling coined the term "gamification" to describe what is also cited as "game-based learning education" in the literature [9]. Audience response systems (ARS) have been shown to increase learner engagement in education literature. The use of ARS has been proposed for emergency medicine education to help combat the estimated learner attention span of 15–20 minutes during lectures [10]. For this reason, the authors of this chapter utilize 25-minute lecture blocks during their residency program's didactics rather than the more traditional 1-h time slot. There is neurobiological evidence that active learner attention leads to functional changes in the brain associated with learning [11]. Gamification builds on learner engagement from traditional ARS by relying on both fun and addicting game elements. These include low-stakes competition and rewards such as audience leaderboards and merit badges [12]. Similar to ARS, game-style learning inherently requires learner engagement.

Gamification often provides immediate feedback as well, which has also been shown to improve learner engagement and educational efficacy [12]. Urh et al.. demonstrated that learners had improved motivation, educational engagement, and learning effectiveness from the use of gamification in higher education [13, 14].

Nevin et al. demonstrated that leaderboards were the most effective game element in their study of internal medicine residents and gamification [15]. Earning ranks or badges was less effective than the leaderboard. Interestingly, their study also showed that retention of knowledge was improved in the gamification group. Over 25% of questions were answered on weekends, demonstrating utility for gamification in asynchronous curricula as well. This is important given the Accreditation Council for Graduate Medical Education (ACGME) allowance for up to 20% asynchronous education in residency curriculums, now termed "individualized interactive instruction" in the 2022 ACGME program requirement update [16].

Although evidence for its usefulness has been growing, the literature is not all positive for gamification of medical education. In a 2010 systematic review, Akl et al. ultimately concluded evidence was mixed and the authors could not promote or negate the utility of gamification as part of an educational curriculum with medical students [17]. Nearly a decade later, a 2018 literature review of gamification in education by Majuri et al. revealed mainly positive results overall, although the authors similarly reported a few mixed and negative studies [18]. Of note, previous literature on gamification in education has mostly focused on the learning habits of Millennials, including many of the studies on gamification cited in this chapter. However, at the time of publication of this text in 2023, the oldest Millennials are entering the fourth decade of life. Generation Z is defined by the Pew Research Center as those individuals born from 1997 to 2012 [19]. Thus, in 2023, the oldest individuals in Generation Z will be entering their late 20 s, and they will likely make up the majority of medical school students. They will soon also overtake Millennials as the main generation educated in emergency medicine residencies. Synaptic architecture has been shown to be structurally different in individuals of Generation Z, with brain areas for visual ability being more augmented than previous generations. This suggests that visual learning and interactive games will be a more effective educational modality than traditional auditory lectures [14, 20]. Hampton et al. found that individuals in Generation Z spend on average over 15 h/week on their smartphones, have an average attention span of 8 s, expect immediate feedback, and communicated preferentially in short bits of information, mirroring Twitter posts [14, 21]. Melero et al. demonstrated that the use of smart phones and their software applications had a significant improvement in student performance due to increased engagement and attention [22]. Rahman et al. published that online software such as Kahoot! and Socrative allow educators to engage and motivate students [14, 23]. Many online educational platforms like Kahoot! have a smart phone application to allow learners to engage and interface with game-style learning from their individual phones during a classroom activity. Kahoot! also utilizes low-stakes competition with a leaderboard updated after each question is answered. Saxena et al. conclude in their 2021 systematic review on gamification in Generation Z that educators should incorporate smart phone technology and gamification in their curriculums for effective learning [14]. Thus, gamification will likely have an increasingly important role in tailoring medical education to learners in Generation Z.

The Flipped Classroom

The flipped classroom is an instructional model that can increase interaction with the learner. In traditional lectures, new content is presented in the classroom, and the learner applies this information in activities outside of the classroom. The flipped classroom model inverts this. New content is initially studied by the learner prior to coming to the classroom. This information could be presented in many ways, including assigned readings, podcasts, or online videos. This allows for classroom time to learn how to apply this knowledge, correct errors, and discuss clinical applications. Studies have shown that flipped classroom methods can improve learning performance, engage learners, and increase learner satisfaction [24].

This model can be effectively applied in emergency medicine. Traditionally, a topic such as asthma might be presented with a PowerPoint lecture discussing the content. The learner would then be left on their own to hopefully apply this content in clinical situations. A flipped classroom approach could be much more effective. For example, the educator would assign material to review in advance, such as a podcast or textbook chapter discussing asthma. Once in the classroom, time is then allotted to discuss clinical cases and clarify any challenging material related to asthma.

It is critical for the advanced material to be carefully selected. Ideally, material would be presented in more than one format to accommodate learners with different preferences. For example, one could offer a podcast, textbook chapter, and online video covering the topic in different ways. Another advantage of this method is that it provides junior learners with multiple high-yield resources for review if the topic is new to them. Learners may struggle to find appropriate ancillary material or references on a topic introduced in a traditional lecture, and there are multiple low-yield or even incorrect resources readily available in the digital age of the Internet and Google. In a flipped classroom model, the educator must ensure that the material is both accurate and as concise as possible. One of the downsides of flipped classroom teaching is that it can potentially require a larger time commitment from the learner.

There are some challenges to the effective use of the flipped classroom technique. The preparatory materials must be carefully curated or created by the teacher. This is partially alleviated by the emergence of numerous free open-access medical education (FOAMed) resources. As previously mentioned, these materials need to be as concise as possible to avoid overly large time commitments from the learner.

Lastly, it is imperative for learners to prepare for these sessions by reviewing the material. If they do not, they will be tasked with applying knowledge that they have not mastered and will learn less than by traditional lectures. Educators may need to assess if materials were properly reviewed if a learner is struggling with this method.

Simulation-Based Healthcare Education

Simulation exercises are yet another example of a nonconventional teaching methodology. The fundamental advantage of using simulation-based healthcare education is to maximize learner participation in a context that mirrors often higher-stakes situations they will likely be confronted with in the emergency department. The use of simulation is by no means unique to healthcare, as it has been employed in the military, in aviation, and even more broadly in engineering, particularly as it pertains to safety and teamwork.

Simulations allow learners to acquire, improve, and maintain clinical competence by practicing cognitive, psychomotor, and social skills in a safe and controlled environment [25]. Recognizing that the emergency physician is expected to possess a great breadth and depth of medical knowledge, demonstrate mastery of procedures performed under significant stress, and build rapport with patients in a matter of minutes, simulations have proven especially useful to the field. Increased recognition of the importance of this mode of education has led to significant advancements in both the technology and curricula that facilitate training. Within emergency medicine, simulations are generally conducted as mock patient encounters with the aim of understanding a particular disease process, improving a technical ability, or developing efficient team-based skills.

Medical simulations range in both appearance and function as it pertains to the learning objectives of a given task. This is often precariously referred to as "fidelity." [26] Simulation training is more than just training with a manikin. The evidence to date overwhelmingly emphasizes the importance of creating tasks designed to support predefined learning objectives. This can come in the form of simple task trainers, computer models, virtual reality, or standardized patients [26, 27].

Significant improvements in learner performance can be achieved with models made of readily available objects. Matsumoto et al. demonstrated that medical students' learning surgical skills saw drastic improvement with simulations, with no significant difference found between those trained with a $3700 high-fidelity model and a $20 homemade model predominately composed of a coffee cup and Penrose drain [28]. This supports the argument that more time with what might be considered a low-fidelity simulation is likely more effective than less time with a high-fidelity simulation when considering cost constraints of curricular planning [27]. One cost-effective approach might be to learn basic skills with lower-fidelity models and use higher-fidelity models such as virtual reality for skill mastery.

Acknowledging that equipment and space are commonly cited needs for this type of training, there are limitations to a simulation-based education which are less obvious. First, the development of a curriculum with clearly defined goals and the supplemental case material to support that curriculum require some degree of expertise in medical education. Second, and perhaps most importantly, is the need for faculty or facilitators that have some understanding of a simple but systematic feedback process. Feedback, and more precisely *debriefing*, is a commonly forgotten component of the training process, but it is undoubtedly the most important aspect of this type of training [29, 30]. A simulated case is simply incomplete if time is not allocated to reflect and discuss both the learner's actions and thought processes that led to those actions. Feedback enables learner introspection and facilitates deliberate practice for educational growth.

Conclusion

Designing a curriculum must both emphasize the knowledge to be covered and maximize learner retention to be effective. We propose that the more attention and participation a teacher can elicit from learners, the more worthwhile the learning opportunity. While selective implementation of PowerPoint or other slide software lectures can be used, we suggest a multimodal didactic approach incorporating low-stakes quizzing and gamification software, flipped classroom activities, and simulations to yield an effective educational curriculum. These educational adjuncts will likely become more important with the learning styles of individuals of Generation Z as they arrive in medical school classrooms and emergency medicine residencies over the next few years. Low-stakes quizzing and gamification increase participation, test previously acquired knowledge, and provide an opportunity to review answers for prompt feedback. The flipped classroom assumes a base level of knowledge from which the learner and educator can work through common sticking points to more efficiently use lecture time. Lastly, simulations offer a protected environment to practice the cognitive, procedural, and social skills needed to successfully navigate the emergency department. Consideration of which topics would be best presented in each didactic style is paramount.

References

1. Amare N. To slideware or not to slideware: students' experiences with Powerpoint vs Lecture. J Tech Writ Commun. 2006;36(3):297–308. https://doi.org/10.2190/03gx-f1hw-vw5m-7dar.
2. Savoy A, Proctor RW, Salvendy G. Information retention from PowerPoint™ and traditional lectures. Comput Educ. 2009;52(4):858–67. https://doi.org/10.1016/j.compedu.2008.12.005.

3. Bartsch RA, Cobern KM. Effectiveness of PowerPoint presentations in lectures. Comput Educ. 2003;41(1):77–86. https://doi.org/10.1016/s0360-1315(03)00027-7.
4. Craig RJ, Amernic JH. PowerPoint presentation technology and the dynamics of teaching. Innov High Educ. 2006;31(3):147–60. https://doi.org/10.1007/s10755-006-9017-5.
5. Freeman S, Eddy SL, McDonough M, et al. Active learning increases student performance in science, engineering, and mathematics. Proc Natl Acad Sci. 2014;111(23):8410–5. https://doi.org/10.1073/pnas.1319030111.
6. van Vliet EA, Winnips JC, Brouwer N. Flipped-class pedagogy enhances student metacognition and collaborative-learning strategies in higher education but effect does not persist. CBE Life Sci Educ. 2015;14:3. https://doi.org/10.1187/cbe.14-09-0141.
7. Michael J. Where's the evidence that active learning works? Adv Physiol Educ. 2006;30(4):159–67. https://doi.org/10.1152/advan.00053.2006.
8. Brown PC. Make it stick : the science of successful learning, vol. xi. The Belknap Press of Harvard University Press; 2014. p. 313.
9. Abd Rahman S, Khalilah K, Mohamad SNA. An integration of game-based learning in a classroom: an overview (2016-2021). Int J Acad Res Progress Educ Dev. 2022;11:1207–21. https://doi.org/10.6007/IJARPED/v11-i1/12347.
10. Toohey SL, Wray A, Wiechmann W, Lin M, Boysen-Osborn M. Ten tips for engaging the millennial learner and moving an emergency medicine residency curriculum into the 21st century. West J Emerg Med. 2016;17(3):337–43. https://doi.org/10.5811/westjem.2016.3.29863.
11. Friedlander MJ, Andrews L, Armstrong EG, et al. What can medical education learn from the neurobiology of learning? Acad Med. 2011;86(4):415–20. https://doi.org/10.1097/ACM.0b013e31820dc197.
12. Singhal S, Hough J, Cripps D. Twelve tips for incorporating gamification into medical education [version 1]. MedEdPublish. 2019;8:216. https://doi.org/10.15694/mep.2019.000216.1.
13. Urh M, Vukovic G, Jereb E, Pintar R. The model for introduction of gamification into E-learning in higher education. Procedia Soc Behav Sci. 2015;197:388–97. https://doi.org/10.1016/j.sbspro.2015.07.154.
14. Saxena M, Mishra D. Gamification and gen Z in higher education: a systematic review of literature. Int J Inf Commun Technol. 2021;17:1–22. https://doi.org/10.4018/IJICTE.20211001.oa10.
15. Nevin CR, Westfall AO, Rodriguez JM, et al. Gamification as a tool for enhancing graduate medical education. Postgrad Med J. 2014;90(1070):685–93. https://doi.org/10.1136/postgradmedj-2013-132486.
16. ACGME Program Requirements for Graduate Medical Education in Emergency Medicine. Accreditation Council for Graduate Medical Education website; 2022. https://www.acgme.org/globalassets/pfassets/programrequirements/110_emergencymedicine_2022_tcc.pdf. Accessed July 2022.
17. Akl EA, Pretorius RW, Sackett K, et al. The effect of educational games on medical students' learning outcomes: a systematic review: BEME Guide No 14. Med Teach. 2010;32(1):16–27. https://doi.org/10.3109/01421590903473969.
18. Majuri J, Koivisto J, Hamari J. (2018). Gamification of education and learning: A review of empirical literature. In Proceedings of the 2nd international GamiFIN conference, GamiFIN 2018. CEUR-WS.
19. Dimock M. Defining generations: Where Millennials end and Generation Z begins. Washington, D.C.: Pew Research Center; 2019. https://www.pewresearch.org/fact-tank/2019/01/17/where-millennials-end-and-generation-z-begins/
20. Rothman D. A Tsunami of learners called Generation Z. 2016. https://mdle.net/Journal/A_Tsunami_of_Learners_Called_Generation_Z.pdf. Accessed 17 Feb 2020.
21. Hampton D, Keys Y. Generation Z students: will they change our nursing classrooms? J Nurs Educ Pract. 2016;12/06:7. https://doi.org/10.5430/jnep.v7n4p111.
22. Melero J, Hernández-Leo D, Manatunga K. Group-based mobile learning: do group size and sharing mobile devices matter? Comput Hum Behav. 2015;44:377–85. https://doi.org/10.1016/j.chb.2014.11.078.

23. Ab. Rahman R, Ahmad S, Hashim UR. A Study on Gamification for Higher Education Students' Engagement Towards Education 4.0. *Intelligent and Interactive Computing*. 2019.
24. Akçayir G, Akçayır M. The flipped classroom: a review of its advantages and challenges. Comput Educ. 2018;126:334–45.
25. Motola I, Devine LA, Chung HS, Sullivan JE, Issenberg SB. Simulation in healthcare education: a best evidence practical guide. AMEE Guide No. 82. Med Teach. 2013;35(10):e1511–30. https://doi.org/10.3109/0142159X.2013.818632.
26. Hamstra SJ, Brydges R, Hatala R, Zendejas B, Cook DA. Reconsidering fidelity in simulation-based training. Acad Med. 2014;89(3):387–92. https://doi.org/10.1097/ACM.0000000000000130.
27. Norman G, Dore K, Grierson L. The minimal relationship between simulation fidelity and transfer of learning. Med Educ. 2012;46(7):636–47. https://doi.org/10.1111/j.1365-2923.2012.04243.x.
28. Matsumoto ED, Hamstra SJ, Radomski SB, Cusimano MD. The effect of bench model fidelity on endourological skills: a randomized controlled study. J Urol. 2002;167(3):1243–7.
29. Savoldelli GL, Naik VN, Park J, Joo HS, Chow R, Hamstra SJ. Value of debriefing during simulated crisis management: oral versus video-assisted oral feedback. Anesthesiology. 2006;105(2):279–85. https://doi.org/10.1097/00000542-200608000-00010.
30. Rudolph JW, Simon R, Raemer DB, Eppich WJ. Debriefing as formative assessment: closing performance gaps in medical education. Acad Emerg Med. 2008;15(11):1010–6. https://doi.org/10.1111/j.1553-2712.2008.00248.x.

Chapter 87
Teaching on a Regional and National Stage

Annahieta Kalantari

We have all fallen victim to a lecture-based didactic that used some kind of presentation software resulting in the death of our interests and attention spans. We went from eagerness to learn about some of the latest and greatest updates in patient care to playing on our phones in a matter of seconds. We have also attended national conferences and sat through engaging, educational, and entertaining didactics that provided valuable, practicing changing tidbits. How do we become the latter? Where do we even begin? The good news is that there are some well-established stepping stones to get you onto this path. You can acquire all the necessary skills to teach on a regional or national stage. The first step, and the most time-consuming, is developing a quality product. This is often what was skipped in the sessions that put us to sleep. Although the most time-consuming, it is not the most challenging.

Develop a Quality Product

There are multiple teaching strategies that educators can use when teaching on a national or regional stage. For this type of setting, the most common format is that of a lecture. Lectures are generally a passive learning experience for the audience, but they accommodate a large number of learners and allow for a structured presentation of complicated topics [1]. As such, they are the most common platform for teaching on a regional or national stage so this section will focus on a lecture as the product.

A. Kalantari (✉)
Department of Emergency Medicine, Penn State Health Milton S Hershey Medical Center, Hershey, PA, USA
e-mail: akalantari@pennstatehealth.psu.edu

R. P. Olympia et al. (eds.), *An Emergency Physician's Path*,
https://doi.org/10.1007/978-3-031-47873-4_87

There are three fundamental components to any lecture-based didactic: a story, the speaker's presence and delivery, and the visual slides [2]. Unfortunately, the first step for most people is to open up the computer and work on the presentation slides before developing their story. This is a fatal flaw in putting a talk together and is destined for a death by PowerPoint experience for your audience. The most important component of any talk is story development. Humans love stories. Histories and lessons have been shared through the exchange of story for centuries [3]. A good story told well eliminates the need for slides. Just watch any of the top ten TED Talks for proof. Developing a story when discussing scientific data may present challenges however.

Thoroughly researching topics will assist with story development. Once a literature search is completed and full texts have been selected, take notes on each of the papers. As you accumulate notes, develop a mind map of the material [4]. Mind mapping allows authors to organize information into headings and subheadings. It also assists with structured writing and story development. See Fig. 87.1 as an example of a mind map on how to structure a talk. Protagonists, such as patient narratives or certain medications, and antagonists, such as disease processes or adverse reactions, can be developed from the information displayed in a mind map. For example, you have been assigned the task of giving a talk on direct oral anticoagulant inhibitor reversal. You can start your presentation by sharing a story of a very active elderly female. You can give her a name and detail her life. In your narrative, she can fall, hit her head, and have a subsequent subdural hematoma. You have now opened the door wide open on providing the scientific data your audience requires to treat this lovely elderly female. You close the presentation with the resolution of the story.

Once your story is developed, you may now work on the multimedia component. The media used should complement and add to the story. Oftentimes, projected slides are a wall of words compelling the audience to read the slides rather than engage with the speaker. This process causes dissonance and is counterproductive to learning. Richard Mayer developed ten multimedia principles grounded in research-based educational theories to foster learning with the use of media technologies [5]. They are:

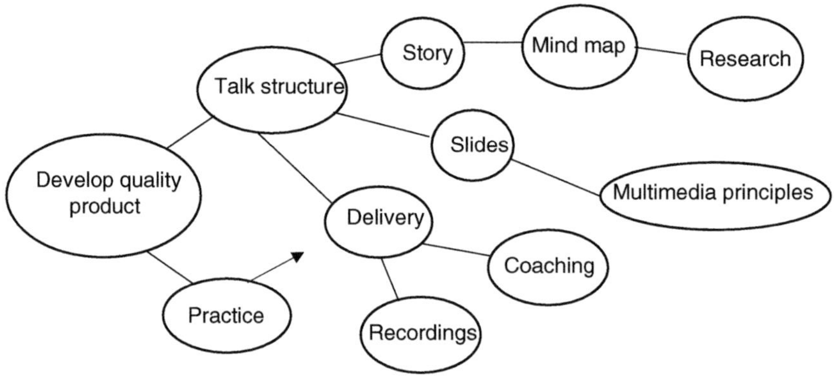

Fig. 87.1 Mind map on structuring a talk

1. Multiple representation principle—Present words and pictures rather than words alone. Example: Put up a picture of the coagulation cascade, and explain the process rather than just explaining it alone.
2. Coherence principle—Exclude extraneous material. Example: Remove the extraneous parts of the coagulation cascade image that are not important to the discussion.
3. Signaling principle—Highlight essential material. Example: Point to the areas of the coagulation cascade that are especially important or make them bold in the image.
4. Redundancy principle—Do not add on-screen text to narrated animation. Example: If using a narrated video to explain the coagulation cascade, do not add text for people to read on the screen as well.
5. Temporal contiguity principle—Present corresponding words and pictures together rather than separately. Example: The coagulation cycle picture should project simultaneously with the verbal explanation of the process.
6. Spatial contiguity principle—Place printed words next to the corresponding graphs. Example: If using a label for the coagulation cascade, it should be next to the photo of it.
7. Pre-training principle—Provide pre-training in names and characteristics of key concepts. Example: Prepare and distribute prereading materials on normal coagulation.
8. Segmenting principle—Break lessons into learner-controlled segments. Example: If using an animation of the coagulation cascade, space out each step and pause in between to allow learners to ask questions.
9. Modality principle—Present words in spoken form. Example: The coagulation cascade should be a picture of the steps rather than sentences explaining the steps.
10. Personalization principle—Present words in conversational or polite style. Example: Be yourself, and just talk to your audience like you would anyone else to whom you would be teaching the coagulation cascade [5].

Image selection is also important. Presentations are projected onto large screens at the regional and national level. Therefore, large images must be selected to avoid pixelation during the projection process. Presenters must also be mindful of copyright laws. Do not use images with copyright stamping. There are several websites that provide free, high-quality images. There are also online subscriptions to images as well. The latter may be a better option for individuals who must prepare multiple different talks per year.

It is now time to move onto the delivery of the presentation. This is the performance aspect of teaching on a stage. Just as actors can evoke audience responses with the use of voice and movement, so can speakers. Movements should be done with intent. For example, pacing back and forth for the sake of movement is distracting to your audience. Leaning in toward your audience when you want them to pause and think about something is movement with intent. Potential speakers may need to adjust the cadence and/or projection of their speech as well. A cadence should be a comfortable listening pace, and volume should be mindful of the presence or absence of a microphone during the presentation. Coaches are available to assist with the delivery of a presentation. Some are formal and require a fee, but informal coaches are an excellent option as well. Many current national speakers are happy to mentor and coach individuals interested in taking the stage as well.

Putting all the components of a lecture didactic together requires hours of practice. Give the talk out loud and record your voice. This will allow you to hear your speech cadence and volume, your pauses, and your fillers such as "um." Once you hear them, you can improve upon them. Do a video recording so that you can see how you move within a room. Do you pace back and forth for no reason? Do you favor one side of the room? Once you have worked through your speech and movement, present your lecture locally. It can be within your own department or another department within your institution. Obtain feedback and adjust your presentation based on the feedback you receive. You have now developed a high-quality product that is ready for marketing.

Seeking Opportunities

There are a variety of speaking opportunities available. First, many organizations at regional and national levels request content from speakers. In medical education, for example, the Accreditation Council for Graduate Medical Education, the Association of American Medical Colleges, and the Council of Residency Directors in Emergency Medicine put out a yearly call for speakers. This is an excellent opportunity to submit a talk. They often request a course description and objectives, and some may or may not request a video. Some conferences also have new speaker competitions. The American College of Emergency Physicians holds a "Drop the Mic" contest at their scientific assembly every year. This is a first-come, first-served opportunity and a great chance to showcase skills in front of members of the education committee who select speakers for future conferences. Some national and regional conferences host clinical pathologic case (CPC) competitions as well. A resident typically presents a case up to a key decision point. The attending physician then works through the case and presents his/her logic in developing a differential and the ultimate diagnosis.

Whether speaking locally, regionally, or nationally, amplification will assist with future invitations. Social media has become a strong platform for marketing [6]. Popularities of different platforms evolve over time, but posts generally have a similar content of visual media with a caption and associated hashtag or key phrase [7]. Ask a colleague to take a well-angled photo as you speak and create a post for social media. As many conferences may require a short video with submissions, you may also consider amplifying that short video on social media as well. Social media is an inexpensive advertisement that has a potentially wide reach.

Networking may also open up speaking opportunities. The world of emergency medicine is small. If you develop the reputation of a reliable, informative, and skilled speaker and have a wide network, your name may be offered as a candidate for speaking openings for different grand round opportunities and conferences at the regional and national level. This will also assist in the promotion process if you choose a career at an academic institution.

Get Gritty With It

Even when everything is done correctly, be prepared to hear "no" and have offers declined. There will be more opportunities. Educating at the regional and national level takes hard work, time, and many attempts before success follows. It takes grit, passion, and perseverance to reach these long-term goals [8]. Do not allow the fear of failure to paralyze you as you venture outside of your comfort zone to reach for new opportunities.

Receiving feedback will also require grit. I have spoken at several conferences, and thankfully, the vast majority of the feedback I receive is positive and constructive. However, there are always negative comments that sometimes feel cruel. It is important to try to find what can be learned from the comments without perseverating on the negative emotions associated with the comments [9]. Educating on a stage can present challenges, but it is absolutely worth it if you love teaching and entertaining the masses.

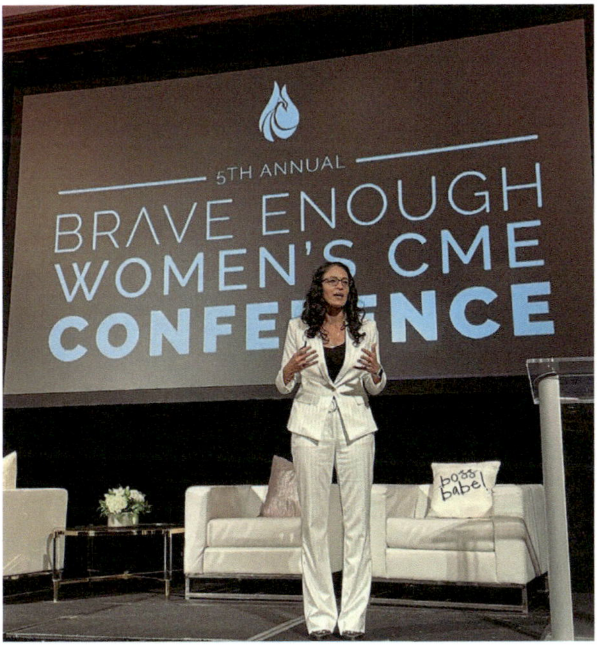

Dr Kalantari speaks about stress growth center stage at the Brave Enough Conference in Scottsdale, AZ

References

1. Thomas PA, Kern DE, Hughes MT, Chen BY. Curriculum development for medical education: a six-step approach. JHU Press; 2016.
2. Reynolds G. Presentation Zen: simple ideas on presentation design and delivery. New Riders; 2011.
3. Gottschall J. The storytelling animal: how stories make us human. Houghton Mifflin Harcourt; 2012.
4. Choudhari SG, Gaidhane AM, Desai P, Srivastava T, Mishra V, Zahiruddin SQ. Applying visual mapping techniques to promote learning in community-based medical education activities. BMC Med Educ. 2021;21(1):1–14.
5. Mayer R. Applying the science of learning to medical education. Med Educ. 2010;44(6):543–9. https://doi.org/10.1111/j.1365-2923.2010.03624.x.
6. Appel G, Grewal L, Hadi R, Stephen AT. The future of social media in marketing. J Acad Mark Sci. 2020;48(1):79–95.
7. Sorensen A, Andrews L, Drennan J. Using social media posts as resources for engaging in value co-creation: the case for social media-based cause brand communities. J Serv Theory Pract. 2017;
8. Duckworth AL, Peterson C, Matthews MD, Kelly DR. Grit: perseverance and passion for long-term goals. J Pers Soc Psychol. 2007;92(6):1087.
9. Stone D, Heen S. *Thanks for the feedback: the science and art of receiving feedback well (even when it is off base, unfair, poorly delivered, and frankly, you're not in the mood)* (no. 10). Penguin, 2015.

Chapter 88
Conducting a Successful Journal Club

Tara Cassidy-Smith and Alexis Pelletier-Bui

Introduction

It's conference day and another journal club (JC) is in progress. The room is packed yet silent. A resident is droning on about a scientific paper. Half the room is checking Instagram while others are catching up on their sleep. There is very poor discussion apart from a few "opinionated" faculty and residents. It is clear from the conversation that very few of the residents (and even faculty) have read the paper. As program leadership, you think to yourself that there must be a better way. Whether you are an individual preparing a JC session or a residency program preparing a JC curriculum, we hope this chapter helps you avoid this common scenario by preparing a successful JC that is well attended and enjoyed and most importantly achieves your teaching goals.

Preparation Is Key

Identifying Goals

The first step to running a successful JC is to determine the objective of your JC, with the two primary goals typically being acquisition of new medical knowledge and/or teaching critical appraisal techniques when reading scientific papers. Secondary goals may include the development of lifelong learning skills, providing a social environment for peer-to-peer learning and improving presentation and

T. Cassidy-Smith · A. Pelletier-Bui (✉)
Department of Emergency Medicine, Cooper Medical School of Rowan University, Camden, NJ, USA
e-mail: cassidy-smith-tara@cooperhealth.edu; pelletier-bui-alexis@cooperhealth.edu

R. P. Olympia et al. (eds.), *An Emergency Physician's Path*,
https://doi.org/10.1007/978-3-031-47873-4_88

communication skills. The goals you define will then help guide subsequent planning, including topic and facilitator selection [1].

Presenter Selection

To facilitate more widespread engagement, we suggest choosing multiple presenters rather than just one for JC. In our residency program, we had difficulty engaging members of all class years with just one senior resident running JC each month. We subsequently developed an approach where multiple levels of learners were involved in leading JC with each advancing year handling a more challenging component of the JC discussion. For example, our interns cover the introduction/background component of the article, and our PGY-2 residents handle the methods and results sections, while our senior residents lead the discussion. Depending on how much time is available, distribution of effort and focus of discussion can be similarly distributed across multiple presenters and even multiple articles.

Topic Selection

Again, the first question to answer when choosing your topic is determining the goal of your JC. An article covering new and upcoming literature may not necessarily be the best to also teach the principles of evidence-based medicine. It may be optimal to have the learner select the article themself based on a specific clinical question to help guide the topic. Allowing the learner to choose can promote better engagement in the discussion process and has the additional benefit of teaching the learner how to search clinical databases to answer a clinical question. Having a faculty mentor assist in, or at least approve this selection, ensures that a high-quality article is chosen. A faculty facilitator overseeing article selection over the course of the academic year helps establish that different types of articles are selected (e.g., retrospective, prospective, observational, randomized controlled trial, systematic review, and meta-analysis).

Number of Articles

The number of articles links back to the primary goal of your JC. Most programs choose between one and four articles to cover in a single JC session [1]. If your goal is to perform an in-depth statistical analysis, you may want to choose one article. If you want to cover a larger breadth of material, you may choose more articles.

Instructing the Leader(s)

Laying out expectations for your JC leader(s) is key to creating a successful JC. JC leaders should be involved in the discussion of goals for JC and selection of the article(s). They should be given deadlines for article choice, well in advance of when the article will be sent to participants, so that the article can be vetted by the faculty facilitator. The faculty facilitator can provide a structured presentation outline to help guide the JC discussion. See Table 88.1 for a sample outline. The facilitator can also help the JC leader(s) identify the salient learning and discussion points for the article and effective teaching strategies to communicate these points.

Table 88.1 Example presentation outline for journal club leaders (adapted from Aztema [2])

General presentation guidelines: Give a *brief* overall assessment of the article and then proceed to address each of the following questions. ***Limit the formal presentation time to a total of 10–15 min, allowing ample opportunity for discussion among participants***
1. **Introduction**
(a) What is the generally accepted current practice in this area?
(b) What question does this paper try to answer?
(c) Is this a question that you think is worth answering?
(d) Who funded the study?
2. **Methods**
(a) What is the study design?
(b) What is the study population?
(c) Is this similar to ours (external validity)?
(d) What were the inclusion/exclusion criteria?
(e) What is the intervention?
(f) Is the control comparison considered the current standard of care?
(g) When was the study conducted?
(h) What outcome measurements do the authors use? Is this a patient-centered outcome?
(i) Could you replicate the study with the information given?
3. **Bias**
(a) Is there evidence of selection bias?
(b) Is there bias in classifications of disease or measurements?
(c) Are there any other forms of bias present?
4. **Results**
(a) Are the outcomes clinically relevant? (Is this a patient-centered outcome?)
(b) What are the results and how are they presented?
(c) Can you identify other results that you might want to see that are not presented?
(d) To what extent does the study establish a causal relationship between two variables (internal validity)?
(e) Was a power analysis performed?
5. **Discussion**
(a) Are limitations addressed?
(b) Have confounding variables been discussed?
6. **Conclusion**
(a) Do the results of the study support the conclusion?
(b) Will this change your clinical practice?
(c) If you were going to do research in this area, what would be your next study?

Critical Appraisal Tool for Participants

To run a stimulating JC with robust conversation, the participants must also prepare in advance. The JC article should be provided 1–2 weeks in advance to allow for ample time for all participants to read the article. Releasing the article more than 2 weeks in advance may cause participants to forget the material before the JC session [1]. Participants should also be provided with a critical appraisal tool to get them thinking more about the article, which could include the following broad questions:

1. What type of study design was used?
2. What was the study population?
3. What intervention or test was studied?
4. What comparison or control was used?
5. What was the primary outcome?
6. What did the study find?
7. What are the strengths and weaknesses of the article?

You can consider having each resident complete this guide prior to JC. You could collect it at the beginning of JC to give credit or utilize it as a tool to increase preparation, engagement, and participation.

Implementation

Setting

While some studies have shown greatest success with JC being held at a faculty member's home in the evening, programs may also choose to utilize conference time at the hospital [1]. Providing food as an incentive is a wise choice—food was found to be associated with increased longevity of the JC and higher attendance, regardless of whether the food was light refreshments versus full dinners [1]. If there are no departmental funds to budget for food, you can consider asking for faculty contributions and alumni fund contributions or have a potluck.

Frequency

The majority of EM residency programs conduct a monthly JC. Less frequent meetings can decrease the retention of evidence-based medicine concepts. Set days and times at regularly scheduled intervals are optimal to allow attendees to schedule accordingly and promote attendance [1].

Length of Time

Most JC sessions run from 1 to 2 h in length. Timing may vary depending on the number of articles chosen and the setting of the JC. If conference time is being utilized, JC may be shorter versus longer for an off-campus event [1].

General Rules

Mandatory attendance is a primary factor associated with JC success [1]. Active involvement of all participants is ideal, which requires all participants to critically read the article in advance with or without a critical appraisal tool as discussed above. A safe learning environment is necessary to facilitate discussion between all levels of learners. Providing defined opportunities for junior learners to contribute may increase their engagement. Consider limiting faculty commentary for at least the first half of the JC session. We found that once the faculty began to debate the merits or limitations of the paper, very few residents remained active in the conversation. To engage our residents early in the discussion, we have asked our faculty not to participate in the discussion until 20 minutes into the conversation. It may be beneficial to have the JC presenters and the faculty facilitator wrap up the session by summarizing the critical appraisal tool answers to affirm comprehension of final concepts.

Taking it to the Next Level

Perhaps your program is already leading a successful JC but you're just looking for a way to spice things up a bit. Here are some ways to add variety to your JC experience:

Gamification

Who doesn't love a little competition? Gamification has the potential to increase engagement and participation from all JC participants. If you choose more than one article for JC, you could create a competition for best presentation. You could choose two articles studying a similar topic but with opposing findings and create a formal debate, allowing participants to elect a winner. In addition, you may consider creating a Jeopardy!®, KAHOOT!®, or other games utilizing your critical appraisal tool or general presentation guideline to create your questions.

Social Media

If you are an individual looking to participate in JC outside of a single residency program, social media is an excellent way to do so. Twitter is one of the most common online platforms utilized for this purpose. It allows learners, content experts, and educators from across the globe to come together and discuss an article. Wiki Journal Club (WJC) is another platform to discuss landmark articles with individuals outside of your institution, with WJC editors choosing the article and any WJC registered member participating in the conversation over a period of 3–4 weeks.

If you are a residency program looking to incorporate social media into JC, there are many ways to do so. If you are simply looking to involve individuals from your residency program who could not be present in person for JC, many video conferencing platforms are easy to incorporate. Even prior to COVID, these platforms were shown to increase attendance at JC [1] and now have become essential for residency program didactics in the realm of COVID. If you want to incorporate others outside of your residency program, including prospective applicants, and do not want/need to be selective regarding other participants, you can choose to livestream your JC via Instagram, Facebook, or other relevant social media platforms as well.

If you are looking to keep the conversation going after an in-person JC, you can ask JC leaders or participants to create social media posts or discussions via various platforms following JC: X, Instagram stories, Facebook groups, curated program websites/blogs, TikTok videos—you can really incorporate anything that is trending!

If contributing to social media is not your thing but you are looking for ways to incorporate already created social media and teach your learners how to critically assess social media, doing so via JC is another excellent option. In the "Flipped Journal Club," created by the EM residency program at Christiana, JC leaders were asked to not only choose a landmark article but also choose a relevant social media piece on the topic. This social media selection was distributed to participants along with the article prior to JC and was critically appraised during JC discussion, along with the JC article choice. The "Flipped Journal Club" was strongly preferred by both residents and faculty at Christiana compared to a "traditional" JC format [3].

Summary

We have attempted to provide a guideline to improve your JC implementation and success. With preparation, you can avoid the cycle of ill-prepared and disengaged trainees and promote a fun, active learning environment.

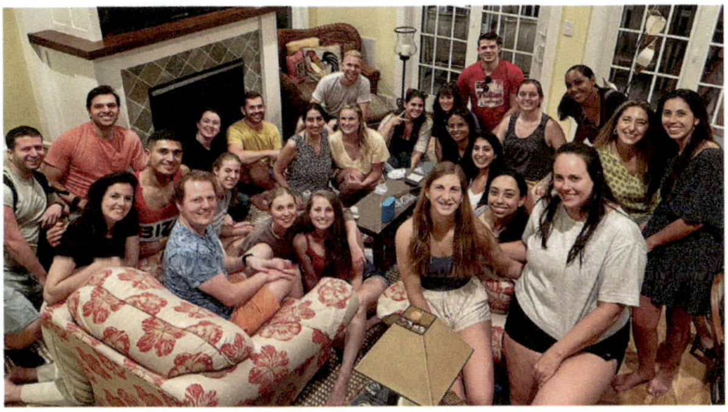

Cooper emergency medicine residents enjoying team building

References

1. Gottlieb M, King A, Byyny R, Parsons M, Bailitz J. Journal Club in Residency Education: an evidence-based guide to best practices from the Council of Emergency Medicine Residency Directors. West J Emerg Med. 2018;19(4):746–55. https://doi.org/10.5811/westjem.2018.4.37507.
2. Atzema C. Presenting at journal club: a guide. Ann Emerg Med. 2004;44:169–74.
3. Bounds R, Boone S. The flipped journal Club. West J Emerg Med. 2018;19(1):23–7. https://doi.org/10.5811/westjem.2017.11.34465.

Chapter 89
Effective Methods of Patient Education

Sapana P. Adhikari

Background

Our healthcare system is becoming increasingly more complex. New technologies, innovative discoveries, and modern treatments are being developed every day. As physicians, we must not only use this new information in our own practice but, just as importantly, make it understandable to our patients. Unfortunately, many patients have poor health literacy. According to a survey by the US Department of Education, about 36% of Americans had a basic or below basic level of health literacy [1]. It is imperative that patients understand medical information as they are increasingly asked to make informed decisions, manage self-care, and take part in complex health decisions. Effective means of patient education are essential when trying to convey health information.

Several factors may contribute to low health literacy (Table 89.1): First, many patients may not have had any formal education on health-related issues since high school. Second, new technologies and medications are being developed at a rapid pace, making it very difficult to keep up with the bombardment of new information. Third, understanding medicine involves much more than just basic anatomy and pathophysiology. Patients need to understand statistics, charts, diagrams, and risk/benefit analysis to make informed medical decisions.

Low health literacy affects everyone, not just the uneducated and poor. Medical instructions can be difficult to understand for even well-educated people with strong reading and writing skills. Currently, most health education is given in the form of pamphlets and written discharge paperwork. However, the National Action Plan to improve health literacy has found that 90% of adults have difficulty understanding health information that is routinely available in healthcare facilities [2]. Information

S. P. Adhikari (✉)
Atrium Mercy Hospital, Charlotte, NC, USA

R. P. Olympia et al. (eds.), *An Emergency Physician's Path*,
https://doi.org/10.1007/978-3-031-47873-4_89

Table 89.1 Factors that contribute to poor patient health literacy

1	Clinicians may not have been taught an effective patient education curriculum in medical school
2	Patient education may be a low priority. Clinicians may perceive that spending time doing physical tasks may seem more important than spending time teaching
3	Patients may not have the readiness or motivation to learn about their health
4	The healthcare system relies heavily on written aftercare instructions. Many patients do not understand these instructions

may be everywhere, but printed health education material is often written at a grade level higher than the reading ability of the majority of patients. Some studies even indicate that patients prefer written material below their school level, especially when ill. Obviously, there is a disconnect between what is available and what patients need.

Poor health literacy can be costly. Studies indicate limited health literacy is associated with worse health outcomes, higher costs, increased use of the health system, and increased health disparities [3]. Informed patients are more likely to follow medical treatment plans that they understand. Health literacy is clearly becoming an important determinant of health. Therefore, effective means of patient education is essential.

Strategies for Effective Patient Education

With over 20 years of clinical practice, I have seen poor health literacy affect patient care firsthand. I have seen patients return to the Emergency Department because they didn't understand aftercare instructions. I have seen patients still confused about their diagnosis even though they may have seen several specialists. Over the years, I have compiled five ways to make patients understand health information effectively:

1. Be concise and limit how much information you give.

   Sometimes, when we describe medical diseases, we tend to go into too much detail. Think of the patient with newly diagnosed pancreatic cancer. Sometimes, we scroll through the CT scan of the abdomen to show a patient their disease or pull up laboratory tests and discuss them. We feel that we should be comprehensive and explain everything. Yet, we forget the health literacy of our patients. Many of our patients may not have looked at an anatomy textbook since high school. They may not understand complicated images or complicated words. I have found it better to try to give the least amount of information that is necessary to convey a diagnosis, not the most. Often, patients will need to explain their medical diagnoses to other family members and friends at home. Imagine trying to convey a detailed description of a medical diagnosis repeatedly. Distortion is bound to happen. In my experience, the simpler the explanation, the better.

Finally, people often remember the first thing and the last thing that they hear. So, it is probably better to start with the most important information and repeat it again and again. Remember, the more information you tell a patient, the less they will likely remember.

2. Use common language, not medical jargon.

Although technical medical terminology is an effective way to communicate with other medical professionals, this language should not be used when we speak with patients. Remember, it took us years of intensive schooling and training to understand these words. We should not expect our patients to understand this highly technical speak. There is a lot of confusion about medical jargon. The same concept can be named in multiple ways. A patient may ask if their bone is broken or fractured, not realizing that it conveys the same thing. Even in highly technical medical speak, there is an ever-increasing way to talk about similar disease processes. For example, the words to describe events related to coronary artery disease have evolved to the term "acute coronary syndrome" as our understanding of its pathophysiology has improved. Similarly, within common lingo, there are multiple ways to say the same thing. For example, a shot is the same thing as an injection. A drug is the same thing as a medication. A meal is the same thing as food or diet. I have found it most helpful to use one word consistently instead of interchanging words that mean the same thing. Also, medical jargon care uses many abbreviations. As we use shorthand to document a patient's UTI or their CHF, sometimes, these words creep into our discussion with the patient. Often, patients may not know what the abbreviations stand for, and this can be confusing.

3. Use visuals at the bedside.

In psychology, there is a theory called picture superiority effect. This concept states that hearing information will lead to 10% retention of content but hearing and seeing information leads to 65% retention of content. Using simplified visuals at the bedside can be an effective way to both make patients understand complicated medical information and remember it. Studies show that many patients benefit from images, but patients with lower literacy skills benefit even more [4]. Visuals need to have the right level of detail. Sometimes, complicated anatomical images with complicated labels are just too detailed and can confuse a patient unnecessarily. These images often require some background knowledge that patients may lack. Also, they take some time to process and may not be ideal to use at the bedside when time is often limited. In the ED, the common diagnosis of kidney stone is much easier for the clinician to explain and for the patient to understand with an image (Fig. 89.1). Visuals are particularly useful for certain demographics: pediatric patients, non-English-speaking patients, and hard-of-hearing patients. And finally, when used at the bedside, simplified visuals can encourage a two-way dialogue between the clinician and the patient, clearing up misconceptions and answering questions in real time. They can also serve as a basic primer for better patient understanding so that patients will then be able to understand aftercare instructions and other information they encounter.

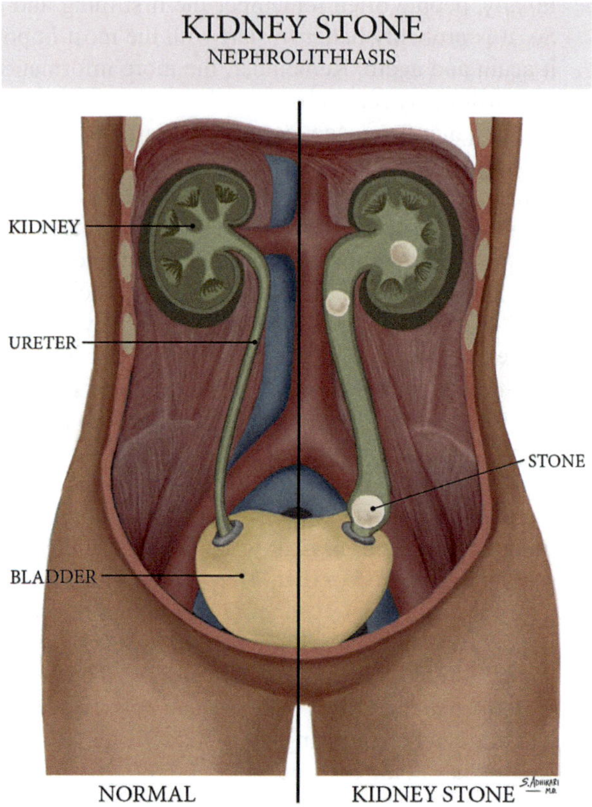

Fig. 89.1 An example of effective visual aid in patient education. Notice the simplified anatomy and minimal labels. Notice, also, the "normal" left side compared with the "abnormal" right side. This image has the right level of detail to convey this diagnosis simply and effectively at the bedside (from Adhikari SP: *Diagnosketch: A Visual Guide to Medical Diagnosis for the Non-Medical Audience*, Oxford University Press, 2022)

4. Focus only on pertinent information.

   Although there is so much information that we may want to tell our patients, it is instead more important to focus on the most pertinent for a specific diagnosis. For example, if a patient presents with a laceration, spend time discussing the proper dressing, the time frame in which it can get wet, and what to look for in an infection. If a patient presents with gastroenteritis, focus on what a patient should eat, how much they should drink, and when they should come back when their symptoms persist. If a patient presents with a gallstone, focus on what foods to avoid, when to return to the ED, and a time frame for follow-up with a general surgeon. As much as we may want to share our knowledge of the disease process, we must remember to focus more on pertinent information that will help our patients get better.
5. Encourage active learning.

   A common technique in patient education that has been studied is the "teach-back method." [5] Here, the clinician explains medical information to the patient and then asks the patient to explain it back to the clinician. Although deemed to be helpful, several barriers to this method exist that include the lack of time, lack of space and privacy, and potential for shame if the patient doesn't demonstrate comprehension. There are other methods of active learning. Telling anecdotes about common scenarios pertaining to a certain diagnosis often helps patients remember important information. Making analogies to nonmedical themes also can be quite helpful. For example, I commonly use an analogy comparing worn-out elastic to discuss the process of diverticulosis. Showing an image of normal vs abnormal anatomy and asking the patient to tell the difference between the two encourage interactive learning.

References

1. Kutner M, Greenberg E, Jin Y, Paulsen C. The Health Literacy of America's adults: results from the 2003 National Assessment of Adult Literacy (NCES 2006–483). U.S. Department of Education. Washington, DC: National Center for Education Statistics; 2006.
2. U.S. Department of Health and Human Services, Office of Disease Prevention and Health Promotion. National action plan to improve health literacy. Washington, DC: Author; 2010.
3. Rasu RS, Bawa WA, Suminski R, Snella K, Warady B. Health literacy impact on national healthcare utilization and expenditure. Int J Health Policy Manag. 2015;4(11):747–55. https://doi.org/10.15171/ijhpm.2015.151.
4. Houts PS, Doak CC, Doak LG, Loscalzo MJ. The role of pictures in improving health communication: a review of research on attention, comprehension, recall, and adherence. Patient Educ Couns. 2006;61(2):173–90. https://doi.org/10.1016/j.pec.2005.05.004. Epub 2005 Aug 24. Erratum in: Patient Educ Couns. 2006 Dec;64(1-3):393-4
5. Use the Teach-Back Method: Tool #5. Content last reviewed September 2020. Agency for Healthcare Research and Quality, Rockville, MD.

Sapana P. Adhikari MD, is an emergency medicine physician and creator and illustrator of *Diagnosketch: A Visual Guide to Medical Diagnosis for the Non-Medical Audience*. Visit her at www.diagnosketch.com.

Part IX
Carving a Path in Emergency Medicine

Chapter 90
Being a Lifelong Learner in Emergency Medicine

Andrew Little

Emergency medicine is a fast-paced and ever-changing field. To be successful, physicians need to update their knowledge and skills continuously. This process of lifelong learning is essential to our clinical careers. There are many ways to stay up-to-date in emergency medicine. We can read journals, attend conferences, and take online courses. Lifelong learning also involves sharing knowledge with colleagues and mentoring others. By engaging in lifelong learning, we ensure that we provide the best possible care for our patients. It is also crucial for our well-being and career.

So how do we go about it? Let's break down some common ways we can approach lifelong learning. First, let us discuss continuing medical education. Continuing medical education (CME) is a type of continuing professional development (CPD) that helps medical professionals keep up-to-date with the latest advances in their field. It can take many forms, including conferences, seminars, workshops, and online courses. CME can be mandatory for some medical professionals, such as those who need to maintain their license to practice medicine. However, CME can still benefit doctors and patients even if it's not required.

CME helps doctors stay up-to-date on the latest medical advances. This is important because discoveries are made all the time in medicine and doctors need to keep up. CME can also help doctors learn about new treatments and technologies they may not be familiar with, leading to better patient care. CME can also be beneficial for patients. When doctors are up-to-date on the latest medical advances, they're more likely to be able to provide the best possible care for their patients. In addition, if a doctor has taken a CME course on a particular condition or disease, they may be able to provide better treatment options for their patients.

So let us review the various ways you can get CME: specifically podcasts, conferences, board reviews, and free open-access medical education (FOAMed).

A. Little (✉)
Advent Health East Orlando, Orlando, FL, USA

R. P. Olympia et al. (eds.), *An Emergency Physician's Path*,
https://doi.org/10.1007/978-3-031-47873-4_90

One of the best ways to stay up-to-date in emergency medicine is to listen to podcasts. These are created by educational companies and also by those who create free open-access medical education (FOAMed), to be covered later, and can be listened to while you commute to work, exercise, work around the house, or do any other activity you like. This flexibility makes podcasts an easy way to integrate staying up-to-date in EM into your daily routine. Compared to other specialties, there are several great podcasts out there that cover a variety of topics related to EM ranging from evidence-based medicine, core content, wellness, professional development, and other topics pertinent to the practice of EM. Numerous studies show that podcasts are an effective way to learn and retain information in EM [1–5]. There are many great podcasts out there that cover a variety of topics related to emergency medicine. If looking to decide which ones you should consider following, visit aliem.com as they have a curated extensive list for you to peruse [6].

Another way to stay up-to-date in emergency medicine is by attending conferences. There are many types of conferences, ranging from small, intimate gatherings to significant, national, and international events. Several benefits will be gained regardless of the size or type of conference you attend. Conferences provide an opportunity to network with other professionals in your field. This can be invaluable when seeking advice or guidance on particular cases or problems you may be facing. Additionally, conferences offer a chance to hear about the latest research and advancements in emergency medicine. They also provide an excellent forum for exchanging ideas and best practices with colleagues worldwide. Of course, not all conferences are created equal, and some may be more beneficial than others, depending on your particular interests and needs. However, all conferences can allow you to learn more about emergency medicine and network with other professionals in the field.

As emergency medicine is a rapidly evolving specialty, it can be challenging to keep up with the latest developments. Board review materials can be a great way to stay current in terms of emergency medicine core content and best practices. Several board review resources are available, including books, online courses, and live events. The best way to use these resources will vary depending on your learning style and needs.

Board review materials can be a great way to supplement your regular continuing medical education (CME). They can also be helpful if you are preparing for initial board certification or recertification exams. When choosing board review materials, look for those that are updated regularly and offer a variety of content formats. Additionally, ensure the materials are relevant to your practice and meet your learning needs.

If you are looking for board review materials (BRM), the following organizations have BRM resources that you may find helpful:

- American College of Emergency Physicians (ACEP).
- American Academy of Emergency Medicine (AAEM).
- Society for Academic Emergency Medicine (SAEM).
- Emergency Medicine Board Review Courses (e.g., RoshReview, BoardVitals).

- Live events (e.g., Essentials of EM, any specialty-specific board review course).
- Online courses (e.g., EM Med Coach, Hippo EM).
- Emergency medicine board review books (e.g., *First Aid for the Emergency Medicine Boards*, *Rapid Review for the Emergency Medicine*).

Remember, there is no one-size-fits-all solution for board review materials. Choose the resources that work best for you and your learning style.

The final way to stay updated that we will highlight, which has become increasingly popular, is using FOAMed [7]. FOAMed is a term used to describe the growing body of medical education resources freely available online. This includes things like blog posts, podcasts, and even video lectures.

One of the great things about FOAMed is that it allows you to learn at your own pace and from anywhere in the world. All you need is an Internet connection and a device (phone, tablet, and computer) to view it on. It can be delivered to your device by subscribing to each FOAMed site individually or using an RSS feed reader app (Feedly is highly recommended).

Another benefit of FOAMed is that it often provides a more "real-world" perspective on medicine than traditional educational resources. This is because many people creating FOAMed content are practicing clinicians who share their experiences and insights. If you're looking for a way to stay up-to-date in emergency medicine, FOAMed is worth checking out. There are lots of great resources available, and new ones are being created all the time.

Outside of the various CME options outlined above, it is important to know of other ways to become a lifelong learner. One other major activity that comes to mind is participating in hospital, company, or organizational physician leadership courses. There are many reasons why someone might want to take a physician leadership course. Perhaps you want to learn how to be a more effective leader in your practice or hospital, or you may be interested in moving into a managerial or executive role within healthcare. Whatever the reason, these courses can provide you with valuable insights and skills for those who wish to assume a leadership position within the medical field.

Some of the topics covered in physician leadership courses include effective communication, teamwork, conflict resolution, and financial management. These skills are essential for any leader, but they are especially important for those in the medical field who must deal with complex issues daily. By taking a course on physician leadership, learners can gain the knowledge and tools they need to be successful in any leadership role they may assume in the future.

Finally, it is worth introducing the idea of creating an active learning group (you could also call it a mastermind group, educational coalition, and other names). There are many reasons why you might want to create an active learning network. Perhaps you want to connect with other educators who share your interest in teaching and learning. Maybe you want to find new ways to engage students in learning. Or maybe you simply want to stay up-to-date on the latest educational research and practices.

Whatever your reason, an active learning network can provide you with a wealth of resources and support. In an active learning network, all members share ideas, resources, and best practices. They also collaborate on projects and activities that provide teaching and learning opportunities for everyone involved.

An active learning network can help you:

- Stay connected with other educators.
- Access resources and support.
- Improve your teaching practice.
- Increase your knowledge of educational research and practices.

If you are interested in creating or joining an active learning network, there are many options available. You can join an existing network or create your own. There are also online platforms that facilitate active learning networks. The key is to find a platform or community that meets your needs and interests. Once you find a good fit, you'll be on your way to reaping the benefits of an active learning network!

If you want to become a lifelong learner, there are numerous resources at your disposal. How and when you initiate this into your daily life is up to you. The question I will pose is as follows: What are you waiting for?

References

1. Cadogan M, Thoma B, Chan TM, Lin M. Free Open Access Meducation (FOAM): the rise of emergency medicine and critical care blogs and podcasts (2002–2013). Emerg Med J. 2014;31(e1):e76–7. https://doi.org/10.1136/emermed-2013-203502.
2. Lin M, Phipps M, Yilmaz Y, Nash CJ, Gisondi MA, Chan TM. A fork in the road for emergency medicine and critical care blogs and podcasts: cross-sectional study. JMIR Med Educ. 2022;8(4):e39946. Published 2022 Oct 28. https://doi.org/10.2196/39946.
3. Colmers-Gray IN, Solis Aguilar L, Gauri A, Ha DJ, Stauffer BA. Keeping up with the literature: a current practice survey and qualitative needs assessment among emergency physicians. AEM Educ Train. 2022;6(3):e10761. Published 2022 Jun 1. https://doi.org/10.1002/aet2.10761.
4. Riddell J, Swaminathan A, Lee M, Mohamed A, Rogers R, Rezaie SR. A survey of emergency medicine residents' use of educational podcasts. West J Emerg Med. 2017;18(2):229–34. https://doi.org/10.5811/westjem.2016.12.32850.
5. Purdy E, Thoma B, Bednarczyk J, Migneault D, Sherbino J. The use of free online educational resources by Canadian emergency medicine residents and program directors. CJEM. 2015;17(2):101–6. https://doi.org/10.1017/cem.2014.73.
6. Social Media index (SMI). ALiEM. https://www.aliem.com/social-media-index/. Published January 5, 2021. Accessed January 1, 2023.
7. Kalnow A, Beck-Esmay J, Riddell J, et al. Continuing medical education delivery preferences among physicians and advanced practice providers in emergency medicine. Cureus. 2021;13(12):e20406. Published 2021 Dec 14. https://doi.org/10.7759/cureus.20406.

Chapter 91
Board Certification and Maintaining Certification

Chaiya Laoteppitaks

Board certification offers an independent evaluation and verification of a physician's skills and expertise. Becoming @@board certified is separate from medical licensure. Medical licensure is not specialty-specific, while board certification is specific to a specialty or subspecialty. Board certification is voluntary, whereas medical licensure is required to practice medicine in a particular state. There are currently three different boards for emergency medicine and EM subspecialties. Founded in 1976, the American Board of Emergency Medicine (ABEM) is the oldest EM board and subsequently has the largest number of board-certified emergency physicians. ABEM is a member board of the American Board of Medical Specialties. In 2021, there were over 39,000 ABEM-certified EM physicians @@ [1]. The American Osteopathic Board of Emergency Medicine (AOBEM) is a member of the American Osteopathic Association Bureau of Osteopathic Specialists. As of 2012, there were 2344 AOBEM board-certified physicians [2]. The third EM board is the Board of Certification in Emergency Medicine (BCEM). BCEM is an affiliated board of certification of the American Board of Physician Specialties (ABPS).

From 1979 until 1988, ABEM offered a pathway for non-EM residency-trained practice track physicians to obtain board certification. In 1988, ABEM closed the practice track pathway. This closure prompted the creation of BCEM. ABEM board eligibility period is time-limited; it begins on the physician's graduation date and ends on December 31st, 5 years after the graduation date. Each board has their own specific requirements to be eligible for board certification (Table 91.1).

Board certification is highly valued by our patients. In 2003, the American Board of Internal Medicine commissioned the Gallup organization to poll the public

C. Laoteppitaks (✉)
Department of Emergency Medicine, Sidney Kimmel Medical College, Philadelphia, PA, USA
e-mail: Chaiya.Laoteppitaks@jefferson.edu

R. P. Olympia et al. (eds.), *An Emergency Physician's Path*,
https://doi.org/10.1007/978-3-031-47873-4_91

Table 91.1 Overview of board certification eligibility requirements

	ABEM	AOBEM	BCEM
Residency training	ACGME[a]- or RCPSC[b]-accredited EM or ABEM-approved combined program	AOA [c]- or ACGME-accredited EM	(1) ACMGE, AOA, RCPSC, or CFPC[d] EM or (2) primary care residency[e] and AAEP[f]-approved EM fellowship or (3) primary care residency[e] and 5 years of full-time EM practice and ≥ 7000 h
Written examination	Yes, after graduating from residency	Yes, after completing at least 80% of residency program	Yes
Oral examination	Yes, after passing written exam	Yes, before or after written exam	Yes
Additional requirements	N/A	N/A	Report on 10 EM case reports in the last 12 months; 3 letters of recommendation
Eligibility period	1. Starts at graduation 2. Ends Dec. 31st, 5 years postgraduation	1. Starts at graduation 2. Ends Dec. 31st, 6 years postgraduation	N/A

[a]Accreditation Council for Graduate Medical Education
[b]Royal College of Physicians and Surgeons of Canada
[c]American Osteopathic Association
[d]College of Family Physicians of Canada
[e]Family Practice, Internal Medicine, Pediatrics, General Surgery
[f]American Academy of Emergency Physicians

regarding their views on board certification and maintenance of certification. Both initial certification and maintenance of certification are highly valued. The public expects that physicians are evaluated frequently. Poll respondents would change their physician if they knew that their current physician or specialist failed to maintain certification. When asked to choose between a nonboard-certified physician who was recommend by a friend of family member or a board-certified physician, the majority of respondents chose the board-certified physician [3]. From a quality standpoint, the relationship between clinical outcomes and board certification is mixed.

Medicine is constantly changing and knowledge degrades over time. All three boards have recertification/maintenance of certification (MOC) programs in place to ensure that their board-certified physicians stay current (Table 91.2).

The vast majority of EM physicians are ABEM certified. Board certification is highly valued by our patients, and the public expects that physicians are evaluated frequently. Each board has continual education requirements to maintain certification. The specific requirements for board certification and MOC vary between the three boards and have changed over the years. EM physicians should refer to their respective board for the most up-to-date requirements.

Table 91.2 Overview of recertification requirements

	ABEM	AOBEM	BCEM
Certification period	5 years	10 years	8 years
Written exam	4 MyEMCert modules	Annual Continuous Osteopathic Recertification Examination (CORE)	Recertification exam
Additional requirements	Maintain licensure, Improvement in Medical Practice activity	Maintain licensure, 2 Practice Performance Assessment and Improvement projects (during years 1–5 and 6–10)	Maintain licensure

References

1. *2020-2021 Annual Report*. 2021, American Board of Emergency Medicine.
2. Moorhead JC, Ludwin F. Number of board-certified emergency physicians. Ann Emerg Med. 2013;62(6):647.
3. Brennan TA, et al. The role of physician specialty board certification status in the quality movement. JAMA. 2004;292(9):1038–43.

Chapter 92
Organizations with an Emergency Medicine Focus: ACEP, AAEM, SAEM, CORD, and EMRA

Joshua Guttman and Eliot Blum

Introduction

Emergency medicine (EM) would not be a recognized specialty today without EM organizations. In 1968, in response to a national push for improved emergency care, the American College of Emergency Physicians (ACEP) was created to educate and train physicians in emergency care [1, 2].

With the outgrowth of EM, new EM organizations began to form, with many focused on specific aspects or niches of EM. EM organizations have been instrumental in bringing together EPs from across the country to collaborate in shared interests. The shared voice of many EPs has been used to successfully advocate congress to enact legislation favorable to EPs and their patients. EM organizations also bring together experts to create clinical guidelines for best practices in EM, educational policies, and research journals to showcase the high level of EM research. Organizations have used fundraising efforts and member dues to provide grants to EPs to conduct research of interest to the EM community.

While membership dues can be costly, becoming a member of an EM organization has multiple advantages for the EP, which include educational content, networking, advocacy, and leadership possibilities. This chapter will discuss the role of EM organizations, why an EP should consider joining one, and the differences between specific prominent EM organizations.

J. Guttman (✉) · E. Blum
Emory University School of Medicine, Atlanta, GA, USA
e-mail: Joshua.guttman@emory.edu; Eliot.h.blum@emory.edu

R. P. Olympia et al. (eds.), *An Emergency Physician's Path*,
https://doi.org/10.1007/978-3-031-47873-4_92

The History of EM Organizations

Into the 1960s, emergency department (ED) visits were increasing across the country. EDs became the entry point of the hospital and the healthcare system for many patients. At that time, EDs were staffed by trainees and physicians with little to no training in emergency care. There were two separate physician groups, one in Virginia and one in Michigan, who independently decided to practice full-time emergency medicine. Dr. John Rupke (who had set up the Michigan group) and Dr. John Wiegenstein (who staffed an ED part time in another part of Michigan) got together to discuss establishing an EM organization. Dr. Rupke had struggled with getting insurers to pay physicians fairly for emergency care, and Dr. Wiegenstein was dismayed at the lack of EM training for physicians staffing EDs and felt that formal training programs were required. They thought that organizing would be the optimal way to accomplish their goals. On August 16, 1968, Dr. Rupke, Dr. Wiegenstein, and six other Michigan physicians met in Lansing, MI, and formed ACEP. Membership was limited to those who "voluntarily devote a significant portion of their medical practice to emergency medicine and surgery." At the same time, Dr. Reinald Leidelmeyer, a physician practicing EM in Fairfax, VA, had also called for a national organization for EM. On November 16, 1968, the Michigan group traveled to Arlington, VA, to meet with Dr. Leidelmeyer and his group. In total, 29 emergency physicians gathered, and together, they became ACEP, with Dr. Wiegenstein serving as the first president. From November 19 to 21, 1970, the first ACEP Scientific Assembly took place in Denver, CO, with 128 practicing emergency physicians attending. This was around 20% of the ACEP membership at the time. ACEP's focus was to develop educational content for emergency physicians, who generally did not have additional training beyond internship, and create the necessary building blocks to establish EM as a specialty [1–3].

Role of Organizations Within Emergency Medicine/Why Join?

Roles of specific organizations within EM and the reasons for joining are broad. Some topics are more specific to a particular organization; however, there is a lot of overlap. Most EPs belong to at least one organization and there are a fair number of EP's who belong to multiple organizations due to the various roles and membership benefits. There are four general roles of EM organizations: networking and collaboration, research and education, advocacy, and improving care and outcomes. Each of these roles parallel specific reasons for obtaining membership and are interrelated. Networking and promoting collaboration are important roles of EM organizations and are a significant reason why EPs join. Annual meetings are a great place for EP's from across the country to meet in person and form relationships with people who have shared interests. These relationships can help individuals with career advancement. For example, finding new job opportunities or collaborating on research or best practices. Each organization also has specific committees/sections that its members can join to foster these relationships and improve the quality of EM.

Research and education are important roles of the academic EM organizations and an important reason why many academic EPs join academic EM organizations. Most organizations have an academic journal, newspaper, and/or online forum where innovative research and clinical information are shared. Grant funding provided by organizations for research helps to advance our specialty and provides another reason to join. There are an abundant number of continuing medical education (CME) courses, both in-person and online, where you can learn the latest research and best practices and get CME credit when needed for state licenses or hospital credentialing. Leadership and teaching workshops are also conducted online and in-person to improve the quality of education.

Advocacy for our specialty, our patients, and our physicians is another important role of EM organizations and reason to join. Legislation occurs at both the federal and state levels that impact EM, and each specific organization has political action committees and other groups that represent our specialty and our patient's best interests. These issues include but are not limited to Medicare/Medicaid, COVID-19, healthcare reform, drug shortages, and surprise billing. By joining interest groups or committees within individual organizations, members can have a greater impact on our specialty than they can as an individual and improve our ability to focus on treating our patients. ACEP has state chapters, and AAEM has state or regional chapters that focus on local issues that have influence and can lead to change at the state level.

Lastly, EM organizations promote the improvement of care and outcomes. As EM physicians, we all strive to provide the best care for our patients; thus, obtaining resources to achieve this goal is an essential reason to join these organizations. Evidence-based clinical practice guidelines are published by several organizations and create a library where EPs can find up-to-date clinical information relating to the treatment of various pathologies.

In summary, there are multiple roles of EM organizations which parallel the many reasons for joining. In the following sections, we will discuss the prominent organizations individually to provide the reader with a closer look into the specific groups that make up our specialty.

American College of Emergency Physicians

ACEP is the oldest emergency medicine organization founded in 1968. While it was initially created to educate and train physicians in emergency care, their mission has expanded to include advocacy for emergency physicians, their patients, and the public. Their vision is "to ensure EPs believe that ACEP is their home and community for career fulfillment and professional identity" [4]. ACEP improves the quality of emergency medical care through multiple avenues including development of clinical policies and practice guidelines, funding research, educating the public on emergency care and disaster preparedness, legislative and regulatory advocacy, CME efforts including educational conferences and online training, and publishing EM's most reviewed scientific journal, *Annals of Emergency Medicine*.

Today, there are over 38,000 members including emergency physicians, residents, medical students, hospital administrators, physician assistants, nurse practitioners, and emergency medical technicians (EMTs). The physician members are comprehensive and include academic faculty at university-based hospitals, faculty at EM residencies based in community hospitals, and nonacademic EPs in varied practice environments. This large constituent base joins the college from multiple backgrounds for multiple reasons and benefits. ACEP has 53 chartered chapters (50 states, Puerto Rico, District of Colombia, Government Services) that advocate for the rights of EPs and their patients on a local level. They are independently incorporated but interact closely with national ACEP.

ACEP's membership offers access to the "#1 peer-reviewed science and research journal in emergency medicine" *Annals of Emergency Medicine*. In addition, members have access to multiple other resources including the *ACEP Now* monthly magazine and *PEER* for EM board prep.

ACEP's Scientific Assembly takes place each fall. The conference focuses on education to promote improved clinical practice of EM. It is a highly interactive and immersive experience, and the goal is to gain knowledge that you can immediately put into practice. The mixed clinical curriculum is complemented by courses on essential practice, risk management, policy development, and new technology. ACEP's *Skills Lab* is one of the highlights of the conference and includes hands-on sessions ranging from ultrasound, advanced airway, and pediatric resuscitation. The conference also includes meetings of the various committees and sections (comprehensive list is available on the ACEP website) to encourage networking and collaboration as this is a vital goal of the conference. The ACEP Council meets yearly during the scientific assembly and votes on resolutions, including changes to the bylaws, College Manual, and the Council Standing Rules, which guide policy development and activities of the college [5].

ACEP offers an abundance of services to their members in the form of education, advocacy, and practice resources. The *ACEP/CORD Teaching Fellowship* is a multipart course to help EPs gain skills and knowledge to become effective medical educators. The course is split into two intensive 5-day seminars that are offered in both summer and fall. There are multiple other educational meetings and courses, and hundreds of free and discounted CME hours are provided online. ACEP advocates for EM federally and locally within your state through the *911 Legislative Grassroots Network* and the *National Emergency Medicine Political Action Committee (NEMPAC)*. ACEP's *Leadership & Advocacy.*

Conference is held annually in Washington, DC, and focuses on advocacy at all levels and building relationships with members of congress [6]. Additionally, the *ACEP Wellness & Assistance Program* offers members access to free counseling and inexpensive legal/financial support.

ACEP also offers research grants, and grants are specifically linked to state chapters and sections. These grants are of varied amounts and help fund projects meant to meet member's needs and educate the public and further the advancement of EM.

Overall, ACEP is the largest and oldest organization within emergency medicine. Its scope is widespread, and thus, any EM clinician interested in improving the quality of the specialty should apply for membership. More information can be found at the ACEP website, http://www.ACEP.org.

Society for Academic Emergency Medicine

SAEM, established in 1989, is the EM society devoted to academic EM. Its stated mission is "to lead the advancement of academic emergency medicine through education, research, and professional development." Its vision is "to be the premier organization for developing and supporting academic leaders and shaping the future science, education, and practice of emergency and acute care." SAEM strives to improve EM, specifically in the areas of medical education, research, workforce development, and professional development [7].

SAEM members are generally EPs who are faculty at a university-based department of EM but also include faculty at EM residencies based in community hospitals. Some members join due to unique interests that have interest groups within SAEM, such as wilderness medicine and critical care.

SAEM membership offers access to two premiere academic EM journals: *Academic Emergency Medicine* (*AEM*) and *Academic Emergency Medicine Education and Training* (*AEM E&T*).

SAEM's annual meeting takes place each May. The SAEM annual meeting is the EM conference most focused on research presentations. Research abstracts are presented in various formats, including oral abstracts, poster sessions, and plenary research presentations. There are also didactic and innovation presentations, with a focus on educational and research aspects of EM, with less focus on clinical medicine. Workshops focused on faculty development and chief resident development cover half-day sessions. Preconference workshops are also offered on academic emergency medicine topics such as grant writing, clinical innovations, and teaching. The conference also includes meetings of the various committees, academies, and interest groups, which allow for networking for those with shared interests. Rounding out the conference are resident competitions such as SimWars and SonoGames as well as fun competitions like a dodgeball tournament.

SAEM offers several services to their members. There is an advanced research methodology course, a research methodology course specific to medical education research, an emerging leader development program, and a chair development program. These courses require an application and have additional tuition. SAEM offers consultation services for academic departments and residency programs, as well as assistance with faculty development. The fellowship approval program takes applications for many fellows who are not approved through the Accreditation

Council for Graduate Medical Education (ACGME). An endorsement of a fellowship by SAEM means the fellowship has met educational and curricular standards acceptable for a fellow in that specific subspecialty. The fellowship approval committee currently accredits ten fellowships, including the newer Social EM fellowship.

The SAEM Foundation offers many grants of varied sizes. These include both research and training grants, including education grants. SAEM Foundation also partners with many of the academies to offer research grants on topics important to those academies.

Overall, SAEM is the premiere EM society for academicians. All those in academic EM should strongly consider membership. More information, including a list of committees, interest groups, and academies, can be found on the SAEM website, http://www.saem.org.

American Academy of Emergency Medicine

AAEM was established in 1993 as a response to the corporatization of medical practice. The founders felt that EPs were being exploited for profits, which included hiring nonboarded EM physicians who would work for less money. The founders felt other organizations either were a part of the problem or were not doing enough to combat perceived unfair business practices. AAEM prides itself on being "the champion of the emergency physician [8]." AAEM believes that every patient presenting to the ED deserves to be evaluated by a board-certified EP and that the only way to become a specialist in EM is through residency training and board certification. As part of this, they are against independent practice of physician assistants (PA) and nurse practitioners (NP) and against employers requiring EPs to cosign the charts of an NP/PA patient whom the EP did not evaluate. AAEM is against the corporate ownership of EM practices. They believe corporations exert undue influence on EPs and the practice of EM and therefore private EM groups should be owned by EPs. They believe all EPs should have due process rights and not have restrictive covenants. They believe that EPs should have full control over their professional fees.

AAEM adheres strongly to their principles and spends significant resources in defending them. AAEM will assist EPs who lose their job without the appropriate due process and assist in finding EM groups that hold to their principles. As of this writing, the AAEM physician group is suing a contract management group in California over the takeover of an ED contract. This is among the many other lawsuits from AAEM to protect against the corporate practice of medicine. AAEM also spends resources in promoting legislation that protects their principles. AAEM is proud of their physician group, AAEM-PG, that supports existing EM democratic groups and assists in the creation of new groups.

AAEM has its scientific assembly in March or April. As AAEM values EP education, the conference fee is refundable for those that attend. The conference focuses on clinical education and updates for EPs. Research poster sessions are also included, as are section meetings, interest group meetings, and state chapter meetings. The conference is much smaller than the ACEP scientific assembly which makes networking and engagement with speakers and leaders much easier. There are many procedural workshops that take place at no extra cost to the attendee but do require advanced registration. The preconference and postconference courses are generally very affordable and run at cost. Social events include a state chapter and section reception, yoga, and a fun run.

Membership benefits include access to the AAEM EM journal, the *Journal of Emergency Medicine*. Additionally, there are online education, board review courses, and discounts on clinical resources. Importantly, AAEM assists EPs who have found themselves victims of corporate practice.

AAEM members believe strongly in the AAEM's stated values and believe it is worthy of both membership dues and donations. AAEM members believe that AAEM truly fights for the EP and understands the experience of "regular" EPs. EPs who share AAEM's values or want a smaller EM society with a greater chance at leadership and advancement should consider joining AAEM. More information, including committees, interest groups, and sections, can be found on the AAEM website, http://www.aaem.org.

Other Organizations (CORD, EMRA)

Council of Residency Directors in EM

CORD was initially formed in 1989 as an organization targeted specifically for residency program directors focused on EM education. Currently, there are 257 EM residency programs that are involved in the organization. Its mission is "to lead the advancement of EM education," and its vision is to "set the global standard for excellence in EM education through fostering innovation, community, professional development, and scholarship" [9]. Since inception, its members have grown to include program directors, assistant/associate program directors, clerkship academic faculty, and anyone interested in fulfillment of its mission.

CORD's academic assembly typically occurs each March. The multi-track conference has topics ranging from leadership development and mentorship; program development and curriculum; research; diversity, equity, and inclusion (DEI); and wellness. There are also specific lectures designed for senior/junior faculty, program coordinators, residents, and chief residents. The *Clinical Pathological Case Competition (CPC)* is one of the highlights where residents present interesting cases, and a faculty member must guess the pathology. CORD offers a preconference workshop and entertaining networking events.

CORD offers several services to their members specific to residents and faculty. They offer two courses: a mini-fellowship in wellness leadership for residents and a residency administration fellowship. CORD offers consulting services pertaining to advising, education, and remediation. They also offer excellent written and oral board review and preparation.

The Emergency Medicine Foundation (EMF)/CORD offers two large grants: One is for education scholarship/starter with a maximum amount of $10,000, and the second is for education research with a maximum amount of $25,000.

Overall, CORD is the premiere organization targeted to residency programs and EM education. All those interested in fulfillment of its mission and vision should strongly consider membership. More information can be found on the CORD website, http://www.cordem.org.

Emergency Medicine Residents' Association

EMRA was formed in 1974 as an organization specifically targeted to EM learners including medical students, residents, and fellows. Currently, there are over 16,000 members involved in the organization. Its mission states that "the EMRA is the voice of EM physicians-in-training and the future of our specialty," and its goal is to create the best doctors and leaders and to help make EM the best specialty [10].

Membership offers access to EMRA's award-winning magazine for EM, *EMResident.*

The first EMRA reception was held in Atlanta in 1979 during the ACEP Scientific Assembly, and now you can find EMRA events and lectures at ACEP, SAEM, and CORD conferences. Topics range from the *EMRA Medical Student Council* meeting, *EMRA Representative Council* meeting, and various committee programming. CORD hosts the *EMRA Quiz Show* and ACEP hosts the *EMRA Resident SimWars Competition*, and typically one evening during the annual ACEP Scientific Assembly, there is a large EMRA party.

EMRA offers several services to their members. For medical students, they offer advising resources to help with rotations, interviews, and the match, a medical student council to gain access to leadership positions, and scholarship opportunities. For residents and fellows, they offer resources to help with career planning (moonlighting, CV prep, job search, contract negotiation), financial planning, and legal/medical malpractice. The *EMRA and ACEP Leadership Academy* provides professional development for emerging leaders in EM. Members also get free access to *EM:RAP* and receive discounts on multiple products related to the in-training exam and board prep. Additionally, the networking opportunities gained through membership are abundant.

EMRA makes a $25,000 annual contribution to EMF in support of resident research and presents multiple awards associated with scholarships.

Overall, EMRA is the oldest and largest resident organization in the world [10]. All learners interested in EM should strongly consider membership. More information can be found on the EMRA website, http://www.emra.org.

Conclusion

EM societies have been instrumental in creating and developing EM as a specialty. Every EP can find an organization that aligns with their values and interests. EPs value these organizations for their advocacy, political action, education, research collaboration, and policy creation. Indeed, many EPs are members of multiple organizations. Every EP should consider joining one or more EM organizations to add his or her voice for the benefit of EM.

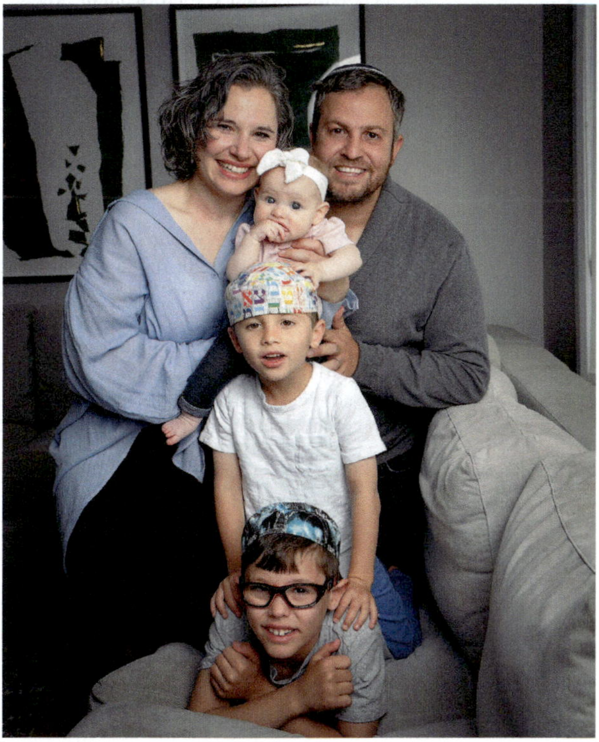

Dr. Joshua Guttman with his wife Rebecca and children Jonah, Dov, and Abigail pictured in April 2022

References

1. American College of Emergency Physicians, ACEP's 50th anniversary. https://www.acep.org/who-we-are/50Years. Accessed 1 Aug 2022.
2. Zink BJ. Creator and keeper of the flame of emergency medicine: John G. Wiegenstein, MD, 1930-2004. Ann Emerg Med. 2005;45(3):241–3.

3. Wagner MJ, Appold K. Emergency medicine training: the Foundation of the Safety net. ACEP Now. 2018; https://www.acepnow.com/article/emergency-resident-training-the-foundation-of-the-safety-net. Accessed 1 Aug 2022
4. American College of Emergency Physicians, ACEP's Strategic Plan. https://www.acep.org/strategicplan/. Accessed 1 Aug 2022.
5. American College of Emergency Physicians, ACEP Council. https://www.acep.org/how-we-serve/council/. Accessed Jan 9, 2023.
6. American College of Emergency Physicians, ACEP's Leadership & Advocacy Conference. https://www.acep.org/lac/. Accessed 9 Jan 2023.
7. Society for Academic Emergency Medicine. About SAEM. https://www.saem.org/about-saem, Accessed August 1, 2022.
8. American Academy of Emergency Medicine. About Us, https://www.aaem.org/about-us/our-values/history. Accessed 1 Aug 2022.
9. Council of Residency Directors in Emergency Medicine, CORD Mission/Vision. https://www.cordem.org/about-cord/mission%2D%2Dvision/, Accessed 1 Aug 2022.
10. Emergency Medicine Residents' Association, About EMRA. https://www.emra.org/about-emra. Accessed 1 Aug 2022.

Chapter 93
Setting and Pursuing SMART Goals—Your 5- and 10-Year Plan

Blake Isom

The SMART acronym was first described in a 1981 article by Dr. George T. Doran to help executives develop objectives for their business teams. Each objective would be accompanied by an action plan. As Dr. Doran wrote, "The establishment of objectives and the development of their respective action plans are the most critical step in a company's management process." In the years since its publication, the SMART method has grown in popularity and usage. Today, it – as well as many of its iterations – can be found in high school classrooms, self-help guides, religious manuals, and business training seminars. By applying these principles to your life, you can develop a clearer sense of direction for your career and self.

SMART Stands for Specific, Measurable, Attainable, Relevant, and Time-Based

Specific When developing your goals, be clear and concise. This is the most important step in goal setting. What do you want to accomplish in the next 5 and 10 years? This step helps focus your attention to your future. Specific goals prioritize a clear vision of what, when, and how you are going to achieve this goal. This focus on a single area for development will increase productivity and success. An example of a specific goal may be to develop an action plan to improve your Press Ganey scores. Your course of action will be to sit down during every patient encounter and make return phone calls to three patients per shift. You will become more mindful of your desire to improve your Press-Ganey score as you follow this method. Changes to

B. Isom (✉)
Department of Emergency Medicine, UPMC Harrisburg, Harrisburg, PA, USA
e-mail: Isombk@upmc.edu

R. P. Olympia et al. (eds.), *An Emergency Physician's Path*,
https://doi.org/10.1007/978-3-031-47873-4_93

specific goals will occur frequently. When reevaluating your goals, you should keep asking yourself, "what steps need to be taken next" to stay on the path to the goal. Being clear and focused will help the journey of reaching your goals easier to tackle.

Measurable How do you assess the achievement of this goal? Your goals should be tracked. Regular performance reviews will help you stay on course. You might decide, for instance, that you want to get healthier physically within the following 5 years. You determine that regular exercise is essential to achieving this goal. As such, you might set the goal to run a 5 K race by the end of the year. A key component to achieving this shorter-term goal will be to develop a specific training regimen. You could then measure your success by conducting a self-evaluation at the end of each week to determine how well you followed your regimen. A weekly check-in may include parameters such as how many times per week you plan to run/walk, distance you will run/walk, and a method to track your time. Each of these parameters is specific and measurable.

How frequently self-evaluations need to be done and what tracking parameters might be used will depend on your specific goal and timeline. The vital point is that they must be frequent and incorporate particular achievement milestones in order to track your progress toward the ultimate objective. Recognize that the plan could change. You may need to adjust the metrics being used to measure your progress to ensure they still align with your end goal.

Attainable You must ensure that the goal is both reasonable and reachable before deciding whether it is feasible. It's fine to set a challenging goal, but it's also crucial to determine its achievability. You shouldn't pick a goal that will lead to an unavoidable failure. While pushing you, these goals shouldn't derail you. Consider the likelihood of achieving this aim when examining your goals. Finding someone who has the expertise you lack could help you achieve a goal that would otherwise be impossible. Working together with colleagues and more experienced leaders may generate fresh ideas to assist you in reaching your objective.

Consider that you want to create a process to enhance the flow of patients from the hospital's emergency room to a particular floor. Those in leadership of internal medicine and nursing may have ideas on how to make this procedure better. The decision-making process will be greatly aided by the participation of the leaders in this process. Working collaboratively to gather information about problem areas and suggestions for improvement will be essential. Finding the source of each department's issues and working together to come up with solutions to increase throughput can help you achieve a target that would otherwise be impossible.

Relevant Every objective needs to be aligned with your 5- and 10-year vision. An important question to ask yourself would be as follows: "Why do I want to do this and how does this fit into my future?" Considering these issues will assist and clarify the overall objective and fit of this goal. This is your "why" for what you are doing. In the book *Start with Why: How Great Leaders Inspire Everyone to Take Action*, Simon Sinek states "All companies start with WHY, but only the best ones maintain their WHY clear year after year." You will need to periodically remind yourself of your "why." This will inspire, drive, and give you the perseverance needed during challenging times.

Time-Based Every goal needs to have a deadline. A time-based goal creates urgency and attention. To accomplish your main goal, there are frequently time-restricted targets. Knowing these deadlines will enable you to establish milestones and begin allocating tasks backward. For instance, you may wish to become a director of an emergency department within the next 5 years. You first may want to increase your education by getting an MBA in the next 2 years. You can then aim to move to the position of assistant director during the following 3 years. These actions will assist in educating you for the role of director. When determining if the goal is time-sensitive, ask this question: "When am I going to achieve this goal?" If you can answer that question, then your goal is time-based.

Life Application

During COVID, I felt myself becoming stagnant and trapped. The stress at work with the unknowns of COVID-19 made work difficult. Coming home to school via zoom and having no social activities made life exhausting. I knew I had to get out of the rut that I was feeling. The only way I thought of breaking through this difficult time was to reevaluate my goals. I needed to make some short-term goals to accelerate my path to who I envisioned myself being. These goals needed to make me feel uncomfortable and demand me to grow. I needed to force myself to be 100% committed with some type of consequence if I did not follow through. A few friends and family members had committed to and achieved goals using a program called 75 Hard. 75 Hard requires a commitment to a series of goals that you do for 75 consecutive days. If you fail even 1 day, you start over. As I read up on this program, I knew that I wanted to do something similar but not precisely like 75 Hard. There were certain aspects of this program that I loved, but there were other areas that, due to time restraints, I knew I could not achieve. I decided to make my own 75 Hard, and I encouraged a few friends to join me on this journey of doing hard things for 75 days.

I decided to analyze my 5- and 10-year goals using the SMART method for every aspect of my life. I felt there were multiple areas that needed a boost or reset. I first focused on my physical health. I had quit exercising and my eating habits were terrible. The first goal was to exercise at least 20 minutes per day for 6 days a week. I also cut out candy and decided to drink 3 L of water per day. I love candy! This was a difficult goal, so I had to decrease this temptation in my house. I got rid of the leftover candy and did not buy any more. Drinking more water has always made me feel more balanced and less moody. I went and bought a 1-L water container to track this goal.

One of my 5-year goals is to maintain a strong relationship with my wife and children. I knew I was wasting a lot of time on social media, and I needed to be present when I was with my family. I decided to put a limit on the amount of time I spent on each app. This would allow me to spend more high-quality time with them. Also, my kids fight with one another, and this was a huge stressor for me. Oftentimes, I would put fuel to the fire by yelling or fighting with them. I decided to not yell at my kids for 75 days. I decided that how I react should not be dictated by my surroundings and that I choose my reactions.

The other aspect of my life that needed attention was the spiritual aspect. With all this extra stress with work and kids, I needed to have more peace in my life. I needed more time to meditate and to get myself right mentally. The goal I made was to pray or meditate for 10 minutes per day.

After coming up with these goals, I shared them with my family and a few friends, and I started my 75 Hard. I ended up restarting my 75 Hard three times due to yelling at my kids. After finishing this journey, I realized that each one of these areas contributed to the other. Meditating for 10 minutes allowed me to be more patient with my children. Eating healthier and exercising helped me feel better which made me less moody and less likely to get mad. I truly had changed from a person who was stressed and mad to someone who was content and at peace. This program ended up taking me about 120 days. I failed a few times and had to get back on the path. That is how your life will be. You will continually need to reevaluate yourself and start over.

Before making your 5- and 10-year goals, decide what you value most. Rank each item from least to greatest in importance. What you value most in your life is the foundation of who you are. These goals should contribute to your foundation. Once you have made this list, think about how each goal can affect your life. Will this goal bring lasting happiness and enjoyment? These goals will give you a blueprint of where you want to be in 5 or 10 years. Now, specify what you want your 5- and 10-year goals to be. After determining these goals, write down your 1-year plan, 6-month plan, 1-month plan, and 1-week plan and then your plan for today. What steps can you make today to help you get on the path to achieving your 5-year plan?

This journey needs to be fun! Be curious about the things you can do and become. Goal setting is a process that should be adventurous. Try doing something easy to achieve. This momentum will give you the confidence to do hard things. Sometimes, you get in your own way. Mentally, you think this will be so hard, but in reality, it's all about starting, trying, failing, and starting again. Life is a process, and you will fall, but it is more important that you get back up with more resolve to accomplish your goals. Hard times can be a springboard to a new and higher level of thinking and achieving. Allow these hard times to change you for the better! Think about why this event is occurring for you instead of to you. Take 100% responsibility. Refuse to play the victim card. You decide how you react to every event in your lives. These reactions help shape who you end up becoming.

By using the SMART method to determine goals, you can develop deliberate action plans for each crucial area. With the help of these techniques, you can continue on the path to becoming the best version of yourself. They won't guarantee that you'll be successful. Your level of success will depend on how well you execute your action plans. To achieve your SMART goals, you will need conviction and perseverance. The SMART method is a tried-and-true way for attaining specific, time-bound goals.

Suggested Readings

Boogaard K. "How to write smart goals (with examples)." *Work-Life by Atlassian*, Atlassian, 17 Feb. 2022, https://www.atlassian.com/blog/productivity/how-to-write-smart-goals.

Frisella A. 75 hard: the 75-day tactical guide to winning the war with yourself. *Andy Frisella*, https://andyfrisella.com/pages/75hard-info.

"Goal." *Wikipedia*, Wikimedia Foundation, 13 July 2022, https://en.wikipedia.org/wiki/Goal.

Hardy, Ben. Make decisions today that will impress your friends in 20 years. *Benjamin P. Hardy*, 19 Sept. 2020, benjaminhardy.com/make-decisions-today-that-will-impress-your-friends-in-20-years/. Accessed 3 Aug. 2022.

Lee S. *What are smart goals?—Ezinearticles.com.* https://ezinearticles.com/?What-Are-SMART-Goals?&id=1843732.

MindTools. SMART goals—how to make your goals achievable. *Mindtools*, Emerald Works, 9 Mar. 2016, www.mindtools.com/pages/article/smart-goals.htm.

Smart Goals for Arts Organizations. *Arts Midwest*, 25 Jan. 2022, https://www.artsmidwest.org/resources/ideas-hub/smart-goals-arts-organizations?gclid=CjwKCAjwx7GYBhB7EiwA0d8oe2KD8pH4qKsdHi6_ijEwbGHkkYuLlnN8fZ8nBG6gUM5_mOgRZ99aMxoC1pY-QAvD_BwE.

The University of California. *SMART goals: a how to guide*. 2017.

There's a S.M.A.R.T. Way to write management's goals and ...—Temple Mis. https://community.mis.temple.edu/mis0855002fall2015/files/2015/10/S.M.A.R.T-Way-Management-Review.pdf.

Chapter 94
Emergency Medicine as a Second Career: Switching Specialties

Faye Pedersen

Introduction: Medicine as a Second Career

Those who change careers have been in alternate careers, some in nonmedical fields and many in a first career for years. They decide to pursue medicine for a variety of reasons which include unrealized aspirations, life-changing events like the COVID pandemic, inspiring mentors, or finally having gotten financial, familial, and professional obligations in order. Nontraditional students come from diverse fields and are usually older than typical medical school applicants given a longer route to the profession. I was 31 when I entered medical school and could count on one hand the number of students in my class over the age of 30. In order to find success, nontraditional students have had to be able to set themselves apart from a pool of qualified premeds by leveraging their backgrounds and unique skillsets.

In my case, I graduated with a degree in Aerospace Engineering, worked for a NASA contractor for the Space Shuttle program, United Space Alliance, as a main propulsion system engineer for 10 years while I completed a master's degree in Materials Science and Engineering, before finally deciding to pursue a medical career. According to the annual Association of American Medical Colleges (AAMC) Matriculating Student Questionnaire (MSQ) from 2020 that invites responses from individuals who accepted admission to schools accredited by the USLCME (US Liaison Committee on Medical Education), many students have a gap after completion of their undergraduate degree to medical school – over half (66.3%) of new matriculants reported that a year or more had passed since graduating from college [1]. For those who have more than a year off between college and medical school, 48.5% reported working at another career, 39.8% worked to improve finances, and

F. Pedersen (✉)
Emergency Physician, (Independent), Pittsburgh, USA

R. P. Olympia et al. (eds.), *An Emergency Physician's Path*,
https://doi.org/10.1007/978-3-031-47873-4_94

23.2% pursued graduated studies, worked or volunteered in research, and fulfilled family obligations (although respondents to this question were able to answer yes to more than one response) [1].

Why Medicine, and Why Specifically Emergency Medicine?

MSQ 2020 notes that most of the matriculants who decide to study medicine decide to do so before college (22.8% before high school, 33.9% before college, 11.9% during college, 7.9% after bachelors, 1.7% after an advanced degree) [1]. I am in the minority as I decided to pursue medicine after an advanced degree to satisfy a lifelong ambition. Is there a common reason why many decide to become a doctor despite how difficult and costly the journey is? President Emeritus of the AAMC Darrell Kirch found that the common theme from nearly everyone he asked is that "they want to help others, and that help is usually driven by a deep sense of compassion" [2].

In addition to the sense of compassion, many unique experiences shape an individual's decision to pursue medicine. For emergency physician Dr. Jessica Zhang, who has a BA in International Relations, she initially worked for a government consulting firm and for a nonprofit for a refugee camp in Ghana. Her experience made her realize how unhealthy most people were, even in industrial nations, and decided to pursue a medical career. Dr. Jodi Galdes, who graduated with a computer science degree, worked 6 years as a software analyst and then project manager. After volunteering at a clinic at Henry Ford Hospital, she was inspired by a mentor, Dr. Greene, a former MIT computer science graduate, who told her that medicine was problem-solving, with humans, and the work was more gratifying. She is currently the emergency department medical director at Trinity Health Livonia and CMIO for Trinity Health Southeastern Michigan.

In the MSQ 2020, although over one-third (35.5%) of new medical students reported plans to enter family medicine, internal medicine, internal medicine/pediatrics, OBGYN, and respective subspecialties, it also notes that when all matriculating students are asked what specialty they will pick, 8.5% chose emergency medicine, third only to undecided and internal medicine [1].

Reflecting on Switching Careers

The decision to change careers has been no small feat, and there were many questions that loomed throughout the application process: Where do I start? What prerequisites do I need? Can I afford this? How much debt will I be in? Am I competitive enough? Will my employer be supportive? Can I do this? Am I going in for the right reasons?

Dr. Kate Lewis graduated with a mathematics and comparative sociolinguistics degree, worked in Japan teaching English, and then returned to the United States and reflected on her life as well as next career while taking classes at the University of California, Berkeley. In her words, "as I considered this, I asked myself what I liked about work and what I didn't like. How did I want to be challenged and grow? Was I willing to go back to school?" She decided on a medical career after discussions with a physician friend and is currently a practicing emergency physician in Alexandria, Virginia.

There are many companies that specialize in counseling nontraditional students, but for me, I was lucky to be able to speak to the premedical advisor of the school where I was pursuing my master's degree. After poring through what I needed to do to fulfill the requirements, my advisor helped fill in the gaps of what I needed to do to be a competitive applicant. This included optimizing opportunities in shadowing and volunteering and working on my MCAT. Throughout this process, I repeatedly self-reflected and had discussions with my partner on whether it was worth it and if after all this work I would reach a goal that would make me happy.

The financial implications are some of the most daunting considerations when it comes to switching to medicine as a second career. According to the AAMC Medical School Graduation Student Questionnaire (GSQ) 2021, 68.7% of responders reported receiving scholarships, grants, and stipends. Of the respondents who graduated with debt, total premedical and medical school debt reported was $200,000 [3]. This is not an insignificant number that continues to accrue interest, not quite offset by average pay for residents which varies by state and institution and is typically around $60,000 for first year residents. The career changer must consider the loss of income, including benefits like retirement contributions and their ability to provide for family. 2.4% of matriculants had more than one dependent not counting their spouse [1]. Dr. Kate Lewis, former teacher, interviewed for medical school while pregnant with her first child and how family-friendly the schools were affected her final choice of medical schools. Dr. Jodi Galdes, former software analyst, already had two small children, one 4 years old and one born during medical school, by the time she graduated medical school, and this greatly affected her choices as well.

Some complete prerequisites including classes, shadowing hours, and studying for the MCAT while continuing to work. Sometimes, due to uncertainty about being able to go to medical school, the applicant may choose to hide their aspirations. Fortunately, for me, the Space Shuttle program that I was part of was wrapping up during my transition to my new career, and I had very supportive co-workers. Additionally, some may continue to work to help offset costs or provide for family. Dr. Scarlett Michael had a circuitous route to becoming an emergency medicine physician including earning a degree in psychology, working as a substitute teacher, earning a Bachelor of Science in nursing, and then working as a nurse during the medical school application process. While in medical school, she even stayed in the pool as an ICU nurse.

For others, many more challenges threaten the transition. Dr. Terry Moy-Brown always aspired to go to medical school but faced an uphill battle. She explained that "I was an immigrant who arrived in the country shortly after graduating high school, was a minority (black and Hispanic), and came from a poor family (I was the first member of my family to graduate college)." She graduated with a master's degree in Public Health and worked on a management information system to process Medicaid claims, before transitioning into banking as a home loan officer and then finally pursuing medical school. She currently works ER locum shifts as well as co-chairing the urgent cares in Vancouver Clinic in Vancouver, Washington.

The Appeal of an Emergency Medicine Career

When asked about career paths after medical school, matriculating students most frequently cited work/life balance (48.3%); having a stable, secure future (44.7%); and ability to pay off debt (44.0%) as essential considerations, and as such, an emergency medicine career has been an attractive option [1]. Interestingly, when graduating students in 2021 were asked about the specialty they intend to practice in, emergency medicine ranks third in popularity, almost 9.8% of respondents, behind internal medicine and pediatrics and their respective subspecialties (recall that matriculating students also ranked emergency medicine as third for area of interest) [3].

For Dr. Jodi Galdes, former software analyst, her first choice was OBGYN. However, as a single parent with two small children, emergency medicine provided the perfect balance. She had the ability to leave work at work and could plan around her children's special days. Dr. Kate Lewis initially aspired to be a pediatrician since she missed teaching and kids, but after some observation shifts in the peds ED, she was encouraged by the ER attendings to consider general emergency medicine. She was drawn to EM by the opportunity to help a variety of patients as well as an attractive opportunity to be able to be at home with her kids for important events, because even if the schedule is not easy, there are often opportunities to be flexible.

For Dr. Jessica Zhang, EM was always the default because she wanted "a broad practice, something fast moving, and something I could practice anywhere. I did not want to be tied to a practice or a patient roster." Similarly, Dr. Mary Schmidt, who graduated with a Materials Science and Engineering degree with second major in Chemistry, worked for 5 years at a powder metallurgy plant, before deciding on a medical career. During med school interviews, she stated she was going to do EM. She explains: "I always knew. I loved the outdoors and wilderness medicine. I taught wilderness first aid. I was briefly a volunteer EMT-Basic and took a wilderness EMT certification course (though my state didn't use that certification, it helped for regional search and rescue operations). I was heavily involved in volunteer search and rescue."

Dr. Emily Miller, former pediatric critical care doctor, explains that "multiple factors including a variety of practice settings, more career options especially the option of an essentially clinically oriented career, and a spouse and sister who are EM physicians drew me into emergency medicine." She currently practices as a community EM and pediatric EM physician. Dr. Scarlett Michael, former nurse, found herself interested in the ER – the pace, the variety of pathology, and getting to know people without getting as attached as when she was an ICU nurse and feeling helpless to stop the dying of loved ones. She enjoyed the variety that comes with ER and that there was not a set order or script. As for me, although I volunteered in the Emergency Room triage at my local hospital emergency room, I wanted to explore other options. When I realized I liked many different things, including procedures and a variety of pathologies, I realized the emergency medicine was my calling.

Given that ability to pay off debt was cited as a consideration in careers, it would be remiss to not talk about compensation. The average emergency physician income was $373,000 with an average incentive bonus of $51,000 in 2021, based on the compensation report surveying 13,000 physicians across multiple specialties, and the same survey found that most emergency medicine physicians (53%) felt fairly compensated (although down from 62% in 2021) [4].

With regard to the stability of emergency medicine, there is some debate about the future of the profession that will be discussed later.

What Do You Enjoy About Practicing Emergency Medicine?

For emergency physicians, the most rewarding part of the job was cited as "being very good at what they do" at 27%, "knowing that I'm making the world a better place" at 27%, "making good money" at 17%, "patient relationships" at 12%, and the rest to a lesser degree including teaching and pride of being a doctor [4].

Dr. Galdes was able to come full circle and incorporate previous education (in computer science) with her current position as a CMIO and notes that "I like the fact that I can still work shifts clinically. I love taking care of patients (still most gratifying part of job) and also help manage my department and make it a great place for my colleagues to work." Dr. Emily Miller, former pediatric critical care attending, says "I love being an emergency physician. I feel at home in the ED and have since the first day of residency. I love the pace, shift work, uncertainty, variety. I love hearing my patients' crazy stories and feeling like I made a little difference for them. I love the people I spend my days (or evenings or nights) with the nurses, the PAs, the other doctors." Similarly, Dr. Terry Moy-Brown noted that what drew her to emergency medicine and keeps her in it was that "we could see all the variety of patients and all comers regardless of their ability to pay, immigration status, and I enjoyed taking care of problems for short periods."

Dr. Mary Schmidt finds that "Most days, there is at least one person that I have truly helped, and that feels good. The EM lifestyle, with rotating shifts, is both a blessing and a curse, and I think you have to live it for a while to understand. I enjoy having random weekdays off with my kids. I was able to homeschool during the first year of COVID without much difficulty." As for me, I do enjoy taking care of people. Like Dr. Jodi Galdes, I feel that when patients come in, they come in with a problem or more to solve, not unlike the engineering problems I was previously faced with, but patients are so much more interesting.

The Challenges of Emergency Medicine

Emergency physicians found that the most challenging aspects of the job are 25% dealing with difficult patients, 22% rules and regulations, 15% worrying about being sued, and 9% long hours [4]. In my interview of the EM physicians already introduced in this chapter, there is an agreement with the above challenges, and several note additional concerns. Burnout, staffing challenges, corporate influence in medicine, oversight of advanced practitioners and scope of specialties, focus on administration, and desire to measure metrics including patients per hour and patient satisfaction, shift work, and disrespect from patients and other physicians are all active concerns in emergency medicine. Dr. Kate Lewis explains that "I don't believe that just because something can be measured that it should be measured. We should aim for a system that really rewards seniority, mentorship, and true patient quality."

The stability of emergency medicine as a profession is also now being questioned. In 2019, projections of physician shortage of 37,800 to 12,400 physicians by the AAMC by 2030 was published and attributed to population growth by 10.6% and age (42.4% increase in aged 65 and above), many physicians nearing traditional retirement age (2/5 of physicians will be older than 65), and an AAMC 2019 national survey, which reported 40% of physician respondents admitted feeling burned out at least once a week before COVID-19, which could cause doctors to reduce hours and retire sooner [5]. Some saw the projections by the shortage reports as driving the oversupply of emergency medicine physicians. The first emergency medicine residency training program began in 1970. There were 145 programs in 2008, which grew to 247 programs by 2019, and the number of residency positions increased by 6% between 2018 and 2019 alone [6]. By 2021, there were 273 residency programs accredited by the ACGME [6]. A study released by Marco et al. in 2021 noted that "increases in telemedicine, urgent care, changes in insurance coverage, and COVID-19 may affect projections; as such, given 2% annual graduate medical education growth, 3% annual emergency physician attrition, and 20% encounters by NP or PA and 11% increase in ED, the report resulted in an expected surplus of 7845 emergency physicians" [7]. However, a review by Gettel et al., based on a cross-sectional analysis from 2013 to 2019 on reimbursement and entry and attrition rates calculated annually, found that the rate of EP attrition is actually more than 5%, well above the 3% suggesting potential overestimation of anticipated future clinician surplus which disproportionally affects vulnerable areas like rural locations [8].

Litigation stress and the perceived threat of malpractice were cited as the third most challenging aspect of emergency medicine. Using data from the AMA's physician practice benchmark survey in 2016, 34% of all physicians have had a claim filed against them during their careers, and 16.8% were sued two or more times. 51.7% of emergency medicine physicians have had a claim filed against them, and 25.7% were sued at least twice (only behind general surgery and obstetrics) [9]. According to this survey, by the age 55, 41.3% of emergency physicians have been sued, and of those older than age 55, 72.2% have been sued [9].

Lastly, my colleagues cite burnout as a challenge. "Burnout negatively impacts physician health and increases the risk of adversely influencing patient outcomes. It is the most common chronic work-related stress exposure and has a high occurrence in EM" [7]. Using the Maslach Burnout Inventory Scale, which is considered the standard assessment of burnout, "the prevalence of burnout in EM is higher than 60%...versus other departments at 38% and the general population at 30%" [17]. Not surprisingly, the factors that my colleagues in this article and this study have cited to contribute to burnout include but are not limited to shift work, often rapid alternating day/night shifts, difficult patients, job strain especially from rapidly changing rules, fear of making mistakes, often blurred scope of practice with non-physicians, disrespect from nonemergency physician colleagues, threats to compensation, fear of becoming ill and not being able to provide for family, and the experience of workplace violence.

Given projections of emergency physician surplus and a likely COVID-19 effect where emergency physicians were thrust into the front lines of combatting an evolving pandemic but had hours (and compensation) and ancillary staff reduced due to declining patient volumes in the beginning of the epidemic, coupled with the threats discussed above including burnout, the threat of litigation, and regulations and corporations creeping into the practice of medicine, emergency medicine has become less desirable. Although emergency medicine remains in the top ten of matching specialties and routinely fills 99% of its positions, in the 2021 Match of allopathic candidates, 219 spots were unfilled (compared to an average of 12 in prior years) [6], although this does not include the SOAP results.

A study by Lall posed the following question: "Are emergency physicians satisfied?" In a study surveying 1102 participants, 863 responders reported satisfaction with their jobs. Despite a lower proportion of female respondents, mean satisfaction for women was 3.699 vs an overall mean of 3.972 [6] based on 5-point Likert scale, with 1 and 5 indicating "least satisfied" and "most satisfied," respectively. Based on prior studies that found that women often carry a large proportion of the responsibility for managing for childcare and household duties, it is likely that these responsibilities might affect career satisfaction. Case in point, when I interviewed Dr. Kay Moody, she apologized because she was also juggling doing taxes while doing laundry, answering questions for her short-term rental reservations, dealing with the plumber, and having to chase after her dogs and pet goats going after the Amazon delivery driver. Going back to the study, Lall et al. conclude that most emergency physicians were satisfied or very satisfied with their career despite significant risk for burnout. However, the study did not include the effect of the pandemic but does align with a 2022 survey result of more than 13 K physicians in over 29 specialties, where 6% of respondents were emergency physicians: the highest rate of burnout was with emergency medicine physicians (60% of emergency physician responders in 2021 responded positively to having burnout, whereas, in 2020, it was 43% of emergency physician responders) [10]; however, 66% of emergency medicine physicians would choose to enter medicine again (versus 69% physician overall), and 74% would choose emergency medicine again, ranking toward the bottom of list of physicians who love their specialties [11].

Advice when Considering Emergency Medicine as a Second Career

Dr. Terry Moy-Brown advises those considering a career transition to "Research all the current challenges we are facing and also really get to see what it is like for someone in similar circumstances to practice EM." Dr. Kate Lewis notes: "It is a great field, but it is a challenging field. You will sacrifice time and energy to get your degree. MD might not be the best path for everyone depending on where they are in life. The field of medicine is becoming harder for most people – burnout is real and likely for most people at some point. Just be honest with yourself about your goals, what you are willing to put up with, and what you are willing to sacrifice. I love being an EP, but I don't think this job is for most people. You need resilience." Her thoughts are echoed by Dr. Jodi Galdes—"We see patients in extreme situations; you have to be Teflon. If you're sensitive, this field would be tough. Multitasking – fast paced with little to no-home responsibilities depending on your group – can be a fantastic lifestyle! You have to like shift work. Being able to sleep easily at any time of day is ideal. Highly recommend shadowing an ED doc if at all possible."

"If you can't get medical school out of your head, you've got to do it! But if you're doing it just for the money, to be the boss, because you think your parents, friends, will think more of you or in any way feel you would be just as happy just moving up the ladder in your current career, do the latter. A career in medicine is great in many ways, but it's a lot of time and money," explains Dr. Scarlett Michael, former nurse. Dr. Kay Moody, former ballet teacher, cautions "never compromise your ethics. Stand true to yourself and advocate for your patients and community even if your job is threatened for doing so. And always be available to help a colleague."

As for myself, I feel incredibly fortunate to be able to practice emergency medicine. There are undoubtedly challenges, but the most satisfying reward of each shift, like Dr. Mary Schmidt earlier said, is being able to help at least one person feel better.

Acknowledgements I would like to thank the following individuals who generously provided their mentorship, stories, and advice about theirEmergency medicine experiences and career for this chapter: Dr. Jodi Galdes, Dr. Jessica Zhang, Dr. K Kay Moody, Dr. Scarlett Michael, Dr. Kate Lewis, Dr. Terry Moy-Brown, Dr. Mary Schmidt, Dr. Emily Miller, and Dr. John O'Neill. I would also like to acknowledge my husband, Hans Pedersen, who has been an incredible support system during this career change.

References

1. Association of American Medical Colleges [Internet]. Matriculating Student Questionnaire 2020 All Schools Summary Report. [December 2020; cited 15 Aug 2022]. Available from: https://www.aamc.org/data-reports/students-residents/report/matriculating-student-questionnaire-msq
2. Kirch D. AAMC insights. [Internet]. That's when I knew I wanted to be a doctor. (Published June 26, 2018, cited 24 Aug 2022). https://www.aamc.org/news-insights/insights/s-when-i-knew-i-wanted-be-doctor
3. Association of American Medical Colleges [Internet]. Medical School Graduation Questionnaire 2021 All Schools Summary Report. [July 2021, Cited 20 Aug 2022]. Available from: https://www.aamc.org/data-reports/students-residents/report/graduation-questionnaire-gq
4. McKenna J. Medscape emergency medicine physician compensation report 2022: incomes gain, pay gaps remain. [Internet]. (Published 13 May 2022, cited 24 Aug 2022). https://www.medscape.com/slideshow/2022-compensation-emergency-medicine-6015138
5. HIS Markit Ltd. The complexities of physician supply and demand: projections from 2019 to 2034. Report for Association of American Medical Colleges. (June 2021, cited 20 Aug 2022). https://www.aamc.org/media/54681/download
6. Shaw G. After years of calling for more EPs, EM finds itself with too many after years of calling for more EPs, EM finds itself with too many. Emergency Medicine News. (Published ahead of print May 24, 2021, cited 27 Aug 2022). https://journals.lww.com/em-news/blog/breakingnews/pages/post.aspx?PostID=586
7. Zhang Q, Mu MC, He Y, Cai ZL, Li ZC. Burnout in emergency medicine physicians: a meta-analysis and systematic review. Medicine (Baltimore). 2020;99(32):e21462. https://doi.org/10.1097/MD.0000000000021462. PMID: 32769876; PMCID: PMC7593073
8. Gettel CJ, Courtney DM, Janke AT, Rothenberg C, Mills AM, Sun W, Venkatesh AK. The 2013 to 2019 emergency medicine workforce: clinician entry and attrition across the US geography. Ann Emerg Med. 2022;80(3):260–71. https://doi.org/10.1016/j.annemergmed.2022.04.031. ISSN 0196-0644 (https://www.sciencedirect.com/science/article/pii/S0196064422002803)
9. Guardado JR. American Medical Association—Policy Research Perspectives, Medical Liability Claim Frequency Among U.S. Physicians [Internet]. (published 2017, cited 26 Aug 2022). https://www.ama-assn.org/sites/ama-assn.org/files/corp/media-browser/public/government/advocacy/policy-research-perspective-medical-liability-claim-frequency.pdf
10. Kane L. Medscape physician burnout and depression 2022 [Internet]. (Published January 21, 2022, cited 26 Aug 2022). https://www.medscape.com/slideshow/2022-lifestyle-burnout-6014664.
11. Marco CA, Courtney DM, Ling LJ, et al. The emergency medicine physician workforce: projections for 2030. Ann Emerg Med. 2021;78:6. https://doi.org/10.1016/j.annemergmed.2021.05.029.
12. Lall MD, Chang BP, Park J, et al. Are emergency physicians satisfied? An analysis of operational/organization factors. JACEP Open. 2021;2:e12546.

Chapter 95
Maintaining Wellness and Work-Life Balance

Al'ai Alvarez

In the last decade, there has been growing emphasis on physician wellness in emergency medicine (EM). This heightened focus is likely because EM continues to lead as the specialty with the highest burnout, as highlighted in the annual Physician Burnout and Depression Report [1]. It is essential to understand that wellness is not simply the absence of burnout, nor is there a one-size-fits-all approach to addressing burnout.

Transitioning out of residency can be stressful, often marked with experiences of impostorism. A recent study shows that physicians experience the imposter phenomenon more than workers from other fields, and it is associated with burnout [2]. An expectation during transitions is identity formation; therefore, it is essential to remember that we are not our job, that the imposter phenomenon is common, and that we are not alone in this experience. This shared commonality is critical as we navigate the tensions inherent in the scarcity of time, energy, and attention.

The National Wellness Institute highlights six distinct dimensions of wellness: emotional, occupational, physical, social, intellectual, and spiritual [3]. Leading the efforts to address burnout, Stanford WellMD/WellPhD pioneered the role of the chief wellness officer and introduced the Professional Fulfillment Model to focus efforts beyond wellness interventions and physician well-being [4]. This model's three core components include having a culture of wellness, the efficiency of practice, and personal resilience.

Discussions on wellness as it relates to personal resilience are often evoke strong negative reactions. In part, the response points to the need for addressing well-being with intentional efforts from the institution to promote the culture of wellness and improve efficiencies in our practice. We simply cannot resilience our way out of

A. Alvarez (✉)
Emergency Medicine, Stanford University, Palo Alto, CA, USA
e-mail: alai.alvarez@stanford.edu

R. P. Olympia et al. (eds.), *An Emergency Physician's Path*,
https://doi.org/10.1007/978-3-031-47873-4_95

burnout, and one study highlights that physicians are already more resilient than the general population [5]. However, resilience allows us to focus on what is within our control. While this chapter will not focus on institutional efforts, it is worth emphasizing that systematic interventions are the cornerstone of promoting professional fulfillment and well-being and reducing burnout [6].

The Designing Your Life framework suggests measuring life using gauges for work, health, love, and play [7]. By adopting this gauge analogy, we can aim to optimize each of these life dimensions instead of limiting it to balancing work and life. The term work-life balance is misleading because it implies a zero-sum game where prioritizing work necessarily detracts from life, and vice versa.

Finding alignment between our values and the values and mission of our work is also critical. The more authentically aligned we are, the more our work gauge is filled. Health includes not just physical but also mental and emotional health. EM as a specialty is exhausting and, at times, traumatic. We often experience vicarious trauma when caring for patients. Because of the constant exposure to trauma, we must prioritize taking care of our health—regular checkups, getting mental health support, and attending to our basic needs [8]. Love refers to relationships and our fundamental need to connect with others and ourselves. Play includes vacations, hobbies, and other non-work-related activities. Referred to as the third thing, those activities are part of a timed detachment from work [9]. Embracing your inner child, being creative, and finding flow are some ways of filling one's play gauge [10].

Work-life integration is another way of looking at the gauges. Instead of the challenge of balancing, integration takes into account the dynamic nature of our attention. We can find time to focus on work while at home and still find moments to take a break. We can see the next patient and still enjoy a moment to eat or take a biobreak or call a loved one. Harmony is when integration finds its flow state [11]. The key is making time for ourselves and holding ourselves accountable for this practice. Using our calendar to integrate the different work and personal activities achieves this approach. Our calendar can be a reflection of our gauges [12].

Addressing time conflicts requires the practice of self-compassion, which according to Dr. Kristin Neff, is comprised of three elements: self-awareness or mindfulness, or the practice of being present; common humanity, or the understanding that suffering is a shared human experience and highlights how we are not alone in our struggles; and most importantly, self-kindness, or the ability to offer the same kindness to ourselves as we would to our loved ones in times of distress [13]. Practicing self-compassion is not easy, although not impossible to train and develop the habit. Developing a mindfulness practice through meditation is one form of training the mind to be more present and more self-aware, which is necessary to break the amygdala hijack of rumination by applying perspectives of shared humanity and practicing self-kindness.

Practicing self-compassion leads to agency and empowerment. It allows us to practice limit setting and creating boundaries. Self-compassion also gives us the perspective to understand what is within and beyond our control. Self-compassion also leads to self-advocacy to not compromise our needs and values. The practice also empowers us to be creative in designing and finding contentment in prioritizing our work, health, love, and play gauges.

It is crucial to acknowledge additional external factors that diminish one's well-being. The COVID-19 pandemic has disrupted our sense of well-being and work-life harmony [14]. The pandemic also highlighted the inequities in caregiving responsibilities, negatively impacting women in medicine further [15]. Those identifying as underrepresented in medicine are also more likely to experience bias, imposter phenomenon, and microaggressions, in addition to the already demanding toll of work [16].

EM is an exciting field and a specialty that is rife with challenges. We have worked so hard to get to where we are, only to experience burnout and not enjoy the fruits of our labor. Let us remember to take the time to prioritize our health, love, and play, instead of focusing solely on our work. May we make a better effort to attend to our needs. Let us find ways to discover and prioritize our values. And may we continue to be reminded to embrace our shared human experience and practice self-kindness as we journey through life after EM residency.

References

1. Physician Burnout & Depression Report 2022: Stress, anxiety, and anger. Medscape. https://www.medscape.com/slideshow/2022-lifestyle-burnout-6014664. Accessed 21 Sept 2022.
2. Shanafelt T, Dyrbye L, Sinsky C, et al. Imposter phenomenon in US Physicians Relative to the US Working Population. Mayo Clin Proc. 2022.;s0025-6196(22):00378-0; https://doi.org/10.1016/j.mayocp.2022.06.021.
3. Six Dimensions of Wellness - National Wellness Institute. Published April 29, 2020. https://nationalwellness.org/resources/six-dimensions-of-wellness/. Accessed 21 Sept 2022.
4. The Stanford Model of Professional Fulfillment™ | WellMD & WellPhD | Stanford Medicine. https://wellmd.stanford.edu/about/model-external.html. Accessed 21 Sept 2022.
5. Resilience and burnout among physicians and the general US working population | Professional Well-being | JAMA Network Open | JAMA Network. https://jamanetwork.com/journals/jamanetworkopen/fullarticle/2767829. Accessed 21 Sept 2022.
6. Shanafelt TD. Physician Well-being 2.0: where are we and where are we going? Mayo Clin Proc. 2021;96(10):2682–93. https://doi.org/10.1016/j.mayocp.2021.06.005.
7. Burnett B, Evans D. Designing your life: how to build a well-lived, joyful life. Knopf; 2016. https://designingyour.life/. Accessed 21 Sept 2022
8. Shapiro DE, Duquette C, Abbott LM, Babineau T, Pearl A, Haidet P. Beyond burnout: a physician wellness hierarchy designed to prioritize interventions at the systems level. Am J Med. Published online December. 2018; https://doi.org/10.1016/j.amjmed.2018.11.028.
9. Cline P. Residue: processing extreme experiences. LinkedIn. Published April 20, 2020. https://www.linkedin.com/pulse/residue-processing-extreme-experiences-preston-cline/. Accessed Sept 21 2022.
10. Csikszentmihalyi M. Flow, the secret to happiness | TED Talk. https://www.ted.com/talks/mihaly_csikszentmihalyi_flow_the_secret_to_happiness. Accessed 21 Sept 2022.
11. Fletcher P. Work-life balance is over: let's talk about work-life harmony. Forbes. 2020; Published November 13. https://www.forbes.com/sites/forbeshumanresourcescouncil/2020/11/13/work-life-balance-is-over-lets-talk-about-work-life-harmony/?sh=172d8c225b48. Accessed 21 Sept 2022

12. Kanapicki J. The 1440 doctor: how to unplug while working from home. ALiEM. 2022; Published January 19. https://www.aliem.com/1440-doctor-unplug-while-working-from-home/. Accessed 21 Sept 2022
13. Neff KD. Self-compassion: theory, method, research, and intervention. Annu Rev Psychol. Published online August 12. 2022; https://doi.org/10.1146/annurev-psych-032420-031047.
14. Shanafelt TD, West CP, Dyrbye LN, et al. Changes in burnout and satisfaction with work-life integration in physicians over the first 2 years of the COVID-19 pandemic. Mayo Clin Proc. Published online September 14. 2022; https://doi.org/10.1016/j.mayocp.2022.09.002.
15. The impact of COVID-19 on the careers of women in academic sciences, engineering, and medicine |The National Academies Press. https://nap.nationalacademies.org/catalog/26061/the-impact-of-covid-19-on-the-careers-of-women-in-academic-sciences-engineering-and-medicine. Accessed 21 Sept 2022.
16. Osseo-Asare A, Balasuriya L, Huot SJ, et al. Minority resident physicians' views on the role of race/ethnicity in their training experiences in the workplace. JAMA Netw Open. 2018;1(5):e182723. https://doi.org/10.1001/jamanetworkopen.2018.2723.

Chapter 96
Dealing with Burnout

Nicole Battaglioli

Burnout is typically defined as the prolonged exposure to stress resulting in emotional exhaustion and depersonalization [1]. To be honest, as the COVID-19 pandemic closed in on its second year, this is exactly how I felt: emotionally exhausted and detached. Each subsequent shift that I worked felt ever harrowing. I was the walking definition of burnout and needed to find my way back.

For a physician, burnout often looks like poor work-life integration and decreased professional satisfaction. For the healthcare system, burnout looks like increased healthcare costs and clinical errors (West). Unfortunately for both, burnout can be closely commingled with substance abuse, depression, and suicidality. Rates of burnout for the emergency medicine physician have been historically high. Typically reported as an increase in emotional exhaustion or an increase in depersonalization, the incidence is estimated at 60–80% of emergency medicine residents and physicians [2–5].

Though some individual factors are attributed to burnout, many systems and organizational-level issues highly influence the level of burnout in the physician workforce. Understaffing and inefficient processes, excessive workload and administrative burdens, organizational support structures, and leadership culture are all drivers of physician burnout [6]. Additionally, it is argued that emergency physicians face a higher intensity to their clinical practice, endure higher risks of litigation, and are negatively impacted by the circadian rhythm disruptions of shift work, likely contributing to higher levels of burnout when compared to other specialties [7].

N. Battaglioli (✉)
Agnes Scott College, Atlanta, GA, USA
e-mail: nbattaglioli@agnesscott.edu

R. P. Olympia et al. (eds.), *An Emergency Physician's Path*,
https://doi.org/10.1007/978-3-031-47873-4_96

So what can be done about the issues of burnout in emergency medicine, and how do you come back from a state of career burnout?

Well, to start, let's look at the following question: "What is happiness?" Consider breaking "happiness" up in three theoretical constructs: affective well-being (feelings of joy and pleasure), eudaimonic well-being (sense of meaning and purpose in life), and evaluative well-being (life satisfaction) [8]. It is safe to say that the majority of physicians took on the practice of medicine with the intent of deriving significant eudaimonic well-being from our careers. Whether our choice was influenced by the promise of helping our many patients, a stable and admirable income, or the hope of community notoriety, we chose to become a physician with a certain outcome in mind. To pursue a career in medicine, many physicians have likely delayed focusing on other aspects of their life that may bring them evaluative well-being: having children, finding a spouse or partner, financial stability, or working on one's personal health and wellness.

Processing Trauma

The first step toward suring up mental health and working past burnout is to continually process past and ongoing trauma. As emergency medicine physicians, we are apt to take on vicarious trauma through the sick and traumatized patients we see and when adverse events are experienced. Additionally, many of us carry unprocessed trauma from our youth. The National Child Traumatic Stress Network looked at the incidence of adverse childhood experiences (ACEs, Table 96.1) and the downstream psychosocial and biological impact of those experiences (Head Start ECLKC).

Researchers found that children who had experienced four or more ACEs were at 10–12× greater risk for intravenous drug use and attempted suicide and had 2–3× greater risk for developing heart disease and cancer. Individuals who experienced a singular ACE such as physical abuse, sexual abuse, or witnessing of maternal battering resulted in higher prevalence of low mental health scores on the Medical Outcomes Scale SF-36 when compared to those who had not experienced any ACEs [9]. Knowing that exposure to childhood trauma can impact both physical and mental health, healthcare workers would benefit from processing these events and their impact due to the nature of our jobs.

Table 96.1 Examples of adverse childhood experiences (ACEs)

Child physical abuse	Child sexual abuse	Child emotional abuse
Emotional neglect	Physical neglect	Mentally ill, depressed, or suicidal person in the home
Drug addicted or alcoholic family member	Witnessing domestic violence against mother	Loss of a parent to death or abandonment by divorce
	Incarceration of any family member for a crime	

The secondary trauma experienced through our work can result in physician feelings of guilt, shame, inadequacy, and incompetence. On top of that, the medical culture in which we work values perseverance and perfectionism and does not always openly tolerate feelings of uncertainty or emotional openness. If these feelings are not addressed, they can morph into a secondary victim syndrome (SVS) that can often result in self-isolation and absenteeism and have a negative impact on clinical work [10]. The recovery process of SVS was found to be fairly predictable [11]. The six stages of this process include (a) chaos and accident response, (b) intrusive reflections, (c) restoring personal integrity, (d) enduring the inquisition, (e) obtaining emotional first aid, and (f) moving on. Moving on takes the form of "surviving," "thriving," or "dropping out," where dropping out can imply leaving a particular practice environment or leaving medicine altogether. While thriving implies that the individual has transitioned from the event successfully, surviving is often associated with persistent emotional baggage [12]. To aid in the recovery process, some organizations have implemented peer support programs with the goal of providing emotional first aid and providing an environment of psychological safety while promoting a culture of patient safety [13]. The challenge with these programs is that the programmatic development and implementation can be varied between institutions and clinicians may be hesitant to engage with them due to persistent mental health stigma.

Setting Boundaries

The second step to working through burnout is to set healthy boundaries that encourage self-care and well-being. Healthy boundaries are limits that you put into place which consider your personal values, wants, and needs. These are crucial as poor boundaries can lead to internal conflict and neglect – leading to feelings of anger, resentment, and burnout. Boundaries help you to make decisions that are in your own best interest or in the interest of your core values instead of in the best interest of those around you. Boundaries work best when you are able to define what your boundary is and communicate that to other involved parties without overexplaining yourself and defining the consequences or why the boundary is important to you (positive psychology). Working on healthy boundaries will help make space for our evaluative well-being and what makes us whole outside of medicine.

Finding Joy

Lastly, reconnect with your eudemonic well-being—figure out what will bring you joy in medicine. This often requires a determined and careful evaluation of your core values and your ikigai—the Japanese concept of your life's worth, meaning, or purpose. Components of ikigai include what you are good at, what you love, what you can get paid for, and what the world needs. When speaking with an emergency medicine colleague about finding joy in her daily practice, she stated, "I don't expect every shift to be amazing, but I make a purposeful choice to try to connect with at least one patient per shift in a positive way."

For some experiencing burnout, this may mean leaving a job that is not personally fulfilling or toxic for your mental health. When speaking to another colleague, they reflected upon a recent job move: "The institution I was working for just wasn't in line with my values. I was miserable, and I knew that I had to make a change, even though it was scary to leave."

Professional and personal burnout is not uncommon among emergency medicine physicians—and it can be difficult to find your way back. It can take time and deliberate work to recover, but I recommend working through your trauma, setting boundaries, and making changes to rediscover the joy in your work as a place to start.

References

1. Friganović A, Selič P, Ilić B, Sedić B. Stress and burnout syndrome and their associations with coping and job satisfaction in critical care nurses: a literature review. Psychiatr Danub. 2019;31(Suppl 1):21–31.
2. Boutou A, Pitsiou G, Sourla E, Kioumis I. Burnout syndrome among emergency medicine physicians: an update on its prevalence and risk factors. Eur Rev Med Pharmacol Sci. 2019;23(20):9058–65. https://doi.org/10.26355/eurrev_201910_19308.
3. Lin M, Battaglioli N, Melamed M, Mott SE, Chung AS, Robinson DW. High prevalence of burnout among US emergency medicine residents: results from the 2017 National Emergency Medicine Wellness Survey. Ann Emerg Med. 2019;74(5):682–90. https://doi.org/10.1016/j.annemergmed.2019.01.037. Epub 2019 Mar 14
4. Mercuri M, Clayton N, Archambault P, Wallner C, Boulos ME, Chan TM, Gérin-Lajoie C, Gray S, Schwartz L, Ritchie K, de Wit K. Network for Canadian emergency researchers. Canadian emergency medicine physician burnout: a survey of Canadian emergency physicians during the second wave of the COVID-19 pandemic. CJEM. 2022;24(3):288–92.
5. Zhang Q, Mu MC, He Y, Cai ZL, Li ZC. Burnout in emergency medicine physicians: a meta-analysis and systematic review. Medicine (Baltimore). 2020;99(32):e21462. https://doi.org/10.1097/MD.0000000000021462. PMID: 32769876; PMCID: PMC7593073
6. West CP, Dyrbye LN, Shanafelt TD. (Mayo Clinic, Rochester, MN; and Stanford University Medical Center, Stanford, CA, USA)Physician burnout: contributors, consequences and solutions (review). J Intern Med. 2018;283:516–29.
7. Stehman CR, Testo Z, Gershaw RS, Kellogg AR. Burnout, drop out, suicide: physician loss in emergency medicine, part I. West J Emerg Med. 2019;20(3):485–94. https://doi.org/10.5811/westjem.2019.4.40970. Epub 2019 Apr 23. Erratum in: West J Emerg Med. 2019 Aug 21;20(5):840-841. PMID: 31123550; PMCID: PMC6526882
8. Steptoe A. Happiness and health. Annu Rev Public Health. 2019;40:339–59. https://doi.org/10.1146/annurev-publhealth-040218-044150. Epub 2019 Jan 2
9. Edwards VJ, Holden GW, Felitti VJ, Anda RF. Relationship between multiple forms of childhood maltreatment and adult mental health in community respondents: results from the adverse childhood experiences study. Am J Psychiatry. 2003;160(8):1453–60. https://doi.org/10.1176/appi.ajp.160.8.1453.

10. Sachs CJ, Wheaton N. Second victim syndrome. 2022 Jun 27. In: StatPearls [Internet]. Treasure Island (FL): StatPearls Publishing; 2022 Jan.
11. Scott SD, Hirschinger LE, Cox KR, McCoig M, Brandt J, Hall LW. The natural history of recovery for the healthcare provider "second victim" after adverse patient events. Qual Saf Health Care. 2009;18(5):325–30. https://doi.org/10.1136/qshc.2009.032870.
12. Ozeke O, Ozeke V, Coskun O, Budakoglu II. Second victims in health care: current perspectives. Adv Med Educ Pract. 2019;10:593–603. https://doi.org/10.2147/AMEP.S185912. PMID: 31496861; PMCID: PMC6697646
13. Shapiro J, Galowitz P. Peer support for clinicians: a programmatic approach. Acad Med. 2016;91(9):1200–4. https://doi.org/10.1097/ACM.0000000000001297.

Chapter 97
Investing in Your Financial Future

Harvey Castro

Student Loans

When a student is in medical school, they inevitably have to take loans to pay for medical studies. Therefore, he must manage this situation in a very healthy and effective way. Some students try to get extra jobs to pay back the amount while still in medical school, but I believe it is a hassle. Medical school is not a walk in the park; it is tough! The sheer pressure of passing your exams is profound. Unlike other professions, one cannot afford to have divided attention. One needs to focus and study well to get through challenging exams. The right time to start paying back your loans is when you're in your residency. You may get your loans postponed, but the interest on your debt will keep on accruing and will hurt you in the long run. During the years of residency, you are earning enough to be able to pay back your loans. The main challenge here is that some people try to live lavishly off these years' earnings. This will have a terrible long-term effect. Even though a resident is earning well, he still needs to pay off his debts; therefore, an intelligent decision is to live like a resident!

Figure 97.1 explains the rising medical school debt from 1978 to 2018, and it is very clear that taking loans is not a privilege anymore but a need of modern society. So, one should not hesitate while deciding if he needs a loan since the numbers say that you're likely to need financial assistance in the form of loans.

You must also have clear thinking and goals about financing your journey. Taking too much money will create all sorts of challenges in the long run. Therefore, you must plan well and take advice from your seniors and colleagues about which debt plan will suit you the most.

H. Castro (✉)
Trusted ER, Coppell, TX, USA

R. P. Olympia et al. (eds.), *An Emergency Physician's Path*,
https://doi.org/10.1007/978-3-031-47873-4_97

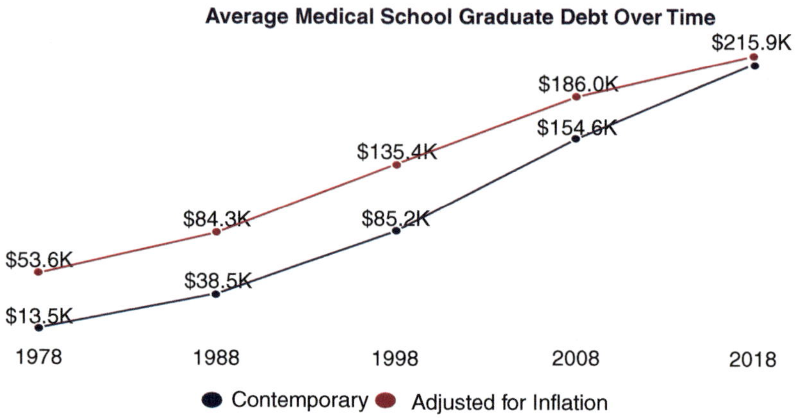

Fig. 97.1 Average medical school debt (Hanson 2021)

Inflation Is Not Always Bad!

Inflation is a grave phenomenon that negatively impacts most consumers; however, since the interest rates on student loans are fixed, inflation will benefit the students as rising inflation devalues the currency. The phenomenon of inflation is indeed out of your hands, but in any case, if you get lucky, this will benefit you. Generally, over a year, it is estimated that around 2% of inflation is average, which will add up yearly. Besides this, it is also crucial that we talk about the emotional aspect of financial challenges and their impact on this journey. I used to get very anxious when I would think about taking loans for my studies and how I would pay them back. It would always make me nervous. I have to add that even though I believe and endorse that every person should have clarity of mind when making decisions, I, too, would get puzzled and emotionally overwhelmed in individual decision-making. Therefore, it is very typical if any of you go through such circumstances. The idea is that we have to manage our challenges and emotions simultaneously. It is important to stick to rules and have objectivity. So, for instance, if you're feeling nervous about taking loans, you should evaluate it and maybe go a step further and ask another person that you feel is credible about the plan you'd need to follow. In my experience, sharing your sentiments with people of similar expertise will always produce better results. Two minds are always better than one.

Postresidency Plans

If you could finally pay back your student loans while in training, life usually does not get any more straightforward by the end of your residency. You now have to worry about maintaining a decent lifestyle. Most people at this stage get married if they haven't already, and they might try to have kids. You must plan well and keep your finances in check. I have always believed that your seniors are the right people to talk to because they have just been through the same challenges and are familiar with all the cliffs of the way.

Passive Income

It is said that if you have only one source of income, you are just one step away from poverty and rightly so. The recent surge of the COVID-19 pandemic has affected jobs worldwide. A lot of students in medical school, as well as in residency, require lectures, notes, and books to get through exams. Yes, there are many sources available for that already, but there is also much room for your expertise. Unlike past, students try to study smart. They want to learn things effectively while also saving time. One of the best ways to invest your expertise is to make online lectures about a subject of your choice. For instance, a doctor specializing in emergency medicine can write a book about it and prepare online lectures. If you just put it on a YouTube channel and invest a small amount into its marketing and your content is good, there can be excellent traffic on your channel, and therefore, you can earn a sizeable sum. This type of work has the potential to make you known, and it is always a plus point on your resume, regardless of which stage of your career you are at. It is a matter of medical knowledge, creativity, and interest. For instance, when I was in medical school, I had a tough time memorizing microbiology and the most delicate details about so many organisms. If you did not have a very sharp memory, it could give you a really tough time. However, sketchy micro videos that are available at "www.sketchy.com" made it ridiculously easy. That is one idea for starters. If your passion is toward media, you can always try and make documentaries and blogs because there are always a lot of stories to tell.

ER Mentality Is Versatile!

I have tried to keep myself focused on one thing at a time. When the stakes are high, it is challenging to make the right decision; however, it is still possible. As a part of emergency medicine, I always think about the worst-case scenario before deciding. What is the worst that can happen from my actions? It is a very effective tool to not only make professional medical decisions, but it is also equally applicable to financial decision-making. When you think about things with this mindset, you get a lot of clarity for decision-making, and from my personal experience, I have always found this method to be very objective. Prioritize things that matter most to you. It would help if you kept your essential household expenditures as a top priority. This includes housing, transportation, clothing, groceries, and more. In my opinion, the benefit of following this strategy is that you get your basics covered, and only after that do you have to worry about keeping up with your lifestyle.

Buying Assets and Not Liabilities

It is also essential that a doctor should buy assets whenever possible. It is also true that there is a slight risk involved in an asset's value going down, but I think, with proper consultation from experts, it is a profitable business. One should never rely on one source of income. Usually, toward the latter half of your career, if the earnings are good and you have paid off your house and your children's schooling, the extra sum can be invested into buying assets. This will help you finance other recurring expenses, including your household and other postretirement plans. Diversification of investments is one of the many things you can choose while building an investment portfolio. So, for instance, if you have decided that you are investing in the stock exchange, it is always better to invest some amount in other areas, such as buying an asset in the form of a house, flat, or other properties. The benefit of this strategy is that if one investment in your portfolio goes down, you can still earn profits from others.

Investing in Your Career Is Always an Option

If you have gone through specialization and still believe that you can take another course, you should go for it. Learning never stops! You can even go from clinical practice to teacher for undergraduate or postgraduate courses. It is always vital in your life to remain proactive and keep all your options available and ready to be explored. Besides this, I have always believed that it is an intelligent decision to extend your career while keeping your profession at the very top as a healthcare worker. If a doctor tries to change fields completely, it would be highly inconvenient and challenging to accomplish. But pivoting and obtaining additional education on something adjacent or relevant to your field can be quite productive. If you are interested in administration, there is always a way to return partially or completely to clinical medicine. Apply for an MBA degree, and you can get yourself inside the public health and administration domain. This way, your touch with your primary profession will be maintained while you enjoy your financial freedom and new opportunities.

There is a beneficial book, and one of my favorites, by Robert T. Kiyosaki, titled *Rich Dad Poor Dad*, which describes how important it is to have financial stability in life. I always recommend my juniors go through it and try to obtain that stage; it is essential to take a bold and intelligent decision about how one wants to manage his earnings. Life is not just about having a job and earning money. It is also about growing and succeeding. The financial aspect of life is one of the most significant spheres, and to have dominant success in this sphere contributes massively to the overall success of your life. You should get all the help and information you need to establish your enterprise.

Some General Recommendations You Should Consider

On a general observation, your wealth directly reflects the state of two financial forces – your income and your expenditure. A combination of high-income and limited expenses will improve your financial state, leaving you with more to invest in your portfolio. In many cases, you will have greater control over your expenditure. Establishing good financial habits early is a recommendation you will have to consider seriously. As your income increases or your expenses decrease, you should adjust your budget to set aside an increasing amount of money to reinvest into your portfolio. You should also consider setting up a plan for financial emergencies. This will include starting an emergency savings plan or buying life/disability insurance. Employers usually have this option ready for your consideration. As your financial outlook improves, you can gradually increase your coverage amount, ensuring you are adequately insured against any financial emergency. While trying to make sure you have the best possible financial plan, you must stay on the right side of the law concerning taxes. Depending on existing laws in your state, the tax laws might be a bit different. Hiring the services of expert lawyers, accountants, or tax managers should be a crucial part of your financial plan. This becomes very important as your assets and portfolio grow.

Do Not Be Afraid of Setbacks

Lastly, I would like to say that there are certain moments when things do not work out in your favor, regardless of how hard you have tried to succeed. A failed exam is not your reality. You can come back stronger! Success is just a painful journey full of failures and setbacks. So do not get disheartened by failures. They are part of your journey. Embrace them with grace. All the successful people in the world have gone through setbacks and heartaches. I want to share one of the personal experiences I had when I was in my third year of medical school. I struggled with pharmacology during that period, and eventually, I could not pass it in the finals and had to reappear in the exams. I eventually passed the supplementary exams, but the mental pressure that I had to endure in this process was enormous. I had this fear of failure that I might not be good enough to grasp the knowledge of this subject and maybe my ability to memorize such a massive volume of information. I had started to have disbelief in my ability. In such situations, when you're in the phase of setbacks, you are often at risk of developing self-doubt; however, if you can convince yourself that your mind is just playing games with you and that the reality is not what you're feeling, your chances of overcoming failures and setbacks increase significantly. I wish you the very best of luck!

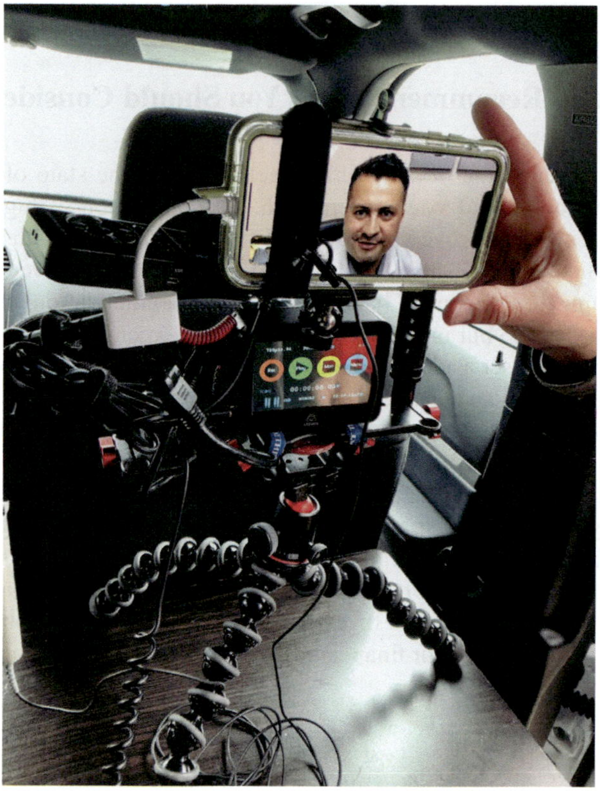

Turning crises into stepping stones: the journey of financial acuity amidst a pandemic. #InvestInYourFuture #Covid19

Suggested Readings

Connelly P, List C. The effect of understanding issues of personal finance on the well-being of physicians in training. WMJ. 2018;117(4):164–6.

Dahle J. Investing and personal finance for doctors. Retrieved from: https://www.whitecoatinvestor.com/

Hanson M. Average medical school debt, 2019 Retrieved from: https://educationdata.org/average-medical-school-debt

Jennings JD, Quinn C, Ly JA, Rehman S. Orthopaedic surgery resident financial literacy: an assessment of knowledge in debt, investment, and retirement savings. Am Surg. 2019;85(4):353–8.

McKillip R, Ernst M, Ahn J, Tekian A, Shappell E. Toward a resident personal finance curriculum: quantifying resident financial circumstances, needs, and interests. Cureus. 2018;10(4):e2540.
Poppler LH, Sharma K, Buck DW, Myckatyn TM. Five financial pearls for medical students, residents, and young surgeons. Plast Reconstr Surg Glob Open. 2019;7(2):e1992.
Ramme AJ, Patel M, Patel KA, Montag WH, Schau AJ, Sabo SI, Bedi A. Personal finance primer for the future orthopaedic surgeon: a starting point. JB JS Open Access. 2021;6(1):e20.00006.

Chapter 98
Life Insurance 101

Mathew Cherian

COVID Pandemic

There was a lot of uncertainty and fear during the March 2020 COVID-19 pandemic shutdowns. Our fear regarding the burgeoning pandemic was coupled with a new type of concern as our son was born 3 days after the New Mexico shutdown. Most of that fear was related to how two extremely educated people with a working knowledge of child development were completely unprepared for a little child. But it was also filled with the joy of looking at his little fingers in wonderment and realizing you are responsible for providing for him.

As I returned to work, after 4 weeks of paternity leave, I participated in organizational meetings within our hospital system discussing the limited amount of PPE. There was a talk of residents who had been sick or hospitalized and attendings who had died resuscitating COVID-19 patients. I was reassured by the fact that my wife and I had obtained life insurance policies that would ensure our child would be financially taken care of if anything were to happen to either of us.

This reassurance lasted until I was transitioning between residency and my attending position. I had planned a larger than usual gap in hopes of traveling abroad. However, with the closing of international borders and the risks associated with travel, I was stuck at home. My financial advisor had asked me to send him copies of my life and disability insurance policy. Once I started looking through the documents, I realized that the policy I had in place was not appropriate! I felt betrayed by the salesman who sold me this policy and my own naivete.

M. Cherian (✉)
Department of Emergency Medicine, Carle Foundation Hospital, Urbana, IL, USA
e-mail: Mathew.cherian@carle.org

R. P. Olympia et al. (eds.), *An Emergency Physician's Path*,
https://doi.org/10.1007/978-3-031-47873-4_98

What Went Wrong?

My wife had graduated from her emergency medicine residency in 2015 while I was still a medical student. Her residency program included financial education for residents, and she understood the need, but not the specifics, of purchasing life and disability insurance. I, while interested in some aspects of personal finance, was not well versed in the details. Someone she knew pointed her toward a "financial advisor." This financial advisor was actually a captive insurance agent and made a lot of promises. He steered us in the direction of obtaining disability insurance but also recommended that since we were getting married and thinking of starting a family in the near future we should also obtain life insurance. I said in no uncertain terms that I just wanted term life insurance based on quick perusal through some personal finance books. However, what I purchased was marketed as term life insurance but ended up being a more expensive less than suitable product. I wished someone had given me a primer or a blueprint on buying life insurance so that I wouldn't have made those mistakes.

Life Insurance 101

The following are the answers to very common basic questions regarding life insurance and what I wish I had known before purchasing:

What Is Life Insurance?

Life insurance is an insurance product that pays a death benefit (payout) for a given premium (payment) over a predetermined length of time (term). You pay an annual premium, and if you die through accident or natural causes over the period of insurance, your named beneficiaries receive a payout. Since the definition of life and death is black and white (unlike *The Princess Bride* where you can be "mostly dead"), term life insurance tends to be fairly inexpensive, but there are other products that are often marketed toward high-income professional such as emergency physicians which can be drastically more expensive and not advantageous.

Do I Need Life Insurance?

Not necessarily. The major reason that you need life insurance is if you have someone who depends on you for income. If you have a wife, partner, significant other, child, sibling, or parent who depends on your income and would have difficulty supporting themselves, then you should have life insurance in place. If you are single with no plans to get married any time soon, then it is unlikely you need life insurance.

Another situation in which you might need life insurance is if you have debts that someone would be wholly responsible for if you were to die. For example, if you bought a house with your parents and they were expecting you to pay the mortgage, they may need you to have insurance so they can pay off the debt in the unlikely eventuality that you die.

If you have a stay-at-home spouse or partner, they, too, may need life insurance. This is especially true if you have young children. Your stay-at-home partner is a primary caregiver, may cook, clean, and take the kids to school. All of these functions would need to be replaced if your partner died, and hiring for this is quite costly. Likely, the policy on this individual does not need to be as large as for the primary earner.

What Type of Life Insurance Should I Get?

There are generally two major categories of life insurance: the life insurance you need and what your insurance salesman will sell you! This is just a joke, but for most people there is only one type of life insurance that makes sense: long-term level premium life insurance [1].

Term life insurance is a type of life insurance that has a set annual cost (premium) which stays in force for a set amount of time (term) with a set dollar value (death benefit) paid out to your beneficiaries in the event of your death. The standard terms for life insurance are 15, 20, and 30 years. Typically, the death benefit is sold in half million dollar or million-dollar increments. Therefore, I could buy a 30-year three million dollar term life policy. Once I purchase this policy, it would stay in force for 30 years, and if I pay the annual premiums, my beneficiaries would receive three million dollars if I expired. At the end of the term, the policy goes away. There is no cash value or investment associated with the policy.

There are several alternate types of insurance, but they are all essentially permanent life insurance. These go under various names including whole life, universal life, cash value, etc. Permanent life insurance combines a life insurance with an investment product. In many instances, part of the annual premium you pay, which could be up to 20 times what a similar term life insurance policy will cost, goes to cover the death benefit. However, the remainder usually remains as cash value with low-yield investment. This insurance policy will be in effect until you die at which point the cash value disappears and the death benefit is paid out to your heirs [2].

Permanent life insurance is marketed by insurance salesmen in a sophisticated way to accomplish a few goals. They will tell you that it is important for estate planning purposes and will help to pass money down tax-free. They will extoll the virtues of the cash value and how you can borrow against this. They will tell you that by paying for term life insurance you are not getting anything at the end of it and your premiums disappear. These are poor arguments. Mixing life insurance and investing makes this needlessly complicated and many times more expensive. The yield on the cash value accounts is minimal, and you would be much better off putting this money in an investment account. You are being told an advantage is that you can borrow your own money! The real benefit is usually that the insurance agent makes a much heftier commission on the sale of permanent life insurance than for term and try to get doctors to buy it because we may not have as much financial sophistication since we have been using most of our time to learn to take care of our patients!

How Much Life Insurance Should You Get?

This is a very good but complicated question because there are innumerable ways you can calculate this. There are several factors that have to be taken into account. Are you married, partnered, or single? Do you have kids? Will these children need additional college savings? Do you have any outstanding large debts?

You can do a quick analysis using freely available online calculators found through a simple Google search. However, precision isn't necessary as term life insurance is generally bought in million to half million-dollar increments. Many financial advisors will use a simple rule of thumb to ballpark the figure. That rule of thumb is 10x annual income. For the median-income-earning emergency medicine, attending that will end up being roughly 2–4 million dollars.

What Affects the Premiums?

Life insurance premiums are determined by several factors including the term and death benefit of the policy as well as actuarial risk. The longer the term of the policy (15 vs 30 years), the more expensive that policy is going to be and the higher the premium. As you can imagine, there is a larger risk but still relatively small risk of the individual dying over the course of 30 years instead of over the course of 15 years. Premiums also tend to be proportionate to the death benefit of the policy. A 500,000 dollar policy is going to be less expensive than a one million dollar policy given the same term.

There are many factors that go into calculating that risk. Your age, sex, smoking history, and health history are all among the things that will be used by the insurance company to determine your premium. For example, my wife pays a far lower-term life insurance premium than I do (roughly half) for the same level of coverage because women are at lower risk of dying. The best thing you can do to keep premiums low is be relatively young and healthy at your initial application.

When Should I Get a Policy?

There is no perfect time to obtain a policy, but there are several factors which might influence your decision to obtain a policy. Realistically, you'd like to get your policy when you are young and healthy, before you develop any medical conditions, and when you have dependents or expect to have dependents. For example, it did not make sense for me to have a policy in medical school when I was unmarried and had no children. However, my classmates in medical school who had three kids (where did they get the time?) needed a life insurance policy in place.

The end of residency training usually marks a reasonable time in which to obtain a life insurance policy. Since you will be applying for disability at the same time, often, you can use the same information to shop for both policies, and underwriting can take place at the same time. Again, this only makes sense if you have or are planning to have dependents or those who depend on your income.

One additional caveat is for female physicians. While women, like my wife, generally pay lower premiums for life insurance, pregnancy can reveal a number of medical conditions which either make it more expensive or less likely obtain life insurance. It may be prudent for those female emergency physicians to apply before getting pregnant.

I Have Insurance Through My Job. Do I Need Another Policy?

My advice is yes. Many hospitals, private groups, or contract management groups provide life insurance as a benefit of employment. The benefit on this policy is usually in the range of 1–2× salary. Unfortunately, as discussed earlier, this is not nearly enough death benefit for the average emergency physician. Also, these policies tend not to be portable so you may not be able to take the policy when you leave your current job or, if you can, it is usually prohibitively expensive to do so. It is better to have a personal insurance policy in place that is portable if you end up leaving your current job.

Blueprint

This is an outline of the strategy I wish I had when first purchasing life insurance. It is the strategy I used the second time, and I hope that it will help to guide you through the process:

1. *Do your research*: I have outlined a lot of the most common information regarding life insurance, but it is just a primer. Before going into an agent's office, it's important to know what you want and state it clearly so that you aren't sold something you neither want nor need. I would recommend reading blogs like

The White Coat Investor or listening to podcasts such as *The Money Guy Show* as places to start for some advice on obtaining life insurance. They have specific articles or clips on life insurance. You should also figure out how much insurance you'll need and for what term.

2. *Consider laddering policies*: This is a sophisticated way to cut down on the cost of life insurance and protect yourself in the unlikely event the life insurance company you choose goes bankrupt. As mentioned earlier, the longer the term and higher the death benefit, the more costly the premium. Laddering means getting policies for different terms. When most people purchase their initial policy, their kids are young, and they don't have much in the way of assets. At this stage, you need a higher death benefit. As you get older, you develop more assets, your house is more likely to be paid off, and the need for life insurance decreases. Therefore, if you want three million dollars of coverage when your kids are young, you can buy three separate one million dollar policies at term lengths of 15, 20, and 30 years each. That way, when your children are young, you have a three million dollar benefit, but as your life insurance policies lapse, you'd have a progressively smaller benefit. So, at 25 years out, you'd be left with one policy for a million dollars. You can also ladder across multiple companies to spread the risk of the life insurance company you choose going bankrupt. You can choose one policy from Company A, another from Company B, and third from Company C.
3. *Find an independent agent*: This is going to be the most challenging. The most important word is *independent*. Many agents, including the one I initially used, were *captive agents* who would only quote from a single insurance company. This limits you and doesn't allow you to compete on price. You may be able to find an independent agent online, in your local area or by word of mouth.
4. *Get quotes*: An independent agent should be able to run your demographic information to obtain quotes from 20–50 companies. They should present you a list of the companies, the quote for the term and death benefit, and their ratings from various agencies. This allows you to compare and choose quotes that make sense for you. The insurance industry is heavily regulated, and, in general, an independent agent should only be quoting you from reliable top-tier agencies.
5. *Go through underwriting*: Once you have selected a quote, you'll need to go through underwriting. This is the process by which the insurance company checks your medical history to make sure that you meet their quoted risk profile. They will ask for things like medical conditions, family history, and potentially dangerous hobbies (scuba, cave diving, etc.). It is important to be honest in this portion of the process because if it is discovered that you lied it is possible for the death benefit not to be paid out. A good agent will walk you through this process. Part of the process usually involves obtaining fasting labs, height, weight, and vitals to ensure that someone is healthy and doesn't have undiagnosed underlying conditions. If issues arise, the insurance company may ask for clarifying information. For example, I had accidently marked I participated in free diving which created a huge red flag. My agent and I were able to go back and work through this with the company and resolve the error.

6. *Wait until your policies are in force*: Once underwriting has taken place, eventually, the policy will be issued, and you will be told the policy is in force after payment of your first premium.
7. *Periodically reconsider your need for life insurance*: Over the course of time, your need for life insurance will change. Many people keep their term life insurance for the full term because it's relatively inexpensive, but if you accumulate enough assets, it may not be worth it to keep it. You can, at any time, cancel the policy by not paying the premium and letting it lapse. You may have the opposite problem and want a larger death benefit for your family realizing your initial policy was too small. Life insurance doesn't need to be something you address annually, but probably something you should think about every few years.

In the end, I was able to obtain appropriate long-term level premium life insurance for my family and have now secured their future. Just remember even if you made this mistake already, it can be undone and corrected but like emergency medicine better to learn from someone else's mistakes.

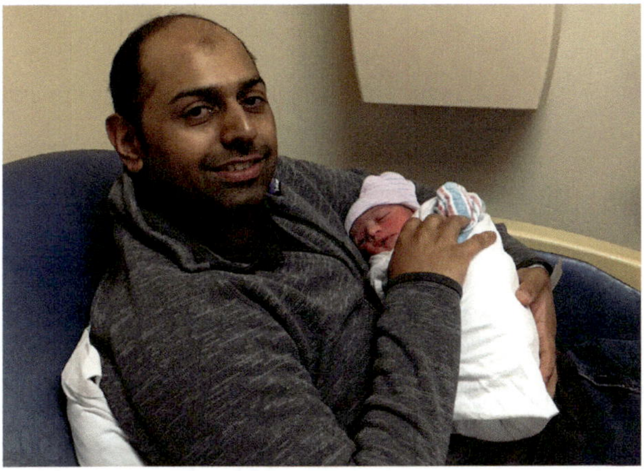

Dr. Mathew Cherian holding his eldest son, Roshan, shortly after birth

References

1. Dahle JM. The white coat investor. Salt Lake City: White Coat Investor LLC; 2014.
2. Steuer T. Questions and answers on life insurance. Alameda: Life Insurance Sage Press; 2010.

Chapter 99
Disability Insurance 101

Chaiya Laoteppitaks

Your greatest asset is your ability to work, to earn income. According to a 2020 report from the Association of American Medical Colleges, the median educational debt of a graduating medical student in 2019 was $200,000 with 73% of graduating students reporting some educational debt [1]. More than one in four 20-year-olds will become disabled before reaching retirement age. A physician has a greater likelihood of suffering from a severe disability that impacts their ability to work than they are to die prematurely [2, 3]. Disability insurance is critical to protecting your income. While life insurance is fairly simple (you are either alive or dead), disability insurance is a much more complicated product. Disability insurance provides you an income if you can no longer work. Disability insurance can cover either short-term or long-term disability; you may obtain coverage through an individual policy, from a group policy, or from an association policy.

The elimination period (also known as the waiting or qualifying period) is the amount of time between the injury and when the injured party (you) can begin to receive payments. Short-term disability insurance is meant to cover temporary, less serious injuries that may prevent you from working for a few months. It can begin paying as soon as you get injured and will cover you for a short time (typically 3–12 months). Many employers offer this type of coverage as an employee benefit. On the other hand, long-term disability insurance has a longer elimination period, anywhere between 1 and 6 months. Once payments begin, you will receive payments until age 65 (or older depending on your policy). Unless you are financially independent, you need to purchase long-term disability insurance.

C. Laoteppitaks (✉)
Department of Emergency Medicine, Sidney Kimmel Medical College,
Philadelphia, PA, USA
e-mail: Chaiya.Laoteppitaks@jefferson.edu

R. P. Olympia et al. (eds.), *An Emergency Physician's Path*,
https://doi.org/10.1007/978-3-031-47873-4_99

Policies offered by your employer or a professional association are often cheaper than individual policies and have generic coverage. Their definitions of disability are typically weaker as well. Additionally, these polices are not portable and cannot be taken with you if you change employers or leave that association, and they are not secured and can be canceled at any time. For tax purposes, if the insurance premium was paid with pre-tax dollars (such as with an employer-provided policy), any benefit payments are taxable. Aside from being less costly, these plans often do not require medical screening exams or long questionnaires.

Exactly what constitutes a disability varies from policy to policy, and the broader the definition, the more expensive the policy. It is helpful to break down disability insurance into three coverage tiers [4]: Tier 1, "any occupation" coverage is the weakest; if you can work in any profession, you are not disabled. Tier 2, "specialty-specific-not working" coverage pays a benefit if you cannot work in your specialty and you are not working in any other capacity. This type of coverage will not consider you disabled if your disability prevents you from working in an Emergency Department, but you are still working in an Urgent Care. Many group plans start off as "specialty-specific-not working," but then convert to "any occupation" after 2 years. Tier 3, "specialty-specific" coverage is the best coverage and what you should seek out whenever possible. "Specialty-specific" coverage pays out if you cannot work in your specialty. It does not matter if you can work in an Urgent Care or any other role; if you are no longer able to perform your specialty, you are disabled. The keywords/phrases you are looking for in a policy are "You are not able to perform the material and substantial duties of your occupation even if you are gainfully employed in another occupation."

There are six insurance companies which offer "specialty-specific" plans to physicians, Ameritas, Guardian, MassMutual, Ohio National Financial Services, Principal, and The Standard. Because it is an insurance product, disability insurance must be purchased for an insurance broker. As with any significant financial decision, it is important to explore your options. You will want to find an independent broker who offers policies from many carriers, who is physician focused and who has experience with their clients filing claims and collecting their benefits.

Disability insurance typically covers 60% of a physician's income, but it is better to think of disability insurance as covering your expenses rather than covering your income. Ideally, your disability benefit money will cover your living expenses and your retirement savings (since you will be receiving payments until age 65). You will have to continue to save for retirement using your disability benefit money. Because you are paying your premium with after-tax dollars, your disability payments will not be taxed. Your insurance plan may offer an optional retirement benefit where additional money is placed into a retirement vehicle for you. If your spouse or partner is also a physician or in another high-earning job, you may be able to live on one income and may not require as large of a disability benefit.

Until what age you will receive payments is known as the benefit period. Often, this is until age 65 or 67. Mental health or substance use-related disabilities often have a much shorter benefit period (2 years). Generally, any preexisting medical conditions will be excluded when applying for disability insurance. Other exclusions may apply as well such as acts of war, normal pregnancy, active military duty, and foreign travel. If you are active military and going to be deployed, talk to your agent or insurance company and see if you are covered during your deployment or if you can place your policy on hold.

Riders are policy provisions that add benefits or amend the terms of the basic policy. Riders may or may not cost an additional premium. One important rider to add or purchase is a residual or partial disability rider. This rider would provide partial disability income until you could return to full-time work. A cost-of-living adjustment (COLA) rider will adjust your benefit based on inflation. This adjustment only occurs after you become disabled. Once you become disabled, your benefit will increase (usually once a year) based on inflation. If your policy offers a noncancelable and guaranteed rider, you should purchase it. A noncancelable and guaranteed renewable policy cannot be changed by your insurance policy; the premiums, the monthly benefits, the benefits period, none of them can be changed. A future purchase rider allows you to buy a larger benefit at a later date without a medical examination or questionnaire. A future purchase rider is especially important early in your career (e.g., during residency) when you anticipate higher future earnings. If you have reached the peak in your earnings, you can forgo this rider. A catastrophic disability rider will pay an additional benefit if you are so severely disabled that you cannot perform your activities of daily living. Depending on the cost of the rider and whether or not you are already at the maximal benefit, you might consider adding this rider.

Disability insurance is usually less expensive to purchase when you are young as you are less likely to have medical conditions that drive up costs. Premiums for females are generally higher because, statistically speaking, females develop more and longer-lasting disabling conditions than males. Some policies offer unisex rates which can offer a significant discount for females. Purchasing disability insurance prior to becoming pregnant is another way to keep costs down. Pregnancy alone is not considered a disability, but complications of pregnancy can be. Increasing the elimination period or decreasing the benefit period can also reduce your premium.

After 8 or more years of postsecondary school education and 3 or more years of residency training, it is critical to protect your ability to earn an income with an individual long-term disability insurance policy that is "specialty-specific." You want a policy that will cover your expenses (including retirement savings), is noncancelable and guaranteed renewable, and has a COLA benefit. Look for an independent insurance agent or broker that has experience working with physicians. Group and association policies can offer additional coverage, but the best protection is with an individual policy.

References

1. Youngclaus JFJ. *Physician education debt and the cost to attend medical school: 2020 Update*. 2020: Association of American Medical Colleges.
2. Association, A.M. *Understanding disability insurance for physicians*. [cited 2022 9/11]; Available from: https://www.ama-assn.org/medical-residents/medical-residency-personal-finance/understanding-disability-insurance-physicians.
3. Administration, S.S. *The faces and facts of disability*. [cited 2022 9/11]; Available from: https://www.ssa.gov/disabilityfacts/facts.html.
4. Group, L.F. *Disability insurance for doctors*. [cited 2022 9/11]; Available from: https://www.larsonfinancial.com/doctor-disability-insurance/.

Chapter 100
Loan Repayment

Brian Freeze and Drew Nyce

The prospects of repaying your student loans may seem like a daunting challenge. Many physicians have borrowed a staggering amount of money to complete their medical education, but historically doctors repay their loans without significant long-term financial hardship. According to the AAMC, the average amount of debt for medical school graduates is between $195,000 and $220,000 depending on location and public versus private school. Those numbers also do not account for any debt already incurred prior to medical school such as undergraduate or postbaccalaureate programs. The keys to managing your financial debt and associated stress are being knowledgeable about the specifics of loan repayment and developing a plan that works for you.

The first step in approaching loan repayment is to gain a fundamental understanding of your loans:

- *Step 1*: There are two big categories of loans, federal and private. Federal loans are monies borrowed from the federal government, but there are so many loans you often deal with a loan management company directly and not the federal government (i.e., Nelnet, FedLoan, Great Lakes, etc.).

  All your federal student loan information can be obtained in a single place, https://nslds.ed.gov/nslds/nslds_SA/, and then look for "financial aid review."

  Anytime you want to know more about your federal student loans, check out www.studentaid.gov. They have answers to many common questions and the most up-to-date information about student loan management, repayment programs, and student loan forgiveness.

  Private student loans are from private companies, usually large financial institutions like banks. Information on your private loans is usually available on their

B. Freeze (✉) · D. Nyce
Cooper University Hospital, Camden, NJ, USA
e-mail: Freeze-brian@cooperhealth.edu; Nyce-drew@cooperhealth.edu

R. P. Olympia et al. (eds.), *An Emergency Physician's Path*,
https://doi.org/10.1007/978-3-031-47873-4_100

websites, but if you are not sure if or who you have a private loan with, the most efficient process is to access your credit report (not your credit score) that lists all the companies you owe money. You can access it once a year for free (www.annualcreditreport.com), but be mindful for ads or sites with similar names or URLS. The information will provide you the name of the company/financial institution you owed money to. Contact the respective institutions for the following information: loan principal (initial amount you borrowed), interest rate, accrued interest, any loan status (repayment plan, etc.), and possibly the loan servicer.

- *Step 2: Definitions*

  There is a specific language used when talking about loans and more confusing and specific language when talking about federal student loans. Understanding of loan verbiage is important to make smart decisions around managing your loans:

  - *Principal*—the initial amount of money you borrowed.
  - *Interest*—the amount of money that you have been charged for borrowing the principal amount. To pay off your debt, you must pay back the interest and principal.
  - *Interest Rate*—the rate at which the interest accrues over the course of your loan. For example, 7% interest on a $100,000 principal loan means you owe an additional $7000 by the end of the year. Interest rates are frequently reported as an APR (annual percentage rate). APR includes the interest but also other additional fees or costs that are charged to the borrower to make it easier to compare loans and costs.
  - *Capitalization*—when the outstanding interest that has accumulated is added back into the principal of the loan. This means that if you had $50,000 in interest on a principal of $100,000, at 10% interest, typically, you would be accruing $10,000 in interest a year. After capitalization, you would now accrue 10% of $150,000 or $15,000 per year. Certain activities with your loans can trigger a capitalization event.
  - *Consolidate*—the process of combing multiple different loans together into a single loan. This process is unique to just federal student loans. This makes managing the paperwork and logistics easier because instead of 8 to 16 (or more) loans you only have one loan. It also allows you to consolidate a loan that was not previously eligible for a federal repayment program into one that has eligibility.
  - *Delinquent*—if you miss a payment, your loan is now considered delinquent (even if only a few days late!). Once you pay back your loan up to current, you are no longer delinquent, but the fact that you were late on a payment will negatively affect your credit score.
  - *Default*—if you fail to make payments for 270 days (~9 months). This has a significant impact on your credit score, making it very difficult to borrow money in the future (i.e., car or house loan).

- *Deferment*—a specific defined period of hardship, during which you are *not* required to make payments. Any *subsidized* federal loans will *not* accrue any interest; however, any *unsubsidized* loans will accrue interest. Matriculation in medical school is an example of a period that qualifies for deferment; you were not making any payments on your student loans while in medical school. To put your loans into deferment, you need to meet specific criteria (see studentaid.gov); this is done through your loan servicer (it should have been done automatically for you while in medical school).
- *Forbearance*—also a time when you are *not* making payments on your loans. However, you did not qualify for a deferment. Your interest is still accumulating. The benefit of forbearance is you are communicating with your loan servicer (usually annually at a minimum), and this would prevent you from going into delinquency or default.
- *Refinance*—when you renegotiate the terms of your loan, either with the same institution or a new one. The purpose of this is generally to get better terms (i.e., lower interest rates). Most commonly, this is done after residency when you no longer benefit from the federal student loan programs and want to pay of your debt with as little interest as possible. Once, you leave the federal student loan program, you cannot refinance back into it, but you can move from one institution to another if they have better deals/rates or terms.
- *Grace Period*—a period usually at the end of a deferral period before you need to start (or restart) making payments. Most federal loans have a mandatory 6-month grace period following graduation.

• *Step 3: Additional Definitions—Income-Driven Repayment.*

Federal student loans, in addition to specific terminology, also have special repayment programs that can sometimes be confusing. Let's review various programs to understand what they mean what a real-world example would like.

Most student loans would enter a standard 10-year repayment plan upon graduation. That means you would make a monthly payment every month for 10 years to pay back your debt. For example, an initial loan principle of $200,000 (at 7% interest) would equate to a monthly payment of over $2430 (over those 10 years, you would pay a total of $291,514 or over $90,000 of interest in addition to the original $200,000 borrowed). This repayment plan is not feasible for most residents because of this situation as well as many other students who recently graduated in similar situations the federal government developed income-driven repayment plans. There are several plans (Income-Contingent Repayment (ICR), Income-Based Repayment (IBR), Pay As You Earn (PAYE), Revised Pay As You Earn (REPAYE)) with slight difference, but all work on the same principles; borrowers are responsible for paying 5–15% (based on which plan) of their discretionary income per month (regardless of the total balance of the loan). Discretionary income is defined as the adjusted gross income (AGI, line 11 on form 1040 of your taxes) minus 150% of the poverty line (based on your family size). For example, in 2022, the poverty line for a single person is $13,590. For a single person with an AGI of $65,000, your discretionary income would be

$65,000–1.50 * ($13,590) or $44,615 which would be $3718 a month. Therefore, your required loan payment would then be 10% (or 5–15% depending on the plan) or $371.80 a month.

The only requirement to qualify for an income-driven repayment plan is to have federal student loans. You can enter the plan in both for profit and not-for-profit jobs and regardless of your employment status (full time, part time, etc.). This is different than the requirements if you are looking for loan forgiveness.

Loan Forgiveness

At the time of writing this chapter, student loan forgiveness is a hot topic that has recently been in the news: from the first wave of public service loan forgiveness to the onetime $10,000 loan forgiveness earmarked for early 2023 (then held up in the court system). Currently, only federal student loans are eligible for these programs, so unfortunately your private loans are not eligible for loan forgiveness; they need to be paid according to the agreement you signed. There are two programs in place to assist with loan forgiveness on your federal loans.

The first program, public service loan forgiveness or often referred to as PSLF, is more restrictive but is very advantageous to the borrower. PSLF is a program to forgive federal student loans after 120 qualified payments. One must be employed full time for a not-for-profit company (or the federal government) and enrolled in an eligible repayment program. If you work for a nonprofit (not necessarily the same one) for 10 years and make monthly payments, the remaining balance (interest + principal) is forgiven federal tax and penalty free.

The second program is less advantageous compared to the PSLF, but it is much easier to qualify for. Eligibility requires you to have federal student loans and enrolled in an income-driven repayment plan. After 20 or 25 years (depending on the program) of payments, the remaining loan balance is forgiven. There is no limitation based on who you work for or if you work full or part time. However, the remaining loan balance (principal + interest) that is forgiven could be considered taxable income in the year it is forgiven. That means when you file your federal income taxes for the year your loans are forgiven; if you made $300,000 and had a $500,000 loan balance forgiven, you would owe federal taxes on an income of roughly $800,000 (an additional tax bill of upward of $100,000). This is often referred to as the "tax bomb." In late 2020, federal legislation was passed to no longer count student loan forgiveness as taxable income. If that ruling doesn't change, then there would be no tax bomb. This does not apply to the PSLF plan as the program specifies the loan forgiveness would not be taxed at the federal level. In almost all situations, this longer forgiveness program is not the preferred option. Working full time for a not-for-profit hospital for 10 years and getting PSLF or simply paying off the loan in a shorter time are far better options. This program is more directed for professions that are harder to find not-for-profit jobs or have a higher-debt-to-income ratio (i.e., veterinarians, dentists).

What to Do as a Medical Student

Your primary objective during medical school is to learn medicine and graduate. Realistically, most students who borrow money do not have the financial resources to repay interest and/or principal toward their loans while matriculated in medical school so don't perseverate about your loans. Remember that you are investing in yourself and your career. Be smart about how much you borrow; you don't have to live super frugally and be miserable, but also don't "live it up" on borrowed money. Some practical ideas to consider reducing costs are to live with roommates and when possible live close to the medical school to cut down on transportation costs. Don't forget to file your taxes, especially as a fourth-year student. Even if you have no income, you may be eligible for a few tax credits and therefore a tax refund.

What to Do as a Resident

Managing private student loans during residency is often very straightforward. When you took the private loans, you agreed to a repayment plan. Therefore, you can start to pay in accordance with that agreement (typically a 10-year payment plan) or refinance to another private lender with different terms.

For federal student loans, you have three decisions to make during residency:

1. Are you entering an income-based repayment plan, refinancing, or entering forbearance?
2. If you're entering a repayment plan, which one?
3. When do you want to start making payments?

Your primary goal in residency is to gain the clinical skills and knowledge to practice excellent Emergency Medicine independently. Becoming a strong clinician who is board certified in EM will help ensure you have a sustained high income that will assist your repayment plan for your loans.

In general, for almost all residents with a single tax filing status, the approach to loan repayment is the same: enroll in REPAYE during residency. However, if you are married especially to a high-income earner, you have more nuanced options to sort through based on your loan amount, your spouse's income, and your plans in the future. See the resources at the end of this chapter to get further guidance on your unique scenarios. Currently, the most advantageous plan for most residents is REPAYE. REPAYE is an income-driven repayment plan that also gives you an extra subsidy (free money) on the loan interest that your payments couldn't cover. This has the impact of lowering your effective interest rate and APR on your loans which means your loan balance grows slower. This subsidy is so good that it likely results in a lower interest rate than you would be able to otherwise obtain if you refinanced your loans instead. So, in most cases, even if you know you will not pursue PSLF or loan forgiveness after residency, the best plan is still to use an income-driven

Table 100.1 Comparison of various repayment plans

	PAYE	REPAYE	Biden-Harris New proposal[a]
Monthly payment % of discretionary income	10%	10%	5%[b]
Qualifies for PSLF	Yes	Yes	Yes
Tax filing status allowed	Single, married filing jointly, married filing separately	Single, married filing jointly	Unknown
Interest subsidy	No	50% of unpaid	100% of unpaid
Example—Single resident earning 65 k, with 200 k student loans at 7% interest			
Monthly payment	$371.80	$371.80	$143.43
Annual accrued interest	$14,000	$14,000	$14,000
Amount paid through the year	$4461.6	$4461.6	$1721.16
End-of-year loan balance before subsidy	$209,538.4	$209,538.4	$211,769.2
Loan balance when factoring in subsidy	$209,538.4	$204,769.2	$200,000
Value of the subsidy	NA	$4769.2	$12,278.84
Effective interest rate	7%[c]	4.7%[c]	0.9%[c]

[a]This plan was announced but specifics have not been released nor officially signed into law
[b]The definition of discretionary income in the new plan is proposed to be 225% of the poverty line (compared to 150% in the current definition)
[c]These effective interest rates are variable based on how much you pay: the less you pay, the more subsidy and the lower the effective interest rate is. But in almost all cases where you are getting a subsidy, the effective interest rate is still less than you could get if you were to refinance your loans

repayment plan during residency to maximize this subsidy. Table 100.1 compares the various repayment plans.

There are a few important factors to remember. Your monthly payment as outlined above is based on your annual income. The most common way to document or prove your income to the federal government is by providing the previous year's tax return. If you are married and file taxes together, the total income (yours + your spouse's) is used to determine your monthly payment which can result in much larger monthly payments necessitating different plans. Additionally, this approach means that when you start this process as an intern and provide your tax return from the prior year (MS4), you will likely report an income of $0. That translates to a monthly payment for intern year as $0. The zero-dollar "payments" still qualify for the interest subsidy and count toward the 120 qualified payments required if you choose to pursue PSLF (hence why it's important to file taxes especially in your last year of medical school).

If you cannot afford the payments dictated by an income-driven repayment plan, your only other option would be to contact your loan servicer and enter into forbearance. This is typically a not ideal situation because you lose out on the interest subsidy and low-cost PSLF qualifying patients and your student loans will grow at a much faster rate.

How Do you Enter a Repayment Plan?

First, you need to log into your loan servicer's website and enroll your loans into your desired repayment plan (PAYE, REPAY, etc.). As explained above, you may have discovered you have multiple loans. Instead of trying to manage the paperwork and details of 5–20 individual loans, it is often beneficial and easier to roll them together into a single loan. This process is called consolidation. You can only do it with your federal student loans. This means moving forward you will only have one loan to manage.

Be aware that there are some downsides to consolidating. First, any interest that accrued will be capitalized (added to the principal), but this will happen at the end of your grace period regardless of consolidation. Second, any payments you had made toward a qualifying PSLF are erased. Obviously, having just graduated should not be a problem but would be a good reason to keep medical school and undergraduate loans separate and why it's important to consolidate at the start. Finally, the interest rate on your final consolidate loans is a weighted average round up to the nearest 1/8th of a percent.

The last decision to make is when to start making payments or when to end your grace period. Essentially, you have two options: start immediately (July) or wait as long as possible (approximately November). There are advantages and disadvantages to both approaches, so choose the option that best fits your financial situation and anticipated future. The long-term difference between the two however is very small, so don't stress about it too much:

Starting immediately: As detailed above, many interns will qualify for zero-dollar payments. Best to start that 120-payment clock going and start counting those payments as soon as possible? The more payments you make, the sooner your loan is forgiven. This is the best strategy for people who plan to pursue PSLF. You should try to consolidate and enroll in a payment plan in June or July of your intern year. It is not possible to enroll sooner as you must wait for your medical school to release your loans upon graduation.

Wait until the end: After you enroll in a repayment plan, you must re-enroll every year (and recertify your income). So, the sooner you enroll, the sooner you must recertify your income. This is a good plan for people who know they will not be eligible for PSLF down the road, plan to enter private practice, and pay off their loans after they graduate. Don't worry if you are not sure; you can always split the difference.

Congratulations. You are essentially done with the tasks of loan repayment. Moving forward, remember to re-enroll your loan into your plan of choice and recertify your income (aka upload last year's taxes) on an annual basis. In addition, it is recommend to verify your employment status annually. The means having your employer fill out the form to make sure your payments are counting toward your 120 qualified payments. Download the form from the student aid website, and ask your employer to fill it out (often either HR or sometimes GME departments can do this for you):

https://studentaid.gov/manage-loans/forgiveness-cancellation/public-service/public-service-loan-forgiveness-application.

What to Do as an Attending

Congratulations on graduating residency and successfully becoming an Emergency Medicine physician! The first months after residency are generally met with many emotions: stress, anxiety, and excitement to name a few. We recommend focusing on developing your clinical skills, learning your healthcare system, and passing your boards during the first few months postresidency. Transitioning to independent practice presents many anticipated and unexpected challenges, so concentrate on your long-term loan repayment plan after you take your written boards.

After adjusting to life as an independent EM physician, in November or December, it is time to develop the final plan for you student loans. Private loans are straightforward; keep paying your monthly payment, or consider refinancing (maybe you can get a better rate by agreeing to a more aggressive monthly payment, etc.).

Your federal loans present more options to consider when deciding on a long-term repayment plan. You can decide to remain in an income-driven repayment plan and pursue PSLF or develop your own repayment plan that fits your budget. Remember if you stay in a federal income-driven repayment plan your monthly payment is based on your income, so when you start making more money as an attending that monthly payment is naturally going to increase significantly (also as a result there will be little to no interest subsidy because your payments will cover all of the accruing interest). When considering what option works best for you, consider the amount of money you will likely pay off over the remaining 120 payments given your income level. As a rule of thumb, if your loan balance is around $100,0000, you will likely pay off your loan under most income-driven repayment plans before the 10-year mark and not benefit from any loan forgiveness. In this scenario, you should strongly consider refinancing the loans with a private company and pay a lower interest rate. The benefit with this approach is paying back less interest with the lower interest rate. However, if you think you will continue to work for a company that meets the criteria for PSLF and have a loan balance over $100,000, then it makes sense to continue federal income-driven payment plans.

Please note that just because you work *at* a hospital that happens to be a not-for-profit does not always mean that you work *for* the hospital. Many times, physicians work for private groups that contract with the hospital, and those groups are for profit and therefore do not qualify for PSLF. This is common in Emergency Medicine.

If you decide to refinance your federal student loans because you will not be eligible for PSLF or don't want to wait for forgiveness, your next step is to refinance your student loans. Likely you will already be inundated with ads for refinance opportunities. Generally, they all offer a 10–15-min process for an initial approximate quote. Fill out the info for a bunch of different companies, then take the top (based on offering the lowest APR) three to four offers, and fill out their full application. Generally, you should be aiming for a 5-year payoff period (from the time you gradated residency) and looking for the best APR (interest rate) from various companies. You likely will have an option between both variable and fixed rates. In just about all scenarios (especially on 5-year repayment plans), it works out to be cheaper to use the variable rate. However, that does mean your payment may change month to month and there's a small chance your rate could increase a lot. It is not wrong to select fixed rate if that makes your budgeting and planning a little easier and less stressful.

If you Need More Help

If you want to learn more about this topic or have a more complex situation, there are another few great sources to read more about all the complexities involved in this topic:

1. *Medical Student Loans: A Comprehensive Guide* by Ben White, MD (also available as a free pdf: download from his website www.benwhite.com/studentloans/).
2. *The White Coat Investor: A Doctor's Guide to Personal Finance and Investing* by James M. Dahle.
3. www.doctoredmoney.com is a website that has a few very helpful interactive tools to help you understand the various income-driven repayment plans and what it would like with your specific situation.
4. Finally, you can consider paying someone for advice. Generally, you want to look for people with specific experience working with physicians and ideally who only deals with student loans. Be wary of taking advice from anyone trying to sell you something else (disability insurance, life insurance, or some other investment product).

Chapter 101
Retirement Planning

Laura H. Mattia and Robert W. Wolford

Many of us consider retirement the ultimate goal of a career. Whatever the motivation (escape stress\burnout, spend time with family, try something new, etc.), it is important to define your expectations in retirement. What excites you about retirement? Everyone's retirement looks different and what excites one person does not excite another. A thoughtful retirement plan includes financial modeling, but, more importantly, it requires you to think about what your postretirement life will look like. This chapter discusses the financial considerations of retirement planning. Chapter 102 will discuss the nonmoney factors to consider in planning an outstanding retirement.

Several steps are required to plan your postretirement financial life:

Step 1. Estimate Your Required Annual Income

The best place to start planning for retirement is to create a vision of what life after emergency medicine looks like. Only then can you determine if you have enough income and resources to successfully achieve your vision.

Your income requirements will depend upon your lifestyle expectation and your goals. To estimate your lifestyle expenses, start with your current budget for expenses (housing\rent, car, food and groceries, utilities, cell phone, insurance, medical, gym and club memberships, taxes, hobbies, etc.). From there, you can determine how your spending will change. Paying off a mortgage and eliminating work-related costs will decrease your expenses. Today's active retirees often have increased expenses due to travel, new hobbies, etc., and these additional

L. H. Mattia
Atlas Fiduciary Financial, LLC, Sarasota, FL, USA
e-mail: Lauram@atlasfiduciary.com

R. W. Wolford (✉)
Department of Emergency Medicine, University of Illinois College of Medicine at Peoria, Peoria, IL, USA

R. P. Olympia et al. (eds.), *An Emergency Physician's Path*,
https://doi.org/10.1007/978-3-031-47873-4_101

expenditures must be planned for. Many preretirees overlook important necessities such as health care (not all covered by Medicare), home maintenance, and car maintenance\replacement.

Future inflation is often overlooked. If a retiree has a fixed retirement income beginning at age 65 and inflation is 3% (the average inflation rate over the past 100 years), the retiree has a loss of purchasing power of 26% in 10 years, 45% in 20 years, and 59% in 30 years. This risk must be factored into your analysis.

Step 2. Estimate How Long You Will Live in Retirement

Knowing your estimated life expectancy and planned retirement age, you can calculate the number of years your money must last. Identifying the age most emergency physicians retire is challenging. A Korean study reported that emergency physicians more than other medical doctors are likely to retire early [1]. In addition, a survey of retired emergency physicians found that 40% retired earlier than they planned [2]. The individual physician must consider the consequence of early retirement on life expectancy and the need for additional savings.

In 2019, men in the United States aged 65 can expect to live 18.2 more years on average, and women aged 65 years can expect to live, on average, 20.8. The IRS estimates life expectancy around age 90 to protect against the risk of outliving retirement money. When estimating your life expectancy, factor in your family history and personal health condition. You may want to assume you will live to 100 or more to be conservative. Retirement life expectancy is the time beginning at retirement and extending until death. Proper planning will protect you from outliving your assets, the number one fear of retirees.

Step 3. Identify Your Retirement Income Sources

After estimating annual expenses and the number of years you will need it, the next is to identify potential income sources. Over the past 30 years, major changes in how individual retirees finance their retirement have occurred. As the future of Social Security becomes more uncertain and pension plans disappear, personal savings must account for a larger share of retirement income.

Some retirees plan to receive income from continued employment. The assumption is that if they do not have enough money to retire when the time comes, they will just keep working. Unfortunately, this may not be feasible due to health issues or unfavorable job conditions.

Social Security

Social Security is a source of guaranteed income to help you meet living expenses. Social Security represents a large financial asset. For example, if you receive $40,000 per year from Social Security, this would be equivalent to $1,000,000 in assets, assuming you follow the widely discussed 4% withdrawal rule. About half of all Americans file for Social Security when they first become eligible for benefits, at age 62. Choosing the best time to claim your benefit is not easy as the system is complex and there are a lot of misconceptions about Social Security.

To avoid errors and get the greatest benefits, it is important to understand how the system works. Americans who have worked for 40 quarters are eligible for benefits as early as age 62, but they could get larger monthly checks by waiting. When you should claim depends on your situation. For every year you wait to claim beyond full retirement age, until age 70, your benefits will increase by 8% (not including the compounding of cost-of-living adjustments). After 70, there are no additional increases, so this is the longest you should wait to claim. How long you should wait after 62 to claim benefits depends on numerous factors, including your health. Coordinating with your spouse to determine the best time to claim your mutual benefits has an impact on your combined benefits while you are both alive and on those of the surviving spouse after one of you dies. Surviving spouses are eligible for benefits beginning at age 60 and disabled spouses at 50, but they can only receive one benefit, so it pays to optimize at least one of your benefits. Divorced people can claim on their ex-spouses' accounts if they were married for at least 10 years. This is only an advantage if your ex-spouse's account would provide greater benefits than your own. Making this claim will not limit the benefits your ex draws. They can still get their full benefit as if you had not made this claim.

Making the right Social Security choices requires investing some time and effort to understand the rules and how they apply to your situation. Visit the Social Security Administration (SSA) website (https://www.ssa.gov), and create your account. With your account established, you ensure you are receiving accurate credit for your annual income, use the site's benefit calculator, claim your benefit, and decrease the ability of others to commit fraud by stealing your identity and claiming your benefits.

Personal Savings Play a Large Role in Retirement

In the past, Social Security and pension plans were depended on to fund an individual's retirement. Unfortunately, this is no longer the case. Personal savings play a central role in funding retirement income needs, and while individuals preparing for retirement recognize this need, many are unable to save enough.

The move from defined benefit plans (i.e., pensions) where the employer takes the risk to 401(k) and 403 (b) plans requires individuals to make their own decisions about how to allocate assets to generate income in retirement. It is essential to take full advantage of employer-provided benefits or retirement contribution-matching programs, if available.

Personal savings available for retirement income consist of the following three categories:

- Brokerage and Bank Accounts—Taxable Accounts.

  These savings are not tax sheltered, so all capital gains and income are realized in real time.

- Traditional Retirement Accounts.

  Investment retirement accounts (IRAs) and defined contribution (DC) plans are the most common retirement accounts. At age 72, you must begin taking distributions from all traditional retirement accounts in the form of required minimum distributions (RMDs).
- Roth Retirement Accounts.

  While there is no tax benefit when you contribute to a Roth account, your earnings grow tax-free, and you can withdraw from them tax-free. Roth accounts are not subject to required minimum distributions (RMDs), but the ability to make contributions to them is limited by your income (check https://www.irs.gov, as this changes annually).

The Distribution Stage

The change from accumulating wealth (preretirement) to the distribution\spending (retirement) phase is often jarring. As a retiree, you must approach your investments differently than how you did as a 40-year-old when you were accumulating wealth. Nearly 60% of emergency physicians are concerned about their financial preparation for retirement [2]. Historically, retirement strategies focused on de-risking and capital preservation. Moving to cash and laddering fixed income is one way to minimize market risk. In recent years, it has become clear that a longevity strategy may be more appropriate, as the retiree's primary risk may now be outliving their money. A longevity strategy calls for a disciplined approach to maintain some equity exposure to keep pace with inflation and taxes and adding some alternative exposure to mitigate the increased risk. With a broad mix of investments, you have a higher probability of weathering any future economic environment and achieving greater security.

An Investment Strategy Will Improve your Chance of Success

One of the most important determinants of success in investing is preparing and sticking to a strategy. For years, successful investors and experienced investment committees have used a documented strategy for managing critical investment decisions. Although you may consider yourself a disciplined and savvy investor, empirical evidence demonstrates that most investors make decisions based upon emotion and often make bad decisions as they attempt to chase yield. Studies have shown consistently that while mutual funds quote excellent long-term track records, the actual performance for average investors is lower because they tend to make buy and sell decisions at the wrong time. Markets by their nature go up and down, never in a straight line. While some investors may be able to overcome behavioral risk, having the discipline to not sell at the worst times, volatility can cause actual losses and result in less money over time. Negative compounding results in lower actual returns and also creates havoc when taking distributions.

Volatility risk and *behavioral risk* are two risks inherent to investing. A third risk, *sequence risk,* is exclusive to retirees due to cash withdrawal needs. With cash inflows, it is better to experience bad returns first as you buy more shares at a lower price, enhancing the effect of compounding. This is the basic tenet of dollar-cost averaging during the accumulation phase. When taking distributions, the opposite is true. Good returns up front help to preserve and grow assets; bad returns up front eat away at your principal, and you can never get it back. Volatile market returns impact your portfolio differently depending upon whether you are in the accumulation or distribution phase which is another reason to maintain a low-volatility portfolio.

Adhering to an investment strategy helps avoid these pitfalls by removing emotions from investment decisions and minimizing risk. The investor's objective is to create a predetermined plan, prior to any investment decisions, so that during the market's move up or down, the preplanned strategy will invoke smarter and timelier decisions void of emotion. There is a simple approach to developing your investment strategy:

1. Determine your risk tolerance

   Some people are risk-takers and others avoid risk. Risk can be a combination of volatility and liquidity. Be honest and do not overthink this. There are various questionnaires available that can help you determine your level of risk tolerance. The success of an investment plan will be determined by one's ability to invest in a portfolio with a suitable amount of risk.
2. Decide on goals, objectives, and strategies.

   Establish investment-performance goals with appropriate benchmarks to monitor results. What is the target rate of return? What are the sources and measurements of risk? How long do you require your savings to last? How much income needs to be withdrawn from the portfolio?
3. Decide on your strategy for managing volatility risk.

   Maximizing return without regard for volatility risk is a major contributor to the failure of most individual investors. All investors want maximum return with the least amount of risk, but how one manages volatility risk will determine success. Most institutional investors adopt a strategy based on science and modern portfolio theory. The "efficient portfolio" relies on blending together different investments, specifically for the purpose of controlling volatility.

   The goal is to preserve your assets and to grow those assets responsibly. The best way to accomplish this goal is to build a diversified portfolio with multiple asset classes. While it may be possible to "outperform" by making a concentrated bet on an attractive investment, to do so entails a level of risk that may be unnecessary. Appropriate asset allocation should enable an investor to achieve attractive compound asset growth in the good years while providing acceptable downside protection during the bad years.

4. Set guidelines for asset classes.

   The investment strategy should provide guidelines to select asset classes. The more specific you are within each class, the better. For example, you may decide to use the following asset classes in your portfolio: large-cap domestic stock, small-cap domestic stock, mid-cap domestic stock, international stock, domestic bonds, international bonds, real estate, convertible securities, natural resource funds, and alternative investments. For each asset class, you should compile a list of all your constraints. For example, you might determine that you will never invest more than 35% in domestic bonds; that you will only invest in individual bonds – never bond funds, that they should be investment grade – AAA bonds; and that you will not hold more than 5% in any issuance. Also, determine what asset classes you will avoid, for example, limited partnerships, junk bonds (average quality BBB and below), aggressive mutual funds, and hedge funds, due to the additional risks associated with these investments.
5. Implement an asset allocation policy.

   Based on the first four steps, you can create an asset allocation – setting up a portfolio that has multiple asset classes. The allocation must consider the need for cash flow, growth, and safety. Studies have shown that 90% of an investor's success comes from asset allocation decisions, not from security selection or timing. This step involves analyzing each new asset in terms of how it will impact the overall portfolio and determining the optimum amount to include.

   The goal of asset allocation is to find asset classes that have a low correlation to each other to reduce volatility while targeting a specific return. Correlation measures the way asset classes move in relation to each other. The ideal mix is chosen with asset classes that move in opposite directions under different economic environments so that combined the overall portfolio is more stable making it easier to withdraw income and less prone to sequential and behavioral risk.
6. Rebalancing

   This might be the most crucial step. Your strategy should clearly delineate how often you are going to monitor performance and when you are going to rebalance. This component is the discipline that most investors lack. The ability to harvest gains as investments are going up and at the same time invest in asset classes when they are out of favor is the greatest tool the investment strategy can offer. Not many investors were savvy enough to sell equity as it grew in 2019, 2020, and 2021 and buy alternative assets, but those who had a strategy may have been some of the few who did and benefited in 2022 when equity plummeted.
7. How to withdraw Your income to maximize efficiency

   Once you have successfully reduced volatility and you are rebalancing on a regular basis, you can withdraw cash generated from dividends, coupons, maturing bonds, and security appreciation captured during the rebalancing process. You should maintain a minimum cash cushion of at least 6 months in addition to your emergency savings.

   The order you withdraw your funds can depend on numerous factors. Usually, it makes sense to withdraw from your taxable account to allow the money in your retirement accounts to grow tax deferred as long as possible. However, if you are older, have a sizeable portfolio, and have low tax basis investments, it might make sense to leave them for an inheritance or charitable gift. Taking withdrawals from a traditional IRA or 401(k) will create a tax liability in the form of ordinary income. You also lose the opportunity to grow your investments tax deferred, but once you turn 72 you are required to begin taking required minimum distributions (RMDs). If you have a sizeable traditional IRA, it might make more sense to begin spreading the tax burden over a longer period but with careful consideration of your marginal tax bracket and Medicare part B and part D premium bracket (known as IRMAA) in each year. Since Roth IRAs are never subject to RMD, it is ideal to let that money continue to grow tax deferred. Your heirs will benefit from the preferential tax treatment if they should inherit your assets in this form. Usually, you will want to use the Roth funds last unless there are specific tax reasons to use them sooner.

Conclusion

The decision to retire is a major life transition requiring deep thought and considerations which are unique for every person. Typically, the average investor's success is not based on choosing the "best" investment but on decisions regarding upfront planning, an investment strategy, and diversification. You would not go on a trip somewhere new without a map (or these days a navigation system). The same should be true as you evaluate your options to navigate the unknown territory of retirement and the capital markets. It might be worth having a professional, independent fee-only, CFP to help you plan. A reliable source to find this type of independent advisor who will sign a fiduciary oath while working with you is NAPFA.org. If you decide to do it yourself, consider conducting further research on the material presented in this chapter to ensure a successful retirement.

References

1. Shin J, Kim YJ, Kim JK, Lee DE, Moon S, Choe JY, Lee WK, Lee HM, Cho KH. Probability of early retirement among emergency physicians. J Prev Med Public Health. 2018;51(3):154–62. https://doi.org/10.3961/jpmph.18.079. Epub 2018 May 17. PMID: 29886711; PMCID: PMC5996188
2. Kuhn GJ, Marco CA, Mallory MNS, Blanda M, Kaplan JA, Schneider SM, Joldersma KB, Martin SI, Choo EK. Financial planning and satisfaction across life domains among retired emergency physicians in the United States. Am J Emerg Med. 2018;36(3):508–10. https://doi.org/10.1016/j.ajem.2017.06.059.

Chapter 102
The Ultimate Career Decision—When Should I Retire?

Timothy J. Schaefer and Robert W. Wolford

Begin with the end in mind! Great advise for many goals or planning tasks and certainly true for retirement planning. Think of retiring as a lifestyle change. For physicians, we can roughly divide our lives into thirds. The first 1/3rd is "learning" (childhood, schooling, residency/fellowship), the second 1/3rd is "earning" (working life, building a home, and building a nest egg, creating a legacy), and the final phase is "yearning," yearning for those golden retirement years of free time and leisure (ok I had to stretch a little to make this rhyme). For most of us, retirement will last 20–30 years, so while many people think of retiring as retiring from something, it is wise to think of retiring as retiring to something [1]. Without some planning, these years might not seem so golden and might feel unfulfilling and boring.

Retirement is a new lifestyle with a new sense of self-identity, a new sense of purpose, new goals, and new priorities. Deciding what retirement will look like for you and when to make this transition is a very personal decision based on a variety of factors and should be based on some thought and planning. One of the first questions people have about retirement is as follows: "Will I have enough money for retirement?" However, a more important initial questions is the following: "What will my retirement look like?" What is the end you have in mind for your retirement years? Once you have that figured out, it becomes something to "yearn" for.

In this chapter, we will discuss the nonfinancial part of retirement planning. We will review some statistics about retirement and review some of the more common factors contributing to the decision of when to retire. We will also discuss some concern of working longer, concerns about entering or being in retirement, and review some common plans/goals/priorities in retirement. Finally, we will make some suggestions helping when deciding to retire and planning for retiring.

T. J. Schaefer · R. W. Wolford (✉)
University of Illinois College of Medicine at Peoria, Peoria, IL, USA
e-mail: Timothy.J.Schaefer@osfhealthcare.org

R. P. Olympia et al. (eds.), *An Emergency Physician's Path*,
https://doi.org/10.1007/978-3-031-47873-4_102

Some Facts/Metric Around Physician Retirement

Physicians as a group usually retire between 60 and 69 years of age. In the past several decades, both the general population and physicians have trended toward later retirement ages. The average retirement age for the general population is close to 66 years old, while for physicians it is close to 69 years old [2]. Emergency physician as a group are younger than medical professional as a group. For all medical specialties, about 45% are ≥55 y/o, while about 35% of emergency physicians are ≥55 years old [3]. However, only 47% of emergency physicians are still active clinically at age 65 [4].

According to the Federal Reserve 2019 data for the general population, the median net worth for 65–74 is $266,400, and the average net worth is $1,217,700 [5]. When compared to physicians ages 65–69, 59% had a net worth between $1 million and $5 million, and 17% had a net worth of > $5 million [6]. For emergency physicians already in retirement, 92% were "moderately or extremely" satisfied with their finances [4].

Why Do Physicians Work Longer?

Physicians have a variety of reasons for working longer. One survey listed the following reasons [7]:

- Enjoyment of the practice (58%)
- Enjoyment of the social aspects of working (56%)
- Desire to maintain existing lifestyle (50%)

Physicians who delay retirement site the following reasons: continued career satisfaction, work flexibility, feelings of responsibility, desire to keep active (socially and intellectually), financial reason, and lack of outside interests [2].

What Are Some Concerns of the Older Working Physician?

As physicians age, new concerns may arise about working longer. Concerns about working past 65 years include [7]:

- Ability to stay competitive with changing healthcare environment (38%)
- Concerns about declining personal health (37%)
- Providing quality patient care (26%)
- Concerns about technology (23%)
- Concern about spouse or partner (21%)

Emergency medicine physicians in the preretirement, age ≥55, had the following concerns [8]:

- Less ability to recover from night shifts (74%)
- Higher level of emotional exhaustion (44%)
- Less ability to handle heavy patient volume (40%)
- Less ability to handle stress of EM (36%)
- Health limitation on ability to practice (28%)
- Memory somewhat or considerably worse (28%)

What Are the Reasons Physicians Retire?

Physicians tend to retire for both positive and negative reasons. One negative reason for early retirement is low job satisfaction. A variety of factors can contribute to low job satisfaction including loss of control, low morale, frustration with colleagues/administration, feeling undervalued, lacking prestige, loss of interest in work, excessive workload, burnout, excessive regulations in medicine, unwelcome changes, bureaucracy, oppressive management, medicolegal concerns, or financial troubles [2]. Personal health concerns including poor general health, cognitive decline, difficulty sleeping, psychological distress, or health concerns of significant others are also common factors in deciding when to retire [2].

For emergency physicians specifically, some more common factors contributing to the decision to retire included [4]:

- Made enough money to retire (47%)
- Personal health issues (34%)
- Physically too demanding (23%)
- Burned out from the job (22%)
- No longer interested in practicing (22%)

What Are Physicians Looking Forward to in Retirement?

While retiring to leave all the negative baggage of an unsatisfying job might seem like a relief, there are things many physicians look forward to [7]:

- Travel more (76%)
- Pursue other interests (66%)
- Time with family/friends (65%)
- Time for hobbies/activities (65%)

What Are Physicians Concerned About in Retirement?

Finally, physicians have some concerns about their new retirement lifestyle including:

- Loss of social dynamics of work
- Loss of purpose, boredom/loneliness/depression
- Unable to maintain desired lifestyle
- Not feeling useful

Emergency physicians overall have high levels of satisfaction in multiple areas of retirement; however, some emergency physicians listed "not at all or slightly" satisfied in [4]:

- Sense of identity (21%)
- Physical health (17%)
- Fulfillment in current work/activities (12%)

An older preretirement group of emergency physicians reported concerns of financial preparations (58%) and loss of identity upon retirement (44%) [8].

Planning Suggestions

Like death and taxes, for that vast majority of us, retirement is inevitable. While saving for retirement should start very early in your career (probably with your first paycheck), the nonfinancial planning can probably wait until later. A majority of physicians start this portion of planning around 50–55 years old [2, 9], but since emergency physician tends to leave clinical practice at a younger age, we'd suggest start thinking about this a little earlier. Broad areas to think about include time, health (mental/emotional/physical), social, and spiritual [10]:

Time—What are you going to do with your time? Retiring frees up a lot of spare time. Sixteen hours a day of awake time for 20–30 years is a lot of time! You won't have enough odd jobs or hobbies to keep you busy [9]. While many people say they stay busy in retirement, it's important to not just be doing things to stay busy but to be thoughtful and proactive doing what you want to do [9]. Just staying busy may contribute to lack of purpose and discontent.

One approach is to ease into retirement. That might mean cutting back on clinical hours or cutting back on nonclinical tasks like teaching, administrative task, committees, editorial boards, etc. Think of this as not just cutting back on work but "practicing retirement." During this time, try out new hobbies, plan different activities, maybe do some volunteer work, contribute to charitable organization, get involve with community activities, or spend time in different areas like teaching or mentoring which can be a great way to share your talents and wisdom with others [9].

If you to decide to do full retirement on a specific date, you can still plan to do the same type of "practice retirement" task mentioned above. The key point we are suggesting is not to putter around the first 1–2 years of retirement trying to come up with meaningful thinks to do; create a plan.

Health – "The greatest wealth is health" (unknown). "If you don't take care of your body, where are you going to live?" (unknown) [11]. While you certainly can't control every unfortunate health event, be aggressively proactive about taking care of yourself and those you plan to share retirement with. What's the point of retirement if you're not able to or not around to enjoy it? Take care of yourself. Get your checkups and screening test and preventative medicines. Stay physically and mentally active.

There is a strong sense of personal identity, sense of value, feelings of purpose, prestige, and ego satisfaction link to being a "doc." Many physicians have a real fear of losing that identity and purpose, and it can be difficult to replace those feelings in retirement [2].

The identity changes associated with retirement are real, and at some point, it will hit you that you "use to be a physician"! Accept it, move on, and decide what the "new you" will be. What will the reinvented you look like?

Social—While it's common to build close relationship with colleague and co-workers, many times, those relationships are more acquaintance or business relationships. Checking in and maintaining contact with colleagues and co-workers will often help with the transition to retirement. Plan to take time to improve current relationships and/or build new relationships and friendships.

Spiritual—For many, this is a deeply personal and important part of who they are, so be sure to include this component in your personal retirement plan.

Make a Plan

There are varieties of planning tools you could use, and as with any plan, the key is to create it and act on it. If you are planning to share your retirement with a spouse or significant other, then you should plan this together.

Here is one simple suggestion to get started: Write down five things you want to see/do/image in your personal retirement. Now next to each item, write down what will be the first step to make that happen [10]. Like with all plans, you'll need to revise, update, and expand your plan regularly, but the key is to get started and commit to it.

After all of this, one final thought, you do not have to retire. If you continue to feel significant purpose and joy in work, if you are physically and mentally able to continue do the job satisfactorily and assuming there are no regulatory requirements about retirement, then go ahead, and continue to work.

References

1. Cronan JJ. Retirement: I's not about the finances! J Am Coll Radiol. 2009;6:242–5.
2. Silver MP, Hamilton AD, Biswas A, Warrick NI. A systematic review of physician retirement planning. Human Resources for Health. 2016;14:67.
3. Active physicians by age and specialty, 2019 in physician specialty data report. AAMC. 2019 at https://www.aamc.org/data-reports/workforce/interactive-data/active-physicians-age-and-specialty-2019
4. Kuhn GJ, Marco CA, Mallory MS, et al. Financial planning and satisfaction across life domains among retired emergency physicians in the United States. Am J of Emerg Med. 2018;36:508–10.
5. Change in U.S. Family finances from 2016 to 2019: evidence from the survey of consumer finances. Federal Reserve Bulletin. 2020;106(5) http://www.federalreserve.gov/publications/files/scf20.pdf
6. Medscape Physician Wealth and Debt Report 2019., http://www.medscape.com/slideshow/2019-compensaton-wealth-debt-6011524#5
7. Survey report—physician views on retirement. CompHealth Blog. July 31, 2017, https://comphealth.com/resources/physician-views-on-retirement-survey-report/
8. Goldberg R, Thomas H, Penner L. Issues of concern to emergency physicians in pre-retirement years: a survey. J of Emerg Med. 2009;40(6):706–9.
9. American Association of Individual Investors. Lifestyle changes: misconceptions about life in retirement. American Association of Individual Investors. https://www.aaii.com/evergreen/article/lifestyle-changes-myths-and-misconceptions-about-life-in-retirement
10. Laura R. Right way retirement. Financial Advisor Mag. July 16, 2021., https://www.fa-mag.com/news/right-way-retirement-63041.html
11. The 50 Best Quotes About Health & Nutrition, Dr. Edward Group https://explore.globalhealing.com/quotes-about-health/ Accessed 17 May 2022.

Chapter 103
Life After Retirement—Paying it Forward

Joan Naidorf

There will come a day for every emergency physician when the excitement, rigor, challenge, and torment of a shift in the emergency department will seem like too much. Every one will reach a time when they will look at themselves and their surroundings with a lot more questions than answers. The technologies and advances introduced over the previous decade get harder and harder to learn. The night shifts and time shifts set you back for hours and days. There is less joy.

The financial advisors will tell you, to the best of their educated guesses, if you have enough money to retire and live comfortably on your nest egg. Sadly, the pattern that I see, repeated all too often, is that hardworking people who worry and plan so carefully for retirement become ill and die before they get a chance to travel, play golf, or pivot to a second career or hobby that interests them.

Many physicians feel that their hard-won knowledge and experiences are at their peak just when they decide, for other reasons, to hang up their stethoscopes. How can emergency physicians, who have learned so much from our patients, mentors, and colleagues, "pay it forward?"

Pay it forward is an expression for when the recipient of an act of kindness does something kind for someone else rather than simply accepting or repaying the original good deed. The phrase is believed to have originated in 1916 by author Lily Hardy Hammond in her novel *In the Garden of Delight,* where she wrote a bit of wordplay: "You don't pay love back; you *pay it forward*." The notion was popularized by an award-winning 1999 novel by Catherine Ryan Hyde that was later made into a movie.

How can emergency physicians give back as they step away from clinical shifts in the emergency department? Seeing and treating patients on a volunteer basis are surprisingly difficult because of the need for malpractice coverage. Some volunteer organizations count on physicians having malpractice coverage through their main jobs.

J. Naidorf (✉)
Alexandria, VA, USA

R. P. Olympia et al. (eds.), *An Emergency Physician's Path*,
https://doi.org/10.1007/978-3-031-47873-4_103

Some overseas opportunities are eager to have US physicians participate in health and wellness missions. Many well-run charities run clinics in Haiti, but I had my own planned experience there interrupted during a period of civil unrest. Many organizations and university-based programs serve in Africa and areas of Central America. Sadly, much international travel was interrupted for 2 years during the COVID-19 pandemic of 2020–2022.

In the area where I live, a clinic that serves the Carpenter's Shelter (a homeless center) in Alexandria and the Arlington Free Clinic both have malpractice insurance that covers physicians while they practice there. Clinics such as these tend toward family and internal medicine concerns and not emergency or urgent care. One physician that I worked with, Corrine Lahti, MD, started volunteering at those two sites after a skiing accident cut short her career in the emergency department. She found it to be a satisfying way to give back to the community.

Another of my dynamic colleagues who figured out how to stay active and vital in emergency medicine was Dr. James Vafier. Jim spent much of his career practicing emergency medicine in Alexandria, Virginia, and as the operational medical director for the Alexandria Fire Department for several years. He loved teaching and interacting with the excellent paramedic staff that serves the City of Alexandria. After retiring from a long career in the emergency department, he took a faculty position at the Northern Virginia Community College to train emergency medical technicians and paramedics.

Jim was actively involved in the training of paramedics and placing them into clinical rotation with community EMS units. He also spent time, like many retired physicians love to do, being with his grandchildren. When Jim passed away in May of 2022, there were some huge shoes left to fill at the community college.

Other mentoring opportunities exist at medical schools which help their students with residency match mock interviews. Through Eastern Virginia Medical School in Norfolk, Virginia, alumni can participate in mock interview sessions with current students by contacting the alumni office. Retiring physicians can check with their alma maters or their local medical schools to see if opportunities are available.

My Own Experience

I became board certified in EM through my residence at the Albert Einstein Health Center in Philadelphia. Went I went through, it was actually based at the Osteopathic Medical Center, a hospital which no longer exists. As residents, we rotated through all the specialty services of emergency medicine with stints at the Children's Hospital of Philadelphia, trauma at the Lehigh Valley Hospital in Allentown, and burn care at St. Agnes Burn Center in South Philadelphia.

I took a job at a suburban hospital in Alexandria, Virginia, near where my husband grew up. In June of 1961, several physicians left private practice in general medicine to staff the emergency room at Alexandria Hospital, according to the website of the American College of Emergency Physicians. These physicians were the first full-time group to provide care exclusively in an ER, a concept referred to as the Alexandria Plan. When I joined the group in 1989, I was the first physician in the group who had done residency training in emergency medicine.

My husband trained in gastroenterology and was starting a solo gastroenterology practice in the Mount Vernon area of Alexandria. I was able to transition to a part-time position during the years that I had three children. Juggling carpools to school, flute lessons, and basketball games became very challenging when both my husband and I were working on weekends. Babies and toddlers require close supervision, and those needs change when they reach school age. Driving to and from school and activities practically takes a full-time transportation person.

I began working as a civilian contractor at a military hospital very close to my house. The staffing at the DeWitt Army Hospital and later the Fort Belvoir Community Hospital was covered by active-duty military personnel, Government Service Administration physicians, and a contract group. The contractors generally had to cover evenings, weekends, and holidays. I found that the military medical system worked much like a big health maintenance organization.

The emergency department was there to cover after hours pediatric visits and general emergency needs of active military personnel and their dependents. That comprises a very large population in Northern Virginia, where many military families live and settle after their careers are over. I worked at the military community hospital for several years and simultaneously took a nonclinical job that became available.

One of the divisions of United Healthcare, later Optum, was using physicians to review admissions to evaluate whether a patient should be placed as an inpatient or outpatient. I worked in section of the company that wrote appeal letters on behalf of various hospitals who had their patients' inpatient admissions denied by the healthcare insurance provider. The appeal process would extend all the way to hearings in front of administrative law judges. As part of that job, I would represent the hospital, in lieu of an attorney, to argue the merits of overturning a denial of service.

After that position ended in 2018, I felt that my insight and the wealth of my experience could still benefit students, residents, and my colleagues. I turned back to one of my first loves, writing. I started writing responses and reflections to various topics and articles that I read in the newspaper or heard through other media. It was easier than ever to find a platform to publish my work. I was able to get my articles published on the Doximity Op-Med page and on KevinMD.com. Through KevinMD.com, Kevin Pho even gives authors the opportunity to be interviewed on his daily podcast.

I opened my mind to other opportunities. A friend told me that she was going to be teaching a college course on medical ethics. Because of the start of the COVID-19 pandemic in 2020, the course was being taught online. I asked her if I could audit the class and she gave a resounding yes, with one caveat. I had to teach one of the classes. I presented the students a class on ethical considerations of medical training. I also offered to mentor some of the premed students which led to some lovely relationships.

Get Back to Your Passions

I met Kathy Kelly, MD, when she was an intern at the Emergency Medicine residency program at the Medical College of Pennsylvania when I was a fourth-year student rotating through that ED on an elective. Kathy went on to do a pediatric emergency medicine fellowship at Children's Hospital of Philadelphia when pediatric fellowships were just getting off the ground. We both moved to the same area of Northern Virginia and have worked at the same and different hospital emergency departments. Kathy stayed in the full-time practice of EM through the COVID-19 pandemic with full PPE and reduced staffing when all the patients returned.

After she retired in 2021, Kathy found her way back to taking the guitar lessons that she could never quite find the time for when she was working full time and raising her daughter, Emma. She also went back out on the golf course and joined a ladies' group to play once or twice weekly. To pay it forward, she continued with urgent care telemedicine visits as long as that opportunity was available.

One of the passions I picked up once again was reading. I read many genres but find myself particularly drawn to medical memoirs and fiction. When I noted the book club column in the DO magazine was looking for physicians to start writing some of the reviews, I jumped at the opportunity. The first book that I reviewed was *The Beauty in Breaking: A Memoir* which is a medical memoir by Michele Harper.

My next review was for Anne Fadiman's prize-winning work of medical sociology: *The Spirit Catches You and You Fall Down: A Hmong Child, Her American Doctors, and the Collision of Two Cultures*. This is a nonfiction book that tells the story of Lia Lee, a Hmong child with epilepsy, whose tragic course reveals the dangers of a lack of cross-cultural communication in the medical profession.

I never made the time to read the book when it came out in 1997. There were Hmong people living in Philadelphia, and there were many misunderstandings around the need for childhood vaccinations. For the review, I read the 20th anniversary edition that includes a valuable Afterword chapter with essential updates by the author. I benefited from going back to read this classic, and I could share that knowledge in an enthusiastic way with the readers of *The DO* online.

Later that year, *The DO* was moved to an editorial structure that featured contributions and columns written exclusively by osteopathic medical students and physicians. I volunteered for the physician advisory board and took an assignment, along with one of my colleagues, as a writer of the book review column. With that opportunity, I get to keep reading and sharing my reviews with other interested readers.

Speaking and Lecturing

Another way to pay it forward is to impart your knowledge to students, residents, and colleagues through lectures. If there is a topic that you have gained expertise in or know really well, this can be a nice way to share with colleagues. I wanted to do this and I reached out to my state medical association. I was able to get on the schedule for one of their continuing medical education courses which, at the time, consisted of recording a lecture for a virtual conference.

At the national meeting of the American College of Osteopathic Emergency Physicians, I met up some of my old friends and attending physicians. My natural network was at the stage of directing emergency medicine residency programs, and one person was even the dean of a medical school. My old friends were more than happy to have me lecture to their students and residents. I did not have to "prove" myself to them. I presented various topics over the following year, and I naturally built up my repertoire of topics.

Writing a Book

One of my first colleagues in the ED at Inova Alexandria Hospital was Dr. Stephen Bednar, who often said when imparting his wisdom "It'll be in my book!". How many of us have a book inside us and don't exactly know how to nurture it and coax it out? One of my friends encouraged me to write a book after reading a few of my online articles.

One topic that I lectured on kept coming up for me as holding an important message that I wanted to put out into the world. Years earlier when I was a clinical faculty member at George Washington University School of Medicine, I researched a sensitive topic so that I could do a better job with it and share what I learned with the residents and students of the emergency medicine program.

The topic was "How to Deal with Difficult Patients." In my own experience as a new attending physician, I noticed that one or two interactions with my patients or their families went so badly that I would feel frustrated, defeated, and cynical. I loved the whole field of emergency medicine with the challenges, the procedures, working with the team, and saying goodbye to my patients. That one aspect of those challenging interactions brought my mood down and placed me into a victim mentality.

I researched the medical literature and found that much had been written about these interactions and how they can raise negative emotions in clinicians. Most of the literature was written by psychiatrists and based on the tendency toward long-term relationships that they would develop with patients over days, months, and years. I adapted the information to the experience of the emergency physician and presented the topic as a grand round presentation. My director liked the presentation so much that he asked me to give the presentation again the next year. I also presented the talk for paramedics and physical therapists.

After revisiting the topic with several residency programs in 2019, I decided to expand my lecture into the form of a book. I decided to write the book that I would have wanted to read while I was in the thick of patient care. This is what Anthony Orsini, DO, did with *It's All in the Delivery.* He saw a deficiency in how physicians were communicating bad news to patients, and he wrote the book he would have wanted to read. Physician authors are writing the books that they wanted to read. They found some of the answers and they want to share them. How many of you have a book inside you with a message that other people need to read or hear? I know that I did.

I decided to expand the lecture on “Dealing with Difficult Patients” into a book manuscript. I already had the basic ideas and many of the references (photocopied articles from the library). I set my weekly goal to complete a chapter every week until I covered the topic to the best of my ability and said what I wanted to say. At 17 weeks and chapters later, I had my first draft. At about this time, one of the articles I had published on KevinMD.com was published, and I had the opportunity to talk with Kevin Pho during the recording of his podcast.

During my prep work, I noticed that Kevin had published a book with co-author Susan Gay entitled *Establishing, Managing and Protecting Your Online Reputation: A Social Media Guide for Physicians and Medical Practices*. I asked Kevin how he went about getting his book published. He most graciously said that he would send an email introducing me to his publisher. The person was Nancy Collins of the publishing arm of the American Association for Physician Leadership (AAPL), formerly Greenbranch Publishing.

What the heck, I figured I might as well ask the very experienced professional publisher what to do with my manuscript. I was hoping for an honest opinion about what I should do with my book draft. I was prepared to self-publish or throw it into the trash bin. Would anyone want to listen to my take on this very common problem? Nancy said the answer was YES. She liked it! She wanted to “take it to the next step?!”

Over the next few weeks, I discovered that comment meant writing the book pitch. Most people pitch the idea of a book to the publisher before writing their book. Nancy had to present the idea to the publishing team at the AAPL and convince them that my book was a worthy project. She was successful, and in May of 2021, I was offered a contract to publish *Changing How We Think About Difficult Patients: A Guide for Physicians and Healthcare Professionals*. Figure 103.1 contains an image of the paperback version printed by the American Association for Physician leadership.

The team wanted me to broaden the scope of the book to include physicians, nurses, and all clinicians who interact with patients in a variety of clinical settings. My initial focus was exclusively on the emergency physicians practicing in emergency departments and urgent care centers. Going back and forth with edits and layout issues took several months. To break up the monotony of the text, several drawings were added by graphic artist Victor Cruceanu. By late autumn of 2021, the copy, layout, and cover designs were finished.

To get some blurbs onto the back cover and the inside of the book, I had to ask total strangers to read my book and send me back a few lines. Next to getting my hair and some makeup applied to get the author head shot, this was the hardest part of writing the book and getting it published. Several busy author physicians were quite kind and charitable with their time so that I could get some terrific lines to endorse the book. The book was launched into the world in January of 2022.

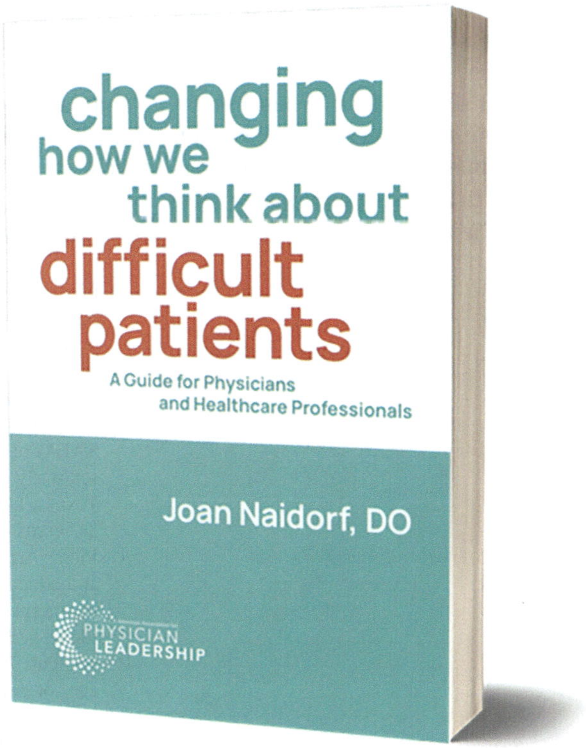

Fig. 103.1 My pay it forward project

The effort to market and promote a book falls quite squarely onto the author. Some authors who are published by the major publishing houses have the power of their marketing department, connections, and influence to get the word out there. I established a website and went about pitching myself to various podcasts and media outlets. In July of 2022, I had a perspective piece published in *The Washington Post*.

The book has a simple premise. If clinicians define what makes a difficult patient, they can be taught how to change their thoughts about what makes some interactions with patients or their families so uncomfortable. I review the predictable fears and challenges of being a patient. The typical patterns of patient response are reviewed. I review the medical literature on the topic of "difficult" interactions. Then I explain many of the typical thought distortions that occur in the minds of clinicians. Awareness of the negative thinking is key and the notion that thoughts create our feelings.

If we can guide our minds to ask better questions and to consider the challenges with intention, we can soften our anger or frustration. We can arouse curiosity and compassion by finding some common ground with the patient and brainstorming solutions. Competent patients have the autonomy to refuse care or to disregard the physician's advice. Someone will always disagree or disapprove of us or our actions. With confidence and self-love, clinicians can whither criticism and stand by their decisions.

I hope that my book will be read by nursing students, medical residents, and anyone who takes care of patients. Some folks find their way to these conclusions by intuition: many need some guidance. I am eager to pay forward the kindness wisdom of my mentors. When I show up someday as a grouchy old lady, I hope some youngster will give me the benefit of the doubt and treat me like a grandma.

I hope that someday when you hang up your stethoscope, you will find a hobby or avenue that lights you up and places some love into the world. When you keep your eyes and ears alert for opportunities, they will actually find you.

Chapter 104
Top Ten Things We Wish We Knew About a Career in Emergency Medicine Before We Embarked on this Journey

Elizabeth Barrall Werley, Jeffrey S. Lubin, and Robert P. Olympia

The Patient Population you Treat and Resources at Your Disposal May Change Dramatically Depending on Where You Work

When you are done with your training, realize that you may see very different patient populations depending on where you work. Urban EDs generally have a very different patient population from suburban EDs. Critical access hospitals have very different resources than academic medical centers. While the medicine is the same, the practice is not. Be sure to balance out what you feel would make the best practice for you.

Sometimes Christmas Is Not on December 25

As obvious as it sounds, the Emergency Department needs to run 24 hours a day, 7 days a week, 365 days a year. That means it needs to be staffed on nights, weekends, and holidays. This can be hard on your home life. Kids may not understand that daddy or mommy needs to sleep after working all night. You might need to celebrate holidays early or late (or not at all). While many physicians in all fields of medicine feel some of this, shift workers like emergency physicians are affected by it the most. You get paid for working when other physicians do not want to.

E. B. Werley · J. S. Lubin · R. P. Olympia (✉)
Emergency Medicine, Penn State Milton S. Hershey Medical Center, Hershey, PA, USA
e-mail: ewerley@pennstatehealth.psu.edu; jlubin@pennstatehealth.psu.edu; rolympia@hmc.psu.edu

R. P. Olympia et al. (eds.), *An Emergency Physician's Path*,
https://doi.org/10.1007/978-3-031-47873-4_104

Changing Paths Can and Does Happen

In the past, it was considered common knowledge that it was difficult to make a switch from community practice to academic practice, and only a small percentage of emergency physicians could accomplish this. However, even if that statement was true a decade or more ago, it is less likely true now. There are plenty of ways to become involved in academics. For instance, if your community site is a teaching site, you can practice your clinical teaching skills or get more involved with academic roles as a rotation director or site director for a medical school or as a rotation director for a residency program. Resident learners appreciate the "real-world" perspective of community physicians, so you provide an asset that the tertiary care academic centers do not have. If there is an open position advertised at an academic location, it doesn't hurt to apply. If you get selected as a clinical physician, there are ways to become more involved either through leadership, education, or scholarship. Even publishing doesn't have to be intimidating with assistance from more seasoned colleagues in your department.

Even When You're Not Traditionally Teaching, You're Still Teaching

There is formal teaching in medicine, through either established medical school or residency curricula. However, you should not forget the importance of clinical bedside teaching or teaching other learners. Clinical bedside teaching involves the day-to-day practice of medicine, and it does not always have to be a medical student or resident. Think about orienting new faculty to your department, onboarding new advanced practice providers either new to medicine in general or new to EM, and overseeing their patient care and giving them feedback. Try explaining to a nurse or tech what you are thinking about a patient or why you are managing them the way you are. You can become involved in the more formal education of others as well, such as being an EMS director and working on more formal and informal educational elements with them.

Don't Be Afraid to Say Yes

New opportunities arise all the time. Even if it is something you do not have tremendous knowledge about, if it interests you, it may be worth trying. If you are stepping up into a role you have not performed before or it is a new role altogether, don't be afraid to ask for mentorship by someone more senior than you, and ask for very clear delineation of expectations for the role.

Don't Be Afraid to Say No

Know your personal boundaries; it's okay to say no from time to time. As emergency medicine physicians, we like to fix things. It is fine to help out your department or hospital in a time of need, by stepping into an interim role or joining a committee or being a liaison. If you agree to help out with something that is less personally interesting to you, make sure you balance that with projects that do interest you to avoid burnout. Also, keep in mind that only you know what is going on in your personal life at any point in time. If there are factors involving you or your family that are otherwise occupying your time and energy, it may be appropriate to not take on additional work responsibilities, both for your own well-being and to ensure that someone else can dedicate the time and effort required of it.

Develop Your Niche Within Emergency Medicine

One of the great things about emergency medicine is that we need to know a lot of information about all kinds of medicine. We will see any patient at any time for any reason. But, sometimes, it is nice to be the "go-to" person on a particular area of emergency medicine. Will you be the departmental expert on prehospital care? On medical education? On head trauma? What are the areas within emergency medicine that you find most rewarding? Giving some extra time to your niche within the field is one way to differentiate yourself and help protect against burnout.

Conflict Management Will Be Part of Your Practice

We see patients during some of the most stressful times in their lives. Anyone from the public can come looking for help. When we call consultants, it always means that we are giving them more work. Add this to the time pressure and realities of staffing shortages and patient boarding, and we are set up for conflict. Whether it is de-escalating an upset patient, managing a difficult patient with a behavioral health crisis, or convincing a specialist to come to the hospital on a holiday, people management skills are crucial for the successful practice of emergency medicine. You will be challenged routinely during heated moments; learning to be ready for them cannot be overstated.

You Work in a Fishbowl, With Everyone Looking in

One of the most exciting challenges in emergency medicine is having the first chance to make a diagnosis and start management of a patient's condition. We often need to do that with limited history, without the benefit of diagnostic testing results, and in a time-pressured environment. Our colleagues in other departments most commonly have the benefit of a more complete story and workup. A diagnosis that might be obvious to them was not so obvious before the blanks were filled in. This sets up an ideal situation for Monday morning quarterbacking. It is easy to take this as a personal attack and become offended; however, it is important to try to reframe these experiences. As physicians, it is important for us to see every opportunity for improvement as a learning opportunity. Put the visceral response aside, and objectively think about how we could have done something better or more efficiently. We owe it to our patients to continually look for ways to do better.

People Can Have a Distorted View of What We Do (Positive or Negative)

On the same idea, people can have a very distorted view of what happens in an ED. For most of the population, going to the ED happens only on the most difficult, emotional, or otherwise challenging days of their lives. What we deal with routinely, such as death, life-changing injuries, life-threatening illnesses, and mental health crises, are things that most people are exposed to only a few times in their lives. When we start an IV and rehydrate a lethargic, dehydrated child, the parents may see us as saving the child's life. Or when we miss a diagnosis, maybe one that would not reasonably be expected to be made in an ED, we may be seen as careless or sloppy.

Most People Do Not Understand our World

That said, most people do not understand what we do. Patients (and even other physicians) are not familiar with our skill set. They will ask you when you are going to be through with your training and open your own practice (take this as a complement). They will question your ability to do things, expecting a specialist to be called to do things clearly within our scope of practice (take this as an opportunity to educate). Some will think you are a trauma surgeon; some will think you are a "triage doctor." They will not understand that every patient with chest pain does not need to be seen by a cardiologist or be admitted to the hospital. Emergency medicine has come a very long way and is a very unique practice within medicine.

We Have Two Ears and One Mouth so that We Can Listen Twice As Much as we Speak

Patients often present to the ED for one of two reasons: they have significant pain, or they (or their parents/family members) are anxious or concerned about something. We as EM physicians are trained well to recognize and treat pain, but at times we aren't so great at recognizing the anxiety or concerns from our patients, or we fail to spend the time or effort to listen to our patients and explain why we choose to do, or not to do, certain things. Whether it is the chaos of the ED, or not having the time or space to communicate well, or because we have preconceived expectations that do not coincide with our patients' expectations, we need to do a better job of listening first and then communicating our thoughts second. I became a better physician when I had children and when my family members presented to the ED over the years with various emergencies – put yourself in your patient's shoes, and treat your patients as if they were your children or family members. I learned compassion being on the other end of the physician-patient relationship.

One of my favorite methods of effective communication was described by Wayne and Mary Sotile in *The Resilient Physician: Effective Emotional Management for Doctors and Their Medical Organizations*:

Be assertive.
Be warm.
Show empathy.
Listen.
Be specific.
Self-disclose with discretion.
Use humor appropriately.
Select positive words.
Match the pace of the person to whom you are speaking.
Check your hearing .

As for listening, I love the mnemonic "LADDER": *l*ook at the other person, *a*sk questions, *d*on't interrupt, *d*on't change the subject (without permission), curb your *e*motions, and ***r***espond (reflect on what is said, validate it, offer support, keep a partnership approach, be respectful, and don't overreact or underreact to what is said).

Conflict and negative emotions can still result after appropriate communication with our patients, so it is important to provide them the risks and benefits of desired interventions and to perform shared decision-making.

Avengers Assemble

I'll admit it. Early in my career, I was a perfectionist. I wouldn't trust others in the department to carry out the orders needed for my patients nor would I trust medical students and residents to write the ED notes on patients we managed together, so I would do it myself. When it came to my first research project, I didn't trust my colleagues to enroll patients, so I did it myself. I slowly learned that "doing it myself" was painful and time-consuming and learned the importance of trusting others, being clear about roles and responsibilities, and delegating the work. Working in the ED is the ultimate team sport – as the ED attending, you are the coach – your job is to define expectations, to educate when education is necessary, to encourage and inspire your team, to be a leader in times of chaos, and at times, to be critical, but constructive, in order to deliver the best care for your patients. In EM, we are trained to roll with the punches – accept a full waiting room with no empty beds in sight and multiple ED boarders, accept less than optimal staffing, accept criticism from patients or other medical colleagues. Asking for help is not a sign of weakness; it is the first step to wellness, which ultimately improves the care of our patients. Lastly, surround yourself with the best team possible. In research, this means collaboration with other departments inside and outside your institution; utilizing medical students, residents, and other support staff as research assistants; and becoming teammates with librarians, biostatisticians, and the IRB.

Take a Breath, and Then Turn the Page

Twenty plus years into my PEM career, I still remember my first "missed" meningococcemia, my first pediatric resuscitation that we couldn't save, the first time I ordered the wrong dose of medication, and the first time that I had to tell parents that their child had cancer. We tend to remember the sad moments and the "mistakes" in our career more than the happy moments and the "saves." Overcoming these sad moments and "mistakes" can be difficult, leading to guilt and many sleepless nights. I decided many years ago that in order for me to provide the best care for my patients and to maintain a healthy well-being, I would consciously focus on "letting go." For me, this meant that I would take a moment to breathe, to allow myself to grieve, to forgive myself, to realize my self-worth, and to leave these moments at work. After a shift, I spend a few minutes in the quiet of my office reflecting on my day, noting both positive and negative aspects, leaving the world of second guessing decisions and questioning my competence at work, and going home with peace and clarity, ready to tackle my next shift with renewed optimism and energy.

"Find Your Passion, and It's No Longer Work"—L.A. Reid (American Record Producer and Executive)

After several years working in EM, I can honestly say that I still love what I do. Don't get me wrong, there are days when I come home from work either in tears or reaching for a few glasses of wine or comatose on the couch questioning my life choices. But I feel blessed to be able to enter the lives of those who need our help the most, and it is this passion for service that has motivated me throughout my career. I challenge you to remember the feeling you had in medical school when you decided to pursue a career in emergency medicine. Although your passions and interests will likely change during your career in emergency medicine, recognizing your passion at each stage of your career is the first step to having a successful and satisfying career. My passion started as a desire to serve ill and injured children and their families and, over the years, transformed into a passion for research, education, and mentorship. Allow your career to grow and transform based on your passions at each stage of your life, and I promise that work won't feel like such a burden.

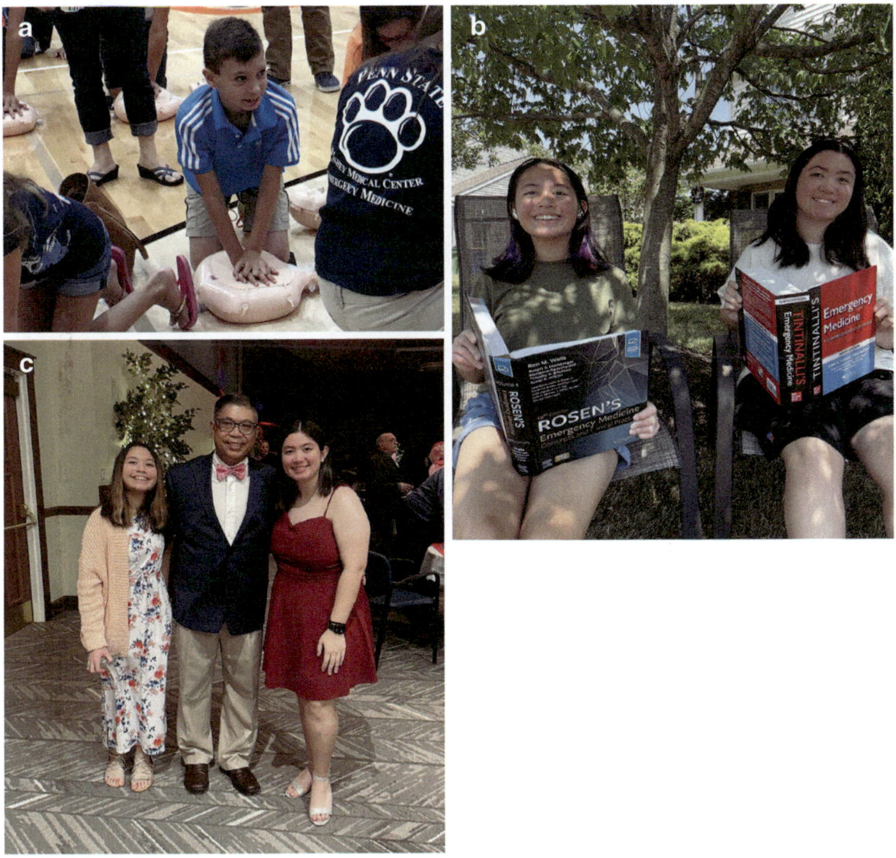

(**a**) Emergency medicine provides countless opportunities for community outreach, evidenced by this mass CPR training event at a local school. (**b**) Emergency medicine requires lifelong learning, at any age. Abigail and Madelyn enjoying a summer day with some "light" reading. (**c**) Work-life balance is one of the keys to success during a career in emergency medicine. Daddy-daughter Dance 2023

Correction to: An Emergency Physician's Path

Robert P. Olympia, Elizabeth Barrall Werley, Jeffrey S. Lubin, and Kahyun Yoon-Flannery

Correction to:
R. P. Olympia et al. (eds.), *An Emergency Physician's Path*, https://doi.org/10.1007/978-3-031-47873-4

The List of Contributors section was missed out by mistake in the original publication of the book. However, it has been included in the corrected version.

The updated version of this book can be found at https://doi.org/10.1007/978-3-031-47873-4

R. P. Olympia et al. (eds.), *An Emergency Physician's Path*,
https://doi.org/10.1007/978-3-031-47873-4_105

Index

R. P. Olympia et al. (eds.), *An Emergency Physician's Path*,
https://doi.org/10.1007/978-3-031-47873-4

clinicians. Awareness of the negative [illegible]

[illegible]

Conflict and negative emotions can [illegible]
with our patients, so it is important to provide them [illegible]

GPSR Compliance

The European Union's (EU) General Product Safety Regulation (GPSR) is a set of rules that requires consumer products to be safe and our obligations to ensure this.

If you have any concerns about our products, you can contact us on ProductSafety@springernature.com

In case Publisher is established outside the EU, the EU authorized representative is:

Springer Nature Customer Service Center GmbH
Europaplatz 3
69115 Heidelberg, Germany

Batch number: 10732117

Printed by Printforce, the Netherlands